Recent Progress in

HORMONE RESEARCH

The Proceedings of the Laurentian Hormone Conference

VOLUME 40

RECENT PROGRESS IN
HORMONE RESEARCH

Proceedings of the
1983 Laurentian Hormone Conference

Edited by
ROY O. GREEP

VOLUME 40

PROGRAM COMMITTEE

G. D. Aurbach	E. E. McGarry
J. D. Baxter	A. R. Means
J. C. Beck	B. W. O'Malley
H. Friesen	J. E. Rall
R. O. Greep	K. Savard
I. A. Kourides	N. B. Schwartz

J. L. Vaitukaitis

ACADEMIC PRESS, INC.
(Harcourt Brace Jovanovich, Publishers)

Orlando   San Diego   San Francisco   New York   London
Toronto   Montreal   Sydney   Tokyo   São Paulo

ACADEMIC PRESS, INC.
Orlando, Florida 32887

United Kingdom Edition published by
ACADEMIC PRESS, INC. (LONDON) LTD.
24/28 Oval Road, London NW1 7DX

LIBRARY OF CONGRESS CATALOG CARD NUMBER: Med. 47-38
ISBN 0-12-571140-9

PRINTED IN THE UNITED STATES OF AMERICA

84 85 86 87   9 8 7 6 5 4 3 2 1

CONTENTS

List of Contributors and Discussants vii

Preface.. ix

1. Promoter Elements of Genes Coding for Proteins and Modulation of
   Transcription by Estrogens and Progesterone
   Pierre Chambon, Andrée Dierich, Marie-Pierre Gaub, Sonia Jakowlev, Jan
   Jongstra, Andrée Krust, Jean-Paul LePennec, Pierre Oudet, and Tim
   Reudelhuber 1
   Discussion by *Chambon, Cohen, Hager, Kelly, Oppenheimer, Rall, and
   Sonnenschein* 40

2. Structure, Expression, and Evolution of the Genes for the Human Glycoprotein
   Hormones
   John C. Fiddes and Karen Talmadge 43
   Discussion by *Chambon, Drouin, Fiddes, Friesen, Gibori, Kourides,
   Littlefield, Marut, Moll, Nicoll, Niswender, Oppenheimer, Raj, Rall,
   Turek, and Weintraub* 74

3. The Regulation and Organization of Thyroid Stimulating Hormone Genes
   Ione A. Kourides, James A. Gurr, and Ofra Wolf...................... 79
   Discussion by *Aurbach, Bancroft, Fiddes, Greep, Kourides, Means, Rall,
   Schwartz, Sterling, Stone, and Oppenheimer*......................... 117

4. Mouse Mammary Tumor Virus Model in Studies of Glucocorticoid Regulation
   Gordon L. Hager, Helene Richard-Foy, Michael Kessel, David Wheeler,
   Alex C. Lichtler, and Michael C. Ostrowski......................... 121
   Discussion by *Bancroft, Chambon, French, Hager, Means, and Rall* 140

5. Role of the Circadian System in Reproductive Phenomena
   Fred W. Turek, Jennifer Swann, and David J. Earnest 143
   Discussion by *Billiar, Bradlow, Callard, Foster, Frisch, Gibori, Goodman,
   Greep, MacDonald, Marut, Peter, Robertson, Schwartz, Slaughter, Turek,
   Werder, Wise, and Ying*... 177

6. Neuroendocrine Basis of Seasonal Reproduction
   Fred J. Karsch, Eric L. Bittman, Douglas L. Foster, Robert L. Goodman,
   Sandra J. Legan, and Jane E. Robinson 185
   Discussion by *Callard, Cohen, Collins, Goodman, Guillemin, Irvine, Karsch,
   Keefe, MacDonald, Merriam, Nicoll, Niswender, Osathanondh, Peter,
   Pomerantz, Robertson, Turek, and Wehrenberg* 225

7. Somatocrinin: The Growth Hormone Releasing Factor
   Roger Guillemin, Paul Brazeau, Peter Böhlen, Frederick Esch, Nicholas
   Ling, William B. Wehrenberg, Bertrand Bloch, Christiane Mougin, Fusun
   Zeytin, and Andrew Baird... 233
   Discussion by *Anderson, Cohen, Donahoe, Friesen, Geller, Guillemin,
   Labrie, Marut, Merriam, Moll, Papkoff, Pearson, Peter, Russell, Saffran,
   Samaan, Schulster, Selmanoff, Sterling, Wehrenberg, Werder, and Zor*.... 286

8. Phospholipid Turnover in Hormone Action
   Yasutomi Nishizuka, Yoshimi Takai, Akira Kishimoto, Ushio Kikkawa,
   and Kozo Kaibuchi.. 301
   Discussion by *Chatterton, Clark, Czech, Friesen, Grandison, Littlefield,
   Means, Nishizuka, Oppenheimer, Peck, Posner, and Zor*................. 342

9. New Perspectives on the Mechanism of Insulin Action
   Michael P. Czech 347
   Discussion by *Aurbach, Czech, Kelly, Nishizuka, Oppenheimer, Posner,
   Samaan, Sonnenschein, and Sterling*................................... 373

10. The Interaction of Prolactin with Its Receptors in Target Tissues and Its
    Mechanism of Action
    Paul A. Kelly, Jean Djiane, Masao Katoh, Louis H. Ferland, Louis-Marie
    Houdebine, Bertrand Teyssot, and Isabelle Dusanter-Fourt 379
    Discussion by *Bancroft, Chatterton, Cohen, Djiane, Donahoe, Friesen,
    Houdebine, Kelly, Nicoll, Posner, Sonnenschein, and Wynn*............. 436

11. The Hypothalamic Control of the Menstrual Cycle and the Role of Endogenous
    Opioid Peptides
    Michel Ferin, Dean Van Vugt, and Sharon Wardlaw 441
    Discussion by *Billiar, Callard, Cohen, Cutler, Foster, Karsch, Martin,
    Murphy, Nekola, Schwartz, Segaloff, Selmanoff, and Turek* 480

12. A Role for Hypothalamic Catecholamines in the Regulation of Gonadotropin
    Secretion
    Charles A. Barraclough, Phyllis M. Wise, and Michael K. Selmanoff 487
    Discussion by *Barofsky, Barraclough, Beattie, Billier, Callard, Cohen, Ferin,
    Goodman, Greep, Keefe, Martin, Peter, Pomerantz, Schwartz, Turek, and
    Van Vugt*.. 521

13. Cell Proliferation in the Mammalian Testis: Biology of the Seminiferous Growth
    Factor (SGF)
    Anthony R. Bellvé and Larry A. Feig 531
    Discussion by *Barofsky, Bellvé, Budzik, Callard, Cohen, Concannon, Dias,
    Donahoe, Foster, French, Huseby, Littlefield, Means, Nicoll, Payne,
    Peter, Pomerantz, Posner, Raj, Rosner, and Ying* 561

14. Endocytosis and Membrane Traffic in Cultured Cells
    Mark C. Willingham and Ira Pastan 569
    Discussion by *Aurbach, Dias, Djiane, Oppenheimer, Posner, Rall,
    Sonnenschein, Sterling, Willingham, and Yoshinaga* 581

15. Hereditary Resistance to 1,25-Dihydroxyvitamin D
    Stephen J. Marx, Uri A. Liberman, Charles Eil, George T. Gamblin,
    Donald A. DeGrange, and Sonia Balsan 589
    Discussion by *Chatterton, Eil, Geller, Liberman, Marx, Moll, Oppenheimer,
    Schulster, Slaughter, Walters, Werder, and Wynn* 616

Index 621

LIST OF CONTRIBUTORS AND DISCUSSANTS

R. N. Anderson
G. D. Aurbach
A. Baird
S. Balsan
F. C. Bancroft
A. L. Barofsky
C. A. Barraclough
C. W. Beattie
A. R. Bellvé
R. B. Billiar
E. L. Bittman
B. Bloch
P. Böhlen
H. L. Bradlow
P. Brazeau
G. P. Budzik
G. Callard
I. Callard
P. Chambon
R. Chatterton
M. R. Clark
S. L. Cohen
D. C. Collins
P. W. Concannon
G. B. Cutler, Jr.
M. P. Czech
D. A. DeGrange
J. A. Dias
A. Dierich
J. Djiane
P. K. Donahoe
J. Drouin
I. Dusanter-Fourt
D. J. Earnest
C. Eil
F. Esch
L. Feig
M. Ferin
L. H. Ferland
J. C. Fiddes
D. L. Foster
F. S. French
H. Friesen
R. E. Frisch
G. T. Gamblin

M-P. Gaub
J. Geller
G. Gibori
R. L. Goodman
L. J. Grandison
R. O. Greep
R. Guillemin
J. A. Gurr
G. L. Hager
L.-M. Houdebine
R. A. Huseby
C. Irvine
S. Jakowlev
J. Jongstra
K. Kaibuchi
F. J. Karsch
M. Katoh
D. R. Keefe
P. A. Kelly
M. Kessel
U. Kikkawa
A. Kishimoto
I. A. Kourides
A. Krust
F. Labrie
J.-P. LePennec
S. J. Legan
U. A. Liberman
A. C. Lichtler
N. Ling
B. A. Littlefield
G. J. MacDonald
E. L. Marut
S. J. Marx
A. R. Means
G. R. Merriam
G. Moll, Jr.
C. Mougin
B. Murphy
M. V. Nekola
C. S. Nicoll
Y. Nishizuka
G. D. Niswender
J. H. Oppenheimer
R. Osathanondh

M. C. Ostrowski
P. Oudet
H. Papkoff
I. Pastan
A. H. Payne
O. H. Pearson
E. J. Peck
R. E. Peter
D. Pomerantz
B. Posner
M. Raj
J. E. Rall
T. Reudelhuber
H. Richard-Foy
H. Robertson
J. E. Robinson
J. F. Roser
S. M. Russell
M. Saffran
N. Samaan
D. Schulster
N. B. Schwartz
A. Segaloff
M. K. Selmanoff

G. Slaughter
C. Sonnenschein
K. Sterling
R. T. Stone
J. Swann
Y. Takai
K. Talmadge
B. Teyssot
F. W. Turek
D. Van Vugt
M. R. Walters
S. Wardlaw
W. B. Wehrenberg
B. Weintraub
K. V. Werder
D. Wheeler
M. C. Willingham
P. M. Wise
O. Wolf
P. Wynn
S.-Y. Ying
Y. Yoshinaga
F. Zeytin
U. Zor

PREFACE

The 1983 Laurentian Hormone Conference, the proceedings of which are published in this volume, was held at Mont Tremblant, Canada on the thirty-eighth anniversary of the first official meeting of that body at Mont Tremblant. The proceedings of that first meeting were published as Volume 1 of this serial publication. At the first meeting an excellent scientific program was presented for a gathering of endocrinologists actively engaged in research. On comparing the first and thirty-eighth conference, the only changes have been in the tools and techniques used to explore the biology and chemistry of hormones and how they act. In the interim, movement has been from anatomy and physiology of hormone-secreting organs and target tissues, to cellular and subcellular endocrine chemistry and biology, to molecular endocrinology and hormonal control of gene expression.

The first article, "Promoter Elements of Genes Coding for Proteins and Modulation of Transcription by Estrogens and Progesterone" by Pierre Chambon, the Gregory Pincus Memorial Lecturer, set the tone of excellence and penetrating insight for the variety of studies at the leading edge of endocrinology that were to follow. These included neuroendocrinology, mechanism of hormone action, reproductive biology, subcellular processing of hormones and their receptors, and last, but intriguingly, "Hereditary Resistance to 1,25-Dihydroxyvitamin D."

For handling the chairmanships of the several sessions of this program with skill, expertise, aplomb, and an occasional touch of humor, we are endebted to Drs. Bruce Weintraub, F. Carter Bancroft, Gordon Niswender, Fernand Labrie, Uriel Zor, Joseph Martin, Frank French, and Brian Little.

For all of her unending year round labors on behalf of the Laurentian Hormone Conference and for the onerous task of readying the proceedings of the 1983 Conference for publication, I am deeply indebted to our Executive Secretary, Martha (Wright) Devin. And to Lucy Felicissimo and Linda Carsagnini for their ever prompt and skillful transcribing of the taped discussion of each paper goes our profound appreciation and admiration of a job well done. The expertise and priorities assigned to the production of this volume by the staff of Academic Press are gratefully acknowledged by me and the Board of Directors of the Laurentian Hormone Conference.

Roy O. Greep

Recent Progress in

HORMONE RESEARCH

The Proceedings of the Laurentian Hormone Conference

VOLUME 40

Promoter Elements of Genes Coding for Proteins and Modulation of Transcription by Estrogens and Progesterone[1]

PIERRE CHAMBON, ANDRÉE DIERICH, MARIE-PIERRE GAUB, SONIA JAKOWLEV, JAN JONGSTRA, ANDRÉE KRUST, JEAN-PAUL LEPENNEC, PIERRE OUDET, AND TIM REUDELHUBER

Laboratoire de Génétique Moléculaire des Eucaryotes du CNRS, Unité 184 de Biologie Moléculaire et de Génie Génétique de l'INSERM, Institut de Chimie Biologique, Faculté de Médecine, Strasbourg, France

I. Introduction

How is gene expression controlled in eukaryotic cells? This question is at the heart of problems and questions which are obviously not new, but their study, at the molecular level, constitutes the new "frontier" in biology. What is the molecular basis for cell determination which leads to the development of embryos? Why is a gene active in one cell, and inactive in another? And how is this imprint of genes maintained stably even after cell division? What are the molecular explanations for differential regulation of gene expression in the differentiated cells? What is turning on the expression of "committed" genes? How could variations in hormonal, nutritional, and even environmental parameters control gene expression? There is no doubt that the answers to these fundamental questions will be of great interest to all biologists, but in addition, it is certain that they will have important consequences in medicine.

It is clear that our picture of the molecular anatomy of genomes of higher eukaryotes, and of how it functions, has changed dramatically over the last 10 to 15 years. In this regard it is interesting to note that of the many new, and sometimes amazing, findings, few have been the result of elaborate theories. Rather, as has been the case in many scientific pursuits, the discoveries have been made possible by the development of powerful new methods. This should not surprise us, because not knowing the molecular logics of evolution, it is impossible to predict how the genome is organized and how it functions. Who could have predicted the

---

[1] The Gregory Pincus Memorial Lecture.

1

existence of split genes? Thanks to the advent of recombinant DNA technology, DNA sequencing, and a number of other related techniques, genes from almost any organisms can now be isolated and made accessible for direct manipulation. A new approach has become possible, aimed at purifying genes of known function, and ultimately at reconstructing the necessary molecular environment in a test tube. Classical *in vivo* genetics has been replaced by *in vitro* genetics (also called genetic biochemistry, surrogate or substitutive genetics), in which the study of the function of a given gene involves first its cloning, then its modification by site-directed mutagenesis, and finally its introduction into a proper cellular environment by DNA transfer with the possible help of appropriate vectors.

Transcriptional control is clearly the principal mechanism for regulation of gene expression in prokaryotes (Rodriguez and Chamberlin, 1982). Although it is today widely accepted that control of most, if not all, eukaryotic genes occurs at the transcriptional level, it is worth recalling that not too long ago the opposite view, namely that of no stringent control of gene expression at the level of transcription, was dominant. Because of the results of some DNA–nuclear RNA hybridization experiments, some people in the field thought that gene expression does not need to be as precisely regulated at the level of transcription in eukaryotes as in prokaryotes! Although I share the general belief that in eukaryotes most, but not all, of the regulation in gene expression is transcriptional, it is important to stress that there are only a few genes for which it has been unequivocally demonstrated that their regulation is indeed at the transcriptional level, and there are well-known examples of posttranscriptional regulation at the RNA processing and translational levels. In this respect, there may be surprises. We certainly should keep an eye open and not be too dogmatic.

Control of the expression of genes transcribed by RNA polymerase class B (II) is obviously of prime importance (which does not mean that other genes, such as tRNA, 5 S, and ribosomal genes are not important), because most of them code for proteins and some of them must play key roles in development. If we believe that the regulation of transcription is one of the crucial mechanisms operating during development, the first step in its study is clearly to determine how genes are turned on and off, and in particular to study how initiation of transcription is controlled at the molecular level. Investigating how a given gene functions in a differentiated cell will eventually lead to the identification of molecules important for its action and, then, by tracing them back during development, to the elucidation of the molecular nature of this process.

The modulation of gene expression by steroid hormones offers a number of useful model systems to study how the expression of a given gene or a set of genes can be positively regulated at the transcriptional level in animal cells (for refs. see Anderson, 1983). It is generally thought that the effect of steroid hormones is mediated by hormone-specific intracellular receptor proteins that associate with specific DNA or chromatin sites upon binding the hormone ligand (Yamamoto and Alberts, 1976; Mulvihill *et al.*, 1982; Schrader *et al.*, 1981). It is assumed that this receptor–genome interaction is the primary event in the induction of transcription of a gene programmed to respond to a given steroid hormone in a given differentiated responsive cell. Since the first step in initiation of transcription of a given gene is the binding of the transcription machinery to the specific DNA elements which constitute the gene promoter, it is further assumed that the hormone–receptor complex facilitates this binding by interacting with a specific region located in the vicinity of the gene. Evidently, the study of the validity of such proposals requires a previous knowledge of the structural and functional organization of the promoter region of the gene in question, and more generally, of promoters of animal genes coding for proteins.

The purpose of this article is to first review the current knowledge of the organization of such promoters, with a special emphasis on some of our studies which may be particularly relevant to steroid hormone action, and then to describe some of our recent work directly pertinent to the problem of regulation of transcription by estrogens and progesterone.

II. Promoter Elements of Genes Coding for Proteins in Eukaryotes

In prokaryotes initiation of transcription is controlled at specific DNA regions, called promoters. Promoters were first defined by Jacob *et al.* (1964) primarily on genetic evidence, as cis-acting initiating regions indispensable for the expression of bacterial structural genes. Subsequent *in vivo* and *in vitro* biochemical studies have demonstrated that prokaryotic promoters are DNA regions, 5' to the structural genes, which can be comprised of multiple functional elements (Rosenberg and Court, 1979; Losick and Chamberlin, 1976; Rodriguez and Chamberlin, 1982; Siebenlist *et al.*, 1980; Fig. 1). A prokaryotic promoter region must contain a basic element required for recognition, binding, and RNA chain initiation by RNA polymerase. This element includes the mRNA start-site (consensus sequence CAT), the AT-rich Pribnow or Schaller box sequence located approximately 10 bp upstream from the startsite (consensus sequence 5'-TATAAT-3'), and very often a third region of homology, the "recognition" sequence, located further upstream in the −35 region (consensus sequence 5'-TTGACA-3'). A fixed spatial relationship between the Pribnow box and the "recognition" site is mandatory, since deletion or addition of a single base pair between these two sequences can

PIERRE CHAMBON ET AL.

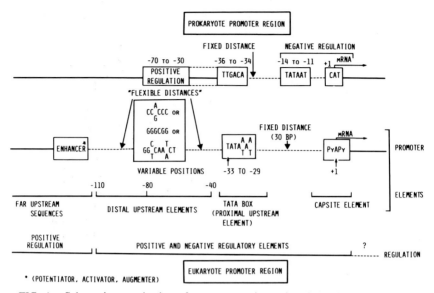

FIG. 1. Schematic organization of promoter regions of prokaryotic (upper line) and eukaryotic (lower lines) genes coding for proteins (see text). The direction of transcription is from left to right (arrows). +1 indicates the location of the mRNA start-site. Positions upstream from the start-site are numbered negatively. BP, base pairs.

lead to a dramatic alteration in the efficiency of transcription by *E. coli* RNA polymerase (Stefano and Gralla, 1982). In addition, one or more regulatory elements, i.e., sequences which interact with protein factors which control positively or negatively the efficiency of transcription initiation, may also be present within the same region (see above for references and Miller and Reznikoff, 1978; Fig. 1). Such specific regulatory proteins, the activity of which can be modulated by interaction with specific ligands, have been characterized in a few cases, but with one exception for positive regulation (Guarente *et al.*, 1982; Hochschild *et al.*, 1983; Hawley and McClure, 1983), the underlying molecular mechanisms are not yet fully elucidated.

In contrast to prokaryotic cells, progress in unraveling the molecular mechanisms involved in control of transcription in eukaryotic cells has been until the late 1970s, extremely slow. The possibility that in eukaryotes these mechanisms may not be identical to those in prokaryotes was first suggested 10 years ago following the discovery of the multiplicity of eukaryotic RNA polymerases by our group and Roeder and Rutter (for reviews, see Chambon, 1975; Roeder, 1976). It was subsequently established that cells of both higher and lower eukaryotes contain three structurally and functionally distinct classes of RNA polymerase which are localized in different subcellular fractions. Class A or I catalyzes the synthesis of ribosomal RNA, class B or II that of mRNA, and class C or III that of transfer RNA (tRNA) and 5 S RNA (for reviews, see Chambon, 1975; Roeder, 1976). Although highly purified preparations of these enzymes, particularly RNA polymerase B, were available shortly after their discovery, their role in the control of transcription remained elusive for several years. This was due in large part to the lack of meaningful *in vitro* cell-free transcription systems. Indeed, because of the complexity of the eukaryotic genome, there was no means to study the transcription of a given gene *in vitro* by incubating the total cellular DNA with purified RNA polymerase. Even when well-defined viral DNA templates such as the Simian virus 40 (SV40) and adenovirus-2 genomes were available, the primary transcription products were unknown, precluding any valid analysis of the factors involved in the control of transcription. Furthermore, intact viral DNAs proved to be very poor templates *in vitro* for the purified RNA polymerase B, which was known to transcribe SV40 and adenovirus genomes *in vivo* (Chambon, 1975). Several technical breakthroughs were required before these problems could be overcome. The discovery of restriction enzymes and reverse transcriptase, followed by the advent of molecular cloning and of methods for separating, visualizing, and rapidly sequencing DNA and RNA molecules, have made it possible to study, at the nucleotide level, the anatomy of eukaryotic cellular and viral genes and of their primary RNA transcripts (Chambon, 1977; Breathnach and Chambon, 1981). It has now been shown in several instances (for example, see Ziff and Evans, 1978; Wasylyk *et al.*, 1980, for the adenovirus major late transcription unit and for the ovalbumin transcription unit, respectively) that the 5' ends of the RNA primary transcripts and of the mature mRNAs coincide and therefore that the start point of transcription corresponds to the base coding for the 5' terminal nucleotide of the mRNAs.

Knowing the molecular anatomy of some genes and of their primary transcripts at the nucleotide level, it became possible to investigate whether eukaryotic genes coding for proteins are flanked on their 5' end side by promoter elements functionally equivalent to those of prokaryotic genes. Studies performed over the last 4 years in our and other laboratories have revealed that the promoter region of eukaryotic protein coding genes contains some "classical" elements similar to those found in prokaryotes, but also some unexpected "baroque" elements which have no known counterparts in bacteria. The term "promoter" is used here in a broad sense to cover any DNA sequence required for accurate and efficient initiation of transcription. The dissection of promoters into their essential elements was made possible mainly because of two complementary technical breakthroughs: (1) the establishment in 1978–1979 of cell-free systems which transcribe accurately purified viral or cellular genes *in vitro* (Wu, 1978; Weil *et al.*, 1979; Manley *et al.*, 1980) (the term accurate is used here to qualify RNA chain initiation occurring at the *in vivo* capsite); and (2) the possibility of introducing genes which have been altered by site-directed mutagenesis into the nuclei of cells in culture or of *Xenopus laevis* oocytes, and to study subsequently their expression (Mulligan and Berg, 1980; Pellicer *et al.*, 1980).

A. TWO "CLASSICAL" PROMOTER ELEMENTS: THE CAPSITE AND THE TATA BOX

Soon after the eukaryotic protein-coding genes began to be sequenced, and the 5' end of their transcription units mapped, comparison of their 5' end flanking regions revealed the presence of an AT-rich region of homology (the Hogness–Goldberg box or TATA box, consensus sequence 5'-TATA$_T^A$A$_T^A$-3') centered approximately 28 bp upstream from the start point of transcription (Gannon *et al.*, 1979; Corden *et al.*, 1980; Breathnach and Chambon, 1981; see Fig. 1). This highly conserved region of homology is present in almost all of the eukaryotic protein-coding genes which have been analyzed up to now; in the few cases where it is absent, it appears to be replaced by a substitute TATA-like sequence which plays the same role (Brady *et al.*, 1982). Studies with TATA box mutants obtained by site-directed mutagenesis have shown that the TATA box element plays, both in *in vitro* and *in vivo*, a qualitative and quantitative role in initiation of transcription. The TATA box is a positioning element which directs the transcription machinery to initiate RNA synthesis approximately 30 bp downstream at the mRNA capsite (Corden *et al.*, 1980; Breathnach and Chambon, 1981; Wasylyk *et al.*, 1983a). It is thus responsible for the accuracy of initiation of transcription. However, its integrity is also required to achieve maximum RNA synthesis from a given promoter region (Wasylyk *et al.*, 1983a). It appears therefore that the eukaryotic TATA box possesses to some extent the same promoter function as the prokaryotic Pribnow box. On the other hand, the Pribnow box is located approximately 10 bp upstream from the RNA startsite (one DNA helix turn), whereas the TATA box is separated from the mRNA startsite by approximately 3 turns of the double helix. In addition, *in vitro* studies have provided some evidence that the TATA box interacts specifically with at least one initiation factor and that this interaction is responsible for the formation of a stable preinitiation complex between the transcription machinery and the promoter sequences (Davison *et al.*, 1983).

No such stable initiation factor binding to the Pribnow box has been found in prokaryotes.

The capsite or mRNA startsite element which contains the base(s) coding for the 5' terminal nucleotides of the mRNA is less conserved than the TATA box element (for reviews, see Corden *et al.*, 1980; Breathnach and Chambon, 1981). Its deletion, which results in RNA chain initiation from new start points located approximately 30 bp downstream from the TATA box, is usually accompanied by a decrease in the amount of RNA initiated from the promoter region. That transcription is nevertheless seen when the wild-type mRNA startsite has been deleted indicates, however, that a degree of flexibility exists in the mechanism of start-point selection.

B. THE DISTAL UPSTREAM PROMOTER ELEMENTS

A second conserved sequence located in some genes upstream from the TATA box at approximately 70–90 bp from the mRNA startsite has the consensus sequence $5'\text{-GGPyCAA}_A^T\text{CT-}3'$, and presents some similarity with the -35 region of some *E. coli* promoters (Benoist *et al.*, 1980). That this and other sequences located further upstream from the TATA box are promoter elements required *in vivo* to ensure the efficiency, but not the accuracy of initiation of transcription, has been recently documented for a number of genes (Dierks *et al.*, 1983; Everett *et al.*, 1983). At the present time, these upstream promoter elements appear to be quite polymorphic. Their number (up to three in the case of the rabbit β-globin gene, see Dierks *et al.*, 1983) and their position in the 40–110 bp region upstream from the mRNA startsite is variable from one promoter to another. Although these elements do not exhibit the clear evolutionary conservation of the TATA box, some homologies are nevertheless apparent and at least two types of homologous sequences can be discerned at the present time (Fig. 1). One of them corresponds to the previously mentioned $5'\text{-GGPyCAA}_A^T\text{CT-}3'$ consensus sequence, whereas the other comprises the sequence $5'\text{-CCPuCCC-}3'$ and the complementary sequence $5'\text{-GGGCGG-}3'$ (McKnight, 1982; McKnight and Kingsbury, 1982; Everett *et al.*, 1983; Dierks *et al.*, 1983; Fromm and Berg, 1983; Baty *et al.*, 1984). How these upstream elements control the efficiency of transcription initiation is unknown (for a discussion of this point, see McKnight, 1982; Everett *et al.*, 1983). In view of their variable position with respect to the TATA box, it is unlikely that they interact directly with the RNA polymerase initiating molecules in the same manner as the prokaryotic -35 region, which is at a fixed distance from the Pribnow box (see above). Observations made *in vivo* with the mouse metallothionine gene (Brinster *et al.,* 1982) and the *Drosophila* heatshock hsp 70 gene (Pelham, 1982; Pelham and Bienz, 1982) suggest that these upstream sequences interact with regulatory factors. *In vitro* studies have also suggested that the effect of these upstream elements is mediated through interaction with initiation factors (Grosschedl and Birnstiel, 1982; Hen *et al.,* 1982). An initiation factor, which specifically binds *in vitro* to the 21 bp repeat upstream element of the SV40 early promoter and which is required for efficient transcription from this promoter, has been recently characterized by Dynan and Tjian (1983a,b). That specific regulatory transcription factors can functionally interact with upstream elements is also suggested by the observation that the silk worm fibroin gene promoter is preferentially activated during *in vitro* transcription by species-specific extracts and that this activation is dependent on the presence of upstream sequences (Tsuda and Suzuki, 1981). Whether the multiplicity of upstream promoter elements within a given promoter region reflects a multiplicity of regulatory factors modulating the level of transcription is presently unknown.

C. THE "BAROQUE" ENHANCER ELEMENTS

The initial finding (Benoist and Chambon, 1981; Gruss *et al.,* 1981) that the SV40 early promoter comprises a crucial, quantitatively determinative promoter element (the 72 bp repeat) located more than 110 bp upstream from the mRNA startsite came as a big surprise, since there was no precedent in prokaryotes for such a far upstream element. The surprise became amazement when it was found that this SV40 promoter element could potentiate initiation of early transcription *in vivo,* not only from the other homologous promoter elements which control RNA chain initiation from the SV40 early mRNA startsites, but also from a number of heterologous viral or cellular promoter elements, all inactive in its absence (Banerji *et al.,* 1981; Moreau *et al.,* 1981). Potentiating elements with similar properties were subsequently found far upstream from the classical promoter elements of a number of viral transcriptional units and termed enhancers (Yaniv, 1982; Khoury and Gruss, 1983; Gluzman and Shenk, 1983; Hen *et al.,* 1983).

In vivo studies on enhancers, mostly on the canonical SV40 72 bp repeat enhancer, have shown that enhancers are cis-acting elements which exhibit the following striking properties. They can potentiate initiation of transcription from any potential heterologous "natural" or "substitute" promoter elements, whether or not they contain a TATA box element, and irrespective of the presence of functional upstream elements (Wasylyk *et al.,* 1983b). In addition enhancer elements appear to function bidirectionally, i.e., their efficiency is independent of their orientation with respect to the activated promoter elements. Enhancers appear to be active even when they are separated from the potentiated promoter elements by several kilobases. However, their enhancing efficiency decreases as the length of interposed sequences is increased and proximal promoter elements are activated in preference to more distal ones. Enhancer elements are not restricted to viral genes which are transcribed "constitutively" by RNA polymerase B early in infection, since they have been recently found in some immunoglobulin genes (Banerji *et al.*, 1983; Gillies *et al.*, 1983; Mercola *et al.*, 1983; Neuberger, 1983; Picard and Schaffner, 1983; Queen and Baltimore, 1983; Stafford and Queen, 1983). Enhancer elements can be "naturally" located upstream (as in the case of the SV40 early promoter), within (for instance in the intron separating the constant and variable regions of the rearranged immunoglobulin heavy chain) or downstream (as in the case of the early promoter of the bovine papilloma virus) from a transcription unit. Finally some enhancers exhibit a marked species or cell specificity (Yaniv, 1982; Khoury and Gruss, 1983; and the above references for immunoglobulin gene enhancer), suggesting that they could interact with specific regulatory proteins (see below).

1. The Entry-Site Hypothesis for Enhancer Function

Any hypothesis aimed at explaining in molecular terms the potentiator effect of enhancer elements has to take into account the observations that proximal potential promoter elements are preferentially activated and that activation of transcription from a given promoter element decreases as the length of interposed sequences increases. A plausible hypothesis is that an enhancer corresponds to a particularly efficient bidirectional entry site for some component of the transcription machinery which may be a transcription factor (for instance that which binds tightly to the TATA box) rather than RNA polymerase B itself. This component could then track the DNA until it finds a potential promoter element which will thus be activated for initiation of transcription (Moreau *et al.*, 1981; Wasylyk *et al.*, 1983b).

Several mechanisms, not mutually exclusive, can be invoked to account for such an "entry site" function (Fig. 2). Enhancer sequences could be specifically recognized by the topoisomerase machinery which controls DNA supercoiling, thereby facilitating local modifications of the template superhelicity. Such modifications are known to affect gene expression *in vivo* in prokaryotes (Liu and Miller, 1981; Sternglanz *et al.*, 1981; Hsieh and Brutlag, 1980) and interactions *in vitro* between the DNA template and proteins of the prokaryotic and eukaryotic transcription

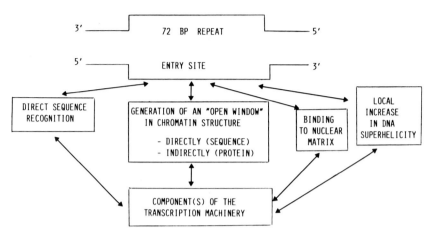

FIG. 2. The entry site model. Current concepts of the mechanism of action of the SV40 72 bp repeat enhancer. See text for comments.

machineries (Chambon,1975; Losick and Chamberlin, 1976; Hossenlopp *et al.*, 1974). Enhancer sequences could also direct the DNA template into a specialized nuclear "compartment" which may contain all factors required for efficient transcription, for instance by providing a DNA attachment site to the matrix onto which actively transcribed genes may be bound (Robinson *et al.*, 1983). At the present time there is no experimental evidence to support either of these two hypothetical mechanisms. However, two other possible mechanisms accounting for an entry site function of enhancers have recently received some experimental support from studies performed in our laboratory on the SV40 72 bp repeat enhancer.

2. Generation of an "Open Window" in Chromatin Structure by the SV40 Enhancer

That the SV40 enhancer could play a role in the generation of an "open window" in chromatin structure was suggested from studies performed late in viral infection, when SV40 DNA is found in the nucleus of infected cells associated with histones in the form of a minichromosome (Griffith, 1975; Bellard *et al.*, 1976; Cremisi *et al.*, 1976), which has a nucleosomal structure similar to that of cellular chromatin (Kornberg, 1977; Chambon, 1977; McGhee and Felsenfeld, 1980). When nuclei of SV40 infected cells or isolated SV40 minichromosomes are treated with DNase I (Scott and Wigmore, 1978; Saragosti *et al.*, 1980), DNAse II (Shakhov *et al.*, 1982), endogenous nucleases (Scott and Wigmore, 1978; Waldeck *et al.*, 1978; Wigmore *et al.*, 1980), micrococcal nuclease (Sundin and Varshawsky, 1979), or restriction endonucleases (Varshavsky *et al.*, 1979), a region

In 10

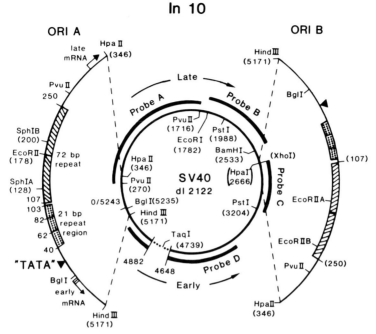

FIG. 3. Schematic representation of the SV40 double origin mutant In10. The inner circle represents the genome of SV40 dl2122 which has a 234 bp deletion around the *Taq* site (dotted line). The position and coordinates of some relevant restriction sites and landmarks are indicated and numbered according to the BBB system (Tooze, 1982). The SV40 ORI region (ORI A) which contains the origin of replication (around the *Bgl*I site) and the early and late gene promoter sequences are shown enlarged at the left side. The three early gene promoter elements ("TATA box," 21 bp repeat region, and 72 bp repeat) are indicated. A similar ORI region from *Hin*dIII to *Hpa*II (5171-346) was inserted at position 2666 in the same orientation with respect to early gene transcription as shown enlarged on the right side (ORI B). The dark bars indicate the restriction fragments used as hybridization probes to map regions of increased DNase I sensitivity at ORI A and ORI B (Jongstra *et al.*, 1984).

extending from the unique *Bgl*I site for approximately 350 bp toward the late side is preferentially cut (the ORI region, Fig. 3, ORI A). In addition, detailed studies of the products of DNAse I digestion early and late in infection have revealed the existence of several discrete hypersensitive sites within this DNA fragment which are separated by relatively resistant segments (Cremisi, 1981; Saragosti *et al.*, 1982) and electron microscopy has shown that approximately 25% of the minichromosomes extracted from nuclei late in infection contain a nucleosome-free region (the nucleosome gap) of approximately 350 bp located in the same position (Saragosti *et al.*, 1980; Jakobovits *et al.*, 1980). Studies with viral mutants in which parts of the ORI region are duplicated indicate that the DNA sequence of this region contains the information required for the generation of the nuclease-sensitive chromatin structure (Wigmore *et al.*, 1980; Chae *et al.*, 1982; Gerard *et al.*, 1982) and for the generation of the nucleosome gap (Chae *et al.*, 1982; Jakobovits *et al.*, 1982).

These findings are of particular interest because the ORI region contains the 72 bp repeat enhancer. They raise the possibility that alteration in chromatin structure as detected by increased sensitivity to endonucleases and the presence of a nucleosome gap, can be induced, at least in part, by the enhancer sequence. Our approach to test the validity of this hypothesis was based on the observation of Shenk (1978) that SV40 mutants with deletions in the large-T intron can accommodate extra DNA sequences in the *Hpa*I site at position 2666 (Fig. 3). Such insertion mutants are viable and have growth characteristics similar to wild-type SV40. Different parts of the ORI region were inserted at this *Hpa*I site using a mutant SV40 strain d12122, which has a deletion of 234 bp between positions 4648 and 4882 (Volckaert *et al.*, 1979) to create SV40 mutants carrying two ORI regions: ORI A, the wild-type origin region which was unaltered in all mutants and ensured viability, and a second wild type or mutated origin region, ORI B.

a. Insertion of a Second ORI Region in SV40 Generates a DNase I Sensitive Chromatin Structure Similar to That of the Wild-Type ORI. Figure 3 represents the SV40 double origin mutant In10. In this mutant, the 418 bp *Hin*dIII–*Hpa*II ORI fragment (5171-346) was inserted as a second ORI (ORI B). To determine the presence of increased DNase I sensitivity at ORI A and ORI B, CV-1 cells were infected with an SV40 In10 virus stock. Nuclei were prepared 40–42 hours later and regions of increased DNase I sensitivity were mapped in SV40 chromatin using the indirect end-labeling technique of Wu (1980). Briefly, after DNase I digestion the DNA was purified and digested with *Eco*RI, fractionated by agarose gel electrophoresis, and transferred to a nitrocellulose filter. The pattern of DNase I digestion at ORI A and B was revealed after hybridization of the blotted DNA to probes A and B, respectively (Fig. 3).

The results of such experiments are schematically summarized in Fig. 4. Two regions of increased DNase I sensitivity can be mapped over the wild-type ORI A region. Region I includes the TATA box of the SV40 early promoter, whereas region II includes the 72 bp repeat enhancer. As shown in the same figure, a pattern of DNase I sensitivity similar to that seen at ORI A was revealed at ORI B of In10. To investigate which sequences were responsible for the induction of region II, mutants In42 and In421 which contain an intact 72 bp repeat or only one 72 bp sequence, respectively, were constructed (Fig. 5). As shown schematically in Fig. 5, the region II of increased DNase I sensitivity was shortened, but

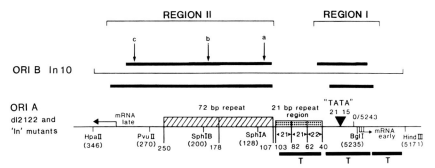

FIG. 4. Diagrammatic comparison of regions of increased DNase I sensitivity at ORI A and ORI B in SV40 mutant In10. The lower line (ORI A) represents the SV40 ORI region with the "TATA box," the 21 bp repeat region, and the 72 bp repeat. The three dark bars below the line indicate the three T-antigen binding sites. The dark bars above the lines ORI A and ORI B In10 indicate the extent of regions of increased DNase sensitivity I and II and are a summary of several mapping experiments using probes A to D to analyze ORI A and probes B and C to analyze ORI B (see Fig. 3) (Jongstra et al., 1984).

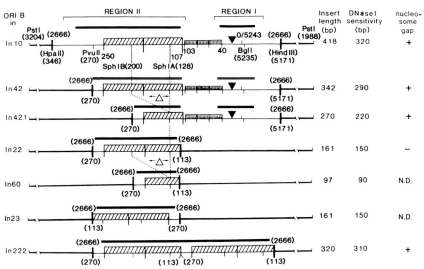

FIG. 5. Diagrammic representation of the results obtained with the various "In" mutants. The small PstI fragments containing ORI B are shown (Fig. 3). For each mutant the insert at ORI B is represented by a thin horizontal line bounded by thick vertical bars. The extent of the regions of increased DNase I sensitivity (I and II) is indicated by a black horizontal bar as in Fig. 4. The column "DNase I sensitivity" gives the distance in base pairs between the outer extremities of the domain of DNase I-sensitive chromatin. The occurrence of minichromosomes with two visible nucleosome gaps is indicated by +. N.D., not determined (Jongstra et al., 1984).

still present in these mutants, indicating a possible involvement of the enhancer sequence in the generation of altered chromatin structure. It is noteworthy that other studies have shown that deletion of one of the two 72 bp sequences has very little effect on the enhancer activity (Benoist and Chambon, 1981; Wasylyk *et al.*, 1983a; Moreau *et al.*, 1981; Gruss *et al.*, 1981; Fromm and Berg, 1982). To further define the sequences necessary to induce the increased DNase I sensitivity over region II, we inserted in both orientations at ORI B a DNA fragment from position 113 to 270, containing mainly the 72 bp repeat (In22 and In23, Fig. 5). Both mutants displayed a DNase I-sensitive region of similar intensity over the inserted fragment. To test the effect of the size of the insert on the extent of the region of increased DNase I sensitivity, a mutant was constructed in which the DNA segment inserted at ORI B of In22 was duplicated (In222). As shown in Fig. 5, this resulted in a duplication of the DNase I-sensitive region seen in In22. We also tested whether a single 72 bp sequence is able to induce an altered chromatin structure by deleting one of the two 72 bp sequences from ORI B at In22 (IN60, Fig. 5). Again a region of increased DNase I sensitivity was found located over the 72 bp sequence. These and other results (Jongstra *et al.*, 1984) demonstrate that a large fraction of the increased DNase I sensitivity in the ORI region of SV40 is critically dependent on the presence of the 72 bp repeat enhancer element. Moreover, and most important, an alteration of chromatin structure is generated at ORI B by insertion of the 72 bp repeat region, in either orientation, and in the absence of other ORI sequences.

b. Insertion of Enhancer Sequences at ORI B Can Generate a Nucleosome Gap. To investigate whether the nucleosomal gap, which is observed over the ORI region in approximately 25% of wild-type SV40 minichromosomes extracted from nuclei late in infection, could be duplicated at ORI B, minichromosomes isolated from cells infected with In10 were examined by electron microscopy. Approximately one-fourth of the minichromosomes had a nucleosome gap (Fig. 6a) which appeared to map preferentially over ORI A when using the single cut restriction enzymes *Eco*RI (Fig. 6b) or *Msp*I (an isoschizomer of *Hpa*II, Fig. 6c; note that the *Hpa*II–*Msp*I site was lost at ORI B). In addition, two diametrically opposed gaps were present in approximately 6% of the minichromosomes (Fig. 6d). These two gaps were mapped over ORI A and ORI B after digestion with *Eco*RI (Fig. 6e) or *Msp*I (Fig. 6f). To determine which ORI sequences were responsible for the generation of the nucleosome gap, we analyzed the "In" mutants described above for the presence of a nucleosome gap at ORI B. Results summarized in Fig. 5 indicate that a similar fraction of the minichromosomes of the two mutants In42 and In421 contained two nucleosome gaps, mapping over ORI A and ORI B,

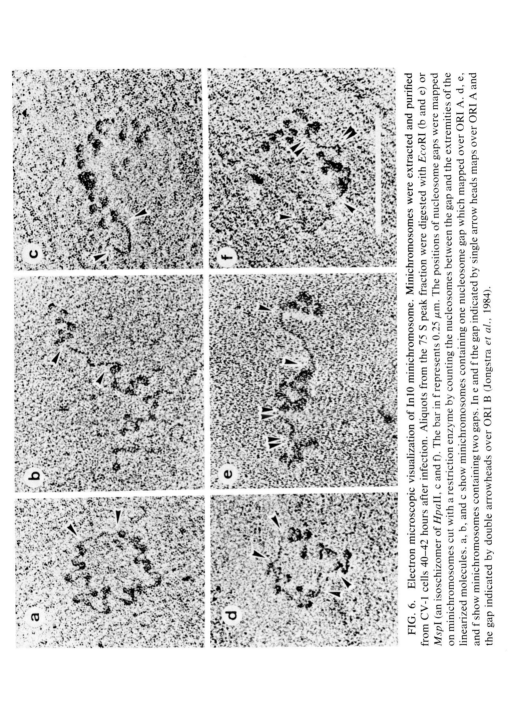

FIG. 6. Electron microscopic visualization of In10 minichromosome. Minichromosomes were extracted and purified from CV-1 cells 40–42 hours after infection. Aliquots from the 75 S peak fraction were digested with *EcoRI* (b and e) or *MspI* (an isoschizomer of *HpaII*, c and f). The bar in f represents 0.25 μm. The positions of nucleosome gaps were mapped on minichromosomes cut with a restriction enzyme by counting the nucleosomes between the gap and the extremities of the linearized molecules. a, b, and c show minichromosomes containing one nucleosome gap which mapped over ORI A. d, e, and f show minichromosomes containing two gaps. In e and f the gap indicated by single arrow heads maps over ORI A and the gap indicated by double arrowheads over ORI B (Jongstra *et al.*, 1984).

while mutant In22 contained a gap only over ORI A. A possible way to account for these results is to postulate that the presence of the DNase I-sensitive region I is a prerequisite for the induction of a nucleosome gap. A second possibility is that the induction of a visible nucleosome gap required the existence of a minimal length of altered chromatin structure. To test these hypotheses we examined minichromosomes extracted from In222-infected cells and found that a similar fraction of them contained two nucleosome gaps (Fig. 5). These results strongly support the conclusion that the total length of increased DNase I sensitivity at ORI B is the crucial factor in determining gap formation and that the increase in nuclease sensitivity and the nucleosome gap occur on the same minichromosomes. But again, the major conclusion is that sequences mostly contained within the 72 bp repeat are sufficient to generate a visible nucleosomal gap.

3. Evidence That the SV40 Enhancer May Interact Specifically with a Transcription Factor

That the SV40 enhancer may be specifically recognized by a transcription factor was recently suggested by the results of *in vitro* studies performed in our laboratory with chimeric recombinant DNA templates containing the SV40 72 bp repeat and heterologous promoter elements (Sassone-Corsi *et al.*, 1984). Such recombinants containing the adenovirus-2 major late promoter element from +33 to −34 and various sequences of the SV40 enhancer inserted 63 bp upstream from the adenovirus-2 major late start site are shown in Fig. 7. Previous *in vivo* studies have shown that no RNA could be detected after short-term transfection of HeLa cells with pSVA34, whereas insertion of the 72 bp repeat (coordinates 113 to 270) in both orientations (pSVBA34, pSVBIA34), in close apposition to the adenovirus-2 major late promoter element, resulted in a dramatic increase, at least 100-fold, of RNA synthesis (Hen *et al.*, 1982). Deletion of exactly one 72 bp sequence (pTBOA34) did not significantly reduce the activity of the SV40 enhancer, whereas deletions affecting the remaining 72 bp sequence (pTB208A34 and pTB101A34) resulted in drastic reductions of the *in vivo* enhancer activity (Hen *et al.*, 1982; our unpublished observations).

The DNA of these chimeric recombinants was used as a template with a cell-free whole cell extract (WCE) (Manley *et al.*, 1980) using either linear or circular templates. Figure 7 shows a comparison of the run-off transcripts obtained with linearized templates (similar results were obtained with circular templates; see Sassone-Corsi *et al.*, 1984). It is clear that the presence of the 72 bp repeat markedly stimulates the synthesis of the

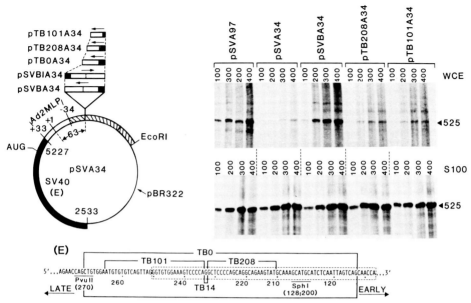

FIG. 7. Structure and *in vitro* transcription of chimeric recombinants containing the wild-type or mutated SV40 72 bp repeat and a promoter element of the Adenovirus major late promoter (Ad2MLP). pSVA34, pSVBA34, pSVBIA34, pTB208A34, and pTB101A34 have been described (Hen *et al.*, 1982). pSVA34 contains the SV40 early coding region [heavy line, SV40 (E), coordinates 5227–2533] downstream from the Ad2MLP region between +33 and −34 which includes the capsite (+1) and the complete TATA box (double line, the replacing Ad2 sequences upstream from −34 are hatched). In pSVBA34 and pSVBIA34 the wild-type (coordinates 113 to 272) segment containing the 72 bp repeat (open boxes) was inserted in both orientations [the arrows indicate the natural orientation with respect to the SV40 (E) sequence] in an *Sst*I site 63 bp upstream from the Ad2MLP capsite. pTBOA34, pTB208A34, pTB101A34 contain the fraction of the 72 bp repeat present in the deletion mutants TBO [one exact 72 bp sequence deleted between the *Sph*I sites at SV40 coordinates 128 and 200, (E)], TB208 and TB101 previously described (E; Moreau *et al.*, 1981; Wasylyk *et al.*, 1983a). E represents the sequence of the 72 bp repeat region present in pTBOA34, pTB208A34, and pTB101A34. The sequence which is boxed corresponds to the 72 bp repeat region (with exactly one 72 bp sequence deleted) inserted in pTBOA34 (the 72 bp sequence is boxed with a dashed line). The effect of the 72 bp repeat on transcription from the adenovirus major late promoter element using a whole cell (WCE) or an S100 extract is shown in the righthand panel; 100, 200, 300, or 400 ng of complete *Taq*I digests were used as indicated, in run-off transcription assays with WCE or S100 (Sassone-Corsi *et al.*, 1984). The size of the run-off RNA initiated at the Ad2MLP capsite is 525 nucleotides.

specific run-off RNA (525 nucleotides in length, compare pSVA34 and pSVBA34). A similar stimulation was observed when the SV40 enhancer was inserted in the reverse orientation (pSVBIA34, not shown; see Sassone-Corsi *et al.*, 1984). No significant decrease in specific transcription was observed when exactly one 72 bp sequence was deleted (pTBOA34), whereas no significant stimulation of transcription over the level observed with pSVA34 was obtained with the deletion mutants pTB101A34 and pTB208A34, in accord with their *in vivo* effect (Hen *et al.*, 1982; Wasylyk *et al.*, 1983a). Other experiments (see Sassone-Corsi *et al.*, 1984) have shown that this *in vitro* activation is a cis-effect which can be observed with other heterologous promoter elements. However, when a cell-free S100 extract (Weil *et al.*, 1979) was used instead of a whole cell extract, no stimulation was observed whether the template was linear (Fig. 7) or circular (not shown).

From these studies we conclude that the characteristics of the *in vitro* stimulation are in keeping with many known properties of the SV40 enhancer *in vivo* (see above), although its magnitude is lower than *in vivo*. Moreover, the fact that this *in vitro* stimulatory effect is observed with a whole cell extract, but not with a S100 extract, suggests the involvement of a specific factor which, in S100 extracts, is either present not at all, or not in an appropriate ratio to other factors modulating transcription *in vitro*.

4. Are Several Mechanisms Involved in the Entry Site Function of the SV40 Enhancer?

From the results presented and discussed above, it appears that at least two mechanisms can be involved to account for the entry site function of the SV40 72 bp repeat. First, the generation of an altered chromatin structure over the enhancer could lead to the formation of an "open window" in the nucleosomal structure, thereby increasing the accessibility of the DNA within the enhancer for binding of macromolecules involved in transcription. Second, sequences within the 72 bp repeat could be specifically recognized by some component of the transcription machinery. One could therefore speculate that both the generation of an open chromatin structure and sequence-specific interactions between the 72 bp repeat and the transcription machinery act in concert to facilitate the activation of promoter elements embedded in the complex genome of higher eukaryotes.

The molecular mechanisms underlying the generation of altered chromatin structures over the 72 bp repeat are unknown. Several possibilities which are not mutually exclusive can be considered. *In vitro* reconstitution experiments showing that nucleosomes form less well on the ORI region than on the rest of the SV40 genome suggest that some DNA sequences within the ORI region cannot easily be folded around the histone octamer core (Wasylyk *et al.*, 1979; Hiwasa *et al.*, 1981). In this respect we note that it has been recently demonstrated that some sequences within and on the late side of the 72 bp repeat can exist in the Z DNA conformation *in vitro* (Nordheim and Rich, 1983) and that nucleosomes cannot be formed over Z DNA (Nickol *et al.*, 1982). The alterations in chromatin structure may also be brought about by the binding of specific proteins, thereby inhibiting nucleosome formation. Interactions between enhancer sequences and specific cellular proteins have been recently suggested by studies demonstrating that the activity of some viral and cellular enhancers is cell- and/or species-specific (see above for references). Such proteins could be component(s) of the transcription machinery (see above) or belong to the class of proteins which specifically recognize form Z DNA (Nordheim *et al.*, 1982).

Obviously the identification of such putative proteins, the further development of *in vitro* systems, and the characterization at the nucleotide level of the sequences within the 72 bp repeat which are responsible for the enhancing activity and for the generation of altered chromatin structures are required to elucidate the molecular mechanisms underlying these important biological functions and their relationship to one another.

D. ARE ENHANCERS WIDESPREAD REGULATORY ELEMENTS OF TRANSCRIPTION OF CELLULAR GENES?

The functional significance of a viral enhancer element activating the transcription of an early viral transcription unit is obvious for the physiology of the virus. It provides a way for efficiently diverting a fraction of the cellular transcription machinery for its own usage, at a time when a single viral promoter, embedded in the highly complex cellular genome, must successfully compete with all of the surrounding cellular promoters. The discovery of viral enhancers immediately raised the question of the possible existence of cellular enhancers which would ensure efficient transcription of cellular genes which are actively transcribed. The finding that viral enhancers could exhibit some cell and/or species specificity (see above) suggested that they may interact with some activating cellular components, the physiological function of which would be to activate some cellular gene enhancers. This suggestion was strongly supported by the discovery of enhancer elements which function only in lymphoid cells and activate the promoter elements of somatically rearranged heavy and kappa light immunoglobulin variable region genes (see above for references). Interestingly enough, the region of the mouse kappa immunoglobulin gene which contains the enhancer element corresponds to a chromatin segment of increased DNase I sensitivity in the lymphoid cells which express this gene (Parslow and Granner, 1983).

It appears therefore that enhancers could correspond to positive regulatory elements which, to be functional, would require the binding of specific regulatory proteins, the presence or absence of which would then determine whether or not an enhancer functions in a given cell type. Incidently, if such specific enhancer binding proteins exist, the protein which binds to the SV40 enhancer should be widespread, since the latter is active in a variety of cell types belonging to different species from man to chicken (our unpublished observations). Although, at the present time, unequivocal evidence for the existence of cellular enhancers has been obtained only in the case of mouse heavy chain and kappa light chain immunoglobulin genes, it is tempting to speculate that enhancers are present in a number of cellular genes and that they serve as a general mechanism for gene regulation in eukaryotes. It is easy to envisage that a particular enhancer-binding protein could activate a given set of genes (a family) which are coordinately and cell specifically expressed at a given stage during the process of cell differentiation. Variations in the distance between the enhancer element and the promoter elements of the various activated genes could determine the actual level of expression of a given gene of the family. Alternatively, or concomitantly, minor variations in the sequences of the enhancers specific to a given family of genes could lead to different binding affinities of a particular enhancer binding protein, which would also result in different levels of expression. Such a possibility is supported by the observation that immunoglobulin enhancers are active only in lymphoid cells, although their sequences present some similarities with those of SV40 and other viral enhancers (Banerji et al., 1983; Hen et al., 1983). Thus, by using these combinatorial possibilities, a large number of genes could be differentially controlled by a small number of enhancer binding proteins.

If such enhancer-based mechanisms of control of gene expression would be operative in eukaryotic cells, one would obviously expect that enhancers activated by binding of receptor–hormone complexes could be involved in the positive regulation of the genes whose expression is induced at the transcriptional level by steroid hormones. In fact, the glucocorticoid response element, which is a far upstream element of the mouse mammary tumor virus (MMTV) promoter region, may be an example of such a regulated enhancer element, since it can enhance transcription from an heterologous promoter element in an apparently orientation-independent manner and does bind the hormone–receptor complex (Chandler et al., 1983). It is however still a matter of controversy whether or not the MMTV glucocorticoid response element possesses all of the characteristics of a bona fide enhancer element (see G. Hager et al., this volume).

The question of whether genes whose expression is controlled at the transcriptional level by estrogen and progesterone possess regulated enhancer elements is discussed below.

III. Toward a Dissection of the Chicken Ovalbumin and Conalbumin Gene Promoter Regions

The mechanism of estrogen and progesterone regulation of gene expression in the chicken oviduct has been extensively studied over the last 10 years (O'Malley et al., 1979; Palmiter et al., 1981; Schrader et al., 1981). In particular, administration of either progesterone or estrogen to "withdrawn" chickens (the so-called secondary stimulation) results in a rapid synthesis of ovalbumin, conalbumin, and the other egg-white proteins (Palmiter, 1973), which is consecutive to an induction of the transcription of their genes (Palmiter, 1975; Chambon, 1977; Mulvihill and Palmiter, 1977, 1980; Nguyen-Huu et al., 1978; McKnight, 1978; O'Malley et al., 1979; McKnight and Palmiter, 1979; Palmiter et al., 1981; Evans et al., 1981; Compere et al., 1981; LeMeur et al., 1981; and references therein). As necessary steps toward the understanding of the hormonal control of transcription, we have previously cloned the ovalbumin gene family (ovalbumin, X and Y genes) (Breathnach et al., 1978; Gannon et al., 1979; Chambon et al., 1979; Royal et al., 1979; Heilig et al., 1980, 1982), the conalbumin gene (Cochet et al., 1979a,b), and the ovomucoid gene (Gerlinger et al., 1982). We have then studied the 5' ends of their transcription units (see also Wasylyk et al., 1980) with the hope that a comparison of the DNA flanking sequences will provide a means of testing the idea that steroid hormones act (at least in part) through interactions of steroid-receptor complexes with the genome (Mulvihill et al., 1982; Heilig et al., 1980, 1982). Unfortunately, these comparisons did not reveal any striking sequence homologies upstream from the capsites of these genes, with the exception of the TATA box sequence. However, Mulvihill et al. (1982), using crude or partially purified preparations of chicken oviduct form A progesterone receptor, observed specific binding of this receptor to several DNA fragments of the ovalbumin, conalbumin, ovomucoid, X and Y genes, notably to fragments located upstream from the RNA startsites of these genes. Based on a comparison of the sequences containing these various binding sites, a consensus sequence that may constitute a region interacting with the progesterone–receptor complex was constructed (Mulvihill et al., 1982; Davison et al., 1982). Moreover, studies performed in our laboratory (Bellard et al., 1982; Kaye et al., 1984) have shown that the chromatin structure of the chicken genome region located upstream from the ovalbumin gene capsite is highly altered for several kilobases and exhibits several zones of nuclease hypersensitivity whose location may correspond, at least for some of them, to steroid hormone–receptor binding sites.

The above results suggest that enhancer elements positively regulated by the binding of hormone-receptor complexes (see Section II,D) could be involved in the hormonal control of transcription of the chicken egg-white protein genes. The establishment of an *in vivo* functional assay for putative enhancer elements is obviously a prerequisite to any study aimed at testing such a possibility. Unfortunately, there is no permanent avian cell line possessing functional estrogen and/or progesterone receptors, into which *in vitro* manipulated ovalbumin or conalbumin gene promoter elements could be introduced to characterize the sequences responsible for the modulation of initiation of transcription by steroid hormones. We have recently circumvented this lack of permanent cell lines by microinjecting chimeric recombinants containing the 5′ upstream regions of the ovalbumin and conalbumin genes into the nuclei of a variety of cells, including chicken oviduct primary cultured cells.

A. CONSTRUCTION OF CHIMERIC RECOMBINANTS TO TEST THE FUNCTION OF THE CONALBUMIN AND OVALBUMIN PROMOTER ELEMENTS AFTER MICROINJECTION INTO CELL NUCLEI

The putative promoter elements located upstream from position +62 of the conalbumin gene (Fig. 8A, the pTCT series) and from position +1 of the ovalbumin gene (Fig. 8B, the pTOT series) were inserted upstream from the SV40 T-antigen coding sequence, in such a manner that T-antigen expression is under the control of these elements. DNAs of the conalbumin pTCT series and of the ovalbumin pTOT series were then microinjected into cell nuclei (using DNA concentrations of either 50 or 100 μg/ml), and 6 or 24 hours after microinjection the cells were scored for T-antigen production by indirect immunofluorescence as previously described (Moreau *et al.*, 1981; Everett *et al.*, 1983). In each series of experiments, the wild-type SV40 early region recombinant pSV1 (Benoist and Chambon, 1981), which possesses the SV40 early promoter region in place of the ovalbumin or conalbumin promoter regions, was also microinjected. The results of the pTCT and pTOT series were expressed relative to the number of immunofluorescent cells obtained with pSV1 taken as 100% (pSV1 was expressed with approximately the same efficiency in all cell types under our experimented conditions).

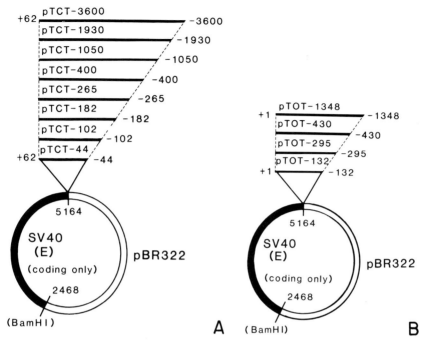

FIG. 8. Schematic representation of the chimeric expression recombinants containing various conalbumin (A, series TCT) and ovalbumin (B, series TOT) promoter regions. The heavy line represents the SV40 T-antigen coding region (see legend to Fig. 7). The coordinates of the various promoter fragments inserted upstream from the SV40 sequence are indicated (see text).

B. THE EXPRESSION OF THE MICROINJECTED OVALBUMIN AND CONALBUMIN GENE PROMOTER REGION RECOMBINANT IS CELL- AND SPECIES-SPECIFIC, BUT THE OVALBUMIN PROMOTER REGION IS FUNCTIONAL IN CHICKEN HEPATOCYTES

Previous studies of our laboratory have shown that the ovalbumin (Breathnach *et al.*, 1980) and conalbumin (Wasylyk and Chambon, 1982; Wasylyk *et al.*, 1983b) gene promoters function very inefficiently in mouse fibroblast LMtk⁻ cells permanently transformed with recombinants containing these promoters. Moreover, most of the ovalbumin and conalbumin RNA produced by these cells is not accurately initiated at the natural capsites. The results summarized in Table I indicate that in the same mouse fibroblast LMtk⁻ cells the promoter regions of these two

TABLE I

Expression of Conalbumin and Ovalbumin Promoter Chimeric Recombinants in Various Cell Types[a]

| | Immunofluorescent cells (percentage of pSV1) (DNA 100 μg/ml, 24 hours) | | | | | |
| | | | | | Primary culture cells | |
Chimeric recombinants	CV1	LMTK⁻	HeLa	MCF-7	Chicken fibroblast	Mouse liver
Convalbumin promoter						
pTCT-44	0 (4)	0 (3)	0 (3)	0 (3)	0 (4)	0 (1)
pTCT-102	0 (4)	0 (3)	0 (3)	0 (3)	0 (4)	0 (1)
pTCT-182	0 (4)	0 (3)	ND	ND	0 (4)	ND
pTCT-265	0 (4)	0 (3)	ND	ND	0 (4)	ND
pTCT-400	0 (4)	0 (3)	0 (3)	0 (3)	0 (4)	ND
pTCT-1050	0 (4)	0 (3)	0 (3)	0 (3)	0 (4)	0 (1)
pTCT-1930	0 (4)	0 (3)	0 (3)	0 (3)	0 (4)	0 (1)
pTCT-3600	0 (4)	0 (3)	0 (3)	0 (3)	0 (4)	0 (1)
Ovalbumin promoter						
pTOT-132	0 (3)	ND	0 (3)	2 (3)	ND	ND
pTOT-295	0 (3)	ND	0 (3)	6.0 (3)	0 (3)	ND
pTOT-430	0 (3)	0 (3)	0 (3)	2 (3)	0 (3)	ND
pTOT-1348	0 (3)	0 (3)	0 (3)	0 (3)	0 (3)	ND

[a] The DNA of the chimeric recombinants of the pTCT and pTOT series (Fig. 8A and B) were microinjected into the cells indicated in the table as previously described (Moreau *et al.*, 1981). T-antigen positive cells were detected by indirect immunofluorescence and the results were expressed in percentage relative to those obtained using the SV40 wild-type pSV1 recombinant (30 to 75% of the pSV1 microinjected cells were T-antigen positive; see text and Moreau *et al.*, 1981). In most cases the figures correspond to average values of several experiments (the number of experiments performed with each recombinant is indicated in parentheses; ND, not determined).

genes also do not function using nuclear microinjection and a transient expression assay. Increasing the length of the inserted segment from −44 to −3600 in the case of the pTCT series, and from −132 to −1348 in the case of the pTOT series, does not change the inactivity of the conalbumin and ovalbumin promoter regions in these mouse cells. Similarly, the promoter regions of these two genes do not function in the monkey kidney-derived CV1 cells, the human HeLa cells or the human breast cancer-derived MCF-7 cells (with the possible exception of the pTOT-132 and pTOT-295 recombinants). The inactivity of the conalbumin and ovalbu-

TABLE II

Expression of Conalbumin and Ovalbumin Promoter Chimeric Recombinants in Primary Culture of Chicken Hepatocytes (Synthetic Medium without Steroid Hormone)[a]

Chimeric recombinants	Immunofluorescent cells (percentage of pSV1)	
	24 hour microinjection DNA (50 μg/ml)	6 hour microinjection DNA (100 μg/ml)
Conalbumin promoter		
pTCT-44	5.5 (3)	7.9 (2)
pTCT-102	28.1 (12)	49.6 (6)
pTCT-182	29.7 (4)	29.5 (4)
pTCT-265	45.3 (7)	30.2 (6)
pTCT-400	48.4 (5)	50.3 (3)
pTCT-1050	62.5 (12)	58.3 (7)
pTCT-1930	48.4 (4)	38.8 (3)
pTCT-3600	18.7 (3)	7.2 (3)
Ovalbumin promoter		
pTOT-132	28.1 (6)	28.8 (3)
pTOT-295	26.5 (4)	32.4 (3)
pTOT-430	37.5 (3)	27.3 (3)
pTOT-1348	40.6 (3)	41.7 (3)

[a] The primary cultured chicken hepatocytes were maintained in a synthetic medium in the absence of steroid hormones. For methods and representation of the results, see text and legend to Table I. Approximately 70% of the cells microinjected with the reference recombinant pSV1 were T-antigen positive.

min promoter regions in the human, monkey, and mouse cells is not primarily related to a problem of species specificity, since they are also inactive in primary cultures of chicken fibroblasts (all of these cells were cultured in the presence of fetal calf serum or calf serum both of which contained steroid hormones).

It is striking that both the pTCT and pTOT series express T-antigen to various extents in chicken liver primary cultured cells (Table II). No T-antigen expression was observed using the corresponding basic recombinant which contains the T-antigen coding region and not the conalbumin or ovalbumin promoter regions (Fig. 8) (not shown). Therefore, it appears that the chicken liver cells may contain a factor(s) responsible for the cell-specific activity of the ovalbumin and conalbumin promoter region. That, in addition, this liver cell specificity is species-specific is indicated by the results obtained by microinjection of the pTCT recombinants in mouse liver primary cultured cells, where the promoter regions are inactive (Table I).

Several points, which deserve further study, are noteworthy in the results shown in Table II. First, it is surprising that the ovalbumin gene promoter region is active in liver cells, since this gene, in contrast to the conalbumin gene, is not expressed in the chicken liver even after steroid hormone administration (McKnight et al., 1980a,b). Thus, it appears that it is not the absence of a specific transcription factor which is responsible for the nonexpression of the ovalbumin gene in the chicken liver, but some developmental event, negatively cis-acting (for example DNA methylation, see Mandel and Chambon, 1979), which can be bypassed by microinjecting the DNA in differentiated hepatocytes. Second, neither estrogen nor progesterone is required for the function of the ovalbumin and conalbumin promoter regions (the hepatocytes were maintained in a synthetic medium free of steroid hormones, and, in addition, the activity of the conalbumin and ovalbumin promoter regions was not inhibited by the addition of an antiestrogen or an antiprogesterone). This is not surprising for the conalbumin gene promoter, since this gene is "constitutively" expressed in chicken liver and its expression is only moderately activated by steroid hormone administration (McKnight et al., 1980a,b). However, the activity of the ovalbumin gene promoter in hepatocytes is intriguing, since the expression of this gene is under strict steroid hormone control in the only chicken cells where it is naturally expressed, i.e., the oviduct tubular gland cells. Third, it is surprising that the conalbumin recombinant pTCT-44 is expressed in a cell-specific manner, since it suggests that some cell-specific factor(s) may interact with the TATA box or the capsite regions, whereas it was assumed up to now that regulatory factors would rather interact with sequences located further upstream (see above). Fourth, sequences located upstream from the TATA box between -44 and -102 are important for the efficiency of the conalbumin promoter region in these assays. Fifth, for both ovalbumin and conalbumin gene promoters, sequences located upstream from position -100 appear to be important to reach maximum expression. However, it is clear that, in both cases, the activity of the promoter elements which are located downstream from position -100 is not crucially dependent on the presence of an upstream enhancer sequence.

C. THE MICROINJECTED OVALBUMIN AND CONALBUMIN GENE PROMOTER RECOMBINANTS ARE EXPRESSED IN CHICKEN OVIDUCT PRIMARY CULTURED CELLS

All of the ovalbumin and conalbumin promoter chimeric recombinants are also expressed to various extents in primary cultures of oviduct cells,

TABLE III

Expression of Conalbumin and Ovalbumin Promoter Chimeric Recombinants in Primary Culture of Chicken Oviduct Cells (Fetal Calf Serum)[a]

Chimeric recombinants	Immunofluorescent cells (percentage of pSV1)	
	24 hour microinjection DNA (50 µg/ml)	6 hour microinjection DNA (100 µg/ml)
Conalbumin promoter		
pTCT-44	15 (4)	28 (5)
pTCT-102	54 (7)	77 (7)
pTCT-182	63 (5)	45 (5)
pTCT-265	28 (10)	43 (5)
pTCT-400	70 (8)	76 (6)
pTCT-1050	70 (6)	103 (6)
pTCT-1930	32 (6)	55 (7)
pTCT-3600	25 (5)	21 (5)
Ovalbumin promoter		
pTOT-132	58 (4)	61 (5)
pTOT-295	46 (4)	55 (6)
pTOT-430	60 (7)	47 (5)
pTOT-1348	43 (3)	45 (4)

[a] The tubular gland primary cultured cells of estrogen-stimulated oviduct were maintained in 10% fetal calf serum. For methods and representation of the results, see text and legend to Table I. Approximately 60 to 70% of the cells microinjected with the reference recombinant pSV1 were T-antigen positive.

isolated from estradiol-stimulated chicken and maintained in the presence of fetal calf serum containing steroid hormones (Table III). Again, it is striking that recombinant pTCT-44, which contains very little conalbumin promoter sequences upstream from the TATA box, is expressed in a cell- and species-specific manner. Once more, the results obtained with both the pTCT and pTOT series do not suggest that sequences located upstream from position $-100/-130$ exert a crucial potentiator (enhancer) role on the activity of the promoter elements located downstream from -100. Finally, it is very interesting to note that, in contrast to the hepatocyte situation (see above), the addition of an antiestrogen or an antiprogesterone, or of both of them, to the culture medium results in a marked decrease in the expression of some conalbumin recombinants and in an even stronger decrease of the expression of some ovalbumin recombinants (our unpublished results).

D. PROSPECTS

The ability to use the nuclear microinjection technique to study the function of the ovalbumin and conalbumin gene promoter region opens the possibility to dissect these regions into their functional elements. It is already clear from the preliminary observations discussed above that the final picture will be much more complicated than anticipated. In this respect, it is certainly puzzling that the promoter of the ovalbumin gene can function specifically and with similar efficiency in cultured hepatocytes (although it is not expressed *in vivo* in the liver) and in cultured oviduct cells. What is even more puzzling, is that its activity in hepatocytes is independent of the presence of steroid hormones, whereas the presence of both estrogen and progesterone is required for its function in the oviduct cells. The observation that some information concerning the cell- and species-specific expression of the conalbumin gene is contained between position $+62$ and -44 is also puzzling. In view of the complexity of the situation, it is clear that much more has to be learned before we will be in a position to answer definitively the question of whether or not enhancer elements, positively regulated by steroid hormones, control the activity of the ovalbumin and conalbumin promoter elements.

IV. A Promising Estrogen-Inducible Gene in Human Breast Cancer Cells

As discussed above, although the chicken oviduct has been an extraordinarily helpful system to study many aspects of regulation of gene expression at the transcriptional level by estrogens and progesterone, the lack of a permanent oviduct cell line containing functional estrogen and progesterone receptors constitutes a serious limitation to its use for *in vitro* genetics studies. In this respect, the development of cell lines derived from human breast cancer that retain most, if not all, of the receptors for steroid hormones (Horwitz and McGuire, 1978; Horwitz *et al.*, 1983; and references therein) may provide an alternative system easier to manipulate *in vitro*. Previous work has indeed shown that the levels of some cellular proteins (including the progesterone receptor) and messenger RNAs are under the control of estrogens in the MCF-7 cell line derived from a human breast cancer containing both estrogen and progesterone receptors (see Horwitz and McGuire, 1978; Westley and Rochefort, 1980; Adams *et al.*, 1980; Edwards *et al.*, 1980; Masiakowski *et al.*, 1982; and references therein). Moreover, another human breast cancer cell line, T47D, has been described which synthesizes high level of progesterone receptor independently of estrogen control (Horwitz *et al.*, 1983; and references therein). These cell lines are thus particularly suited for studies of the molecular bases of steroid hormone control of gene expression; once cloned, the hormone-responsive genes can be easily reintroduced into the parent cell line and *in vitro* mutagenesis techniques used to define control regions at the DNA level. The availability of cloned hormone-responsive genes from MCF-7 cells may also lead to a better understanding of the role of estrogen in breast cancer: tumors which contain estrogen and progesterone receptors may often be treated successfully by antiestrogen administration (for reviews, see Pike *et al.*, 1981). However, the human breast cancer cell lines present one disadvantage when compared to the chicken oviduct; the steroid hormone-induced proteins are present in low amounts in these cell lines, which makes the cloning of the responsive genes more difficult than in the oviduct case. Nevertheless, we have recently cloned a double-stranded cDNA (ds-cDNA) corresponding to a MCF-7 mRNA (termed pS2 RNA) whose synthesis is induced at the transcriptional level by addition of estradiol to the culture medium (Masiakowski *et al.*, 1982). Moreover, we have found that this mRNA, which cannot be detected in any other cell of human origin, is present in biopsies of some breast tumors.

A. pS2 RNA, WHICH IS INDUCED BY ESTRADIOL IN MCF-7 CELLS, IS NOT PRESENT IN OTHER HUMAN CELLS

We have previously reported the accumulation of pS2 RNA after addition of estradiol to MCF-7 cells grown in estradiol-stripped medium (Masiakowski *et al.*, 1982). That this induction is highly specific is shown in Fig. 9A and B, where the same RNA blot was hybridized with the pS2 ds-cDNA probe (Fig. 9A) or with the ds-cDNA probes 36B4 and 3A5 which correspond to polyadenylated RNAs which appear to be expressed in all human cells.

Starting from the RNA of cells grown in estradiol-stripped medium (lanes 1, W), there is a clear increase in pS2 RNA at 3 hours (lanes 5), 8 hours (lanes 6), and 24 hours (lanes 7) after addition of estradiol, whereas very little increase occurs during the first 15 minutes (lanes 2), 30 minutes (lanes 3), and 1 hour (lanes 4) periods. After 24 hours of estradiol exposure, the amount of pS2 RNA is similar to that found in cells which are permanently grown in nontreated fetal calf serum (compare lanes 7, 8, and 9). In marked contrast, there was no modification in the amount of the 36B4 and 3A5 RNAs during the same periods of time (Fig. 9B).

Total or poly(A)$^+$ RNA from a variety of human cells was similarly analyzed. No pS2 RNA could be detected in other human cells in culture (HeLa, cell, human fibroblasts), nor in human cells or tissues (lympho-

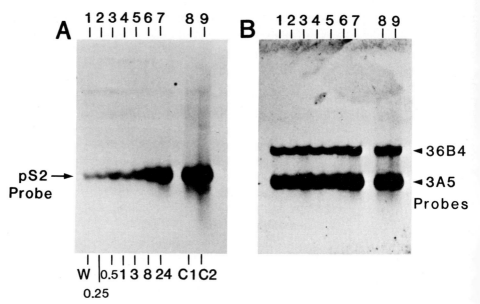

FIG. 9. Accumulation of pS2 RNA in MCF-7 cells following addition of estradiol to an estradiol-stripped culture medium (Masiakowski *et al.*, 1982). Ten micrograms of cytoplasmic RNA was electrophoresed in each lane and, after transfer to DBM-paper, hybridization was performed with either pS2 (A) or 36B4 and 3A5 (B) ds-cDNA probes. Slots 1–7: RNA from cells exposed to estradiol for 0, 15, 30 minutes, 1, 3, 8, and 24 hours. Slots 8 and 9: 10 μg of cytoplasmic or total RNA from cells maintained in 10% fetal calf serum, respectively (Krust and Chambon, 1984).

cytes, placenta, liver, endometrium, normal breast tissue), whereas the presence of 36B4 and 3A5 RNAs was readily revealed in the same cells or tissues (Krust and Chambon, 1984). Moreover, pS2 RNA is not present in the RNA extracted from the human breast cancer cells T47D (see Fig. 10), which contain the estrogen receptor, but in which the synthesis of the progesterone receptor does not require the presence of estrogen (see above). In contrast, 36B4 and 3A5 RNAs were present in T47D cells (Fig. 10). It appears therefore that the induction of accumulation of pS2 RNA by estrogen could be specific to a subset of estrogen receptor-containing human breast cancer cells (see also below). Other studies from our laboratory (not shown; Brown *et al.*, 1984) demonstrate that the addition of estradiol to MCF-7 cells grown in estradiol-stripped medium triggers transcription of the pS2 gene within 15 minutes after addition of hormone. Moreover, this induction of transcription is not inhibited by pretreatment of the cells for 1 hour with the protein synthesis inhibitor cycloheximide (Brown *et al.*, 1984). Thus, induction of transcription of the pS2 gene by

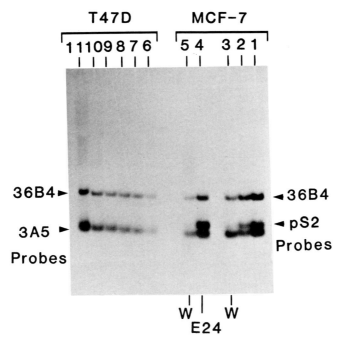

FIG. 10. pS2 RNA is not present in the T47D breast cancer cell line: 4.3, 8.6, 12.9, 17.3, 21.6, and 43.2 μg of total RNA extracted from T47D cells grown in 10% fetal calf serum was electrophoresed in slots 6 to 11, respectively. Slots 1 and 2 contained 23.2 and 10 μg of total RNA extracted from MCF-7 cells grown in fetal calf serum; slots 3 and 5 contained 10 μg of total RNA extracted from MCF-7 cells grown in estradiol-stripped medium; slots 4: 10 μg of total RNA extracted from MCF-7 cells grown first in estradiol-stripped medium and then for 24 hours in the presence of estradiol (Krust and Chambon, 1984). The probes were as indicated in the legend to Fig. 9.

estradiol appears to be a primary effect of the hormone, which makes the pS2 gene a very attractive model system to study regulation of initiation of transcription by estrogens. Studies along these lines are in progress using the promoter region of the pS2 gene which has been recently cloned in our laboratory (Jeltsch et al., 1984).

B. THE PRODUCT OF THE pS2 GENE IS A LOW-MOLECULAR-WEIGHT PROTEIN WHICH MAY BE SECRETED

A full ds-cDNA copy of pS2 RNA has been sequenced in our laboratory (Jakowlew et al., 1984). The sequence of the putative protein encoded by

```
             I                                   II
 ┌─────────────────────────┐ ┌──────────────────────────┐┌──────────────────┐
 MET ALA THR MET GLU ASN LYS VAL ILE CYS ALA LEU VAL LEU VAL SER MET LEU ALA LEU
 1                          10        II                      III            20
                III
 ┌──────────────────────────┐
 GLY THR LEU ALA GLU ALA GLN THR GLU THR CYS THR VAL ALA PRO ARG GLU ARG GLN ASN
                          30                                                40

 CYS GLY PHE PRO GLY VAL THR PRO SER GLN CYS ALA ASN LYS GLY CYS CYS PHE ASP ASP
                          50                                                60

 THR VAL ARG GLY VAL PRO TRP CYS PHE TYR PRO ASN THR ILE ASP VAL PRO PRO GLU GLU
                          70                                                80

 GLU CYS GLU PHE
```

FIG. 11.   Amino-acid sequence of the putative pS2 protein (Jakowlew *et al.*, 1984). See text.

pS2 RNA is shown in Fig. 11. It comprises only 84 amino acids and could be a secreted protein, since it has at its amino end some features which are characteristic of presecretory polypeptides (Perlman and Halvorson, 1983). First, a hydrophobic core (labeled II in Fig. 11) is preceded by a sequence (labeled I), which contains a charged residue (Lys) at its carboxyl-end and is followed by a sequence (labeled III) which contains the putative peptidase recognition sequence Ala-X-B↓ . Furthermore the preferred peptidase cleavage site ↓ located after the sixth amino acid following the core sequence, is preferentially an Ala, Gly, or Ser residue (Perlman and Halvorson, 1983). As shown in Fig. 11, it cannot be decided from the sequence alone whether the cleavage would occur after the glycine at position 21 or the alanine at position 26. However, in both cases, the predicted mature polypeptide would correspond to a small protein, either 63 or 58 amino acids in length. A direct study of the protein, in progress in our laboratory, is obviously required to distinguish between these two possibilities, and to further characterize the pS2 protein. In any case, the low molecular weight of the pS2 protein leads to the very attractive suggestion that it could correspond to a growth factor molecule, perhaps to one of the somatomedin-like estromedins which have been recently found in some estrogen-responsive tissues (Ikeda *et al.*, 1982).

C. THE pS2 GENE IS SPECIFICALLY EXPRESSED IN SOME HUMAN BREAST CANCERS

The observation that pS2 RNA is expressed in the human breast cancer cell line MCF-7, but not in line T47D, raises the interesting possibility that

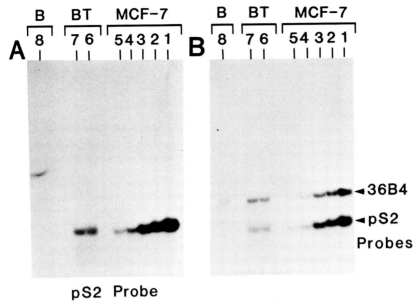

pS2 Probe

FIG. 12. Presence of pS2 RNA in a breast cancer biopsy from an estrogen and progesterone receptor-positive patient. Slots 1 to 5 contained 5.8, 2.9, 1.2, 0.6, and 0.3 μg of total RNA extracted from MCF-7 cells grown in fetal calf serum. Slots 6 and 7 contained two aliquots of the total RNA extracted from the biopsy, whereas slot 8 contained the total RNA extracted from a biopsy of healthy breast tissue. After electrophoresis the DBM-paper was hybridized to the pS2 dis-cDNA probe alone (A) or to a mixture of pS2 and 36B4 ds-cDNA probes (B) (Krust and Chambon, 1984).

it could be used as a probe to identify subsets of estradiol-dependent breast cancers. Previous studies have indeed shown that patients whose breast cancer biopsies are positive for estrogen and progesterone receptors have responsive rates to endocrine therapy approaching 80% (Osborne et al., 1980). However, measurements of progesterone receptors in breast tumor biopsies is often difficult for several reasons (see for instance Saez et al., 1978; Horwitz et al., 1983). Thus, the assay of an additional estrogen-inducible product in breast cancer biopsies would certainly be helpful. In addition, the assay of pS2 RNA in breast cancer biopsies presents the advantage of containing its own internal control (the assay of the universally expressed 36B4 and 3A5 RNAs—see above), whereas no such internal control is available for receptor assays.

A blot containing RNA extracted from a breast cancer biopsy of an estrogen and progesterone receptor-positive patient was hybridized, along with MCF-7 RNA, to pS2 and 36B4 ds-cDNA probes (Krust and Chambon, 1984). As shown in Fig. 12A and B (lanes 6 and 7), pS2 RNA was present in this breast cancer biopsy. However, it was absent in the

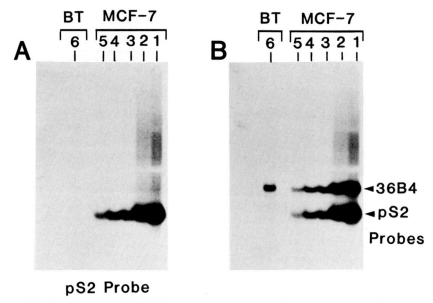

pS2 Probe

FIG. 13. Absence of pS2 RNA in a breast cancer biopsy from an estrogen and progesterone receptor-positive patient. Slots 1 to 5, as described in Fig. 12. Slot 6, total RNA extracted from the tumor biopsy. After electrophoresis the DBM-paper was hybridized as described in the legend to Fig. 12 (Krust and Chambon, 1984).

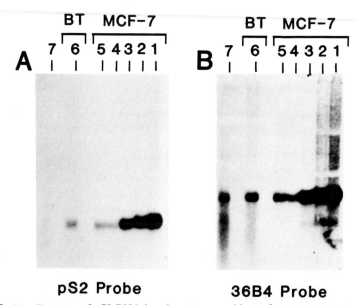

pS2 Probe   **36B4 Probe**

FIG. 14. Presence of pS2 RNA in a breast cancer biopsy from an estrogen receptor-doubtful and progesterone receptor-negative patient. Slots 1–5, as described in Fig. 12. Slot 6, total RNA extracted from the tumor biopsy. Slot 7, total RNA extracted from a breast fibroadenoma. After electrophoresis the DBM-paper was hybridized as described in the legend to Fig. 12, but the 36B4 ds-cDNA probe only was used in B.

biopsy of another estrogen and progesterone-receptor positive patient (Fig. 13, lanes 6), which is reminiscent of the T47D cell line pattern. On the contrary, the biopsy of a patient who was barely positive for estrogen receptor and negative for progesterone receptor, was positive for pS2 RNA (Fig. 14, lanes 6). Such a case may correspond to an hormone-dependent cancer, the diagnosis of which cannot be made by simple estrogen and progesterone receptor assays. We are analyzing at the present time a large number of receptor-positive and -negative biopsies to study the possible predictive value of the presence of pS2 RNA in breast cancers.

V. Conclusions

Although enormous progress has been made during these last 4 years in the characterization of the promoter elements which control initiation of transcription of eukaryotic protein-coding genes, it is clear that many problems remain to be solved before it will be possible to account, in molecular terms, for the control of gene expression by estrogen and progesterone. Regulation of transcription appears to be even more complicated in eukaryotes than in prokaryotes, and the mechanism of action of control elements, like the enhancers, remains largely hypothetical at the present time. Progress with *in vitro* transcription systems is imperatively required to elucidate the major unsolved problems. There is little doubt that the pace at which our knowledge increases in the field of regulation of transcription will become slower, because it is unfortunately technically much more difficult to purify a transcription factor or to reconstruct a specific chromatin template than to construct an additional chimeric recombinant and then to transfect it into HeLa cells. "Elegant" molecular genetics will have to give way to "trivial" biochemistry! At the present time, the newly characterized human breast cancer MCF-7 cell line system appears particularly attractive to solve some of the problems which are more difficult to tackle with the chicken oviduct system. As we have seen, it may even prove useful to the progress of our knowledge of the biology of breast tumors themselves.

ACKNOWLEDGMENTS

We thank our colleagues R. Breathnach, T. Brown, J. M. Jeltsch, and M. Roberts for communication of their unpublished results and A. Wildeman for an excellent critical reading of the manuscript. We are grateful to B. Chambon and C. Kutschis for help in the preparation of the manuscript and to C. Werlé and B. Boulay who made the illustrations. The original work described in this paper was supported by grants from the Centre National de la Recherche Scientifique, the Institut National de la Santé et de la Recherche Médicale, the Association pour le Développement de la Recherche sur le Cancer, the Fondation pour la Recherche Médicale, and from the Fondation Simone et Cino del Duca.

REFERENCES

Adams, D. J., Edwards, D. P., and McGuire, W. L. (1980). *Biochem. Biophys. Res. Commun.* **97,** 1354–1361.

Anderson, J. E. (1983). *In* "Biological Regulation and Development" (R. F. Goldberger and K. R. Yamamoto, eds.), Vol. 3B. Plenum, New York, in press.

Banerji, J., Rusconi, S., and Schaffner, W. (1981). *Cell* **27,** 299–308.

Banerji, J., Olson, L., and Schaffner, W. (1983). *Cell* **33,** 729–740.

Baty, D., Barrera-Saldana, H. A., Everett, R. D., Vigneron, M., and Chambon, P. (1984). *Nucleic Acids Res.* **12,** 915–932.

Bellard, M., Oudet, P., Germond, J. E., and Chambon, P. (1976). *Eur. J. Biochem.* **70,** 543–553.

Bellard, M., Dretzen, G., Bellard, F., Oudet, P., and Chambon, P. (1982). *EMBO J.* **1,** 223–230.

Benoist, C., and Chambon, P. (1981). *Nature (London)* **290,** 304–310.

Benoist, C., O'Hare, K., Breathnach, R., and Chambon, P. (1980). *Nucleic Acids Res.* **8,** 127–142.

Brady, J., Radonovich, M., Vodkin, M., Natarajan, V., Thoren, M., Das, G., Janik, J., and Salzman, N. P. (1982). *Cell* **31,** 625–633.

Breathnach, R., and Chambon, P. (1981). *Annu. Rev. Biochem.* **50,** 349–383.

Breathnach, R., Benoist, C., O'Hare, K., Gannon, F., and Chambon, P. (1978). *Proc. Natl. Acad. Sci. U.S.A.* **75,** 4853–4857.

Brinster, R. L., Chen, H. Y., Warren, R., Sarthy, A., and Palmiter, R. D. (1982). *Nature (London)* **296,** 39–42.

Brown, A., Krust, A., Jeltsch, J. M., Roberts, M., and Chambon, P. (1984). Submitted.

Chae, C. B., Mathis, D. J., Jongstra, J., Oudet, P., Benoist, C., and Chambon, P. (1982). *J. Cell. Biochem. Suppl.* **6,** 328.

Chambon, P. (1975). *Annu. Rev. Biochem.* **44,** 613–633.

Chambon, P. (1977). *Cold Spring Harbor Symp. Quant. Biol.* **42,** 1209–1234.

Chambon, P., Benoist, C., Breathnach, R., Cochet, M., Gannon, F., Gerlinger, P., Krust, A., LeMeur, M., LePennec, J. P., Mandel, J. L., O'Hare, K., and Perrin, F. (1979). *Proc. Miami Winter Symp., 11th* pp. 55–81.

Chandler, V. L., Maler, B. A., and Yamamoto, K. R. (1983). *Cell* **33,** 489–499.

Cochet, M., Gannon, F., Hen, R., Maroteaux, L., Perrin, F., and Chambon, P. (1979a). *Nature (London)* **282,** 567–574.

Cochet, M., Perrin, F., Gannon, F., Krust, A., Chambon, P., McKnight, G. S., Lee, D. C., Mayo, K. E., and Palmiter, R. D. (1979b). *Nucleic Acids Res.* **6,** 2435–2453.

Compere, S. J., McKnight, G. S., and Palmiter, R. D. (1981). *J. Biol. Chem.* **256,** 6341–6347.

Corden, J., Wasylyk, B., Buchwalder, A., Sassone-Corsi, P., Kédinger, C., and Chambon, P. (1980). *Science* **209,** 1406–1414.

Cremisi, C., (1981). *Nucleic Acids Res.* **9,** 5949–5963.

Cremisi, C., Pignatti, P. F., Croissant, O., and Yaniv, M. (1976). *J. Virol.* **17,** 204–211.

Davison, B. L., Mulvihill, E., Egly, J. M., and Chambon, P. (1982). *Cold Spring Harbor Symp. Quant. Biol.* **47,** 921–934.

Davison, B. L., Egly, J. M., Mulvihill, E. R., and Chambon, P. (1983). *Nature (London)* **301,** 680–686.

Dierks, P., van Ooyen, A., Cochran, M., Dobkin, C., Reiser, J., and Weissmann, C. (1983). *Cell* **32,** 695–706.

Dynan, W. S., and Tjian, R. (1983a). *Cell* **32,** 669–680.

Dynan, W. S., and Tjian, R. (1983b). *Cell* **35,** 79–87.

Edwards, D. P., Adams, D. J., Savage, N., and McGuire, W. L. (1980). *Biochem. Biophys. Res. Commun.* **93**, 804–812.

Evans, M. I., Hager, L. J., and McKnight, G. S. (1981). *Cell* **25**, 187–193.

Everett, R. D., Baty, D., and Chambon, P. (1983). *Nucleic Acids Res.* **11**, 2447–2464.

Fromm, M., and Berg, P. (1982). *J. Mol. Appl. Genet.* **1**, 457–481.

Fromm, M., and Berg, P. (1983). *J. Mol. Appl. Genet.* **2**, 127–135.

Gannon, F., O'Hare, K., Perrin, F., LePennec, J. P., Benoist, C., Cochet, M., Breathnach, R., Royal, A., Cami, B., and Chambon, P. (1979). *Nature (London)* **278**, 428–434.

Gerard, R. D., Woodworth-Gutai, M., and Scott, W. A. (1982). *Mol. Cell. Biol.* **2**, 782–788.

Gerlinger, P., Krust, A., LeMeur, M., Perrin, F., Cochet, M., Gannon, F., Dupret, D., and Chambon, P. (1982). *J. Mol. Biol.* **162**, 345–364.

Gillies, S. D., Morrison, S. L., Oi, V. T., and Tonegawa, S. (1983). *Cell* **33**, 717–728.

Gluzman, Y., and Shenk, T., eds. (1983). "Enhancers and Eukaryotic Gene Expression." Cold Spring Harbor Lab., Cold Spring Harbor, New York.

Griffith, J. D. (1975). *Science* **187**, 1202–1203.

Grosschedl, R., and Birnstiel, M. L. (1982). *Proc. Natl. Acad. Sci. U.S.A.* **79**, 297–301.

Gruss, P., Dhar, R., and Khoury, G. (1981). *Proc. Natl. Acad. Sci. U.S.A.* **78**, 943–947.

Guarente, L., Nye, J. S., Hochschild, A., and Plashne, M. (1982). *Proc. Natl. Acad. Sci. U.S.A.* **79**, 2236–2239.

Hawley, D. K., and McClure, W. R. (1983). *Cell* **32**, 327–333.

Heilig, R., Perrin, F., Gannon, F., Mandel, J. L., and Chambon, P. (1980). *Cell* **20**, 625–637.

Heilig, R., Muraskowsky, R., and Mandel, J. L. (1982). *J. Mol. Biol.* **156**, 1–19.

Hen, R., Sassone-Corsi, P., Corden, J., Gaub, M. P., and Chambon, P. (1982). *Proc. Natl. Acad. Sci. U.S.A.* **79**, 7132–7136.

Hen, R., Borrelli, E., Sassone-Corsi, P., and Chambon, P. (1983). *Nucleic Acids Res.* **11**, 8747–8760.

Hiwasa, T., Segawa, M., Yamaguchi, N., and Oda, K. I. (1981). *J. Biochem.* **89**, 1375–1389.

Hochschild, A., Irwin, N., and Plashne, M. (1983). *Cell* **32**, 319–325.

Horwitz, K. B., and McGuire, W. L. (1978). *J. Biol. Chem.* **253**, 2223–2228.

Horwitz, K. B., Mockus, M. B., Pike, A. W., Fonnessey, P. V., and Rebecca, L. (1983). *J. Biol. Chem.* **258**, 7603–7610.

Hossenlopp, P., Oudet, P., and Chambon, P. (1974). *Eur. J. Biochem.* **41**, 397–411.

Hsieh, T., and Brutlag, D. (1980). *Cell* **21**, 115–125.

Ikeda, T., Liu, Q-F., Danielpour, D., Officer, J. B., Ho, M., Leland, F. E., and Sirbasku, D. A. (1982). *In Vitro* **18**, 961–979.

Jacob, F., Ullman, A., and Monod, J. (1964). *C. R. Acad. Sci.* **258**, 3125.

Jakobovits, E. B., Bratosin, S., and Aloni, Y. (1980). *Nature (London)* **285**, 263–265.

Jakobovits, E. B., Bratosin, S., and Aloni, Y. (1982). *Virology* **120**, 340–348.

Jakowlew, S., Breathnach, R., Jeltsch, J. M., Masiakowski, P., and Chambon, P. (1984). *Nucleic Acids Res.*, in press.

Jeltsch, J. M., Brown, A., Roberts, M., Garnier, J. M., and Chambon, P. (1984). Submitted.

Jongstra, J., Reudelhuber, T. L., Oudet, P., Benoist, C., Chae, C. B., Jeltsch, J. M., Mathis, D. J., and Chambon, P. (1984). *Nature (London)* **307**, 708–714.

Kaye, J., Bellard, M., Dretzen, G., Bellard, F., and Chambon, P. (1984). *EMBO J.*, in press.

Khoury, G., and Gruss, P. (1983). *Cell* **33**, 313–314.

Kornberg, R. D. (1977). *Annu. Rev. Biochem.* **46**, 931–954.

Krust, A., and Chambon, P. (1984). Submitted.

LeMeur, M., Glanville, N., Mandel, J. L., Gerlinger, P. Palmiter, R. D., and Chambon, P. (1981). *Cell* **23**, 561–571.

Liu, L. F., and Miller, K. G. (1981). *Proc. Natl. Acad. Sci. U.S.A.* **78**, 3487–3491.

Losick, R., and Chamberlin, M. (1976). *In* "RNA Polymerase," pp. 285–329. Cold Spring Harbor Lab., Cold Spring Harbor, New York.

Mandel, J. L., and Chambon, P. (1979). *Nucleic Acids Res.* 7, 2081–2103.

Manley, J. L., Fire, A., Cano, A., Sharp, P. A., and Gefter, M. L. (1980). *Proc. Natl. Acad. Sci. U.S.A.* 77, 3855–3859.

Masiakowski, P., Breathnach, R., Bloch, J., Gannon, F., Krust, A., and Chambon, P. (1982). *Nucleic Acids Res.* 10, 7895–7903.

McGhee, J. D., and Felsenfeld, G. (1980). *Annu. Rev. Biochem.* 49, 1115–1156.

McKnight, G. S. (1978). *Cell* 14, 403–413.

McKnight, G. S., and Palmiter, R. D. (1979). *J. Biol. Chem.* 254, 9050–9058.

McKnight, G. S., Lee, D. C., Hemmaplardh, D., Finck, A., and Palmiter, R. D. (1980a). *J. Biol. Chem.* 255, 144–147.

McKnight, G. S., Lee, D. C., and Palmiter, R. D. (1980b). *J. Biol. Chem.* 255, 148–153.

McKnight, S. L. (1982). *Cell* 31, 355–365.

McKnight, S. L., and Kingsbury, R. (1982). *Science* 217, 316–325.

Mercola, M., Wang, X. F., Olsen, J., and Calame, K. (1983). *Science* 221, 663–664.

Miller, J. H., ad Reznikoff, W. S., eds. (1978). "The Operon." Cold Spring Harbor Lab. New York.

Moreau, P., Hen, R., Wasylyk, B., Everett, R., Gaub, M. P., and Chambon, P. (1981). *Nucleic Acids Res.* 9, 6047–6068.

Mulligan, R. C., and Berg, P. (1980). *Science* 209, 1422–1427.

Mulvihill, E. R., and Palmiter, R. D. (1977). *J. Biol. Chem.* 252, 1060–1068.

Mulvihill, E. R., and Palmiter, R. D. (1980). *J. Biol. Chem.* 255, 2085–2091.

Mulvihill, E. R., LePennec, J. P., and Chambon, P. (1982). *Cell* 28, 621–632.

Neuberger, M. S. (1983). *EMBO J.* 2, 1373–1378.

Nguyen-Huu, M. C., Sippel, A. A., Hyness, N. E., Groner, B., and Schutz, G. (1978). *Proc. Natl. Acad. Sci. U.S.A.* 75, 686.

Nickol, J., Behe, M., and Felsenfeld, G. (1982). *Proc. Natl. Acad. Sci. U.S.A.* 79, 1771–1775.

Nordheim, A., and Rich, A. (1983). *Nature (London)* 303, 674–679.

Nordheim, A., Tesser, P., Azorin, F., Kwon, Y. H., Möller, A., and Rich, A. (1982). *Proc. Natl. Acad. Sci. U.S.A.* 79, 7729–7733.

O'Malley, B. W., Roop, D. R., Lai, E. C., Nordstrom, J. L., Catterall, J. F., Swaneck, G. E., Colbert, D. A., Tsai, M. J. Dugaiczyk, A., and Woo, S. L. C. (1979). *Recent Prog. Horm. Res.* 35, 1–46.

Osborne, C. K., Yockmowitz, M. G., Knight, W. A., and McGuire, W. L. (1980). *Cancer* 46, 2884.

Palmiter, R. D. (1973). *J. Biol. Chem.* 248, 8260.

Palmiter, R. D. (1975). *Cell* 4, 189–197.

Palmiter, R. D., Mulvihill, E. R., Sheperd, J. J., and McKnight, G. S. (1981). *J. Biol. Chem.* 256, 7910–7916.

Parslow, T. G., and Granner, D. K. (1983). *Nucleic Acids Res.* 11, 4775–4792.

Pelham, H. R. B. (1982). *Cell* 30, 517–528.

Pelham, H. R. B., and Bienz, M. (1982). *EMBO J.* 1, 1473–1477.

Pellicer, A., Robins, D., Wold, B., Sweet, R., Jackson, J., Lowy, J., Roberts, J. M., Sim, G. K., Silverstein, S., and Axel, R. (1980). *Science* 209, 1414–1422.

Perlman, D., and Halvorson, H. O. (1983). *J. Mol. Biol.* 167, 391–409.

Picard, D., and Schaffner, W. (1984). *Nature (London)* 307, 80–82.

Pike, M. C., Siiteri, P. K., and Welsch, C. W., eds. (1981)." Hormones and Breast Cancer" (Bambury Report), Vol. 8. Cold Spring Harbor Lab., Cold Spring Harbor, New York.

Queen, C., and Baltimore, D. (1983). *Cell* 33, 741–748.

Robinson, S. T., Small, D., Idzerba, R., McKnight, G. S., and Vogelstein, B. (1983). *Nucleic Acids Res.* **11**, 5113–5130.

Rodriguez, R. L., and Chamberlin, M. J., eds. (1982). "Promoters: Structure and Function" Praeger, New York.

Roeder, R. G. (1976). *In* "RNA Polymerase," pp. 285–329. Cold Spring Harbor Lab., Cold Spring Harbor, New York.

Rosenberg, M., and Court, D. (1979). *Annu. Rev. Genet.* **13**, 319.

Royal, A., Garapin, A., Cami, B., Perrin, F., Mandel, J. L., LeMeur, M., Bregegere, F., Gannon, F., LePennec, J. P., Chambon, P., and Kourilsky, P. (1979). *Nature (London)* **279**, 125–132.

Saez, S., Martin, P. M., and Chouvet, C. D. (1978). *Cancer Res.* **38**, 3468–3473.

Saragosti, S., Moyne, G., and Yaniv, M. (1980). *Cell* **20**, 65–73.

Saragosti, S., Cereghini, S., and Yaniv, M. (1982). *J. Mol. Biol.* **160**, 133–146.

Sassone-Corsi, P., Dougherty, J., Wasylyk, B., and Chambon, P. (1984). *Proc. Natl. Acad. Sci. U.S.A.* **81**, 308–312.

Schrader, W. T., Birnbaumer, M. E., Hughes, M. R., Weigel, N. L., Grady, W. W., and O'Malley, B. W. (1981). *Recent Prog. Horm. Res.* **37**, 583–633.

Scott, W. A., and Wigmore, D. J. (1978). *Cell* **15**, 1511–1518.

Shakhov, A. N., Nedospasov, S. A., and Georgiev, G. P. (1982). *Nucleic Acids Res.* **10**, 3951–3965.

Shenk, T. (1978). *Cell* **13**, 791–798.

Siebenlist, U., Simpson, R. B., and Gilbert, W. (1980). *Cell* **20**, 269–281.

Stafford, J., and Queen, C. (1983). *Nature (London)* **306**, 77–79.

Stefano, J. E., and Gralla, J. D. (1982). *Proc. Natl. Acad. Sci. U.S.A.* **79**, 1069–1072.

Sternglanz, R., DiNardo, S., Voelkel, K. A., Nishimura, Y., Hirota, Y., Becherer, K., Zumstein, L., and Wang, J. C. (1981). *Proc. Natl. Acad. Sci. U.S.A.* **78**, 2747–2751.

Sundin, O., and Varshavsky, A. (1979). *J. Mol. Biol.* **132**, 535–546.

Tooze, J., ed. (1982). "DNA Tumor Viruses." Cold Spring Harbor Lab., Cold Spring Harbor, New York.

Tsuda, M., and Suzuki, Y. (1981). *Cell* **27**, 175–182.

Varshavsky, A. J., Sudin, O., and Bohn, M. (1979). *Cell* **16**, 453–466.

Volckaert, G., Feunteun, J., Crawford, L. V., Berg, P., and Fiers, W. (1979). *J. Virol.* **30**, 674–682.

Waldeck, W., Föhring, B., Chowdhury, K., Gruss, P., and Sauer, G. (1978). *Proc. Natl. Acad. Sci. U.S.A.* **75**, 5964–5968.

Wasylyk, B., and Chambon, P. (1982). *Cold Spring Harbor Symp. Quant. Biol.* **47**, 921–934.

Wasylyk, B., Oudet, P., and Chambon, P. (1979). *Nucleic Acids Res.* **7**, 705–713.

Wasylyk, B., Kédinger, C., Corden, J., Brison, O., and Chambon, P. (1980). *Nature (London)* **285**, 367–373.

Wasylyk, B., Wasylyk, C., Matthes, H., Wintzerith, M., and Chambon, P. (1983a). *EMBO J.* **2**, 1605–1611.

Wasylyk, B., Wasylyk, C., Augereau, P., and Chambon, P. (1983b). *Cell* **32**, 503–514.

Weil, P. A., Luse, D. S., Segall, J., and Roeder, R. G. (1979). *Cell* **18**, 469–484.

Westley, B., and Rochefort, H. (1980). *Cell* **20**, 353–362.

Wigmore, D. J., Eaton, R. W., and Scott, W. A. (1980). *Virology* **104**, 462–473.

Wu, C. (1980). *Nature (London)* **286**, 854–860.

Wu, G. J. (1978). *Proc. Natl. Acad. Sci. U.S.A.* **75**, 2175–2179.

Yamamoto, K. R., and Alberts, B. M. (1976). *Annu. Rev. Biochem.* **45**, 722–746.

Yaniv, M. (1982). *Nature (London)* **297**, 17–18.

Ziff, E. B., and Evans, R. M. (1978). *Cell* **15**, 1463–1475.

DISCUSSION

J. E. Rall: Thank you very much for an extraordinarily interesting talk. Those 72 base pair repeats are a worry extraordinarily interesting. The lovely EM slide showing the gaps makes me wonder whether you have tried to reconstitute nucleosomes from the 72 base pair repeats and see whether you can use that as an affinity column to pull out a protein. There must be some reason why in the area of the 72 base pair repeats there is DNase I sensitivity.

P. Chambon: Very schematically there are two possibilities (which are not mutually exclusive) to explain the generation of the nucleosome gap. First, the DNA of the 72 bp repeat region could possess the intrinsic property of not being able to be folded in a nucleosome. Second, there may be a protein which binds to the 72 bp repeat and prevents the formation of a nucleosome. With respect to the first possibility, it is worth mentioning that the group of Alex Rich has recently reported [*Nature* (*London*) **303**, 674–678 (1983)] that there are short segments of alternating purine-pyrimidine in the 72 bp repeat which can adopt the Z-DNA conformation, known to not be favorable for the formation of nucleosomes. Along the same lines, I also want to mention an experiment which was done several years ago in our laboratory by B. Wasylyk *et al.* [*Nucleic Acids Res.* **7**, 705–713 (1979)] who showed that *in vitro* reconstruction of minichromosomes from "naked" SV40 DNA and purified histone octamers resulted in a specific lack of nucleosome formation in the SV40 origin region which contains the 72 bp repeat. It certainly would be worth repeating these experiments with SV40 DNA molecules mutated in the 72 bp repeat sequences which are known to affect the enhancer activity. With respect to the second possibility the only protein which up to now has been found associated with the gap region in SV40 minichromosomes isolated from infected cells is the T-antigen (E. Weiss, P. Oudet, and P. Chambon, in preparation). Of course this does not exclude that other proteins are not bound *in vivo* to this region and lost during minichromosome preparation. For instance it is known from the work of A. Rich's laboratory that some proteins (from *Drosophila*) have a high affinity for Z-DNA. However such a protein has not been found associated to the 72 bp repeat region, and to answer your very question, I do not think that affinity chromatography on a DNA (72 bp repeat) column would be of great help, because the protein, if it does exist, is evidently not tightly bound to the 72 bp repeat DNA *in vivo*. However our *in vitro* transcription results (P. Sassone-Corsi *et al.*, submitted) do suggest that a transcription factor does recognize the 72 bp repeat, and it is not excluded that the formation of a nucleosome is prevented by the binding of this factor. More *in vitro* work is clearly required before a satisfactory answer could be given to the problems raised by your question.

J. E. Rall: Thank you. The second question is, you have looked at the sequence of all the 5 genes controlled by estrogen and progesterone and I am sure you have looked for some kind of repeat. Are here any even unrelated to the 72 base pair sequence that you can find anywhere upstream?

P. Chambon: No, there is no sequence similar to the SV40 72 bp repeat enhancer in the sequence of the ovalbumin, X, Y, conalbumin, and ovomucoid genes. In fact we have no evidence at the present time supporting the existence of enhancer-like sequences within or upstream from these genes. This is mainly because there is no chicken cell line containing estrogen and/or progesterone receptors in which we could introduce these genes after mutation of the sequences which bind specifically the receptor molecules *in vivo* [see Mulvihill *et al.*, *Cell* **28**, 621–632 (1982)], in order to investigate whether these sequences exhibit the properties of enhancer elements.

G. Hager: In your discussion about the 72 base pair repeat reconstitution effect *in vitro*, you mentioned that it only worked in whole cell extract and you alluded briefly to the concept of nucleosome formation in those extracts. Could you elaborate on that. Can you see nucleosome formation on naked DNA added to whole cell extracts.

P. Chambon: We have no evidence for nucleosome formation when we incubate our templates in a whole cell extract transcription system [see Hen *et al., Proc. Natl. Acad. Sci. U.S.A.* **79**, 7132–7136 (1982)].

G. Hager: You have still suggested the possibility that chromatin structure could be involved in that effect. Does that mean that the efficiency you are seeing with the 72 base pair repeat is so low *in vitro* that it might be occurring on a population of molecules that are at very low concentration in those extracts; is that your interpretation?

P. Chambon: Obviously, we cannot exclude that the stimulatory effect of the 72 bp repeat observed *in vitro* using a whole-cell extract is due to transcription from a minor subpopulation of template molecules organized in a chromatin structure. However, as I told you before there is no evidence for significant nucleosome formation and nucleosome assembly is not known to be a cooperative event. In addition we have obtained the same stimulations using circular or linear templates. It may be that, in fact, we should not expect a stimulation of *in vitro* transcription by the 72 bp repeat higher than 5- to 10- fold. It is known from *in vivo* experiments that the stimulatory effect of the SV40 enhancer decreases as the template copy number increases. In other words the effect of the SV40 enhancer is best seen (up to several 100-fold stimulation) when the DNA molecules which contain the 72 bp repeat are present into the cells at low copy number. Obviously, the *in vitro* conditions for transcription do not correspond to a low copy number of template molecules, and we cannot decrease the template concentration too much because transcription would not be measurable. But we do know that, as we increase the template concentration, the extent of the *in vitro* stimulatory effect decreases. It may be that the effect of the enhancer can be best seen when the template molecules are in the form of minichromosomes, and preferentially when these minichromosomes are present in low concentration and surrounded by DNA molecules organized in inactive chromatin. In any case, the results that we have obtained *in vitro* with mutants known to decrease the enhancer effect *in vivo*, give us confidence that we are not looking at *in vitro* artifacts. *In vitro* experiments with templates organized in a chromatin structure and purified transcription factors will tell us whether chromatin is essential for achieving maximum stimulation with enhancer elements.

P. Kelly: It was interested in your estrogen-sensitive protein and wondered if you could tell us how it compares with the two different estrogen-induced proteins reported by McGuire's group and by Rochfort's group?

P. Chambon: As far as I know, there is no similarity between the protein that I have described and those reported by the two groups you mentioned. The molecular weights are very different.

C. Sonnenschein: In your excellent presentation of the view that you hold about the control of initiation of the transcriptional process, you mentioned the presence of a receptor in this whole affair as an afterthought. That is to say that you did not have to claim a prominent role for the receptor; I wonder whether you could briefly elaborate on what is your current thought about the role of the estrogen receptor.

P. Chambon: If I did not mention the role of estrogen or progesterone receptor molecules in initiation of transcription, it is not because I believe that they do not play an important role in this process, but because I have no direct evidence supporting it. It is clear from our published work that steroid hormones have a marked effect on the chromatin structure of the ovalbumin gene over more than 3 kb upstream from the initiation site [Bellard *et al. EMBO J.* **1**, 223–230 (1982)]. It is also clear that some of these chromatin structure alterations occur at sequences where specific binding of the progesterone receptor occurs *in vitro* [Mulvihill *et al. Cell* **28**, 621–632 (1982)]. As I already said, what we are missing is the direct demonstration that these sequences are in fact involved in initiation of transcription under hormonal control. And the frustration is that the decisive experiments are difficult to perform because there are no chicken cell lines which can be used to study the effect of mutations in these sequences. Microinjection in the nuclei of oviduct cells in primary culture may be an alternative, but as I told you, the level of hormonal induction that we have obtained in these cells is much lower than what is observed in the whole animal. There are the very reasons why we switched to the MCF-7 cell system, but I may be overpessimistic and we may be fortunate enough to establish in the coming years a faithful *in vitro* transcription system mimicking the known *in vivo* effects of hormone–receptor complexes.

S. L. Cohen: I have a story I would like to tell you and a question I would like to ask. The story concerns the fact that I am a steroid chemist and my knowledge of genetic structure is very, very, limited. There are more steroid chemists in this audience and I would not like to say that they are all in my boat. I think some of them may be much more intelligent than I am. This is a story I heard in San Diego this Spring from Alan Layne. If any of you have heard it, before, I apologize to you. But for the rest of you, I am sure you will enjoy it. Three men were discussing what was their earliest memory, one of them said his earliest memories were very bad because he remembers being born. He said they pushed him and they squeezed him and they pushed him some more and they squeezed him some more and when he finally was out they turned him over and they spanked him and he hadn't done anything wrong. The second one said his memories were much more pleasant and go further back. He remembers being in the amniotic sac. He said it was very comfortable, everything was just hunky dory. The third one said his memories go even further back than that. He remembers going to a picnic with his father, and coming home with his mother. This is a summary of my knowledge of genes. I understand how one measures the ER and the PR, how about the RNA? Is that difficult to measure. Will it be any more difficult than estrogen and progesterone receptors?

P. Chambon: With respect to your story, don't ask me how this genetic transfer occurred. No, within 2 or 3 years, it will not be more difficult than doing a radioimmunoassay.

J. H. Oppenheimer: You started off your discussion with the assumption of the overriding importance of events at the transcriptional level. Do you have any conclusive evidence that processing and stabilization of mRNA may not play an equally important role in raising the level of mRNA?

P. Chambon: Although I am convinced that in most cases control of gene expression is exerted at the transcriptional level, I did not mean that posttranscriptional events do not contribute to regulation of gene expression. There are in fact well established examples of hormone effect on mRNA stability (see for instance the study of R. Palmiter on ovalbumin mRNA stability in chicken oviduct in the presence and absence of steroid hormones) and examples of cell- or tissue-specific alternative processing (splicing) have also been reported. What I do not believe is that 10–30% of the genome is transcribed at any time in any given cell (as it was proposed 10 years ago on the basis of RNA–DNA hybridization results) and that the mRNAs which will ultimately be used in a given cell are sorted out from all of these original transcripts. All of the experimented evidence which has been recently obtained with specific gene probes, and not only in the case of hormonally regulated genes, indicates that regulation at the transcriptional level is in most cases the key step. This does not mean that the regulations which can be subsequently exerted at the processing step or on mRNA stability or on efficiency of mRNA translation do not play any role, and even in some cases a crucial one.

Structure, Expression, and Evolution of the Genes for the Human Glycoprotein Hormones

JOHN C. FIDDES AND KAREN TALMADGE

California Biotechnology, Inc., Mountain View, California

I. Introduction

There are four members of the glycoprotein hormone family: chorionic gonadotropin (CG), luteinizing hormone (LH), follicle stimulating hormone (FSH), and thyroid stimulating hormone (TSH). These hormones have been studied extensively in terms of their biosynthesis, mode of action, and physical structure, but until recently no information has been available on the genes encoding the hormones. In this article, we will review the features of the glycoprotein hormones which make them of interest to molecular biologists, and then describe our recent results on the structure, expression, and evolution of the human glycoprotein hormone genes.

II. The Glycoprotein Hormones

Three of the glycoprotein hormones, LH, FSH, and TSH, are synthesized in the anterior pituitary of a wide range of species, while the fourth, CG, is made in the syncytiotrophoblast of the placenta of certain mammals. LH, FSH, and CG have very similar functions, and are collectively termed the gonadotropins. The two pituitary gonadotropins, LH and FSH, act together to promote the synthesis of steroids by the testes and ovaries and are required for spermatogenesis and ovulation. The placental gonadotropin, CG, is made by the placenta very shortly after conception and reaches a peak level of synthesis at the end of the first trimester of pregnancy. This production of CG by the placenta is essential for the maintenance of pregnancy. CG is functionally most like LH in that it binds to the same ovarian receptors as LH does and results in the synthesis and secretion of the steroids which are needed for fetal development. In contrast, TSH acts on the thyroid gland to produce thyroid hormone.

All four glycoprotein hormones are structurally related. They are dimeric, consisting of two dissimilar subunits, α and β, which are associ-

43

ated noncovalently. The α subunit is common to all four hormones while the β subunits are unique and confer biological specificity. This has been demonstrated by switching experiments in which α and β dimers from two different hormones were dissociated, mixed, and reassociated. The individual subunits had no biological activity while the activity recovered on reassociation was a feature of the β subunit.

All of the β subunits show amino acid sequence homology. In humans, the most closely related pair, with a homology of 82%, is β CG and β LH, which is in keeping with their similar biological function. The other β subunits when compared in pairs have homologies ranging from about 25 to 40%. All of the β subunits have 12 cysteines located in identical places in the amino acid sequence. One interesting feature of the β hCG : β hLH comparison is that β hCG has a carboxy-terminal extension of 24 amino acids which has no homologous counterpart in β hLH. The function of this region is not known but has been suggested to be related to the much greater stability of CG than LH in the circulation. The physiology and biochemistry of these hormones have been reviewed in detail by Canfield *et al.* (1978) (biochemistry), Henderson (1979) (physiology), Lincoln (1979) (physiology), and Pierce and Parsons (1981) (biochemistry).

On the basis of the amino acid sequence homologies and the presence of CG only in certain mammals, it has been proposed (Dayhoff, 1976) that all the β subunits have a common evolutionary ancestor, that the most recently evolved β subunit is that of CG, and that the β subunit of CG evolved from β LH or a β LH-like sequence. There is also a very limited homology between the common α subunits and the individual β subunits. In this case, the location of 6 of the 12 cysteines is conserved. On the basis of this homology, it has been proposed that both the α and β subunits have a common evolutionary origin but that the two subunits diverged very early in the evolution of the glycoprotein hormones (Dayhoff, 1976).

Several questions about the glycoprotein hormones can be answered by a recombinant DNA approach. For example, it would be interesting to know if the common α subunit is encoded by a single gene which is expressed in both the pituitary and the placenta or if, instead, each glycoprotein hormone has its own subunit gene which is regulated differently. Also, we would like to know whether the similarities in the β subunit amino acid sequences are reflected in similarities in the structures of the genes and to find out whether the β subunit genes are linked to each other on the chromosome. Information on the structural organizations of these genes and on their DNA sequences will be useful in understanding the evolution of the glycoprotein hormones as a multigene family and can answer specific questions such as how β hCG evolved from β hLH and how, in the process of doing this, β hCG acquired the 24 amino acid carboxy-terminal extension. Finally, isolation and characterization of the genes encoding the glycoprotein hormones are necessary for understanding the tissue-specific, developmentally regulated expression of these polypeptide hormones.

III. The Gene Encoding the Common α Subunit

Human first trimester placenta is a good source of the mRNA species which encode the α and β subunits of human chorionic gonadotropin (hCG). At about 12 weeks of placental development, substantial quantities of hCG are being synthesized and secreted into the urine. We therefore isolated mRNA from first trimester placenta and used an *in vitro* wheat germ translation system (Roberts and Paterson, 1973) to synthesize ^{35}S-labeled placental proteins. These translation products were immunoprecipitated with an antiserum directed against mature hCG and the products fractionated on a 15% acrylamide:SDS gel (Laemmli, 1970). The results of this are shown in Fig. 1 (Fiddes and Goodman, 1979). Two major products of molecular weights 13,000 and 16,000 are synthesized (Fig. 1, lane 4) and can be specifically precipitated with the hCG antiserum (Fig. 1, lane 3). These are the α and β subunits of hCG, respectively.

Double-stranded cDNA was synthesized by reverse transcription (Efstradiatis *et al.*, 1976) of first trimester mRNA and the resulting products cloned into the unique *Hin*dIII site of the plasmid cloning vector pBR322. Individual cDNA clones were then examined by restriction enzyme analysis to look for characteristic fragments which were detected on restriction enzyme analysis of total, uncloned placental cDNA. One clone was identified and shown by DNA sequence analysis to encode the α subunit of hCG. The complete nucleotide sequence of this 621 base pair clone was determined by the chain termination method (Sanger *et al.*, 1977) and is presented in Fig. 2 (Fiddes and Goodman, 1979).

This cDNA clone has the sequence coding for the 92 amino acid long mature α subunit and allows the prediction of a 24 amino acid signal peptide. The hydrophobic signal peptide is cleaved from the precursor protein when the mature protein is secreted. In addition, the cDNA clone has 220 bases of the 3'-untranslated region and 50 bases of the 5'-untranslated region.

In order to determine whether there are multiple α subunit genes or whether the common α subunit is encoded by a single gene, we isolated a cloned chromosomal α subunit gene. The cloned α subunit cDNA was used as a hybridization probe to screen (Benton and Davis, 1977) a human genomic library in the bacteriophage λ vector charon 4A (Lawn *et al.*,

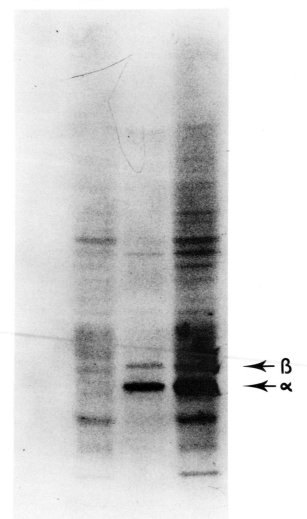

FIG. 1. Immunoprecipitation of wheat germ products by hCG antiserum. The wheat germ translation products generated by first-trimester placental RNA were immunoprecipitated by an antiserum directed against native hCG and the antigen–antibody complex collected by formaldehyde-treated *S. aureus* cells. The products were fractionated on an SDS–15% polyacrylamide gel and visualized by autoradiography of the dried gel. Lane 1, immunoprecipitation of endogeneous wheat germ products; lane 2, endogenous wheat germ translation products; lane 3, immunoprecipitation of wheat germ translation products directed by first-trimester placental polyadenylated RNA; lane 4, wheat germ products of first-trimester placental polyadenylated RNA. The proposed identification of the pre-forms of the α and β subunits of hCG are indicated. Details are given in Fiddes and Goodman (1979).

```
                                                            -24
                                                            met asp tyr
CAGTAACCGCCCTGAACACATCCTGCAAAAAGCCCAGAGAAAGGAGCGCC          ATG GAT TAC
1                                30                    HhaI
    -20                                               -10
tyr arg lys tyr ala ala ile phe leu val thr leu ser val phe leu
TAC AGA AAA TAT GCA GCT ATC TTT CTG GTC ACA TTG TCG GTG TTT CTG
60              AluI                90
                 1                                              10
his val leu his ser ala pro asp val gln asp cys pro glu cys thr
CAT GTT CTC CAT TCC GCT CCT GAT GTG CAG GAT TGC CCA GAA TGC ACG
110                      130
                              20
leu gln glu asn pro phe phe ser gln pro gly ala pro ile leu gln
CTA CAG GAA AAC CCA TTC TTC TCC CAG CCG GGT GCC CCA ATA CTT CAG
    160                          HpaII  190
      30                                        40
cys met gly cys cys phe ser arg ala tyr pro thr pro leu arg ser
TGC ATG GGC TGC TGC TTC TCT AGA GCA TAT CCC ACT CCA CTA AGG TCC
                  220    XbaI                              250
                         50
lys lys thr met leu val gln lys asn val thr ser glu ser thr cys
AAG AAG ACG ATG TTG GTC CAA AAG AAC GTC ACC TCA GAG TCC ACT TGC
60                               280            70   HinfI
cys val ala lys ser tyr asn arg val thr val met gly gly phe lys
TGT GTA GCT AAA TCA TAT AAC AGG GTC ACA GTA ATG GGG GGT TTC AAA
    AluI
              80                          330                 90
val glu asn his thr ala cys his cys ser thr cys tyr tyr his lys
GTG GAG AAC CAC ACG GCG TGC CAC TGC AGT ACT TGT TAT TAT CAC AAA
                  360            PstI                  390
  92
ser OC
TCT TAA ATGTTTTACCAAGTGCTGTCTTGATGACTGCTGATTTTCTGGAATGGAAAATTAA
   400                          430

GTTGTTTAGTGTTTATGGCTTTGTGAGATAAAACTCTCCTTTTCCTTACCATACCACTTTGAC
   460                          490
                   AluI
ACGCTTCAAGGATATACTGCAGCTTTACTGCCTTCCTCCTTATCCTACAGTACAATCAGCAGT
       530    PstI                          560
                                  AluI
CTAGTTCTTTTCATTTGGAATGAATACAGCATTAAGCTT
    590                          HindIII
```

FIG. 2. Nucleotide sequence of the 621 base pair cloned cDNA fragment which codes for the α subunit of hCG. The amino acid sequence of the 92 residue long mature protein is shown as well as the 24 residue presequence deduced from the cDNA sequence. The nucleotides and amino acids are numbered. Restriction enzyme sites for *Pst*I, *Hin*dIII, *Xba*I, *Hpa*II, *Alu*I, *Hin*fI, and *Hha*I are marked. Details are given in Fiddes and Goodman (1979).

1978). A single recombinant was isolated which has an insert of about 17 kilobases (kb). A restriction enzyme map of this recombinant was established and is shown in Fig. 3 (Fiddes and Goodman, 1981). The cloned gene encompasses a total of about 9.4 kb and is split at three locations by introns.

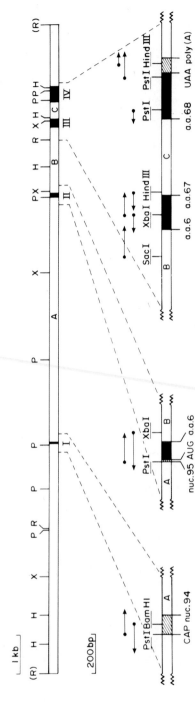

FIG. 3. Restriction endonuclease map of the cloned sequence encoding the common α subunit gene and its flanking regions. The upper section shows the map obtained for the enzymes *Eco*RI, R; *Xba*I, X; *Pst*I, P; and *Hind*III, H. The artificial *Eco*RI sites generated by linker ligation at the ends of the cloned sequences are indicated by (R). The shaded regions in the upper section (I, II, III, and IV) correspond to the four coding regions. These are separated by the three introns, A, B, and C, which are 6.4, 1.7, and 0.4 kb long, respectively. The lower section shows the regions I, II, III, and IV on a scale expanded five times. In the expanded region, solid shading indicates translated regions while cross hatching indicates untranslated regions. Intron A separates nucleotide 94 (nuc. 94) from nucleotide 95 (nuc. 95) in the 5'-untranslated region; intron B is within codon 6 (a.a.6) and intron C is between codons 67 (a.a.67) and 68 (a.a.68). The locations of the predicted gap site (CAP), the initiation codon (AUG), the termination codon (UAA), and the approximate position of the polyadenylation site [poly(A)] are marked. The arrows indicate the restriction enzyme sites which were labeled for sequence analysis and the extent of the sequences determined. Details are given in Fiddes and Goodman (1981).

DNA sequencing was used to confirm the restriction enzyme map, to identify the precise locations of the introns, and to define the 5' and 3' ends of the gene. A partial DNA sequence for the α subunit gene was determined by the chemical sequencing method (Maxam and Gilbert, 1977) and is presented in Fig. 4 (Fiddes and Goodman, 1981). Intron A, which is about 6.4 kb long, is positioned in the 5'-untranslated region seven nucleotides before the ATG initiator codon. The other two introns, B and C, are 1.7 and 0.4 kb long, respectively, and are located within codon number 6 and between codons 67 and 68, respectively. The location of the 5' end of the mature transcript has been identified by priming placental mRNA with a restriction enzyme fragment obtained from the cloned cDNA. In common with many other eukaryotic genes, the sequence TATAAA, which is considered to be a signal involved in the initiation of transcription, is found at about 25 nucleotides before the transcriptional start (Breathnach and Chambon, 1981; Corden et al., 1980).

From an examination of the restriction enzyme map of the cloned α subunit gene, it is possible to predict which EcoRI, HindIII, XbaI, and PstI restriction fragments in total human DNA should hybridize to the α subunit cDNA probe. If no additional fragments are detected, one may reasonably assume that there is a single α subunit gene. This analysis is complicated by the fact that we found three polymorphic types of human DNA using the α subunit cDNA as a hybridization probe. DNA from all three polymorphic types was therefore digested with either HindIII, PstI, or XbaI, and hybridized to the α subunit cDNA probe by the filter method of Southern (1975). The results of this are shown in Fig. 5 (Fiddes and Goodman, 1981). The hybridization patterns with these enzymes and the three different DNA types are consistent with those predicted from the cloned gene and strongly support the conclusion that there is a single α subunit gene which is expressed for hCG, hLH, hFSH, and hTSH. No additional unexplainable fragments are observed with any of the enzymes. It is not however possible to rule out the existence of multiple copies of identical, or very similar sequences, with homologous flanking regions. We do not however consider this to be likely.

We have found a single human α subunit gene, which thus must be expressed in the placenta for the production of hCG, and in the pituitary for the production of hLH, hFSH, and hTSH. It has been observed (see Pierce and Parsons, 1981, for a review) that there is free α subunit in both the pituitary and the placenta. One inference of this may be that the α subunit is expressed constituively. It seems likely, therefore, that the control of glycoprotein hormone expression resides in the different β subunit genes.

tcattggacggaatttcctgttgatcccagggcttagatgcaggtggaaacactctgctgg⸤tataa⸥agca
                        -60   -30

                        PstI   BamHI
ggtgaggacttcattaactG̲C̲A̲GTTACTGAGAACTCATAAGACGAAGCTAAAATCCCTCTTCGGATCCACA
                        1   30

GTCAACCGCCCTGAACACATCCTGCAAAAAGCCCAGAGAAAG gtaatatgaatgaaataattttggggga
        60   90
                                        IVS A 6.4kb
ctttaattgaggagtaagatatttgagaata::::::::::::::::ttttttttttttttttttgccatg

                -24   -20
        PstI   Met Asp Tyr Tyr Arg Lys Tyr Ala Ala Ile Phe Leu Val
tctgtctgcag GAGCGCC ATG GAT TAC TAC AGA AAA TAT GCA GCT ATC TTT CTG GTC
                    Primer   120
        -10   -1   1
Thr Leu Ser Val Phe Leu His Val Leu His Ser Ala Pro Asp Val Gln A
ACA TTG TCG GTG TTT CTG CAT GTT CTC CAT TCC GCT CCT GAT GTG CAG G gtgcg
                150   180
                                        IVS B 1.7kb
tgaccaaatttgtggttcaagtaataaggacaacacacattt:::::::::::::::::::::ttcttttttga

                                        sp Cys Pro Glu Cys Thr Leu
gtcttttttggatattttactctgcctttttttttttccctgatag AT TGC CCA GAA TGC ACG CTA

                        20
Gln Glu Asn Pro Phe Phe Ser Gln Pro Gly Ala Pro Ile Leu Gln Cys Met Gly
CAG GAA AAC CCA TTC TTC TCC CAG CCG GGT GCC CCA ATA CTT CAG TGC ATG GGC
                                        240
                        40
Cys Cys Phe Ser Arg Ala Tyr Pro Thr Pro Leu Arg Ser Lys Lys Thr Met Leu
TGC TGC TTC TCT AGA GCA TAT CCC ACT CCA CTA AGG TCC AAG AAG ACG ATG TTG
        270   **XbaI**   300
                                60
Val Gln Lys Asn Val Thr Ser Glu Ser Thr Cys Cys Val Ala Lys Ser Tyr Asn
GTC CAA AAG AAC GTC ACC TCA GAG TCC ACT TGC TGT GTA GCT AAA TCA TAT AAC
                330   360
Arg   **IVS C 0.4kb**
AGG gtaagaacctcaagatccccagaagcttt:::::::::::::::::::ataatatgtttttttttcc
        HindIII

                                                        80
        Val Thr Val Met Gly Gly Phe Lys Val Glu Asn His Thr Ala Cys
ttcccctttag GTC ACA GTA ATG GGG GGT TTC AAA GTG GAG AAC CAC ACG GCG TGC
                                390

                                92
His Cys Ser Thr Cys Tyr Tyr His Lys Ser OC
CAC TGC AGT ACT TGT TAT TAT CAC AAA TCT TAA ATGTTTTACCAAGTGCTGTCTTGATGA
        PstI   450

CTGCTGATTTTCTGGAATGGAAAATTAAGTTGTTTAGTGTTTATGGCTTTGTGAGATAAAACTCTCCTTTT
                510   540

CCTTACCATACCACTTTGACACGCTTCAAGGATATACTGCAGCTTTACTGCCTTCCTCCTTATCCTACAGT
                570   **PstI**   600

ACAATCAGCAGTCTAGTTCTTTTCATTTGGAATGAATACAGCATTAAGCTTGTTCCACTGCA⸤AATAAA⸥GCC
        630   660   **HindIII**   690

TTTTAAATCATCattcaatcactgaattatcatttttcttcaaagtaag
        704

IV. Structure of a β Subunit Gene

First trimester human placental mRNA was also used as a source for cloning the β subunit of hCG. In this case, the correct recombinants were identified by making use of the known amino acid sequence of β hCG. The restriction enzyme *Sau*96I recognizes the sequence GGNCC. As glycine is coded for by the four codons GGN, and proline by the four codons CCN, every Gly-Pro dipeptide must be represented by an *Sau*96I site in the corresponding gene. In β hCG, there are Gly-Pro dipeptides at positions 102–103 and 136–137. Placental cDNA recombinants were therefore analyzed with *Sau*96I to find those with a restriction enzyme fragment pattern consistent with the position of the two Gly-Pro dipeptides. Two such clones were identified. Both chemical (Maxam and Gilbert, 1977) and chain termination (Sanger *et al.*, 1977) methods were used to obtain the complete nucleotide sequence of one of them, which is 579 nucleotides long, and is shown in Fig. 6 (Fiddes and Goodman, 1980). As with the α subunit cDNA, we can identify the sequence encoding the entire 145 amino acids of the mature protein and can predict a 20 amino acid long signal peptide.

The β hCG cDNA was used as a hybridization probe to screen two separate libraries of human genomic DNA—one in bacteriophage λ charon 4A (Lawn *et al.*, 1977) and one in charon 28 (E. Fritsch and C. Sabourin, unpublished results). This cDNA should detect β hCG genes and, since the β hCG and β human luteinizing hormone (hLH) amino acid sequences are 82% homologous (Pierce and Parsons, 1981), might be expected also to detect β hLH genes. The homology with β hFSH and β hTSH is not sufficient to allow any cross-hybridization to occur. As will be discussed in more detail in the next section, β hCG and β hLH form a

---

FIG. 4. Partial nucleotide sequence of the gene for the α subunit of the human glycoprotein hormones. Coding sequences are shown as capital letters, the intervening sequences are shown in boldface, and the sequences at the 5′ and 3′ ends of the gene which are not included in the mature transcript are indicated by lower case letters. The nucleotides are numbered as they would appear in the mature transcript of the gene and intron nucleotides are therefore not included in the numbering system. Negative numbers refer to nucleotides preceding the proposed 5′ end of the mRNA. The approximate lengths of the three introns (IVS) A, B, and C are indicated. The sequences TATAAA and AATAAA, characteristic of the promoter and the polyadenylation site, respectively, are boxed, and the approximate polyadenylation site is marked at nucleotide 704 by lower case letters. Restriction endonuclease sites for the enzymes *Pst*I, *Hin*dIII, *Bam*HI, and *Xba*I, which were used in the sequence analysis, are indicated. The position of the 29 nucleotide *Alu*I–*Hha*I cDNA fragment used as a primer to identify the transcriptional start is shown. The two nucleotides corresponding to the ends of the primed synthesis products are circled. The amino acids are numbered above the sequence. Details are given in Fiddes and Goodman (1981).

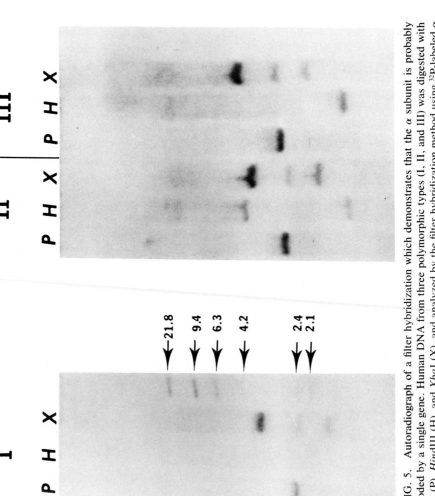

FIG. 5. Autoradiograph of a filter hybridization which demonstrates that the α subunit is probably encoded by a single gene. Human DNA from three polymorphic types (I, II, and III) was digested with PstI (P), HindIII (H), and XbaI (X), and analyzed by the filter hybridization method using ³²P-labeled α hCG cDNA as a probe. The sizes of a ³²P-labeled EcoRI digest of wild-type bacteriophage λ DNA are given in kilobases. Details are given in Fiddes and Goodman (1981).

```
                                    -20
                                    met glu met phe gln gly leu leu leu
AGACAAGGCAGGGGACGCACCAAGG           ATG GAG ATG TTC CAG GGG CTG CTG CTG
1                                       30
     -10                                                         1
leu leu leu leu ser met gly gly thr trp ala ser lys glu pro leu
TTG CTG CTG CTG AGC ATG GGC GGG ACA TGG GCA TCC AAG GAG CCG CTT
         60                                         90
                    10                                      20
arg pro arg cys arg pro ile asn ala thr leu ala val glu lys glu
CGG CCA CGG TGC CGC CCC ATC AAT GCC ACC CTG GCT GTG GAG AAG GAG
    HaeIII                  120
                                        30
gly cys pro val cys ile thr val asn thr thr ile cys ala gly tyr
GGC TGC CCC GTG TGC ATC ACC GTC AAC ACC ACC ATC TGT GCC GGC TAC
150                                             180
         40                                             50
cys pro thr met thr arg val leu gln gly val leu pro ala leu pro
TGC CCC ACC ATG ACC CGC GTG CTG CAG GGG GTC CTG CCG GCC CTG CCT
            210                    PstI    Sau96I  HaeIII/Sau96I
                            60
gln val val cys asn tyr arg asp val arg phe glu ser ile arg leu
CAG GTG GTG TGC AAC TAC CGC GAT GTG CGC TTC GAG TCC ATC CGG CTC
                            270            TaqI/HinfI
70                                          80
pro gly cys pro arg gly val asn pro val val ser tyr ala val ala
CCT GGC TGC CCG CGC GGC GTG AAC CCC GTG GTC TCC TAC GCC GTG GCT
            300                                 330
                    90                                      100
leu ser cys gln cys ala leu cys arg arg ser thr thr asp cys gly
CTC AGC TGT CAA TGT GCA CTC TGC CGC CGC AGC ACC ACT GAC TGC GGG
    PvuII                   360
                                110
gly pro lys asp his pro leu thr cys asp asp pro arg phe gln asp
GGT CCC AAG GAC CAC CCC TTG ACC TGT GAT GAC CCC CGC TTC CAG GAC
Sau96I      Sau96I                         420                Hin
        120                                         130
ser ser ser ser lys ala pro pro pro ser leu pro ser pro ser arg
TCC TCT TCC TCA AAG GCC CCT CCC CCC AGC CTT CCA AGC CCA TCC CGA
fI          HaeIII/Sau96I                               480 Hin
                            140             145
leu pro gly pro ser asp thr pro ile leu pro gln OC
CTC CCG GGG CCC TCG GAC ACC CCG ATC CTC CCA CAA TAA AGGCTTCTCAAT
fI/SmaI/Sau96I/HaeIII        MboI                        530
```

CCGC(A)₄₀
539

FIG. 6. Nucleotide sequence of the 579 base pair cloned cDNA fragment which codes for the β subunit of hCG. The amino acid sequence of the 145 residue long mature protein is shown as well as the 20 residue presequence predicted from the cDNA sequence. The nucleotides and amino acids are numbered. Restriction enzymes sites for *Pst*I, *Pvu*II, *Sau*96I, *Taq*I, *Hae*III, *Hinf*I, *Mbo*I, and *Sma*I are marked. Details are given in Fiddes and Goodman (1980).

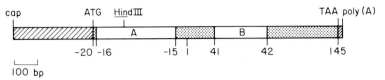

FIG. 7. Composite structure of β hCG and β hLH genes. Dotted areas represent coding regions while the cross-hatched areas represent the 5' and 3'-untranslated regions. The positions of the two introns (A and B) are shown. The locations of the predicted cap site (cap), the initiation codon (ATG), termination codon (TAA), and the polyadenylation site [poly(A)] are marked. Numbers at the bottom of the diagram refer to amino acids (negative numbers refer to the signal peptide). The location of the single HindIII site present in all of the genes is shown. Details are given in Boorstein *et al.* (1982).

multigene family with eight members. These eight genes have a very similar structure which is shown in Fig. 7 (Boorstein et al., 1982).

Unlike the common α subunit gene, the genes for β hCG and β hLH are more compact with a total length of about 1.45 kb. There are two introns, A and B, which are 352 and 233 nucleotides long, respectively. Intron A separates codon −16 of the signal peptide from codon −15, while intron B separates codon 41 from codon 42 of the mature protein. The fact that the β subunit genes have a different number of intervening sequences from

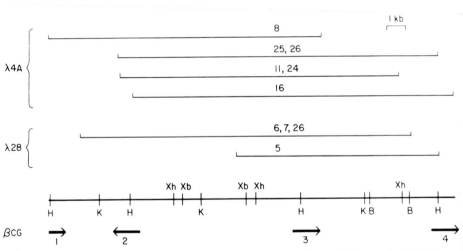

FIG. 8. Organization of one group of cloned sequences that hybridize to the β hCG cDNA probe. The positions of the four genes (1–3 and 4, which is β hLH) are shown by heavy arrows pointing in the proposed direction of transcription. Each number above a line indicates the length of cloned human DNA in an independent recombinant phage isolate. The phages are grouped by whether they were isolated from a charon 4A or charon 28 library. B, BamHI; H, HindIII; K, KpnI; Xb, XbaI; Xh, XhoI. Details are given in Boorstein et al. (1982) and Talmadge et al. (1983).

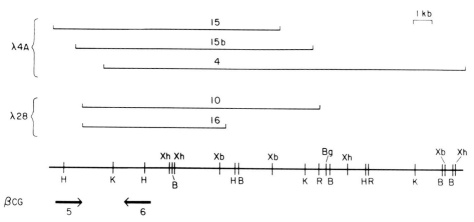

FIG. 9.   Organization of a second group of cloned sequences that hybridize to the β hCG probe. The positions of the two genes (5 and 6) are shown by heavy arrows pointing in the proposed direction of transcription. Bg, *Bgl*II; R, *Eco*RI. Other details are as in Fig. 8. Details are given in Boorstein *et al.* (1982) and Talmadge *et al.* (1983).

the α subunit gene and that they are located in different positions argues against the common evolutionary origin of the α and β genes.

V. There Are Seven β hCG Genes or Pseudogenes and One β hLH Gene

We used the β hCG cDNA as a hybridization probe to isolate a total of 16 phage recombinants from the two independent human genomic libraries described in the previous section. Restriction enzyme maps were determined for each of these recombinant phage. The maps of these phage showed that they belong to three different groups of overlapping recombinants. These are shown in Figs. 8–10 (Boorstein *et al.*, 1982; Talmadge *et*

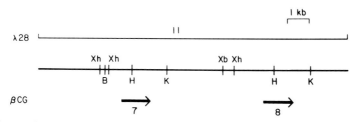

FIG. 10.   Organization of a third group of cloned sequences that hybridize to the β hCG probe. The positions of the two genes (7 and 8) are shown by heavy arrows pointing in the proposed direction of transcription. Other details are as in Fig. 8. Details are given in Boorstein *et al.* (1982) and Talmadge *et al.* (1983).

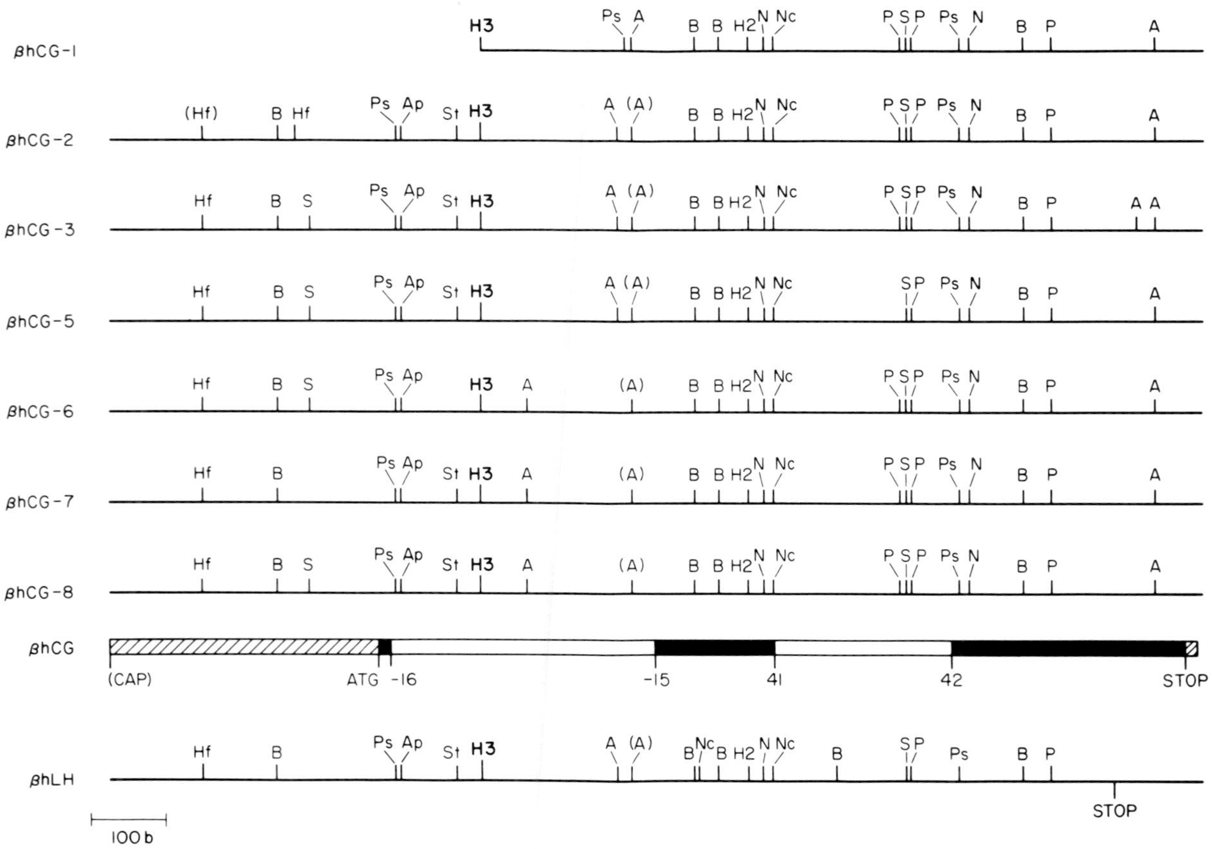
βhCG-1
βhCG-2
βhCG-3
βhCG-5
βhCG-6
βhCG-7
βhCG-8
βhCG
βhLH
(CAP)
ATG -16
-15
41
42
STOP
100 b

al., 1983). The first group, Fig. 8, contains four genes, numbers 1–4, the second group, Fig. 9, contains genes 5 and 6, while the third group, Fig. 10, contains genes 7 and 8.

These genes show an unusual structural organization. Four of the genes, numbers 1 and 2 and numbers 5 and 6, form inverted pairs. In each case, transcription of both genes, if both members of the pair were active, would be convergent. The 3' ends of the two genes in each pair are separated by 2.25 kb. In contrast, the other four genes are arranged in two tandem pairs (3 and 4; 7 and 8) and are separated by 5.5 kb.

As mentioned in the previous section, it is possible that the β hCG fragment used as a hybridization probe is sufficiently homologous to β hLH to allow cross-hybridization between the two sequences. By a combination of DNA sequence analysis and restriction enzyme analysis, we have shown that this is the case. One of the eight isolated genes, gene number 4, Fig. 9, codes for β hLH (Talmadge *et al.*, 1983). The other seven genes, numbers 1–3 and 5–8, code for β hCG or are β hCG pseudogenes. Until all of the genes are sequenced completely, it is not possible to exclude that some of them contain features such as altered splice sites or in-frame termination codons which make then pseudogenes.

We have obtained a complete DNA sequence for two of the β hCG genes, numbers 5 and 6, and for the single β hLH gene (Talmadge *et al.*, 1984). These sequences and their evolutionary implications are discussed later. In order to compare all of the eight genes, we isolated them as separate subclones from the bacteriophage recombinants. A partial restriction enzyme map was established for each of these genes to look for similarities and differences among them. This map is shown in Fig. 11. The details of the mapping strategies have been described in Talmadge *et al.* (1983). We would like to emphasize however that this is not a com-

---

FIG. 11. Comparative restriction enzyme analysis of the β hCG genes 1–3 and 5–8 and the single β hLH gene. The following abbreviations are used for restriction enzymes: A, *Ava*I; Ap, *Apa*I; B, *Bgl*I; H2, *Hinc*II; H3, *Hind*III; Hf, *Hinf*I; N, *Nae*I; Nc, *Nco*I; P, *Pvu*II; Ps, *Pst*I; S, *Sac*I; St, *Stu*I. The common *Hind*III site used to separate the 5' and 3' moieties of the genes is shown in bold type. Sites shown in parentheses were identified by partial digestion. The restriction enzyme maps are lined up with the structure of a composite β hCG gene. The cross-hatched areas are untranslated regions, solid shaded areas are coding sequences, and unshaded areas are introns. The positions of the cap site (CAP) and initiation codon (ATG) are shown. The termination codon for β hCG (STOP) is shown on the composite map while the termination codon for β hLH, which is shorter than β hCG, is shown under the β hLH map. The numbers refer to the amino acids located at the splice junctions; negative numbers refer to the signal peptide. This is a partial restriction enzyme map. Details are given in Talmadge *et al.* (1983).

plete restriction enzyme map for all the enzymes used but in several cases is a partial map designed for comparative purposes only.

Comparing each of the genes by pairs we find that none of the genes is identical. Restriction site differences can be observed between any two genes. However, the overall distribution of sites is very similar among all seven β hCG genes or pseudogenes and the single β hLH gene, showing that they have the same basic structure. This comparative map also shows, as will be discussed in more detail later in the section on DNA sequences, that β hLH is very similar to β hCG. All of the sites present or absent in the β hLH gene are also present or absent in at least one of the β hCG genes, with only three exceptions. The two DNA sequences therefore seem to be more closely related than the amino acid sequences might predict.

It is important to establish whether we have cloned the entire complement of β hCG and β hLH genes found in the human chromosome and to be able to distinguish β hCG from β hLH genes. To demonstrate this, human chromosome DNA was digested with several restriction enzymes and analyzed by filter hybridization (Southern, 1975). Both a β hCG and β hLH fragment were used as hybridization probes because although the two sequences are very similar, it should be possible under stringent hybridization conditions to distinguish the two sets of sequences by the relative intensities of hybridization to each of the probes. An autoradiograph of such a hybridization is shown in Fig. 12 (Talmadge *et al.*, 1983). Differences in the intensity of hybridization with the β hCG and β hLH probes can clearly be seen. For example, with the combined HindIII–KpnI digest (Fig. 12b), a 2.2 kb fragment hybridizes much more strongly to the β hLH than to the beta hCG probes.

In Table I we have correlated the hybridizing fragments seen using both these probes with the restriction enzyme maps of the cloned genes. The results of this correlation demonstrate that the human genome contains seven β hCG genes, or pseudogenes, and a single β hLH gene (Talmadge *et al.*, 1983). No hybridizing fragments were found that do not correspond to the cloned genes. We therefore believe that we have cloned the complete complement of β hCG and β hLH genes from the human genome.

There is evidence to suggest that these eight genes are all linked (N. Vamvakopoulos and J. C. Fiddes, unpublished data). With the enzymes SalI and EcoRI, we observe a single, very large, hybridizing band which is consistent with linkage of all the genes, although this is not conclusive as we cannot exclude the possibility that there are two or more large hybridizing fragments not resolved by electrophoresis.

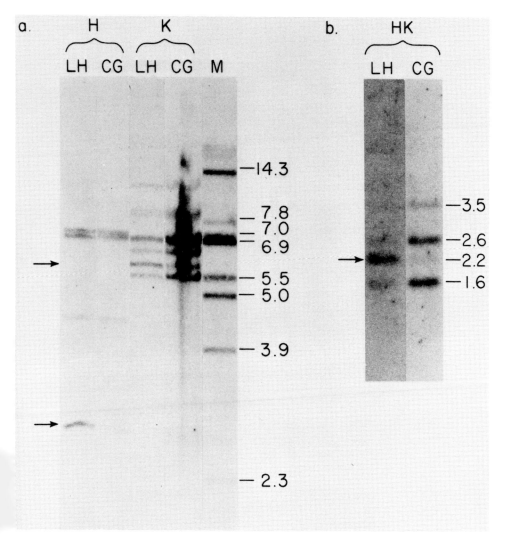

FIG. 12. Autoradiograph of filter hybridizations of human placental DNA. Human DNA was digested with (a) *Hin*dIII (H), *Kpn*I (K), or with (b) both enzymes, and hybridized to the β hCG- or β hLH-specific probes by the filter hybridization method using stringent hybridization and wash conditions. CG, hybridization to the β hCG-specific probe; LH, hybridization to the β hLH-specific probe. Sizes of market fragments (M) are given in kilobases and the positions of the fragments which hybridize more strongly with the β hLH probe are identified at the sides with arrows. Details are given in Talmadge *et al.* (1983).

TABLE I
*Correlation of Cloned β hCG and β hLH Gene
Fragments with Digests of Human DNA[a]*

Enzyme	Fragment size (kb)	Gene
HindIII–KpnI	3.5	3
	2.6	1, 5
	2.2	LH
	1.6	2, 6, 7, 8
HindIII	7.2	3
	7.0	7
	4.3	1, 2, 5, 6
	2.8	LH
KpnI	10.0	6
	8.8	3
	8.6	(1/5/7)
	7.0	8
	7.0	(1/5/7)
	6.5	(1/5/7)
	6.0	LH
	5.3	2

[a] Identification of the HindIII, KpnI, and combined HindIII–KpnI fragments in the human genome containing β hCG or β hLH sequences. These data are a correlation of the results shown in Figs. 8–10 and 12. Genes which are at the ends of the bacteriophage λ recombinants and therefore cannot be assigned a particular fragment are in parentheses. No HindIII fragment has been assigned to β hCG 8. Details are given in Talmadge *et al.* (1983).

VI. Nucleotide Sequence of Two β hCG Genes and the Single β hLH Gene

We have established, using both the chemical and the chain termination methods (Maxam and Gilbert, 1977; Sanger *et al.*, 1977), the complete nucleotide sequence of two of the β hCG genes, numbers 5 and 6, and of the single β hLH gene. A comparison of these nucleotide sequences is shown in Fig. 13 (Talmadge *et al.*, 1984). We chose to sequence β hCG 5 and 6 since they form one of the inverted pairs (Figs. 8 and 9) and we were interested in the possible implications of this symmetrical arrangement for gene expression.

The locations of the introns in the β hCG genes were identified by comparison with the β hCG cDNA sequence. Although we do not have a β hLH cDNA, we were able to locate the introns in β hLH by analogy with β hCG. The sequences at the intron–exon boundaries show the expected homologies with other genes (Breathnach *et al.*, 1978; Catterall *et al.*, 1978).

The β hLH amino acid sequence derived from the nucleotide sequence differs at three locations from the previously published beta hLH amino acid sequence. There is a Met-Met and a Val-Val at positions 41–42 and 55–56, respectively, rather than the single methionine and valine previously reported (Shome and Parlow, 1973). This brings the β hLH sequence into register with the β hCG sequence. Also, we have determined the carboxy-terminal sequence to be His-Pro-Gln-Leu-Ser-Gly-Leu-Leu-Phe-Leu$_{COOH}$ rather than the His-Pro-Gln$_{COOH}$ previously reported (Keutmann *et al.*, 1979). These changes make the β subunit of hLH 121 amino acids long rather than 112, and also make it more homologous to the ovine, bovine, and porcine sequences (Liu *et al.*, 1972; Sairam *et al.*, 1972; Maghuin-Rogister and Hennen, 1973).

The amino acid sequence predicted from the nucleotide sequence of β hCG 5 agrees completely with the previously established amino acid sequence (Morgan *et al.*, 1975; Birken and Canfield, 1977; Keutmann and Williams, 1977). However, with β hCG 6, there is a single coding change. Instead of having aspartic acid at position 117, β hCG 6 has alanine. This position is aspartic acid in both the published amino acid sequence from two groups (Keutmann and Williams, 1977; Birken and Canfield, 1977) and in our cDNA sequence (Fiddes and Goodman, 1980). We have preliminary evidence that genes with the coding change are not expressed, as we will discuss in the next section. In addition, there is a single silent change between β hCG 5 and 6 in codon number 4. In this case, again, β hCG 5 has the same sequence as the previously established cDNA.

We have determined the point of initiation of transcription of the β hCG genes as shown in Fig. 13. This was established (Boorstein *et al.*, 1982) by a combination of SI nuclease mapping and primer extension analysis. The 5′-untranslated region of β hCG is therefore 340 or 341 nucleotides long, although the initial cDNA clone (Fig. 6, Fiddes and Goodman, 1980) only contains 25 of these nucleotides. We do not know whether β hLH initiates transcription in the same position, as the SI analysis was carried out with placental and not pituitary mRNA.

The canonical sequence, TATA$_A^T$A$_A^T$, has been identified in many eukaryotic genes at about 25 to 30 nucleotides before the start of transcription (see Breathnach and Chambon, 1981, for a compilation). This sequence is thought to have an important role in directing the initiation of transcription. In β hCG 5 and 6, the best match to this "TATA box" sequence is TCAAGTA (nucleotides 161–167) in which only three out of

```
                                                    50                                                  100
LH   AAGGGAGAGGTGGGCTCCGGCTTAATCCTCTTGGGGGGCATCTGGCTCAAGTGGCTTCCTCCTGGCAGCACAGTCACGGGAGGAGACCCTCTTCACTGGG
CG5  AAGGGAGAGGTGGGCTCCGGCTGAATCCTCGTTGGGGGGCATCTGGCTCAAGTGGCTTCCTCCTGGCAGCACAGTCACGGGAGGAGACCCTCTTCATTGGG
CG6  AAGGGAGAGGTGGGCTCCGGCTGAATCCTCGTTGGGGGGCATCTGGCTCAAGTGGCTTCCTCCTGGCAGCACACTCACGGGAGGAGACCCTCTTCACTGGG

                                                   150                                   **           200
LH   CAGAAGCTAAGTCGAAGCAGCGCCCCCTCCTGTTAGTTGGACTGTGGTGCAGGAAAGCTCAAGT   GGAGGGTTGAGGCTTCAGTCCAGCACTTTCC
CG5  CAGAAGCTAAGTCCGAAGCCGCGCCCCCTCCTGTTAGTTGGAGGTTGACTGTGGTGCAGGAAAGCCTCAAGTAGAGGAGGGTTGAGGCTTCAATCCAGCACTTTGC
CG6  CAGAAGCTAAGTCCGAAGCCGCGCCCCCTCCTGTTAGTTGGAGGTTGACTGTGGTGCAGGAAAGGCTCAAGTAGAGGAGGAGTTGAGGCTTCAGTCCAGCACTTTCC

                                                   250                                               300
LH   TCGGGTCATGGCCTCCTCCTGGCTCCCAAGACCCCACAATTGGCAGAGCAGGCCTTCTCACCCTACCTCCTGCTTCCAGCCTCGACTAGTCCCTA
CG5  TCGGGTCACGGCCTCCTCCTGGCTCCCAGGACCCCATAGGCAGAGCAGGCCTTCTCACACCCTACCTACCTCTGTGCCTCAGGCTCGACTAGTCCCTA
CG6  ACACTCGACGACTGAGTCTCAGAGTCACAGTGTCCTGGTCTCCGCTGGTCTCCGCCTCATCCTGGCGCTAGACCCTGAGGGGCACTCTGCTGAGC

                                                   350                                               400
LH   GCACTCGACAACTGAGTCTCTGAGTCACTTCACCGGTCTCTGCCTCTGCTCTCGGCGCTAGACCCCTGAGGGGCACTCTGCTGAGC
CG5  GCACTCGACGACTGAGTCTCTGAGTCACTTCACCGGTCGTCTGCCTCGTGTCTACCTTGCTCTCGGCGCTAGACCCTGAGGGGGCTGGGGCGCTGGGGTGCTCGGTGAGC
CG6  ACACTCGACGACTGAGTCTCAGAGTCACTTCACCGGTCGTCTGCCTTCTCGCCCGAAGGGTCACATCCTACAACCTCCTGGCCTGGGGGCACTCTGCTGAGC

                                                   450                                               500
LH   CACTCCTGCGCCTCCCTGGCCATGGCCACTTCACCCTCTCGCCCCGGGGATTAGTGTCCAGGTTACCCCAGGCATCCTATCACCCTCCTGGCCTTGCCGCCGC
CG5  CACTCCTGCGCCCCCCTGGCCTTGTCTACCCTTGCTACCTCTGCCCCCGGGGATTAGTGTCCAGGTTAGTGTCGAGTCACCCAG CATCCTACAACCTCCTGGCCTGTGCCGCCCC
CG6  CACTCCTGTGCCTGGCCTTGTCTACTTCTCGCCCCCGAAGGGTTAGTGTCGAGTCACTCAG CATCCTACAACCTCCTGGCCTGTGCCGCCCC

                                           -20  MetGluMetLeuGln        -16                             600
LH   CCACAACCCCGAGTATAAAGCCAGATACACGAGGCCAGGGGATGCACCAAGGATAGATGTCCAGTAAGACTGCAGGGCCCCTGGGCACCTTCCACC
CG5  CCACAACCCCGAGTATAAAGCCAGGTACACCAGGGACCAGGGACCAGATGTTCCAGTGAGATGTGCAGCGCCCCCCAGTAAGCTTCCAGTG
CG6                                                                                         Phe
```

62

```
                 AsnThrIleGlnAlaValGlyLysGluGlyGluGlyLysCysProValCysIleThrValAsnThrThrIleCysAlaGlyTyrCysProThrMet
                                                                                                  *  1                                           1100
LH    AATGCCATCTGTGTGACAAGAGGTGCCGGTGCACCGTGCCCACCATGTGAGCTGCCCGG
CG5   AATGCCACCTGCTGTGGAGAAGAGGCTGCCGGTGCACCGTGCCCACCATGTGAGCTGCCCGG
CG6   AATGCCACCTGCTGTGGAGAAGAGGCTGCCGGTGCACCGTGCCCACCATGTGAGCTGCCCGG
                                                          Thr

                                                                                                                1200
LH    GGCCGGGGCAGATGCTGCCACCTCAGGGCCAGACCCACAGACCCACAGACCCTCCTGGCCTTCGGGAATGGGGTGTG
CG5   GGCCGGGGCAGTGCTGCCACCTCAGGGCCAGACCCACAGAGACCCACAGACCCTCCTGGCTTCAGGGCTGCGGAATGGGGTGTG
CG6   GGCCGGGGCAGGTGCTGCCACCTCAGGGCCAGACCCACAGAGACCCACAGACCCTCCTGGCTTCAGGGCTGCGGAATGGGGTGTG

                                                                                              60
                                                  MetArgValLeuGlnAlaValLeuProProLeuProGlnValValCysThrTyrArgAspValArgPheGluSerIleAla          1300
LH    GGAAGGCAGGAACAGAGGGCTTCCTGGCTCCTGAGCTCTGAACCTGTGGGTCAGCTTGGGAGCTCAGCTGGCTGCCTAGCCACATGCTCATTC
CG5   GGAGGGCAGGAACAGAGGGCTTCCGGAGCCTGACCCTGAGCTCTGAACCTGTGGGGCAACTCAGCTCAGCTGAGGGCGTGGCCCAGCCACATGCTCATTC
CG6   GGAGGGCAGGAACAGAGGGCTTCCGGAGCCTGACCCTGAGCTCTGAACCTGTGGGGCAACTCAGCTCAGCTGAGGGCGTGGCCCAGCCACATGCTCATTC

              42
              MetArgValLeuGlnAlaValLeuProProLeuProGlnValValCysThrTyrArgAspValArgPheGluSerIleAla
LH    CCCACTCACACGGCCTCCAGATGCCGGTGCTGCAGGCGGTCCTGCCGCCCCTGCCTCAGGTGGTCTGCACTTACCGTGGTTGCCTTCAGTCCATCC
                                                                                                    Asn
CG5   CCCACTCACACGGCTTCCAGACCCGTGCTGCAGGCGGTCCTGCCGGGGTCCTGCCTCAGGTGGTGCAACTACCGGCGATGTGCGCCTTCAGTCCATCC
                                                           Thr      Gly    Ala
CG6   CCCACTCACACGGCTTCCAGACCCGTGCTGCAGGCGGTCCTGCCGGGGTCCTGCCTCAGGTGGTGCAACTACCGGCGATGTGCGCCTTCAGTCCATCC

                                                                                                100
              rgLeuProGlyCysProArgGlyValAspProValSerPheProValAlaLeuSerCysArgCysGlyProCysArgArgSerThrSerAspCysGl
LH    GGCTCCCTGGCTGCCCGCGGGGCGTGGACCCCGTCTCTTTCCCGGTGGCCCTGTCATGCCGCTGCGGACCCTGCAGGTGTCG
                                                                             Gln    AlaLeu
CG5   GGCTCCCTGGCTGCCCGCGGGGCGTGGACCCCGTGAACCCGGTGTCTTCCTACGCCGTGCTCTCAGTGCAATGTGCACTCTGCCCGCCGCAGCCACCACTGACTGCGG
                                                                             TyrAla            Thr
CG6   GGCTCCCTGGCTGCCCGCGGGGCGTGGACCCCGTGAACCCGGTGTCTTCCTACGCCGTGCTCTCAGTGCAATGTGCACTCTGCCCGCCGCAGCCACCACTGACTGCGG

                                                                                                  121
              yGlyProLysHisAspHisThrCysAspHisProLeuThrGlnLeuSerGlyLeuLeuPheLeuTer
LH    GGGTCCCAAAGACCACCCCTTGACCTGACCACACCCCAACTCTCAGCCTCCTCTTCTTCTAAAGACCCCTCCCCCAGCCTTCCCAAGTCCATCCCGACT
                                                                      TAAAGAC
CG5   GGGTCCCAAGACCACCCCTTGACCTGTGATGACCCCCGCTTCCAGGCCTCCTCTTCCTCCTCCAAAGGCCCCTCCCCCCAGCCTTCCCAAGTCCATCCCGACT
                                                                 Asp    Ar    gPheGlnAspSerSerSerLysAlaProProProSerLeuProSerProSerArgLe
CG6   GGGTCCCAAGACCACCCCTTGACCTGTGATGACCCCCGCTTCCAGGCCTCCTCTTCCTCCTCCAAAGGCCCCTCCCCCCAGCCTTCCCAAGTCCATCCCGACT
                                                                        Ala

                                                                        1650
LH    CCTGGAGCCCT  GACACCCCGATCCTCCCACAATAAAGGTTCTCAATCCGCACTCTGGCAGTATC
CG5   CCCGGGGCCCTCGGACACACCCGACCCGATCCTCCCACAATAAAGGTTCTCAATCCGCACTCTGGAGGTGTC
CG6   CCCGGGGCCCTCGGACACACCCGACCCGATCCTCCCACAATAAAGGTTCTCAATCCGCACTCTGGCGGTGTC
              uProGlyProSerAspThrProIleLeuProGlnTer
                                             145                                          *
```

FIG. 13. The complete nucleotide sequences of β hCG 5 and 6 and β hLH. The three sequences have been aligned with gaps where there are deletions and insertions, and the nucleotide sequence numbers, immediately above the nucleotide sequences, are not adjusted for deletions. In the alignment of the nucleotide sequences, boldface letters indicate positions where one of the three sequences differs from the other two. The two asterisks at nucleotides 190 and 191 identify the proposed transcriptional start for β hCG and the single asterisk at nucleotide 1654 marks the polyadenylation site. The amino acid sequence for β hLH is shown above the nucleotide sequence. For β hCG 5 and 6, only the amino acids which differ from those of β hLH are shown below the nucleotide sequences. Amino acid numbers are placed immediately above amino acid names, and negative numbers refer to amino acids in the signal peptide. Details are given in Talmadge et al. (1984).

63

seven nucleotides match the canonical sequence. A second sequence, the "CAAT box" (Corden *et al.*, 1980; see Breathnach and Chambon, 1981, for a compilation), occurs at about 80–100 nucleotides before the start of transcription. In this case, the canonical sequence is GGCAATCT while in the β hCG genes the best match is GCTAAGTCC (nucleotide 106–114) with only five out of nine nucleotides matching. Interestingly there are the sequences TATAAAG and TATGAAG within the 5′-untranslated region of β CG 5 and 6, respectively (positions 515–521) at about 35 nucleotides before the translational initiation codon. We have no evidence that these sequences are part of a functional promoter as we have not detected a shorter β hCG transcript.

We do not know if the initiation of transcription of β hLH is located at the equivalent position as the SI nuclease mapping and primer extension analysis was done with placental but not with pituitary mRNA. A definitive answer to this question will require the analysis of pituitary RNA, but there is suggestive evidence that the 5′-untranslated region of β hLH may be shorter. In eukaryotic DNA, there are usually no initiation codons (ATGs) within the 5′-untranslated region (Kozak, 1978). Mutant insulin genes have been created (Lomedico and McAndrew, 1982) that contain out of frame ATGs within the 5′-untranslated region, but in each case it was shown that the authentic ATG was still used for the initiation of translation. However, in keeping with the general observation that ATGs are not naturally found upstream from the start of translation, the long 5′-untranslated regions of β hCG 5 and 6 do not contain any ATG sequences. On the other hand, the corresponding region of β hLH contains three such sequences at nucleotides 208, 422, and 542 before the probable initiation codon, all of which are out of frame with the coding sequence. The 5′-untranslated region of β hLH is therefore either unusual in containing ATG sequences or is actually considerably shorter than that of β hCG. Like β hCG 5, β hLH contains the TATAAAG sequence about 35 nucleotides before the proposed initiation codon, but we do not know if this is involved in transcription initiation. We also note that there are no sequence differences as far as 550 bases from the initiation codons of the β hCG and β LH genes that might account for the fact that β hCG is expressed in the placenta while β hLH is expressed in the pituitary.

VII. Expression of the β hCG Genes

We have shown that genes 1–3 and 5–8 (Figs. 8–10, Talmadge *et al.*, 1983) are β hCG genes or pseudogenes. Sequence analysis (Fig. 13) shows that β hCG 5 appears to code for the established β hCG amino acid sequence whereas β hCG 6 has a single amino acid change at position 117. We would like to know specifically whether these two genes are expressed *in vivo* and in general which of the other five genes are functional. Analysis of the sequence upstream from the initiation of transcription of β hCG 5 and 6 gives no indication as to which of the genes, if any, are actively expressed in the placenta. Neither of the genes, as discussed previously, has sequences which are a good match to the canonical promoter sequences, although other functional genes have been sequenced and shown also to lack classic TATA and CAAT box sequences (Baker *et al.*, 1979). Gene 5 encodes the normal protein while gene 6 contains a single amino acid difference not detected in the amino acid sequence analysis of two groups (Keutmann and Williams, 1977; Birken and Canfield, 1979) or in our cDNA sequence (Fiddes and Goodman, 1980).

We have preliminary evidence from two separate approaches which suggests that only a limited number of the β hCG genes are functional. This conclusion comes from an analysis of several placental β hCG cDNA clones and from experiments in which the β hCG genes have been reintroduced into mammalian cells in culture (K. Talmadge, M.-J. Gething, and J. C. Fiddes, in preparation).

In β hCG 5, amino acids 117 and 118 are coded for by GAC (Asp) TCC (Ser) (see Fig. 13). This corresponds to a recognition site for the restriction enzyme *Hin*fI (GANTC). In β hCG 6 the corresponding sequence is GCC (Ala) TCC (Ser), which does not correspond to a *Hin*fI site. We have analyzed all of the seven β hCG genes for the presence or absence of a *Hin*fI site at this position and found the site to be present only in genes 1, 3, and 5. The loss of the site in the other four genes, 2, 6, 7, and 8, could mean that they too have Ala at position 117 (although other nucleotide changes at this site could also cause the loss of the *Hin*fI site). A total of 15 independently isolated β hCG gene clones have been analyzed by digestion with *Hin*fI and all were found to have a *Hin*fI site at this position, implying that they would be derived from the transcription of β hCG genes 1, 3 or 5.

The comparative restriction enzyme analysis presented in Fig. 11 (Talmadge *et al.*, 1984) identified β hCG 3 as having a unique *Ava*I site at the position corresponding to amino acids 124–126. None of the other six β hCG genes have this site. The presence of an *Ava*I site in β hCG 3 is caused by a silent third position change in codon 125. Among the same 15 placental cDNA clones analyzed previously, two were found to contain an *Ava*I site at this position, showing that they came from β hCG 3 transcription.

We have also used transient expression in COS cells (Gluzman, 1980; Mellon *et al.*, 1981) to determine whether the β hCG genes are potentially functional. Expression of a foreign gene in this cell system does not tell whether the gene is actively expressed in its normal cell type, but serves as an assay to establish whether the genes have a functional promoter. The COS cell line was established from African green monkey kidney cells and permits replication of plasmids containing an SV40 origin of replication (Gluzman, 1980). All of the β hCG genes, with the exception of β hCG 1 for which we have not yet isolated the 5' end, were subcloned into a vector containing the SV40 origin of replication. These plasmids were than transfected into COS cells and RNA was isolated after 60 hours. This RNA was analyzed by SI nuclease mapping by the method of Berk and Sharp (1977), as modified by Weaver and Weissmann (1979), to search for correctly initiated transcripts of the β hCG genes starting from their own promoters. Preliminary results from these experiments indicate that genes 3 and 5 express in COS cells but genes 2, 6, 7, and 8 do not.

The results of the cDNA clone analysis and the transient expression experiments are therefore consistent and suggest that beta hCG genes 3 and 5, and probably 1, are functional genes encoding the correct β hCG amino acid sequence, while genes β hCG 2, 6, 7, and 8 probably encode an altered amino acid sequence and are not functional.

The β hCG gene structures are exceedingly similar (Fig. 11), yet only three of the seven genes are expressed; in the specific comparison of genes 5 and 6 (Fig. 13), there are no obvious nucleotide changes that explain why gene 5 is expressed but gene 6 is not. Further sequencing of the β hCG gene family members may reveal the early steps in the generation of pseudogenes.

VIII. Evolution of β CG from β LH by Readthrough into the 3'-Untranslated Region

LH is synthesized in the pituitaries of a wide range of species. In contrast, CG is found only in the placenta of certain mammals such as horses, baboons, and humans (Canfield *et al.,* 1978; Pierce and Parsons, 1981; Ward *et al.,* 1982), and is thus considered to be the most recently evolved member of the glycoprotein hormone gene family. Due to the strong structural and biological similarity between LH and CG, it has been proposed previously that CG arose directly from LH or an LH-like ancestral gene (Dayhoff, 1976).

The β subunit of hCG is 24 amino acids longer than the β subunit of hLH. Alignment of the two β subunit amino acid sequences shows that the extra 24 amino acids of the hCG β subunit form a carboxy-terminal extension that is unique to β hCG. We proposed initially (Fiddes and Goodman, 1980) that this carboxy-terminal extension resulted from the readthrough event in which the β CG gene evolved from its β LH ancestor by incorporating the 3'-untranslated region into coding sequence. This proposal was based on the observation that the cDNA for the β subunit of hCG had a particularly short 3'-untranslated region of 16 nucleotides and that the termination codon of β hCG was the TAA sequence of the polyadenylation signal, AATAAA (Proudfoot and Brownlee, 1976).

We can now identify the nucleotide changes that caused the read-through. A single base deletion in the β hCG sequence (nucleotide 1540, Fig. 13, Talmadge *et al.*, 1984) puts the β hCG sequence out of frame with the last seven codons of β hLH and allows the 3'-untranslated region to become incorporated into the coding region. In addition to this, a two base insertion in the β hCG sequence (nucleotides 1612 and 1613, Fig. 13) allows the carboxy-terminal extension to continue to the termination codon, TAA, which is part of the AATAAA polyadenylation site. Without this two base insertion, the β hCG carboxy-terminal extension would be eight amino acids shorter, ending with a TGA termination codon (nucleotides 1611, 1614, and 1615, Fig. 13). If the two base insertion occurred first, this would be a neutral mutation since the inserted bases would still be part of the 3'-untranslated region. If the single base deletion occurred first, β hCG has had two carboxy-terminal extensions read in two different frames. We think the latter is unlikely. Nevertheless, by either mechanism, the primary event which led to the incorporation of the 3'-untranslated region into the coding region was the single base deletion. We note that the β hLH termination codon, put out of frame in β hCG, has been lost by a single base change. We do not think that the change in that termination codon was the initial event leading to the carboxy-terminal extension because there is no other terminator in the 3'-untranslated region in frame with it.

Thus, the β subunit of hCG has acquired 8 amino acids by translation in a new reading frame, and 24 amino acids from a previously untranslated region. This has occurred without any substantial change other than the frameshift mutations since β hCG genes 5 and 6 are 90% homologous with β hLH (11/92 and 10/92 changes, respectively) over the region encoding the carboxy-terminal extension, nucleotides 1541–1634. The function of this carboxy-terminal extension is not known since hCG appears to bind to the same membrane receptors and to elicit the same response (see Pierce and Parsons, 1981, for a review). However, hCG is 10 times more stable than hLH, and it has been proposed that the carboxy-terminal extension plays a role in this (see Canfield *et al.*, 1978, for a review).

IX. Nucleotide Changes in the Evolution of β CG from β LH

As described in the previous section, CG is a more recently evolved function than LH. On the basis of the gene organization shown in Figs. 8–10, we propose that the β hCG gene arose by a duplication of an ancestral β LH gene, followed by a series of changes that created the β CG function. This ancestral β CG gene has subsequently duplicated and rearranged to give the complex organization seen in Figs. 8–10. We do not believe the original ancestral β LH gene duplication occurred at the same time as the ancestral β CG gene rearrangements because it seems highly unlikely that such a mechanism would result in seven β hCG genes but only one β hLH gene. In contrast to CG, the FSH, TSH, and LH functions are very ancient, existing during most of vertebrate evolution, with TSH the oldest and LH the youngest of the three (Dayhoff, 1976). We propose, therefore, that the β subunits of hFSH and hTSH will, unlike β hCG, not be encoded by a complex, multigene family. We have no evidence that suggests whether the β hFSH and hTSH genes will be linked to each other or to β hLH genes.

The nucleotide sequences which we have established for β hCG 5 and 6 and β hLH provide information on the series of changes which took place as the newly duplicated ancestral gene evolved into β hCG. To compare the nucleotide sequence differences between the β hLH gene and each of the two β hCG genes 5 and 6, we have calculated the percentage divergence between the introns, and between replacement and silent substitution sites across the homologous coding region. These data are shown in Table II (Talmadge et al., 1984). We also present in Table II similar calculations for a selection of other gene pairs, including the two β hCG genes themselves, human growth hormone (hGH) and human placental lactogen (hPL) (Goodman et al., 1980; DeNoto et al., 1981; Seeburg, 1982), the two rat preproinsulin genes, I and II (Lomedico et al., 1979), and the rabbit and mouse β globins (Efstradiatis et al., 1977; van den Berg et al., 1978).

Striking differences emerge. For the two preproinsulin (Table II, line e) and beta globin (Table II, line f) gene pairs, the rates of intron and silent position divergence is similar within each pair, and is four to seven times greater than the rate of replacement changes. For example, the rat preproinsulin genes (Table II) have diverged by 3% at replacement sites but by 19% in silent and 21% in intron sites. Similar results have been obtained with six other gene pairs that encode identical functions (three β globin gene pairs and three preproinsulin gene pairs), as well as a gene pair encoding different functions (an α and β globin gene pair) (Perler et al., 1980). Similar results were also found comparing rates of replacement versus silent substitutions in another 36 gene pairs encoding different functions (Miyata et al., 1980). In marked contract, the replacement and silent sites of the two β HCG genes have diverged from those of β LH at similar rates, between 6 and 8%, while the introns of each pair have diverged slightly less, between 4 and 6% (Table II). Thus, unlike most other gene pairs, the replacement, silent and intron changes have all occurred at approximately equal rates. The introns and silent sites of the hGH:hPL gene pair have also diverged at rates (10 and 11%, respec-

TABLE II

Gene Sequence Comparisons[a]

	Replacement		Silent		Intron	
	No./Nucs	%	No./Nucs	%	No./Nucs	%
LH : CG5	19/296.7	6 ± 2	7/101.3	7 ± 3	25/545	5 ± 1
LH : CG6	19/296.7	6 ± 2	8/101.3	8 ± 3	33/545	6 ± 1
CG5 : CG6	1/369	0.3 ± 0.3	1/123	1 ± 1	19/545	3 ± 1
hGH : hPL	33.5/482	7 ± 1	18.5/161	11 ± 3	74/726	10 ± 1
RI : RII	8/249.2	3 ± 1	15/80.8	19 ± 5	21/99	21 ± 5
RBG : MBG	35/330	11 ± 2	49/110	44 ± 6	120/267	45 ± 4

[a] LH, β LH; CG5, β HCG gene 5; CG6, β HCG gene 6; hGH, human growth hormone; hPL, human placental lactogen; RI, rat preproinsulin gene I; RII, rat preproinsulin gene II; RBG, rabbit β globin; MBG, mouse β globin. We calculated the values in the first four lines by the method of Lomedico *et al.* (1979) as follows. To calculate the rate of replacement and silent changes, we classified every coding base (except the initiation codon) as to whether each of the three possible codon substitutions was silent (not altering the encoded amino acid) or replacement (altering the encoded amino acid), and then divided the replacement and silent totals by three (Nucs). We also totaled each actual replacement and silent change (No.). In codons with two changes, half values were assigned when one nucleotide was either replacement or silent with respect to the other change. The fractions shown (%) are the number of actual substitutions divided by the number of potential substitution sites. For introns, we eliminated from consideration the first and last 10 nucleotides, and, for the hGH : hPL comparison, counted each gap as a single change. The values shown in the last two lines are taken from Lomedico *et al.* (1979). The standard deviations were estimated as the square root of [%/Nucs]. These data are not corrected for multiple substitutions. The comparisons between the individual β hCG genes and the β LH gene have been made over their homologous coding regions from the start codons at nucleotide 553 and up to but not including the single base deletion in the β hCG genes at nucleotide 1540 that creates the frameshift. The comparison between the two β hCG genes is over their 164 amino acid signal sequence and mature protein coding regions. The comparison between the hGH : hPL genes is over their 210 amino acid signal sequence and mature protein coding regions. Details are given in Talmadge *et al.* (1984).

tively, Table II) that are only slightly higher than the rate of replacement changes (7%, Table II), and it is thus similar to the β CG : β LH gene pairs in that the relative rates of replacement to neutral changes are high compared to other gene pairs. It is interesting that the hGH : hPL protein pair is analogous to the β CG : β LH protein pair; both proteins in each of the pairs have similar functions, but one (hGH/hLH) is synthesized in the pituitary while the other (hCG/hPL) is synthesized in the placenta. A relatively high rate of replacement over neutral change has been observed in a pair of rabbit globin alleles (Efstradiatis *et al.*, 1977; Hardison *et al.*, 1979; van Ooyen *et al.*, 1979) and a pair of immunoglobulin light chains (Bernard *et al.*, 1978), as well as a relatively high rate of replacement over slight substitutions in cDNA fragments encoding the carboxy-terminal third of two mouse H2^d antigens (Bregegere *et al.,* 1981).

How can we explain the relatively high rate of replacement changes and the relatively low rate of neutral changes between the β hLH and β hCG gene pairs as well as between the hGH and hPL gene pairs? One theory of evolution holds that observed changes in protein structure are spread through the population by selection (Clarke, 1970; Blundell and Wood, 1975; Richmond, 1975). In support of this hypothesis, Perler *et al.* (1980) cited the two rabbit β globin alleles, where there are 4 replacement changes with no silent changes and only 2 intron changes, as a clear example of selection. They assumed that these changes were fixed so rapidly by selection that there was no opportunity for neutral changes to appear. This could be true for the light chain and H2^d antigen gene pairs, although the generation of polymorphisms in these systems is a specialized and, at least in the case of the light chains, perhaps separate mechanism. The selection argument of Perler *et al.* can also be applied to the evolution of the new functions in the β hCG : β hLH and hGH : hPL gene pairs. By this hypothesis, the new function, hCG, whose gene has fewer silent and intron changes compared to its related gene, β hLH, than the hPL gene has compared to its related gene, hGH, was so favorable that it became fixed more rapidly than hPL.

An alternate interpretation of the relatively high rate of replacement changes and relatively low rate of neutral changes in the evolution of β hLH to β hCG is that genes evolve first by fixation of the new function (selection), followed by accumulation of neutral changes (drift). By this hypothesis, the evolution of β hCG is the most recent event yet analyzed, more recent than the evolution of hPL. Like the β CG and β LH genes, the GH and PL genes diverged late in mammalian radiation (Niall, 1972), but which gene family diverged first is not known because systematic cross-species protein comparisons either for CG or for PL have not yet been done.

The neutral mutation-random drift theory (Kimura, 1968; Kimura and Ohta, 1971, 1974), an alternative theory to explain evolution, holds that almost all observed changes in amino acid sequence are neutral and are fixed in the population by random drift. Unless the β CG genes duplicated very recently, it is difficult to envision a mechanism where so many replacement changes in β hCG relative to β hLH are neutral, when there are very few replacement changes (0.3% Table II) allowed between the two β hCG genes. It is unlikely that the β CG genes duplicated recently compared to the original β LH gene duplication, because the rates of β hCG genes 5 : 6 intron divergence (3%, Table II) approaches those of the β hLH : β hCG gene pairs (4 and 6%, Table II).

It is widely supposed that gene conversion maintains gene sequences within a multigene family (for a review see Baltimore, 1981; Dover, 1982). If gene conversion occurs in this locus, it might be expected to include the 93% homologous β hLH gene as well. However, assuming that gene conversion is restricted to the β hCG genes, it would not be a separate evolutionary process, but should act as a mechanism for spreading selective change (if selection is occurring), or neutral change (if most of the observed changes are the product of random drift), or both.

From the rapid rate of replacement over neutral change in the evolution of β hCG from β hLH, and from the low level of replacement versus intron change between the two β hCG genes, we conclude that selection of a new function is the mechanism most consistent with the observed sequence differences. If stability is truly the only difference between CG and LH, then the changes across the homologous coding region, and not just the carboxy-terminal extension, must be involved in this. However, on the basis of the large number of replacement relative to neutral changes in the evolution of β hLH to β hCG, as well as the constraint on the two β hCG coding sequences, we believe that there are other, as yet unidentified, biological functions of CG beyond the observed difference in CG and LH stability that require these coding differences. Moreover, because the divergence between the two β hCG introns approaches the divergence between the introns of the two β hLH : β hCG gene pairs, we propose that the β CG gene duplications and rearrangements occurred soon after the establishment of the new β CG function.

X. Summary

We have used the recombinant DNA technology to begin to understand the tissue-specific, developmentally regulated expression of the four different glycoprotein hormones.

Our isolation of a full-length cDNA encoding the common α subunit has allowed us to demonstrate that there is a single human gene for this protein, expressed in the placenta for production of hCG and in the pituitary for the production of hLH, hFSH, and hTSH. From this, we conclude that the control for the expression of glycoprotein hormones probably resides in the β subunit genes.

Our isolation of a full-length cDNA encoding the β subunit of hCG allowed us to isolate the full human complement of seven hCG β subunit genes or pseudogenes and, by cross-hybridization, the single β hLH gene. The β hLH gene is linked to at least three of the β hCG genes, and together, they show a complex organization of inverted and tandem pairs. We find from an analysis of independently isolated β hCG cDNA clones and from transfection of six of the seven β hCG genes into mammalian tissue culture cells that only three of the seven hCG genes are expressed.

Nevertheless, restriction enzyme analysis of the seven β hCG and single β hLH genes reveals that the genes are all extremely similar, with the same basic structure of three exons and two introns at the same positions. From this we conclude that the β hCG gene family is very early in the evolution of pseudogenes and nucleotide sequencing may elucidate some of the steps.

From a comparison of the nucleotide sequence of two of the β hCG genes and of the single β hLH gene, we show that β hCG arose from β hLH by a series of selected changes with very little neutral drift. The nucleotide sequence of the β hCG cDNA allowed us to predict that the carboxy-terminal extension of hCG arose by readthrough of a β hLH-like gene, incorporating the 3′-untranslated region. The gene sequence comparison reveals that the readthrough event was caused by a single base deletion. From the amino acid differences maintained between β hCG and β hLH, not just in the carboxy-terminal extension but throughout the homologous coding region as well, we conclude that hCG and hLH, which bind to the same receptor and elicit the same response, have distinct functions, beyond an observed difference in protein stability, that require these amino acid changes.

ACKNOWLEDGMENTS

The work described in this review was carried out at the University of California, San Francisco, Cold Spring Harbor Laboratory, and California Biotechnology Inc., and was supported in part by grants from the NIH. We would like to thank our colleagues at these institutions for their encouragement, and, in particular, M.-J. Gething, N. C. Vamvakopoulos and W. R. Boorstein for their collaboration and unpublished data, M. DeLuca, D. Keller, and J. Kloss for technical assistance, and G. Rodgers for preparation of this manuscript.

REFERENCES

Baker, C. C., Heriss, J., Courtois, G., Galibert, F., and Ziff, E. (1979). *Cell* **18**, 569–580.
Baltimore, D. (1981). *Cell* **24**, 529–594.
Benton, W. D., and Davis, R. W. (1977). *Science* **196**, 180–182.
Berk, A. J., and Sharp, P. A. (1977). *Cell* **12**, 721–732.
Bernard, O., Hozumi, N., and Tonegawa, S. (1978). *Cell* **15**, 1133–1144.
Birken, S., and Canfield, R. E. (1977). *J. Biol. Chem.* **252**, 5386–5392.
Blundell, T. L., and Wood, S. P. (1975). *Nature (London)* **257**, 197.
Boorstein, W. R., Vamvakopoulos, N. C., and Fiddes, J. C. (1982). *Nature (London)* **300**, 419–422.
Boothby, M., Ruddon, R. W., Anderson, C., McWilliams, D., and Boime, I. (1981). *J. Biol. Chem.* **265**, 5121–5127.
Breathnach, R., and Chambon, P. (1981). *Rev. Biochem. A* **50**, 349–383.
Breathnach, R., Benoist, C., O'Hare, K., Gannon, F., and Chambon, P. (1978). *Proc. Natl. Acad. Sci. U.S.A.* **75**, 4853–4857.
Bregegere, F., Abasto, J. P., Kvist, S., Rask, L., Lalanne, J. L., Garoff, H., Cami, B., Wiman, K., Larhammar, D., Peterson, P. A., Gachelin, G., Kourilsky, P., and Dobberstein, B. (1981). *Nature (London)* **292**. 78–81.

Canfield, R. E., Birken, S., Morse, J. H., and Morgan, F. J. (1978). In "Peptide Hormones" (J. A. Parsons, ed.), pp. 299–315. Univ. Park Press, Baltimore, Maryland.

Catterall, J. F., O'Malley, B. W., Robertson, M. A., Staden, R., Tanaka, Y., and Brownlee, G. G. (1978). Nature (London) 275, 510–513.

Clarke, B. (1970). Science 168, 1009.

Corden, J., Wasylyk, B., Buchwalder, A., Sassone-Corsi, P., Kedinger, C., and Chambon, P. (1980). Science 209, 1406–1414.

Dayhoff, M. (1976). In "Atlas of Protein Sequence and Structure," Vol. 5, Suppl. 2, p. 122. (Nat. Biomed. Research Foundation), Washington, D.C.

DeNoto, F. M., Moore, D. D., and Goodman, H. M. (1981). Nucleic Acids Res. 9, 3719–3730.

Dover, G. (1982). Nature (London) 299, 111–117.

Efstradiatis, A., Kafatos, F. C., Maxam, A., and Maniatis, T. (1976). Cell 7, 279–288.

Efstradiatis, A., Kafatos, F. C., and Maniatis, T. (1977). Cell 10, 571–585.

Fiddes, J. C., and Goodman, H. M. (1979). Nature (London) 281, 351–356.

Fiddes, J. C., and Goodman, H. M. (1980). Nature (London) 286, 684–687.

Fiddes, J. C., and Goodman, H. M. (1981). J. Mol. Appl. Genet. 1, 3–18.

Gluzman, Y. (1980). Cell 23, 175–182.

Goodman, H. M., DeNoto, F. M., Fiddes, J. C., Hallewell, R. A., Page, G. S., Smith, S. S., and Tischer, E. (1980). In "Mobilization and Reassembly of Genetic Information" (Miami Winter Symposium), (W. A. Scott, R. Werner, D. R. Joseph, and J. Schultz, eds.), pp. 155–179. Academic Press, New York.

Hardison, R. C., Butler, E. T., III, Lacy, E., Maniatis, T., Rosenthal, N., and Efstradiatis, A. (1979). Cell 18, 1285–1297.

Henderson, K. H. (1979). Br. Med. Bull. 35, 161–166.

Keutmann, H. T., and Williams, R. M. (1977). J. Biol. Chem. 252, 5393–5397.

Keutmann, H. T., Williams, R. M., and Ryan, R. J. (1979). Biochem. Biophys. Res. Commun. 90, 842–848.

Kimura, M. (1968). Nature (London) 217, 624–626.

Kimura, M., and Ohta, T. (1971). Nature (London) 229, 467–469.

Kimura, M., and Ohta, T. (1974). Proc. Natl. Acad. Sci. U.S.A. 71, 2848–2852.

Kozak, M. (1978). Cell 15, 1109–1123.

Laemmeli, U. K. (1970). Nature (London) 227, 680–685.

Lawn, R. M., Fritsch, E. F., Parker, R. C., Blake, G., and Maniatis, T. (1978). Cell 15, 1157–1174.

Lincoln, G. A. (1979). Br. Med. Bull. 35, 167–172.

Liu, W.-K., Nahm, H. S., Sweeney, C. M., Holcomb, G. N., and Ward, D. N. (1972). J. Biol. Chem. 247, 4365–4381.

Lomedico, P., Rosenthal, N., Efstradiatis, A., Gilbert, W., Kolodner, R., and Tizard, R. (1979). Cell 18, 545–558.

Lomedico, P. T., and McAndrew, S. J. (1982). Nature (London) 299, 221–226.

Maghuin-Rogister, G., and Hennen, G. (1973). Eur. J. Biochem. 39, 235–253.

Maxam, A., and Gilbert, W. (1977). Proc. Natl. Acad. Sci. U.S.A. 74, 560–564.

Mellon, P., Parker, V., Gluzman, Y., and Maniatis, T. (1981). Cell 27, 279–288.

Miyata, T., Yasunaga, T., and Nishida, T. (1980). Proc. Natl. Acad. Sci. U.S.A. 77, 7328–7332.

Morgan, J. F., Birken, S., and Canfield, R. E. (1975). J. Biol. Chem. 250, 5247–5258.

Niall, H. D. (1972). In "Prolactin and Carcinogenesis" (K. Griffiths, ed.), pp. 13–20. Alpha Omega Alpha Press, Cardiff, Wales.

Perler, F., Efstradiatis, A., Lomedico, P., Gilbert, W., Kolodner, R., and Dodgson, J. (1980). Cell 20, 555–566.

Pierce, J., and Parsons, T. F. (1981). Annu. Rev. Biochem. 50, 465–495.

Proudfoot, N. J., and Brownlee, G. G. (1976). *Nature (London)* **263**, 211–214.

Richmond, R. C. (1975). *Nature (London)* **225**, 1025.

Roberts, B. E., and Paterson, B. M. (1973). *Proc. Natl. Acad. Sci. U.S.A.* **70**, 2330–2334.

Sairam, M. R., Samy, T. S. A., Papkoff, H., and Li, C. H. (1972). *Arch. Biochem. Biophys.* **153**, 572–586.

Sanger, F., Nicklen, S., and Coulson, A. R. (1977). *Proc. Natl. Acad. Sci. U.S.A.* **74**, 5463–5467.

Seeburg, P. H. (1982). *DNA* **1**, 239–249.

Shome, B., and Parlow, A. F. (1973). *J. Clin. Endocrinol. Metab.* **36**, 618–621.

Southern, E. M. (1975). *J. Mol. Biol.* **98**, 503–517.

Talmadge, K., Boorstein, W., and Fiddes, J. C. (1983). *DNA,* **2**, 279–287.

Talmadge, K., Vamvakopoulos, N. C., and Fiddes, J. C. (1984). *Nature (London)* **307**, 37–40.

van den Berg, J., van Ooyen, A., Mantei, N., Schambock, A., Grosveld, G., Flavell, R., and Weissmann, C. (1978). *Nature (London)* **276**, 37–44.

van Ooyen, A., van den Berg, J., Mantei, N., and Weissmann, C. (1979). *Science* **206**, 337–344.

Ward, D. N., Moore, W. T., Jr., and Burleigh, B. D. (1982). *J. Protein Chem.* **1**, 263–280.

Weaver, R. F., and Weissmann, C. (1979). *Nucleic Acids Res.* **6**, 1175–1193.

DISCUSSION

B. Weintraub: Perhaps Dr. Fiddes and others may comment on the evolution of different mechanisms for the biosynthesis of polypeptide hormones. The first mechanism is a prepro-hormone where the initial gene product contains both an amino-terminal signal peptide as well as another more basic peptide which can be located anywhere in the molecule. There is a cotranslational cleavage of the signal peptide and then a posttranslational cleavage of the propeptide. This is the classic biosynthetic mechanism that holds for insulin, parathyroid hormone, and many other hormones of molecular weight less than 15,000. Subsequently the second mechanism shown for growth hormone, prolactin, and placental lactogen is a prehormone where there is no prohormone at all and solely a cotranslational cleavage of a signal peptide. The third mechanism that we are now discussing is a presubunit which is the opposite of the preprohormone mechanism. Instead of the active hormone being cleaved from a large precursor it is assembled from two smaller inactive subunits with only co-translational cleavages of the signal peptides. I should like to ask Dr. Fiddes his thoughts concerning why this particular mechanism evolved for glycoprotein hormones.

J. C. Fiddes: The glycoprotein hormones are really unusual in having two different subunits, one which is common, and one which defines the receptor specificity. These must be something very similar among the receptors for all of the glycoprotein hormones and something very important in the role of the α subunit in holding the individual β subunits in the right configuration for receptor interaction. This may put constraints on the evolution of the system as the α subunit is presently used for four different hormones. Probably the evolutionary origin of the system was a single glycoprotein hormone but now a multihormone family exists and has had to evolve along with the evolution of the receptor. It is possible that the single glycoprotein hormone was the α subunit and that the α subunit gene duplicated and then one of the genes diverged.

F. Turek: I have a comment on your last few statements with regard to the functional significance, or the lack of functional significance, of the genes that are not expressed. Do you think these genes may have been expressed as an evolutionary carryover that look at these lower mammals that would not be found as many unexpressed genes. Is this the way you are looking at that system?

J. C. Fiddes: Yes, I think that what we may be seeing here is a very early stage in the development of pseudo-genes. There is already a single protein change detected in β hCG 6 (alanine at position 117 instead of aspartic acid). Looking at the sequences, however, there are no other obvious changes consistent with pseudo-genes. Maybe we are seeing an early step in what has developed in other systems into very marked pseudo-genes with, for example, deletious and in frame termination codons. We are therefore very interested in looking back through various species to see where this multigene family arose and are in the process of doing that just now in collaboration with Dr. James Roberts. It would certainly be intriguing to find species with different numbers of genes and with different genes active. There are no data as yet but I would predict a situation where we go all the way from a single LH gene to a complex β hCG multigene family without too many intermediate stages. We know that baboon has a CG which is very similar to the human one, but CG is not just a primate function as there is a well-characterized horse CG. Amino acid sequence for this is available and shows that it has a C terminal extension in the same sort of way as human CG. This shows that the development of CG from LH took place before the evolution of the horse and certainly doing a series of Southern blots with genomic DNA from many species will be interesting.

J. E. Rall: You mentioned rather casually that there were a lot of repetitive sequences in the CG genes which gave you some problems. Could you say anything more about them, are they Alu sequences and could they possibly be related to the lack of expression of the 2, 4, 6, and 7 genes?

J. C. Fiddes: There are Alu sequences in this gene region though I haven't mapped them in detail. The repeats I was thinking of are related to the duplications which are present in this family. If you remember the slides in which I showed the groups of phage isolates there is a considerable clustering of the endpoints of the individual phage inserts. We failed to isolate phage extending to the right or left of group A or B and my interpretation of this is that there are some repeat structures which are not stable in *E. coli*. I do not think that Alu repeats are responsible for this or for the lack of expression of genes 2, 6, 7, and 8 because our restriction maps show that the structural genes or any of the regions nearby are not interrupted by Alu sequences.

C. S. Nicoll: Since different genes apparently code for the α and β subunits, and they seem to be located on different chromosomes, do you think that in earlier times these proteins had different functions than they do now? Perhaps they came together later on to aquire their present gonadotropic actions.

J. C. Fiddes: That is difficult to say, but my feeling is that because of the complete lack of biological activity in the individual subunits, maybe they have always had to be present as dimers to be functional.

C. S. Nicoll: I think we would have to study some primitive animals to look for possible separate functions of the individual α and β subunits. Perhaps looking at the protocorbates or even invertebrates would be informative in this regard.

J. C. Fiddes: Right.

I. A. Kourides: Coming back to the point of when in mammalian evolution CG genes evolved or duplicated from LH, we have data suggesting that there is no CG gene expression in rodents; this has been demonstrated by looking for α messenger RNA in the placentae of rodents and being unable to find any α mRNA. If there were a chorionic gonadotropin in the rodent, it would be expected to have a two-subunit nature and, therefore, an α subunit. In addition, I believe that Dr. James Roberts' laboratory also has negative data for the existence of CG genes in rodents; they have only been able to demonstrate a single β LH gene in rodents.

J. C. Fiddes: Yes, I am familiar with that data that Jim has. His rat LH probe, which was obtained using our human LH gene, shows no sign of rat CG genes. Dr. William Chin has the same sort of result.

I. A. Kourides: In any case, these data do support your comment that CG gene duplication is an event late in mammalian evolution.

G. Moll, Jr.:   There is considerable evidence for the existence of bioactive LH and inactive LH from the pituitary gonadotroph. I wonder if other organs could possibly transcribe this LH region differently to produce more than one LH molecule at the transcriptional level.

J. C. Fiddes: Yes, I think that we have just described the present situation in the human and that we have to investigate other species in more detail.

G. D. Niswender: I would like to congratulate you on a very nice presentation. We have recently began to study the details of the mechanism of action of LH versus hCG and have been amazed that although these hormones both stimulate steroidogenesis they are processed by the receptor in quite a different fashion. hCG initiates a much more prolonged steroidogenic response, is internalized at least 50 times slower, and recent data suggest that the hCG–LH receptor complex migrates much slower in the luteal cell membrane. This reduced lateral mobility of the hCG–LH receptor complex is probably an important factor for both slower rate of internalization of the hormone–receptor complex and the prolonged steroidogenic response. I find your speculations regarding the evolution of the LH and CG molecules quite interesting and wonder if you feel that the receptors evolved to fit the hormones or whether the hormones evolved as a result of changes in receptor.

J. C. Fiddes: No necessarily. I was arguing that there was a very strong selection for the development of CG and that this could be the requirement for CG in placental development. This could be brought about by changing the receptor or by the sort of mechanism you are describing.

G. D. Niswender: One of the sidelights is that we have done all this work using the sheep luteal cell model where in fact there is no CG that anyone has been able to detect, at least during early pregnancy, yet the two hormones have a very different effect at the level of the receptor in this species.

J. C. Fiddes: Do you think then that this is the main difference between CG and LH?

G. D. Niswender: When comparisons are made between the rates of internalization of hCG and LH the hCG is internalized with a half time on the nebrae ($t_{1/2}$) of 18 hours while oLH exhibits a $t_{1/2}$ of 18 minutes. The property responsible for this different rate of internalization resides in the β subunit since α oLH recombined with β hCG has a $t_{1/2}$ of 18 hours while α hCG recombined with β oLH is internalized rapidly. We have used lazer photobleaching procedures to measure the lateral mobilities of the hormone–receptor complexes in the plasma membrane and the difference constant of the LH–LH receptor complex was 1 to 2×10^{-10} cm^2/second while for hCG–LH receptor complexes the diffusion constant was less than 1×10^{-12} cm^2/second and could not be measured reliably.

J. C. Fiddes: And you believe that to be the same receptor molecule?

G. D. Niswender: I think there is little doubt that it is the same receptor.

H. Friesen: Do you think it is possible that there may be differential expression of the individual hCG genes at various stages of placental development? Second, have you had an opportunity to examine whether this possibility may exist in patients with choriocarcinoma?

J. C. Fiddes: Basically, I haven't done these experiments. All of the cDNA clones examined were from first trimester placenta. I have not looked at later stages or at choriocarcinomas. It would be interesting to do as it may show differences in expression. The amino acid sequence as determined for β hCG corresponds to the small number of genes which seem to be expressed but a small level of altered sequence might not have been detected in the protein analysis.

B. A. Littlefield: You indicated that the eight β hCG-like genes are located on three different segments which you termed A, B, and C. I was wondering if there is a relationship between those three segments: are they arranged colinearly?

J. C. Fiddes: I think that they are all linked but I don't have the right evidence. The main evidence is that a genomic Southern blot with *Eco*RI or *Sal*I gives a single hybridizing band of about 60 kb. This suggests that the genes are linked but at that size there would be no resolution between two bands of similar size. Also the unique chromosomal localization supports linkage of the groups A, B, and C.

B. A. Littlefield: How about the α subunit?

J. C. Fiddes: It is from a different chromosome.

G. Gibori: I was very interested by the comments made by Dr. Kourides that rodent placenta do not have a mRNA for chorionic gonadotropin. Yet rat placenta produces a chorionic gonadotropin which binds to LH receptor and stimulates testosterone synthesis by Leydig cells.

I. A. Kourides: I think I should reply to this statement. I did not mean to imply that rodents do not have placental luteotropic activity. All I am saying is that the bioactivity is not due to a chorionic gonadotropin with two subunits. It is possible that some other hormone, either described or not yet described, is responsible for rodent placental luteotropic activity.

J. C. Fiddes: Again this is another example of the analogy with placental lactogen and growth hormone. There is no sign of a rodent placental lactogen which is homologous to growth hormone, but obviously the placenta develops adequately.

G. Gibori: The rat placenta does indeed secrete a placental lactogen.

J. C. Fiddes: It is not homologous to growth hormone in the same way that there is no rat CG which is homologous to rat LH. The activity may be present but not coded for by a homologous gene.

P. Chambon: Is there anything drastically different in the 5' upstream region of the CG genes which are not expressed? Did you always insert the same length of 5' upstream sequence in your "expression" experiments and did you make chimeric recombinants taking the promoter region of one gene and inserting it upstream from the coding region of another gene in an attempt to learn where the block in expression could be?

J. C. Fiddes: There is no obvious sequence difference between genes 5 and 6 to account for their different expression. Neither of them has more than 3 out of 7 bases homologous with the TATA sequence. Also the homology between the genes upstream from the cap site is in the 90% range. The constructions for the switching experiments you suggested have been completed by Dr. Karen Talmadge and are about to go on COS cells. These involve switching the two halves of genes 5 and 6. In answer to your third question, no, the genes put in COS cells have different lengths of sequence to their 5' sides. These were our first experiments and we relied simply on the disposition of the *Kpn*I sites.

P. Chambon: Have you made any construction in which the SV40 enhancer was not present in your "expression" chimeric recombinants?

J. C. Fiddes: We have not yet done an experiment without the enhancer. We are using a poisonless derivative of pBR322, pXf3, into which is inserted the SV40 *Hin*dIII C fragment which contains the enhances and origin. We have been cloning into the unique *Kpn*I site in the SV40 fragment. It worked so we haven't gone to other constructs yet.

J. H. Oppenheimer: How do you visualize the coordinate regulation of the $\alpha\beta$ subunits which are located in the genes of different chromosomes?

J. C. Fiddes: This is difficult to answer because they are coordinately regulated and expressed in different tissues. The α gene in the pituitary and placenta but β CG only in the placenta and β LH only in the pituitary. I would assume therefore that there has to be some regulatory sequence which activates the genes and another that determines tissue specificity. Also since there always seems to be an excess of free α subunit over β subunit in the pituitary and placenta then presumably the closer regulation is going to be with the β subunit, with the α subunit being constitutively expressed in comparison.

E. L. Marut: We have mentioned the bioactive forms of the glycoproteins only a few times. The two processes which are associated with bioactivity are the synthesis of the polypeptide chain as well as the glycosylation of the chain, and both these processes are at least in some circumstances under the control of steroid hormones. Are the genomes which encode both these functions related in any way? That is, what is the location of the information for the sequencing of the amino acids in regard to that for the glycosylation?

J. C. Fiddes: There are characteristic sequences in the glycoprotein hormones, and in other glycosylated proteins, which indicate glycosylation. For example the sequence Asn-X-Thr indicates that an asparagine-linked sugar should be added. This is encoded in the primary sequence of the protein and is recognized by the cells glycosylation mechanisms.

U. Zor: I would like to confirm what Dr. Niswender noted with regard to a difference existing between the mechanism of action of LH and hCG. We (together with Drs. Sairam and Amsterdam) used either antagonist of LH or hCG, namely, deglycosylated LH (DGLH) or hCG. We found a huge difference between the effect of these two antagonists on the regulation of the LH receptor. While the DGLH induced about 50–90% disappearance of the receptors from cell surface of granuloma cells during 20 hours of incubation, the DG hCG induced only 15% down-regulation of the receptors. In other words, we recovered most of the cell surface receptors after the interaction of DG hCG with LH receptors, while only a small fraction of the LH receptors were recovered after treatment with DGLH. It seems therefore that although both hormones interact with the same receptor and quite certainly cause the same similar response, namely stimulation of cyclic AMP and steroid hormone production, the internalization of the hormone and the down-regulation of the receptor is quite different between LH and hCG.

J. C. Fiddes: Do you think that the C terminal extension is anything to do with this? Is that the significant change in the structure as it is one region where CG is obviously very different from LH?

U. Zor: There is no doubt there are differences in the affinity of LH or hCG. hCG has much higher affinity to the receptor than LH, but I really do not know why there is so huge a difference between the behavior of LH and hCG.

J. C. Fiddes: It might be interesting to express cloned β hCG without the C terminal extension or to make defined changes in the region which is homologous to LH. This could be done by a recombinant DNA approach using site-specific mutagenesis. The altered proteins could then be examined to see how they function.

J. Drouin: John, wouldn't you think that in considering the evolution of gene families like this one encoding hLH and hCG of the gene duplication and/or rearrangements that one may postulate are not necessarily the limiting step but rather that selective advantage only becomes a reality after changes in tissue specificity of expression? In this case, the various hCG genes probably arose by duplication of an ancestral LH gene but it is only when one or a few of these genes (duplicate or not) started being expressed in the placenta that it acquired meaning and began to evolve in an evolutionary beneficial direction. I would speculate that expression of a gene in a new tissue is really the critical step in the establishment of a gene family. This could, however, be closely related to DNA rearrangements.

J. C. Fiddes: I think that the real selection was initially there as you say and that there was something very significant for placental development in the production of CG. The duplications and rearrangements are secondary events and I don't think there is any selection pressure there.

M. Raj: As you know, during pregnancy, especially in the first trimester, hCG levels reach an all time peak and then taper off. My question is whether there is any information as to at what level the expression of this protein is controlled?

J. C. Fiddes: We have no information on that. Not much is known as to what turns on CG in placental development.

The Regulation and Organization of Thyroid Stimulating Hormone Genes

IONE A. KOURIDES, JAMES A. GURR, AND OFRA WOLF

Laboratory of Molecular Endocrinology, Memorial Sloan-Kettering Cancer Center, and Cornell University Medical College and Graduate School of Medical Sciences, New York, New York

I. Introduction: The Family of Glycoprotein Hormones

Thyroid stimulating hormone (TSH) is one member of a family of glycoprotein hormones which also includes the gonadotropins, luteinizing hormone (LH) and follicle stimulating hormone (FSH), synthesized in the pituitary, and chorionic gonadotropin (CG), synthesized in the placenta (Pierce and Parsons, 1981). Each of these four hormones is composed of two dissimilar, noncovalently bound subunits, called α and β. Within an individual species, the amino acid sequence of the α subunit is identical in all four hormones, whereas each β subunit is structurally sufficiently distinct to confer biologic and immunologic specificity to the complete hormone (Fig. 1). The amino acid sequence of the α subunit is also highly conserved among species. Thus, any α subunit can be combined with a β subunit to give a complete hormone with immunologic and biologic specificity of the β subunit (Pierce, 1971; Pierce and Parsons, 1981). There are areas of strong homology in amino acid sequence among the β subunits of the same species and also between species. Human CG-β and LH-β are the most closely related structurally, with an amino acid sequence homology of 82% (Shome and Parlow, 1973; Morgan *et al.*, 1975; Keutmann and Williams, 1977; Birken and Canfield, 1977; Keutmann *et al*, 1979). This is in keeping with their very similar biologic activities. LH has an important role in stimulating the gonad, whereas CG appears to be important in stimulating the corpus luteum of the ovary to synthesize steroids important in the maintenance of early pregnancy (Catt and Pierce, 1978; Canfield *et al.*, 1976). The other glycoprotein hormone β subunits, when compared, have lower amino acid sequence homologies, in the range of 25–40% (Pierce and Parsons, 1981). These homologies are consistent with the suggestion that all glycoprotein hormone β subunits have evolved from a common ancestral peptide (Pierce and Parsons, 1981; Pierce *et al.*,

79

PLACENTA   PITUITARY

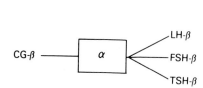

FIG. 1. The family of glycoprotein hormones includes chorionic gonadotropin (CG), synthesized by the placenta, and the three pituitary peptides, luteinizing hormone, follicle stimulating hormone, and thyroid stimulating hormone (LH, FSH, and TSH). Within a species, each hormone contains an identical α subunit and a unique β subunit. These subunits interact noncovalently, and both are needed for biological activity.

1973; Dayhoff, 1976). Homologies between α and β subunits show a less distinct relationship. However, it has been suggested that α and β subunits also evolved from a common ancestral peptide (Dayhoff, 1976; Fontaine and Burzawa-Gerard, 1977).

Although CG is synthesized in the placentas of primates, we do not find CG in rodent placentas. We have been unable to detect α mRNA in rodent placentas, which would be expected to be present if there were a two subunit chorionic gonadotropin in the placentas of these animals (Wurzel et al., 1983). Moreover, Tepper et al. (1983) find only one LH-β gene in rodents and no CG-β genes.

The α subunits of the glycoprotein hormones each contain two N-linked carbohydrate side chains, attached at asparagines 56 and 82 (Pierce and Parsons, 1981). The β subunits of the glycoprotein hormones contain one or two asparagine-linked carbohydrate side chains, except for CG-β which includes also four serine-linked carbohydrate side chains attached to the 24 amino acid carboxyl extension of the molecule, making CG-β distinct from LH-β. Asparagine-linked oligosaccharides are synthesized as a preformed group and transferred en bloc to the peptide, whereas the serine-linked sugars are added one at a time (Tabas et al., 1978; Choi et al., 1971). Glycosylation is required for subunit combination and protection from intracellular degradation, but not for secretion (Weintraub et al., 1980, 1983). Isolated α and β subunits appear to have no thyrotropic or gonadotropic activity (Catt et al., 1973; Rayford et al., 1972).

II. Subunits of TSH: Clinical Studies

After dissociating human TSH and purifying the α and β subunits, we developed highly sensitive and specific radioimmunoassays for each subunit (Kourides et al., 1973, 1974, 1975). Since these assays were specific for free subunits rather than complete hormone, we were able to study subunit secretion and regulation in clinical studies in humans (Kourides *et al.*, 1975, 1978, 1979).

In patients with primary hypothyroidism, free α and TSH-β are secreted directly into the circulation both basally and after the administration of thyrotropin releasing hormone (TRH), rather than arising by the peripheral dissociation of secreted TSH (Kourides *et al.*, 1973, 1975). Moreover, after hypothyroid patients received replacement thyroid hormone, either L-T4 or L-T3, both basal and TRH-stimulated subunit concentrations decreased (Kourides *et al.*, 1975, 1979). We also determined the metabolic clearance rates of both α and TSH-β subunits in humans and then calculated the daily secretion rates of free α and TSH-β relative to complete TSH. We found a higher normal daily secretion rate for α than TSH-β. In primary hypothyroidism, there was a twofold increase in α and TSH-β secretion rates, but a 50-fold increase in the complete TSH secretion rate. Thus, increased subunit synthesis, particularly of the unique β subunit, appeared to be utilized for production of TSH (Kourides *et al.*, 1977a).

In addition, we have prepared extracts of normal human pituitary glands obtained postmorten, fractionated them by gel chromatography on Sephadex G-100, and looked at the content of free α and the three pituitary β subunits. In spite of variability in subunit content among normal pituitaries, a consistent excess of free α subunits relative to the sum of all free pituitary β subunits was demonstrated in each normal pituitary, with an α to β subunit ratio ranging from 1.3 to 8.3 (Fig. 2). These studies supported the concept that biosynthesis of the unique β subunits was limiting in the production of complete glycoprotein hormones (Kourides *et al.*, 1980a,b).

Intrigued by the excess α subunit in normal human pituitaries, we also studied patients with pituitary tumors looking for tumors that might demonstrate α hypersecretion (Kourides *et al.*, 1976). We have now found about 20 α-secreting pituitary tumors. A few have secreted only α subunits; many have also hypersecreted complete TSH; a couple have secreted LH or LH and FSH. About one-third have also secreted the unrelated peptides, growth hormone or prolactin. No tumor we have studied has hypersecreted a pituitary β subunit. Alpha levels have been impressively elevated, as high as 100 ng/ml, much higher than the elevations seen in primary hypothyroidism or primary hypogonadism, but in the range seen in uremia, pregnancy, or with malignant tumors ectopically secreting α subunit. Alpha secretion from these pituitary tumors was relatively autonomous, as evidenced by little increase in α subunit levels after TRH or luteinizing hormone-releasing hormone (LHRH) administra-

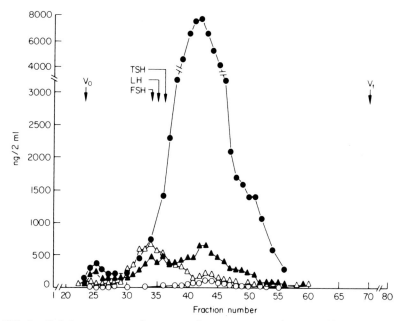

FIG. 2. Gel chromatogram of an extract from a representative normal human pituitary gland fractionated on Sephadex G-100. Two-milliliter fractions were collected, counted, and measured in radioimmunoassays for α subunit, TSH-β, LH-β, and FSH-β. The elution volumes for TSH, LH, and FSH are shown by the arrows; they were determined by measuring the fractions in a radioimmunoassay for each of the complete pituitary glycoprotein hormones. ●, α; ○, TSH-β; ▲, LH-β; △, FSH-β (Kourides et al., 1980a).

tion (Kourides et al., 1976, 1977b; Peterson et al., 1981; Weintraub et al., 1981; Kourides, 1984).

III. The Biosynthesis of TSH

Since clinical studies had shown various situations of α subunit excess, we wished to investigate whether subunits of the glycoprotein hormones, particularly TSH, were independently synthesized, as suspected by us and others, or whether the subunits of TSH were both synthesized within a single large-molecular-weight precursor (Prentice and Ryan, 1975). Through these studies we hoped to explain the α excess in normal pituitary glands and α subunit hypersecretion by pituitary tumors and certain malignancies (Blackman et al., 1980).

For these biosynthetic studies, we elected to use mouse TSH-secreting pituitary tumors. These tumors, first described by Dr. Jacob Furth (Furth et al., 1973), are transplantable into the flanks of hypothyroid mice of the same strain. Thereby, large amounts of tissue are provided. These are relatively benign tumors displaying qualitatively normal hormonal regulation (Blackman *et al.*, 1978; Gershengorn, 1978; Vale *et al.*, 1972; Marshall *et al.*, 1981; Cacicedo *et al.*, 1981; Ross *et al.*, 1983b; Gurr and Kourides, 1983). Thus, they are a better tissue for the study of biosynthesis of TSH than the normal pituitary gland which contains only a small percentage of thyrotrophs and also contains gonadotrophs, which produce α subunits indistinguishable from those in TSH. These tumors do not make the structurally related gonadotropins, nor do they synthesize growth hormone, prolactin, or other pituitary hormones (Furth *et al.*,1973; Blackman *et al.*, 1978). During early passages, these tumors usually synthesize large quantities of TSH. With repeated passage, however, the amount of TSH decreases, and eventually these tumors produce predominantly α subunit. Tumors that synthesize little or no TSH, but small quantities of α subunit, may grow in euthyroid rather than hypothyroid mouse recipients. The TSH and subunits synthesized by these tumors appear identical to those synthesized by normal mouse pituitary glands, as evidenced by similar immunoreactivity of the peptides and similar gel chromatographic characteristics (unpublished observations).

Messenger RNA has been extracted from TSH-secreting tumors and purified by oligo(dT)-cellulose chromatography for poly(A)-enrichment (Aviv and Leder, 1972), in some cases followed by centrifugation through a 5 to 20% sucrose gradient. The messenger RNA has been translated in wheat germ (Roberts and Paterson, 1973) or reticulocyte lysate (Pelham and Jackson, 1976) cell-free systems, devoid of the enzymes necessary for proteolytic cleavage of precursor signal sequences or for core glycosylation. Translation has also been performed in the presence of microsomal membranes, allowing for pre-peptide cleavage and core glycosylation (Kourides *et al.*, 1979; Vamvakopoulos and Kourides, 1979; Giudice and Weintraub, 1979). The *in vitro* protein synthesis has been performed in the presence of [^{35}S]methionine; the labeled peptides synthesized have been analyzed by sodium dodecyl sulfate (SDS)–polyacrylamide gel electrophoresis (Laemmli, 1970), with immunoprecipitation using antibodies to ovine LH-α or bovine TSH-β (Kourides and Weintraub, 1979; Kourides *et al.*, 1979; Vamvakopoulos and Kourides, 1979). The major cell-free translation product, in both the wheat germ and reticulocyte lysate systems had an apparent molecular weight of 14,000 by SDS–polyacrylamide gel electrophoresis (Fig. 3, lane 3). Since treatment with α-mannosidase did not change the apparent molecular weight of this peptide (Fig. 3, lane 9), it presumably did not contain carbohydrate, i.e.; mannose, although its molecular weight was at least 3000 greater than the protein core of the α subunit (11,000) (Kourides *et al.*, 1979). This sug-

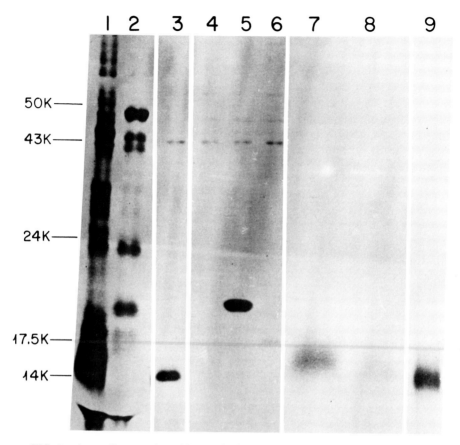

FIG. 3. Autoradiogram of peptides synthesized by translation of mouse TSH-secreting tumor mRNA in rabbit reticulocyte lysate without or with dog pancreatic microsomal membranes. Lanes 1 and 2, total proteins synthesized without and with microsomal membranes. Lane 3, 14,000 MW pre-TSH-α. Lanes 4–6, peptides synthesized with microsomal membranes and precipitated with nonimmune serum, α antibody, and TSH-β antibody, respectively. Lanes 7 and 8, processed α and TSH-β after treatment with α-mannosidase. Lane 9, pre-TSH-α after treatment with α-mannosidase (Kourides et al., 1979).

gested that the peptide synthesized contained a signal sequence, as has been shown for other secretory proteins (Blobel and Dobberstein, 1975a,b; Kreil, 1981). This pre-α subunit could be cleaved of its signal peptide and core glycosylated by the translation of messenger RNA in the presence of dog pancreatic microsomal membranes (Fig. 3, lane 5) or by translation in frog oocytes (Kourides et al., 1979). The processed α subunit had an apparent molecular weight of 21,000, after leader sequence removal and core glycosylation. The signal peptide is important in the translocation of the nascent peptide through the membrane of the endoplasmic reticulum (Blobel and Dobberstein, 1975a,b; Kreil, 1981). The 21,000 α subunit became smaller after treatment with α-mannosidase, implying that the peptide had indeed been core glycosylated (Fig. 3, lane 7) (Kourides et al., 1979). Pre-TSH-β has also been identified in cell-free translation systems, but it has been more difficult to detect because of the smaller amounts of [^{35}S]methionine-labeled pre-TSH-β synthesized compared to pre-α (Giudice and Weintraub, 1979; Kourides et al., 1979). We have found pre-TSH-β to have an apparent molecular weight of 17,000; it is precipitable with antibodies to TSH-β. This 17,000 pre-TSH-β can be processed to a peptide of 18,500 when mouse TSH-secreting tumor mRNA is translated in the presence of microsomal membranes (Fig. 3, lane 6). Treatment of processed TSH-β with α-mannosidase also decreased its molecular weight, implying that it had been core glycosylated (Fig. 3, lane 8). TSH-β of similar apparent molecular weight was also synthesized in the whole cell system, the frog oocyte (Kourides et al., 1979). Our experiments consistently showed excess α to β synthesis in these in vitro systems, using different TSH-secreting pituitary tumors' mRNA. This was true whatever the concentration of magnesium or potassium added to the system, although it is true that variation in magnesium or potassium concentration changes the ratio of α to TSH-β protein synthesized (Kourides et al., 1979). These studies showed that each subunit of TSH was synthesized independently and that there was no large-molecular-weight form synthesized from which both α and TSH-β could be derived.

The use of cell-free translation systems has allowed the identification of the initial precursor forms of TSH subunits, since such forms are rapidly processed before the release of the newly synthesized subunit from the ribosomes. However, study of TSH biosynthesis in whole cells has added considerable insight into posttranslational events such as carbohydrate addition and processing, subunit combination, and secretion (Weintraub et al., 1980, 1983; Chin et al., 1981a; Magner and Weintraub, 1982). The addition of a carbohydrate side chain to both the TSH-α and -β subunits occurs in the rough endoplasmic reticulum (RER), during translation. Addition of a second oligosaccharide moiety to the α subunit occurs later in the RER and the smooth ER (Magner and Weintraub, 1982; Chin et al, 1981a). The oligosaccharide glucose$_3$-mannose$_9$-N-acetylglucosamine$_2$ is preassembled in the microsomal membrane attached by phosphates to a dolichol carrier. This core oligosacchride moiety is then transferred en bloc from the dolichol carrier to the appropriate asparagine residue in the polypeptide chain. Such asparagine residues always occur in the se-

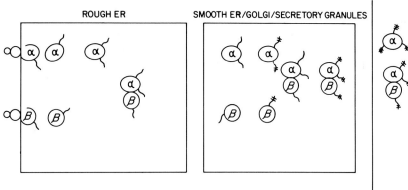

FIG. 4. Model for glycosylation of subunits of TSH. Both α and β subunits of TSH are initially glycosylated during translation of mRNA on the ribosome. Following translocation into the rough endoplasmic reticulum and cleavage of the signal peptide, a second asparagine-linked carbohydrate side chain is added to the α subunit. Crossed lines represent a core sugar side chain containing glucose, mannose, and N-acetylglucosamine. Subunit combination begins in the rough endoplasmic reticulum with core glycosylated subunits. Processing of core sugars with addition of terminal sugars occurs in all later compartments prior to secretion. Double crossed lines represent terminal glycosylation. Terminal phosphorylation can occur on the α subunit; moreover, addition of a third serine-linked carbohydrate side chain has been noted on free, but not combined, α subunits.

quence asparagine-X-serine or threonine (Waechter and Lennarz, 1976; Hubbard and Ivatt, 1981). Combination of glycosylated subunits occurs in the RER, the smooth ER, the Golgi apparatus, and the secretory granules. Carbohydrate side chains are also modified posttranslationally by removal of glucose residues and addition of terminal sugars such as galactose, fucose, N-acetylglucosamine, and sialic acid. Apparently the TSH-β subunit achieves its fully processed form more rapidly than the α subunit, possibly because of the addition of a second oligosaccharide to the α subunit (Magner and Weintraub, 1982, 1984). Recently, Parsons and Pierce (1980) have shown that the oligosaccharide moieties of some glycoprotein hormone subunits, such as bovine TSH-α, are sulfated. Human TSH is probably partly sialylated and partly sulfated (Pierce and Parsons, 1981), the negatively charged sulfate and the negatively charged sialic acid perhaps playing a similar functional role in the molecule. Additionally, various investigators have shown that the secreted free TSH-α subunit had a slightly higher molecular weight than α forms combined with β

either intra- or extracellularly (Weintraub *et al.*, 1975, 1980; Kourides *et al.*, 1980a). Parsons *et al.* (1983) have reported that the free α subunit derived from bovine pituitaries is glycosylated at an additional site, the threonine at position 43, with an O-linked oligosaccharide. This α subunit with a third carbohydrate side chain appears to be incapable of combination with a β subunit. Tunicamycin, an antibiotic that inhibits the formation of the oligosaccharide-lipid intermediate involved in glycosylation at asparagine residues (Struck and Lennarz, 1977), has been shown to totally inhibit subunit glycosylation (Weintraub *et al.*, 1980). The unglycosylated subunits caused by tunicamycin pretreatment of cells did not combine to form TSH but were secreted (Weintraub *et al.*,1980). Thus, glycosylation appears necessary for subunit combination and protection of the subunit from intracellular degradation (Weintraub *et al.*, 1983), but is not important for secretion. A model showing the sites and types of glycosylation in TSH subunits is shown in Fig. 4 (Magner and Weintraub, 1982).

IV. Identification of Separate mRNAs Coding for the α and β Subunits of TSH

Previous investigations had shown that α and β subunits of TSH were independently synthesized as presubunits, implying that biosynthesis of subunits of TSH was from separate mRNAs (Chin *et al.*, 1978; Kourides and Weintraub, 1979; Vamvakopoulos and Kourides, 1979; Kourides *et al.*, 1979; Giudice and Weintraub, 1979). We fractionated mouse TSH-secreting tumor mRNA by sucrose gradient centrifugation and selected 9 S mRNA, which showed maximal synthesis of TSH-α and TSH-β in cell-free translation systems. This 9 S mRNA was iodinated with ^{125}I and yielded two major labeled bands of RNA when analyzed by urea/polyacrylamide gel electrophoresis. These major bands were eluted from the gel and used as markers in a similar electrophoretic separation of unlabeled 9 S mRNA. The unlabeled RNA comigrating with each marker was then translated in a reticulocyte lysate system in the presence of microsomal membranes. Band I mRNA directed the synthesis only of α subunit and not TSH-β, whereas band II mRNA directed the synthesis only of TSH-β and not α subunit (Fig. 5). These studies directly showed that TSH was synthesized from separate mRNAs. It has subsequently been shown, either directly or indirectly, that the α and β subunits of all the glycoprotein hormones are synthesized utilizing separate mRNAs (Landefeld, 1979; Landefeld and Kepa, 1979; Godine *et al.*, 1980, 1981; Alexander and Miller, 1981; Counis *et al.*, 1982; Daniels-McQueen *et al.*, 1978).

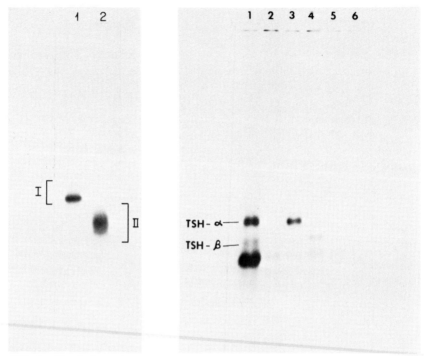

FIG. 5.   Urea/polyacrylamide gel electrophoresis of unlabeled mouse TSH-secreting pituitary tumor mRNA together with gel electrophoretically purified ^{125}I-labeled 9 S mRNA, purified first by sucrose gradient density centrifugation (left panel). Unlabeled mRNAs migrating with labeled RNA I and II were eluted from the gel. The peptides synthesized by translation of mRNAs I and II were evaluated. Lane 1, total peptides synthesized in reticulocyte lysate with microsomal membranes by translation of 9 S mRNA. Lane 3, α subunit synthesized by translation of mRNA I and immunoprecipitated with α antiserum. Lane 4, TSH-β synthesized by translation of mRNA II and immunoprecipitated with TSH-β antiserum. Lanes 5 and 6, the other subunit was not synthesized by translation of the mRNAs and immunoprecipitation with the other antiserum. Lane 2, no peptide was specifically precipitated with nonimmune serum. A small amount of pre-TSH-α was nonspecifically precipitated in lanes 2–4, bottom band (right panel) (Vamvakopoulos and Kourides, 1979).

V. Cloning of cDNAs Encoding the α and β Subunits of Mouse TSH

The finding that the α and TSH-β subunits are encoded by separate mRNAs suggested that these mRNAs may be transcribed from separate genes. We wished to address the question of whether the molecular mechanism underlying the production of unbalanced α and TSH-β subunits involved the unbalanced synthesis of α and TSH-β mRNAs from these

```
     HaeⅢ                        BalI                      DdeI  HaeⅢ
   60                                                    
TCG GAG GCC ACA TGC TGT GTG GCC AAA GCA TTT ACT AAG GCC ACA
SER GLU ALA THR CYS CYS VAL ALA LYS ALA PHE THR LYS ALA THR

                              HinfI
                      80    
GTA ATG GGA AAT GCC AGA GTG GAG AAT CAT ACG GAG TGC CAC TGT
VAL MET GLY ASN ALA ARG VAL GLU ASN HIS THR GLU CYS HIS CYS

                            AluI
                  96    
AGC ACT TGC TAC TAC CAC AAG TCG TAG CT
SER THR CYS TYR TYR HIS LYS SER ✱✱✱
```

FIG. 6.   The nucleotide sequence of a portion of the protein-coding region of an α cDNA is shown with the predicted amino acid sequence for mouse α subunit (Schorr-Toshav *et al.*, 1983a).

genes. To facilitate the study of both the structure of the mouse α and TSH-β genes and the regulation of their expression, we, therefore, synthesized and cloned DNAs complementary to the mRNAs encoding the presubunits of α and TSH-β (Schorr-Toshav *et al.*, 1983a; Gurr *et al.*, 1983).

Poly(A) mRNA from mouse thyrotropic tumor was fractionated by sucrose density gradient centrifugation; the fractions enriched in α and TSH-β mRNA sequences, sedimenting at about 9 S, were used as a template for the synthesis of double-stranded cDNA using reverse transcriptase. The double-stranded cDNA was inserted into the *Pst*I site of the plasmid pBR322 after G · C tailing, and the hybrid plasmid was used to transform *E. coli* RRI (Gurr *et al.*, 1983). Plasmids containing cDNAs encoding α mRNA were identified initially by screening for the presence of characteristic restriction enzyme sites. These were deduced from the known nucleotide sequence of the mouse pre-α subunit cDNA, which was determined by Chin *et al.* (1981b) while this work was in progress. The identity of one such putative α cDNA was confirmed by nucleotide sequencing using the method of Maxam and Gilbert (1980). The nucleotide sequence of a 120 bp fragment of this 520 bp cDNA (Fig. 6) was identical to that determined by Chin *et al.* (1981b). This α cDNA (pTSH-αF) has subsequently been used to screen our mouse cDNA library for other plasmids containing α cDNA inserts, with a yield of about 6%. The plasmid pTSH-αF has also been shown to select α mRNA from mouse tumor poly(A) mRNA in hybridization–selection–translation experiments (Fig. 7).

The colonies in our cDNA library which remained after elimination of plasmids containing α cDNA inserts by colony hybridization with pTSH-αF (Grunstein and Hogness, 1975) were screened for TSH-β cDNA inserts by hybridization–selection and cell-free translation (Fig. 8) (Parnes *et al.*,

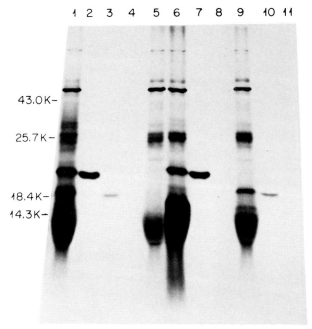

FIG. 7. Identification of TSH-α and TSH-β cDNAs by hybrid-selection and cell-free translation. Plasmid DNA on nitrocellulose filters was hybridized with mouse tumor mRNA. Hybridized mRNA was eluted from the filters and translated in a reticulocyte lysate system with microsomal membranes. Lanes 1–4: proteins synthesized with mouse tumor mRNA (lane 1) and precipitated with α antiserum (lane 2), TSH-β antiserum (lane 3), and nonimmune serum (lane 4). Lane 5: proteins synthesized by mRNA selected by plasmid pBR322 (background). Lanes 6–8: proteins synthesized by mRNA selected by plasmid pTSH-α$_F$ (lane 6) and precipitated by α antiserum (lane 7) and nonimmune serum (lane 8). Lanes 9–11: proteins synthesized by mRNA selected by plasmid pTSH-β$_H$ (lane 9) and precipitated with TSH-β antiserum (lane 10) and nonimmune serum (lane 11). Molecular weight markers (×10^{-3}) are shown on the left (Gurr *et al.*, 1983).

1981). Plasmids were screened in groups of seven by immobilization of DNA on nitrocellulose filters and hybridization with thyrotropic tumor poly(A) mRNA. Hybridized mRNA was then eluted from the filters, translated *in vitro,* and the protein products analyzed for immunoprecipitability with TSH-β antibody. Plasmids from a positive pool were then analyzed individually. About 1% of plasmids contained cDNA hybridizing with TSH-β mRNA (Fig. 7). The complete nucleotide sequence of one of these cDNAs (pTSH-β$_H$) was determined (Fig. 9); the strong homology of the deduced amino acid sequence of mouse pre-TSH-β with the known amino acid sequences of TSH-β subunits from several other species (Sairam and Li, 1977; Pierce *et al.*, 1971; Maghuin-Rogister *et al.*, 1976)

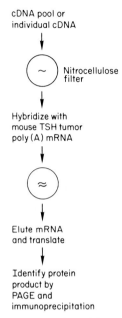

cDNA pool or
individual cDNA

(~) Nitrocellulose
        filter

Hybridize with
mouse TSH tumor
poly (A) mRNA

(≈)

Elute mRNA
and translate

Identify protein
product by
PAGE and
immunoprecipitation

FIG. 8.   Hybridization–selection–translation with mouse tumor poly(A) mRNA. First pools of cDNAs and later individual cDNAs were baked to nitrocellulose filters and hybridized with mouse tumor poly(A) mRNA; then the specifically hybridized mRNA was eluted and translated in the reticulocyte lysate translation system supplemented with microsomal membranes. The protein product was identified by polyacrylamide gel electrophoresis and immunoprecipitation.

confirmed the identity of the mouse TSH-β cDNA (Fig. 10). Sequencing showed that the mouse TSH-β subunit contained 118 amino acids, compared to 112 or 113 found in human or porcine and bovine TSH-β, respectively. To confirm the mouse TSH-β sequence, a cDNA library was constructed from a different mouse tumor, and TSH-β plasmids were isolated. Sequencing of the 3′-region of one of these cDNAs confirmed that mouse TSH-β has an extended carboxyl terminus.

VI. Homologies among the Amino Acid and Nucleotide Sequences of the α and β Subunits of TSH and the Other Glycoprotein Hormones

It has been proposed, based on a comparison of amino acid sequences, that the β subunits of the different glycoprotein hormones have evolved from a common β ancestral gene and that this β ancestral gene, in turn, evolved by duplication from an even more primordial gene from which the

```
ATCCTGCAGTAGTGGGTGGAGAAGAGTGAGCGCATACGAGTGGAGAGAGAAAAATATTCTGCTTCAGTGAGAGCTGGGGTTGTTCAAAGC
         10        20        30        40        50        60        70        80

-20                                              -10                         -1  +1
Met Ser Ala Ala Val Leu Leu Ser Val Leu Phe Ala Leu Ala Ala Ser Cys Ile Pro Thr Glu Tyr
ATG AGT GCT GCC GTC CTC TCC GTG CTT TTT GCT CTT GCT GCA GCA TCC TTT TGT ATT CCC ACT GAG TAT
 90        100        110        120       130        140       150       160        170

 10                    20                             30
Thr Met Tyr Val Asp Arg Arg Glu Cys Ala Tyr Cys Leu Thr Ile Asn Thr Thr Ile Cys Ala Gly Tyr Cys Met Thr Arg
ACA ATG TAC GTG GAT AGG AGA GAG TGC GCC TAC TGC CTG ACC ATC AAC ACC ACC ATC TGT GCT GGG TAT TGT ATG ACA CGG
         180        190        200        210        220        230        240        250

 40                     50                               60
Asp Ile Asn Gly Lys Leu Phe Leu Pro Lys Tyr Ala Leu Ser Gln Asp Val Cys Thr Tyr Arg Asp Phe Ile Tyr Arg Thr
GAT ATC AAT GGC AAA CTG TTT CTT CCC AAA TAT GCA CTC TCT CAG GAT GTC TGT ACA TAC AGA GAC TTC ATC TAC AGA ACG
         260        270        280        290        300        310        320        330

 70                             80
Val Glu Ile Pro Gly Cys Pro His Val Thr Pro Tyr Phe Ser Phe Pro Val Ala Val Ser Cys Lys Cys Gly Lys Cys
GTG GAA ATA CCA GGA TGC CCG CAC CAT GTT ACT CCT TAT TTC TCC CCT GTC GCC GTA AGC TGC AAG TGT GGC AAG TGT
         340        350        360        370        380        390        400        410

 90                             100                           110
Asn Thr Asp Asn Ser Asp Cys Ile His Glu Ala Ile Arg Thr Asn Tyr Cys Thr Lys Pro Gln Ser Phe Tyr Leu Gly Gly
AAT ACT GAC AAC AGT GAC TGC ATA CAC GAG GCT ATA AGA ACC AAC TAC TGC ACC AAG CCG CAG TCT TTC TAT CTG GGG GGA
         420        430        440        450        460        470        480        490

Phe Ser Val ***
TTT TCT GTT TAA CTTCAATAGCAGTGCAATCTGGTTAAATGTGTTTACCTGGAATAGAACGAATAAAATACCATTGAGACGTCTA17
         500        510        520        530        540        550        560        570
```

FIG. 9. The nucleotide sequence of the mRNA-equivalent strand of a cloned cDNA encoding mouse pre-TSH-β. The derived amino acid sequence is shown above the nucleotide sequence. The amino acids in the leader sequence are numbered −20 to −1; those of the mature TSH-β are numbered +1 to 118 (Gurr et al., 1983).

FIG. 10. Comparison of the amino acid sequence of mouse TSH-β, derived from the nucleotide sequence, with the known amino acid sequences of human, bovine, and porcine TSH-β. The determination of some amide groups is uncertain as shown by Asx and Glx. —, Amino acid identical to that in mouse TSH-β (Gurr *et al.*, 1983).

Positions 1–28:

	1									10											20								
Mouse	Phe	Cys	Ile	Pro	Thr	Glu	Tyr	Thr	Met	Tyr	His	Val	Asp	Arg	Arg	Glu	Cys	Ala	Tyr	Cys	Leu	Thr	Ile	Asn	Thr	Thr	Ile	Cys	Ala
Human	—	—	—	—	—	—	—	—	—	His	—	—	Glu	—	Lys	Glx	—	—	—	—	—	—	—	—	—	—	Val	—	—
Bovine	—	—	—	—	—	Met	Thr	—	—	His	—	—	Glu	—	Glu	—	—	—	—	—	—	—	—	Ser	—	—	—	—	—
Porcine	Leu	—	—	—	—	Met	—	—	—	His	—	—	Glu	—	Glu	—	—	—	—	—	—	—	—	—	—	—	—	—	—

Positions 29–56:

			30										40									50							
Mouse	Gly	Tyr	Cys	Met	Thr	Arg	Asp	Ile	Asn	Gly	Lys	Leu	Phe	Leu	Pro	Lys	Tyr	Ala	Leu	Ser	Gln	Asp	Val	Cys	Thr	Tyr	Arg	Asp
Human	—	—	—	—	—	—	Asx	—	—	—	—	—	—	—	—	—	—	—	—	—	Asx	—	—	—	—	—	—	—
Bovine	—	—	—	—	—	—	Asx	Val	Asx	—	—	—	—	—	—	—	—	—	—	—	—	—	—	—	—	—	—	—
Porcine	—	—	—	—	—	—	—	Phe	Asx	—	—	—	—	—	—	—	—	—	—	—	—	—	—	—	—	—	—	—

Positions 57–84:

			60										70									80							
Mouse	Phe	Ile	Tyr	Arg	Thr	Val	Glu	Ile	Pro	Gly	Cys	Pro	His	His	Val	Thr	Pro	Tyr	Phe	Ser	Phe	Pro	Val	Ala	Val	Ser	Cys	Lys
Human	—	—	—	—	—	Glx	—	—	—	—	—	—	Leu	—	Ala	—	—	—	—	—	—	—	—	—	Leu	—	—	—
Bovine	—	—	—	Lys	Ala	—	—	—	—	—	—	—	Leu	—	—	—	—	—	—	—	—	—	—	—	Ile	—	—	—
Porcine	—	—	—	Lys	—	—	—	—	—	—	—	—	Arg	—	—	Tyr	—	—	—	—	—	—	—	—	Ile	—	—	—

Positions 85–112:

			90										100									110							
Mouse	Cys	Gly	Lys	Cys	Asn	Thr	Asp	Asn	Ser	Asp	Cys	Ile	His	Glu	Ala	Val	Arg	Thr	Asn	Tyr	Cys	Thr	Lys	Pro	Gln	Ser	Phe	Tyr
Human	—	—	—	—	Asx	—	Asx	Tyr	—	—	—	—	—	—	—	Ile	Lys	—	Asx	—	—	—	—	—	Glx	Lys	Ser	—
Bovine	—	—	—	—	Asx	—	Asx	Tyr	—	—	—	—	—	—	—	Ile	Lys	—	—	—	—	—	—	—	—	Lys	Ser	—
Porcine	—	—	—	—	Asp	—	Asp	Tyr	—	—	—	—	—	—	—	Ile	Lys	—	—	—	—	—	—	—	Glu	Lys	Ser	—

Positions 113–118:

Mouse	Leu	Gly	Gly	Phe	Ser	Val
Human						
Bovine	Met					
Porcine						

93

α subunit gene also evolved (Pierce *et al.*, 1973; Dayhoff, 1976; Fontaine and Burzawa-Gerard, 1977; Pierce and Parsons, 1981). It is now becoming possible to test this hypothesis at the nucleotide level, as α and β subunit nucleotide sequence data become available.

The nucleotide sequences of the pre-α subunits from mouse, rat, cow, and man have been determined (Chin *et al.*, 1981b; Godine *et al.*, 1982; Nilson *et al.*, 1983; Fiddes and Goodman, 1979). Each protein has an amino terminal leader or signal sequence of 24 amino acids, rich in hydrophobic residues and characteristic of secreted proteins (Blobel and Dobberstein, 1975a,b). The mouse and rat leader sequences differ by only three conservative amino acid substitutions, each of which is the result of a single base change; the mouse and human sequences differ in five positions, and four of these differences can be accounted for by single base changes. The nucleotide sequence of 17 of the 24 amino acids of the bovine leader sequence is known, and the four amino acid differences with the mouse sequence are the result of single base changes. Figure 11 shows that there is considerable homology among the leader sequences of the α subunits of the glycoprotein hormones of these species at both the amino acid and nucleotide level. Alignment of the amino acid sequences of the mature α subunits from several species with respect to the positions of their completely conserved cysteine residues also shows a high degree of homology (Pierce and Parsons, 1981). The mouse α amino acid sequence shows strong similarity to rat (94%), ruminant (bovine, 93%; ovine, 91%), and porcine (98%) α subunits, as well as moderate homology with the equine (82%) and human (75%) α subunits. The nucleotide sequences of the mouse and rat pre-α subunits are 94% homologous in both the leader and mature protein sequences, whereas the mouse and human sequences show 85 and 77% nucleotide sequence homology in the leader and mature sequences, respectively (Chin *et al.*, 1981b; Godine *et al.*, 1982). As might be expected, there is less homology in DNA sequence in the untranslated 5'- and 3'-regions of the α subunit mRNAs. Although the phylogenetically closely related rat and mouse α sequences show a comparatively high homology of about 80% in these regions, between the mouse and human untranslated regions there is homology of only 20–30% (Chin *et al.*, 1981b; Godine *et al.*, 1982). Interestingly, Nilson *et al.* (1983) found that there is 79% homology between the 3'-noncoding region of the bovine and human α subunits, as well as between their coding sequences. The bovine and human 3'-sequences, thus, have almost the same homology as the rat and mouse 3'-untranslated region. This conservation of 3'-untranslated sequences suggests functional significance (Nilson *et al.*, 1983).

A

Mouse
-24 -20   -10   -1 +1
Met Asp Tyr Tyr Arg Lys Tyr Ala Ala Val Ile Leu Val Met Ser Met Phe Leu His Ile Leu His Ser Leu
ATG GAT TAC TAC AGA AAA TAT GCA GCT GTC ATT CTG GTC ATG TCC ATG TTC CTG CAT ATT CTT CAT TCT CTT

Rat
Met Asp Cys Tyr Arg Arg Tyr Ala Ala Val Ile Leu Val Met Ser Met Leu His Ile Leu His Ser Leu
ATG GAT TGC TAC AGA AGA TAT GCG GCT GTC ATT CTG GTC ATG TCC ATG CTG CAT ATT CTT CAT TCT CTT

Human
Met Asp Tyr Tyr Arg Lys Tyr Ala Ala Ile Phe Leu Val Thr Leu Ser Val Phe Leu His Val Leu His Ser Ala
ATG GAT TAC TAC AGA AAA TAT GCA GCT ATC TTT CTG GTC ACA TTG TCG GTG TTT CTG CAT GTT CTC CAT TCC GCT

Bovine
Met Asp - Tyr Arg - - Tyr Ala Ala Val Ile Leu Ala Ile Leu Ser Leu Phe Gln Ile Leu His Ser Phe
ATG - - GCA GCT GTC ATT GCC ATT TTG TCT CTG TTT CTG CAA ATT CTC CAT TCC TTT

B

-20   -10   -1 +1
Mouse TSH-β
Met Ser Ala Ala Val Leu Leu Leu Ser Val Leu Phe Ala Leu Ala Cys Gly Gln Ala Ala Ser Phe
ATG AGT GCT GCC GTC CTC CTC CTG TCC GTG CTT TTT GCT CTT GCT TGT GGG CAA GCA GCA TCC TTT

Rat LH-β
Met Glu Arg Leu Gln Gly Leu Leu Leu Trp Leu Leu Leu Ser Pro Ser Val Val Trp Ala Ser
ATG GAG AGG CTC CAG GGG CTG CTG CTG TGG CTG CTG CTG AGC CCA AGT GTG GTG TGG GCC TCC

Human CG-β
Met Glu Met Phe Gln Gly Leu Leu Leu Leu Leu Leu Leu Ser Met Gly Gly Thr Trp Ala Ser
ATG GAG ATG TTC CAG GGG CTG CTG CTG CTG CTG CTG CTG AGC ATG GGG GGG ACA TGG GCA TCC

FIG. 11. Leader sequences of α subunits (A) of the four species in which they have been determined. Leader sequences are shown for mouse TSH-β, rat LH-β, and human CG-β. They are currently the only known leader sequences of the β subunits (B) of the glycoprotein hormones.

The complete nucleotide sequence of a cDNA insert encoding mouse pre-TSH-β cDNA was determined in this laboratory (Gurr et al., 1983) by the chemical degradation method of Maxam and Gilbert (1980). The cDNA was 595 base pairs long and contained an open reading frame of 137 amino acids after the initiation codon AUG. The first 20 amino acids constituted a leader or signal sequence; a leader sequence of the same length has also been found for the rat LH-β and human CG-β subunits (Fig. 11). Although 14 of the 20 amino acids (70%) and 48 of the 60 nucleotides (80%) of the human CG-β sequence are in an equivalent position in rat LH-β, there is insignificant homology between the leader sequence of mouse TSH-β and either rat LH-β or human CG-β. There is a strong homology between the 118 amino acid sequence of mature mouse TSH-β and the TSH-β subunits from other species: the mouse sequence shows 89% homology with human TSH-β and 85% homology with bovine and porcine TSH-β. The position of all 12 cysteine residues has been conserved. The majority of changes preserve the hydrophobic or hydrophilic character of the amino acid, and all but one could be accounted for by a single alteration in nucleotide sequence. The mouse TSH-β subunit is unique in having a carboxyl-terminal region which is 6 and 5 amino acids longer than the human and pig and the cow TSH-β subunits, respectively (Gurr et al., 1983). The rat LH-β (Chin et al., 1983), human CG-β (Fiddes and Goodman, 1980), and mouse TSH-β (Gurr et al., 1983) subunits all contain the conserved sequence Cys-Ala-Gly-Tyr-Cys at approximately the same position, and, thus, this region of the protein has been implicated as an area of α–β subunit interaction (Pierce and Parsons, 1981). This conserved sequence is the longest homologous nucleotide sequence found between human CG-β and rat LH-β (Chin et al., 1983) although overall there is 73% nucleotide homology between these two nucleotide sequences.

Alignment of the human α and CG-β subunit amino acid sequences shows a very low overall homology (16%), but conservation of the position of 6 out of 12 cysteine residues (Fiddes and Goodman, 1980). Nucleotide homology between these α and β subunits is still very low (31%), but there are areas of higher homology in the regions of the conserved cysteine residues. We have noted a similar phenomenon in a comparison of mouse α and TSH-β nucleotide sequences.

The strong homology among the β subunits of the different glycoprotein hormones at the nucleotide level provides evidence that the β genes have evolved from a common β ancestral gene. The evidence for an evolutionary relationship between the α and β genes is less convincing at present, but the existence of a common ancestor for the α and β genes remains tenable.

VII. Size of α and TSH-β mRNA

Mouse α mRNA has been estimated to be 800–900 nucleotides in length by Northern blotting (Thomas, 1980) of glyoxal-denatured (McMaster and Carmichael, 1977) thyrotropic tumor poly(A) mRNA and hybridization with pTSH-α_F (Gurr *et al.*, 1983) labeled with [α-^{32}P]dCTP by nick translation (Rigby *et al*, 1977) (Fig. 12). This is similar to the value of approximately 800 nucleotides reported for α mRNA from rat (Godine *et al.*, 1982) and human (Fiddes and Goodman, 1981). Similarly, mouse TSH-β mRNA (Gurr *et al.*, 1983) and rat LH-β mRNA (Chin *et al.*, 1983) are

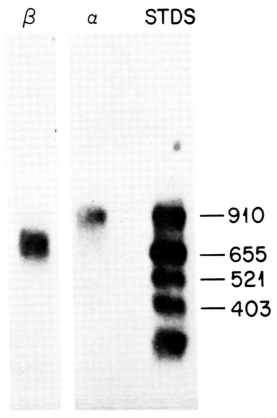

FIG. 12. Estimation of sizes of α and TSH-β mRNAs. Poly(A) mRNA from mouse TSH-secreting tumor was denatured with glyoxal, fractionated by electrophoresis on a 2% agarose gel, transferred to nitrocellulose paper, and hybridized with ^{32}P-labeled α or TSH-β cDNA. The hybridized mRNA was detected by autoradiography. Molecular size markers (number of nucleotides) are from an *Alu*I digest of plasmid pBR322, also treated with glyoxal (Gurr *et al.*, 1983).

about 750 and 700 nucleotides long, respectively. Although the human CG-β protein has a 24 amino acid carboxyl-terminal extension compared to other β subunit proteins (Pierce and Parsons, 1981), its mRNA is also about 750 nucleotides in length (Fiddes and Goodman, 1980) since this extension has arisen by readthrough into the existing 3'-untranslated region following a mutational event, rather than by insertion of additional coding sequences.

VIII. Assignment of α and TSH-β Genes to Different Mouse Chromosomes

Two human chromosomes appear to be necessary for the synthesis of complete CG (Bordelon-Riser et al., 1979). Two groups of investigators agree that α and CG-β genes reside on different human chromosomes, but they disagree as to which chromosomes these are. Since the human LH-β gene is linked to some of the seven CG-β genes (Boorstein et al., 1982; Talmadge et al., 1983), LH-β and CG-β genes must reside on the same chromosome. Whether TSH-β and FSH-β genes reside on the same or different chromosomes from LH-β and CG-β in humans remains unknown. However, we have been able to show that, in the mouse, the genes for α and TSH-β can be assigned to two different chromosomes and the gene for LH-β to a third mouse chromosome (Kourides et al., 1984).

For our studies we have used a series of mouse × hamster somatic cell hybrids, containing reduced numbers of mouse chromosomes and a complete set of hamster chromosomes. The chromosome composition of each hybrid was determined by cytogenetic and isoenzyme analysis (D'Eustacio et al., 1981a,b). DNA isolated from parental mouse cells, parental hamster cells, and somatic cell hybrids was digested with the restriction endonuclease BamHI, fractionated by agarose gel electrophoresis, blotted to nitrocellulose (Southern, 1975), and hybridized (Wahl et al., 1979) to either a ^{32}P-labeled mouse α or TSH-β cDNA probe.

Two fragments in mouse DNA hybridized with the mouse α probe: 10 and 8 kb in certain mouse parental cells and 10 and 6.5 kb in other mouse parental cells, showing that there is an α gene polymorphism between inbred mouse strains (Fig. 13). One fragment of 9 kb in hamster DNA cross-hybridized with the mouse α probe, was always present in the hybrids since they contained a complete set of hamster chromosomes, and, thus, was used as a control for the hybridization procedure. The 10-kb DNA fragment was present in five of the fourteen cell hybrids tested (Fig. 13). The 8- or 6.5-kb DNA fragment was also present in the same five cell hybrids depending on which strain of mouse was the parent. The absence of the mouse 10-kb DNA fragment in the other cell hybrids was used as

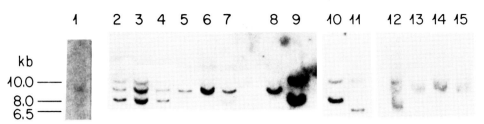

FIG. 13.   Chromosomal localization of the mouse α gene in mouse × hamster cell hybrids. *Bam*HI-digested DNA was electrophoresed on an agarose gel, transferred to nitrocellulose, and hybridized to ^{32}P-labeled mouse α cDNA. Lane 1, hamster parent; lanes 9–11, mouse parents; all other lanes show mouse × hamster cell hybrids (Kourides *et al.*, 1984).

proof of the absence of the mouse α gene and of the chromosome on which it resides. By this analysis the only mouse chromosome to which the α gene could be assigned was chromosome 4.

With the mouse TSH-β cDNA probe, one fragment of 22 kb in mouse DNA hybridized; one fragment of 14 kb cross-hybridized in the hamster DNA and served as a hybridization control. The 22-kb mouse DNA fragment was present in 7 of 15 cell hybrids (Fig. 14); the absence of this fragment in the other 8 cell hybrids was used as proof of the absence of the mouse TSH-β gene and of the chromosome on which it resides. The 22-kb mouse DNA fragment always segregated with mouse chromosome 3.

Using a ^{32}P-labeled rat LH-β cDNA probe, kindly provided by Dr. Mark Tepper and Dr. James Roberts of Columbia University Medical School (New York, NY), and the same somatic cell hybrids, we have also assigned the mouse LH-β gene to another chromosome, number 7. Thus, even though the genes for β subunits of the glycoprotein hormones may have arisen from a common ancestral gene, these genes do not all reside on the same chromosome (Kourides *et al.*, 1984).

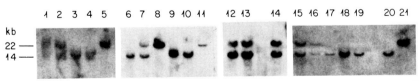

FIG. 14.   Chromosomal localization of the mouse TSH-β gene in mouse × hamster cell hybrids. The preparation of autoradiograms was the same as that used in Fig. 13 except the probe was ^{32}P-labeled mouse TSH-β cDNA. Lanes 5, 8, 11, and 21, mouse parents; lanes 9 and 10, hamster parent; all other lanes show mouse × hamster cell hybrids (Kourides *et al.*, 1984).

IX. Mouse TSH Gene Structure

Human DNA has been shown to contain only one α gene for the α subunits of all four glycoprotein hormone (Boothby et al., 1981; Fiddes and Goodman, 1981). However, there are seven CG-β genes and one LH-β gene in the human (Boorstein et al., 1982; Talmadge et al., 1983), but only one LH-β gene in the rat (Tepper et al., 1983). The human CG-β/ LH-β genes are similar but not identical and arranged in tandem or inverted pairs. Some of the genes are definitely linked, and probably all of them are located on the same chromosome in an area <50 kb in length (Talmadge et al., 1983). Several of the CG-β genes appear to be expressed (Fiddes et al., 1984). The human α gene is 9.4 kb long and contains three introns, 6.4, 1.7, and 0.4 kb long (Fiddes and Goodman, 1981), whereas the human CG-β and LH-β genes are short (about 1.4–1.5 kb long) and contain two introns 350 and 230 base pairs in length (Boorstein et al., 1982; Talmadge et al., 1983).

To elucidate the number and structure of mouse α and TSH-β genes, we have isolated these genes from a DNA genomic library; we have partially characterized their structure to date. A mouse genomic library was obtained from Dr. Leroy Hood of California Institute of Technology (Pasadena, CA), which was made from BALB/c mouse sperm DNA, partially digested with HaeIII and AluI, and cloned in Charon 4A λ (Davis et al., 1980). The screening was done by hybridization to ^{32}P-labeled mouse α and TSH-β probes, according to the method of Benton and Davis (1977). The 520 base pair α cDNA (pTSH-α_F), described earlier, was used to screen our cDNA library for plasmids containing longer α cDNAs. pTSH-$\alpha_{14,1,1}$ was selected and codes for essentially the entire α mRNA sequence. This plasmid and 5'- and 3'-fragments derived from it were used to characterize the α gene. The 595 base pair TSH-β cDNA (pTSH-β_H), also described earlier, contained essentially the whole TSH-β mRNA sequence and was used as a probe to characterize the TSH-β gene fragments.

About 10^6 phages were screened, the equivalent of 5 genomes (Fig. 15). Initial screening using a combination of α and TSH-β probes showed 15 positives, of which one hybridized to α cDNA only (Fig. 16) and 14 hybridized to TSH-β cDNA. Restriction mapping has shown that the TSH-β phages consist of two types: 12 identical phages, represented by C4A/β-24, and two phages of a second type, represented by C4A/β-90 (Fig. 17).

We found only one α gene fragment out of the 10^6 phages screened. The α gene is at least 3.8 kb long and includes three exons and two introns (Fig. 16). Since the first exon is close to the left arm of the Charon 4A

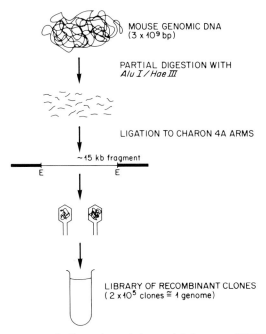

FIG. 15.   A mouse genomic library is made by partial cleavage of DNA with restriction enzymes and insertion of these fragments into phage that are then propagated in *E. Coli.* Screening of 2×10^5 clones or plaques is equivalent to one genome.

vector, this phage may not contain the entire gene. The two introns are about 0.8 and 2.4 kb long and are located in similar positions to the 3'-introns in the human α gene, although they are of different sizes. If homology with the human α gene is conserved we would expect to find a third

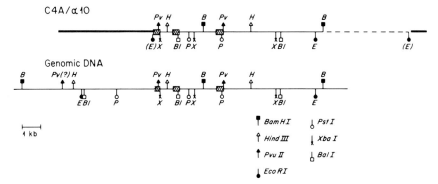

FIG. 16.   Partial restriction map of an α gene fragment in Charon 4A (C4A/α10) and of the α gene in total genomic DNA.

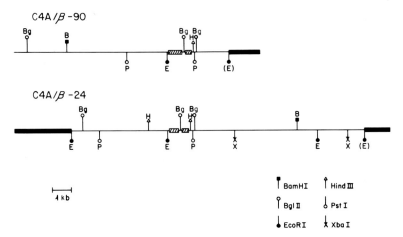

FIG. 17.   Partial restriction maps of two different TSH-β gene fragments in Charon 4A (C4A/β-90 and C4A/β-24).

intron in the 5′-region of the mouse α gene. We are now screening a different mouse library in order to isolate more α phages. We also isolated genomic DNA from normal BALB/c mouse livers and constructed a restriction map. The map obtained from the total DNA is the same as the map obtained from the recombinant phage; each fragment in the genomic map can be accounted for by fragments in the phage map (Fig. 16). These data, combined with the finding of only one α recombinant phage, strongly suggest that there is only one α gene in the mouse.

In contrast, we have isolated two types of recombinant TSH-β phages. The genes are less than 1.5 kb long, similar in structure, and contain at least one intron (Fig. 17). Although the restriction enzyme sites of the gene fragments are similar, there are several distinct differences in the 5′-flanking regions. These data suggest that there is more than one TSH-β gene in the mouse. Further characterization of these two TSH-β genes is currently being pursued in our laboratory. We do not yet know whether one or both are expressed. Neither of these genes is an LH-β gene since there is no hybridization with a rat LH-β cDNA probe obtained from Dr. Mark Tepper and Dr. James Roberts.

X. Extrapituitary TSH

Hormones classically felt to be pituitary in origin have been found in the brain (Krieger and Martin, 1981). The question has arisen as to whether these hormones are transported to these extrapituitary sites or are synthesized there. Since the presence of TSH in extrapituitary rodent brain had previously been reported (Hojvat *et al.*, 1982; Moldow and Yalow, 1978; Ottenweller and Hedge, 1982; Devito and Hedge, 1982), we investigated whether TSH and α subunit were present in the central nervous system outside the pituitary gland (Schorr-Toshav *et al.*, 1983a). Using specific radioimmunoassays, TSH was detected at 2.0 ± 0.4 ng-eq/g in brain, 23 ± 3.1 ng-eq/g in hypothalamus, and $10,500 \pm 1,800$ ng-eq/g in the pituitary gland. For α subunit, levels were 39 ± 0.9 ng/g in brain, 419 ± 144 ng/g in hypothalamus, and $154,000$ ng/g in the pituitary. Posthypophysectomy, hypothalamic levels of TSH fell to the level detected in brain, whereas α levels, although decreased, were still above those in brain. To determine if α subunit was actually synthesized outside the pituitary gland, we assayed poly(A)-containing mRNA from hypothalamus and brain for the presence of mRNA coding for the α subunit. Poly(A) mRNA was electrophoresed on agarose gels, transferred to nitrocellulose, and hybridized with ^{32}P-labeled α subunit cDNA probe. We could detect no mRNA coding for the α subunit in brain or hypothalamus under conditions capable of detecting 3 copies and 14 copies per cell of α subunit in the brain and hypothalamus, respectively. α mRNA was detectable in the pituitary under these conditions. Our findings are consistent with the hypothesis that TSH and α subunit reach the brain by diffusion from the pituitary though they do not exclude totally the possibility that TSH is synthesized in a very small proportion of brain cells. In order to exclude localized biosynthesis of TSH or α subunit, we also sectioned the entire mouse brain and stained it with antisera to ovine α and bovine TSH-β subunits using an immunoperoxidase method. The only specific staining was for α subunit in the pericapillary areas of the median eminence of the mouse hypothalamus. Since such staining did not include fibers or cell bodies, it supported the concept that α subunit in brain occurred by retrograde flow from the pituitary gland rather than localized biosynthesis (Schorr-Toshav *et al.*, 1983b).

XI. Regulation of TSH by Thyroid Hormones in TSH-Secreting Tumors

TSH synthesis and secretion appear to be regulated primarily in a negative fashion by thyroid hormones at the level of the pituitary. Acute administration of thyroid hormone to thyroidectomized rats causes a rapid fall in serum TSH levels, with a concomitant increase in pituitary TSH content (D'Angelo *et al.*, 1976; Spira *et al.*, 1979; Silva and Larsen, 1978, 1979; Lemarchand-Beraud and Berthier, 1981). Both synthesis and release of TSH are, in fact, markedly inhibited by thyroid hormone, but since suppression of synthesis is slower in onset than suppression of release, there is an initial net increase in pituitary TSH content (Spira *et al.*, 1979). TSH synthesis begins to decrease after TSH secretion has already reached a nadir (Spira *et al.*, 1979); thus, prolonged thyroid hormone treatment also results in very low pituitary TSH levels (Harada *et al.*, 1975).

We have shown that treatment of hypothyroid mice bearing thyrotropic tumors with L-T_3 markedly decreases tumor TSH and TSH-β content, but may affect tumor α subunit levels differently depending on the length of treatment. Serum TSH and TSH-β levels are suppressed by L-T_3, but serum α decreases less (Gurr and Kourides, 1983). Ross *et al.* (1983a) have also reported a decrease in serum TSH, α, and TSH-β levels after thyroxine treatment of hypothyroid mice. Additionally, although the pituitary content of TSH and TSH-β decreased, pituitary α content was either unchanged or decreased, depending on the duration of hypothyroidism in the animals.

We have studied the molecular basis for this discordant effect of thyroid hormones on α and TSH-β subunit levels using the mouse thyrotropic tumor system. These tumors synthesize and secrete intact TSH and free α and TSH-β, but do not synthesize the structurally related gonadotropins (Furth *et al.*, 1973; Blackman *et al.*, 1978). In addition, in the tumors, TSH and its subunits can be regulated by TRH, T_3, and somatostatin, as is true for normal pituitary TSH (Blackman *et al.*, 1978; Gershengorn, 1978; Vale *et al.*, 1972; Marshall *et al.*, 1981; Cacicedo *et al.*, 1981; Ross *et al.*, 1983b).

Groups of male LAF$_1$ mice, radiothyroidectomized at the same time at 2–3 months of age, were injected with the same TSH-secreting tumor at 3–4 months of age. The experiments were begun when each tumor had been growing for about 6 months. Animals were treated with L-T_3 (20 μg/ 100 g body weight) for 4 or 10 days or with saline. Levels of TSH and subunits were measured by specific radioimmunoassays. The level of TSH in serum decreased to 3 and 0.3% of control, respectively, after 4 and 10 days of treatment; serum levels of free α subunits were reduced to 60 and 11% of control, respectively; free TSH-β subunits were reduced to undetectable levels (<0.2% of control) at both 4 and 10 days. The decrease in mean tumor TSH content was not statistically significant at 4 days, but at 10 days TSH content was 15% of the level in control animals. There was no significant change in tumor α content after either 4 or 10 days of L-T_3 treatment. However, tumor TSH-β content was reduced to 29 and 10% of control levels after 4 and 10 days, respectively. Thus, although L-T_3 treatment caused a marked decrease in the levels of TSH, free α, and TSH-β subunits in serum, there was a discordant effect of L-T_3 on tumor α and TSH-β content (Fig. 18) (Gurr and Kourides, 1983).

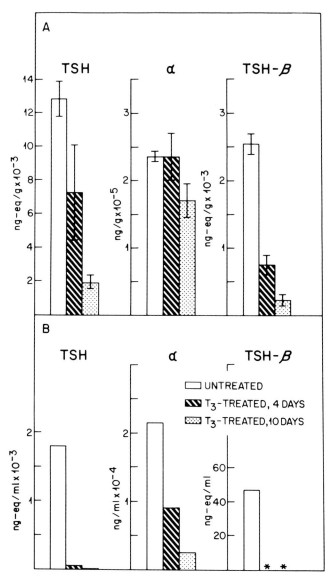

FIG. 18.   Effect of L-T$_3$ treatment on tumor content (A) and serum levels (B) of TSH, α, and TSH-β. Hypothyroid mice bearing tumor TtT 108B were treated with L-T$_3$ (20 μg/100 g body weight) for 4 or 10 days. TSH, α, and TSH-β were determined by radioimmunoassay in tumor extracts and in pooled serum. TSH and TSH-β are expressed in ng-eq since mouse TSH and TSH-β are immunologically distinct from the rat standard TSH and β. Values are mean $\pm$ SE for 2–4 tumors. *, TSH-β concentration <0.1 ng-eq/ml (Gurr and Kourides, 1983).

To address the question of whether there were similar discordant changes in the tumor content of α and TSH-β mRNAs, the effect of L-T$_3$ treatment on both translatable and hybridizable α and TSH-β mRNAs was examined. When poly(A) mRNA from control and L-T$_3$-treated tumors was translated *in vitro* in reticulocyte lysate with microsomal membranes and the translation products analyzed for α and TSH-β protein by immunoprecipitation, it was found that L-T$_3$ treatment, for either 4 or 10 days, reduced the synthesis of TSH-β protein directed by tumor mRNA to undetectable levels. In contrast, α mRNA was not affected at 4 days, and, at 10 days, translatable α mRNA was only markedly decreased in

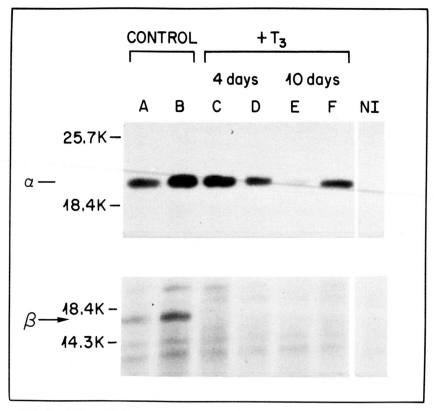

FIG. 19.   Effect of L-T$_3$ treatment on translatable α and TSH-β mRNA. Equal amounts of mRNA from tumors of untreated animals (A, B) and from animals treated with L-T$_3$ for 4 days (C, D) and 10 days (E, F) were translated in reticulocyte lysate with microsomal membranes. [^{35}S]Methionine-labeled translation products were analyzed by SDS–polyacrylamide gel electrophoresis. Top, protein precipitated with α antiserum (lanes A–F) and nonimmune serum (lane NI). Bottom, protein precipitated with TSH-β antiserum (lanes A–F) and nonimmune serum (lane NI). Autoradiograms were developed after 2 days (α) or 13 days (TSH-β). Molecular weight markers are on the left (Gurr and Kourides, 1983).

one of the two animals (Fig. 19). Changes in α and TSH-β mRNA content were examined by Northern blotting of glyoxal-denatured mRNA and hybridization with ^{32}P-labeled α or TSH-β cDNA probes. After both 4 and 10 days of L-T$_3$ treatment there was a dramatic decrease in TSH-β mRNA content, to less than 10% of control. As with mRNA translatability, there was a noticeable decrease in α mRNA content only in one of the animals at 10 days (Fig. 20) (Gurr and Kourides, 1983).

The divergent response of tumor α and TSH-β protein content is consistent with the hypothesis that the availability of the TSH-β subunit is limiting in the production of complete TSH. The fact that serum levels of TSH, α, and TSH-β were suppressed approximately in parallel and to a

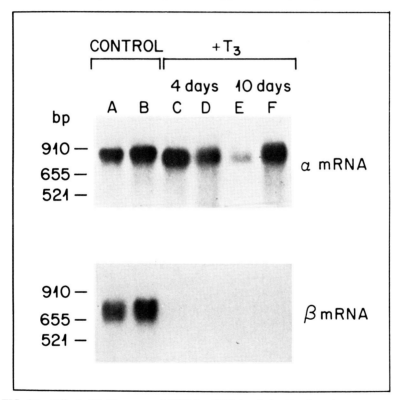

FIG. 20. Effect of L-T$_3$ on α and TSH-β mRNA levels by Northern blotting. Poly(A) mRNA (5 μg) from tumors of untreated animals (A, B) and from animals treated with L-T$_3$ for 4 days (C, D) and 10 days (E, F) was denatured with glyoxal, fractionated by electrophoresis on a 2% agarose gel, and transferred to nitrocellulose. The blot was then hybridized with ^{32}P-labeled pTSH-α_F (top) or pTSH-β_H (bottom). Films were exposed for 3 hours (α) or 5 hours (β). The molecular size markers (nucleotides) are from an AluI digest of pBR322 (Gurr and Kourides, 1983).

greater extent than their tumor content suggests that L-T_3 has a rapid, posttranslational effect on subunit secretion, which is independent of effects on subunit synthesis. The dramatic effects of L-T_3 treatment on tumor levels of both translatable and hybridizable mRNA suggests that L-T_3 acts primarily on TSH-β biosynthesis and at a pretranslational level.

Although the effect of L-T_3 on α mRNA was more variable between animals, reductions in α mRNA were clearly less pronounced and independent of those in TSH-β mRNA. The specific regulation of the biosynthesis of several proteins by L-T_3 has been correlated with modulation of their mRNA levels (Dobner *et al.*, 1981; Miksicek and Towle, 1983; Winberry *et al.*, 1983); it has been directly demonstrated that L-T_3 increases the rate of growth hormone gene transcription (Spindler *et al.*, 1982; Evans *et al.*, 1982). Our results are consistent with a model in which thyroid hormone regulates TSH-β mRNA levels by inhibition of TSH-β gene transcription. However, we have not ruled out mechanisms involving changes in specific mRNA turnover or in the processing of nuclear mRNA precursors. Nevertheless, the discordant effects of thyroid hormone on α and TSH-β subunit protein content are clearly paralleled by similar divergent effects on α and TSH-β mRNA levels.

XII. Hormonal Regulation of TSH in Hypothyroid Pituitary

There have been many studies of the regulation of TSH production at the protein level in the hypothyroid rat and mouse pituitary (D'Angelo *et al.*, 1976; Silva and Larsen, 1978, 1979; Spira *et al.*, 1979; Lemarchand-Beraud and Berthier, 1981; Ross *et al.*, 1983a), but little is known about the mechanism of action of potential physiological effectors. We have initiated studies in non-tumor-bearing LAF$_1$ mice, made hypothyroid 1–2 months prior to the experiment, with L-T_3, TRH, and the dopamine agonist bromocriptine. We have focused on the effects of these modulators on TSH, α, and TSH-β secretion and pituitary α and TSH-β mRNA levels. The dose–response relationship between L-T_3 and TSH protein and mRNA levels has been examined in mice made hypothyroid 2 months before L-T_3 hormone treatment. Mice were treated daily for 4 days with varying doses of L-T_3, and serum levels of intact TSH and free α and TSH-β subunits were measured by radioimmunoassay (Table I). Total RNA was isolated from pituitary tissue by a proteinase K method (Rowe *et al.*, 1978), and equivalent amounts of RNA were applied to nitrocellulose paper by the dot-blot procedure (Thomas, 1980); the blots were separately hybridized with ^{32}P-labeled α and TSH-β cDNA probes. Table I shows that at low doses of L-T_3 there was no effect on TSH or subunit secretion, but α and TSH-β mRNAs were decreased modestly, particu-

TABLE I

Effect of Increasing Doses of L-T₃ on TSH and Subunit Secretion (Serum Levels) and α and TSH-β mRNA Content in the Pituitary

μg L-T$_3$/100 g body weight × 4 days	Protein			mRNA (percentage of control)	
	TSH (ng-eq/ml)	α (ng/ml)	TSH-β (ng-eq/ml)	α	TSH-β
Untreated	13	7.8	1.2	100	100
0.05	21	3.4	1.8	61	61
0.1	22	7	1.4	88	55
0.5	<1.6	<2	<0.1	76	21
1.0	<1.6	<2	<0.1	48	14

larly TSH-β mRNA. At the higher doses, TSH and subunit protein levels were greatly reduced; there was a further decline in α mRNA and an even more marked decline in TSH-β mRNA. These data obtained with hypothyroid pituitaries substantiate the conclusion drawn from experiments using thyrotropic tumors (Gurr and Kourides, 1983) that the effects of L-T₃ are more pronounced on TSH-β mRNA than on α mRNA and that their regulation is not coordinate.

The effects of TRH and bromocriptine on pituitary TSH biosynthesis were also studied in similar experiments (Table II). Groups of hypothyroid mice were treated with TRH, which would be expected to increase TSH and subunit release (Blackman *et al.*, 1978; Vale *et al.*, 1972; Mar-

TABLE II

Effect of TRH and Bromocriptine on TSH and Subunit Secretion (Serum Levels) and α and TSH-β mRNA Content in the Pituitary

	Protein			mRNA (percentage of control)	
	TSH (ng-eq/ml)	α (ng/ml)	TSH-β (ng-eq/ml)	α	TSH-β
Untreated	15	55	2.5	100	100
TRH (10 μg/100 g body weight every 12 hours × 4 days)	18	46	2.1	205	190
Bromocriptine (1 mg/100 g body weight × 4 days)	12	60	1.7	19	48

shall *et al.,* 1981; Cacicedo *et al.,* 1981), and bromocriptine, a dopamine agonist, which we have found to decrease TSH and subunit secretion (Bajorunas *et al.,* 1984). After treatment with either TRH (1.0 μg/100 g body weight, twice daily) or bromocriptine (1 mg/100 g body weight for 4 days), there was little effect on protein secretion. However, TRH treatment elicited a doubling of both α and TSH-β mRNA levels, whereas bromocriptine caused a decrease in both α and TSH-β mRNA, the decrease in α mRNA being more marked. The more striking decrease in α mRNA after bromocriptine might suggest an effect of bromocriptine also on gonadotrophe α mRNA. Thus, it appears that thyroid hormone exerts tight negative feedback particularly on TSH-β mRNA levels. The effects of other hormones on TSH mRNA levels appear more modest.

XIII. α/TSH-β mRNA Ratios in Pituitaries and TSH-Secreting Tumors

It is well established that mouse thyrotropic tumors secrete free α and TSH-β subunits both *in vivo* and *in vitro* and that these tumors contain a molar excess of α over TSH-β subunits (Blackman *et al.,* 1978; Marshall *et al.,* 1981; Ross *et al.,* 1983b; Gurr and Kourides, 1983). The pituitaries of euthyroid and short-term hypothyroid mice also contain an excess of α subunits, although in long-term hypothyroid animals the α/TSH-β ratio is more balanced (unpublished observations). There has been disagreement, however, as to the origin of the imbalance in α and TSH-β levels. Chin *et al.* (1981a) have concluded, from the results of pulse-chase studies of TSH biosynthesis using tumor minces *in vitro,* that α and TSH-β proteins are initially synthesized in equal amounts and that the subsequent excess of α subunits is the result of selective β subunit degradation. In contrast, Magner and Weintraub (1982), using similar methodology, found α/TSH-β ratios always greater than one, with no evidence of β degradation.

The availability of α and TSH-β cDNA probes has allowed us to approach this problem by determining the relative amounts of α and TSH-β mRNA by hybridization and comparing the α/TSH-β mRNA ratio with the α/TSH-β protein content of the tissue. We have looked at the actual ratio of α to TSH-β subunits in various TSH-secreting pituitary tumors. Interestingly, both the absolute amounts of α and TSH-β and the ratios were very variable. The tumor with the greatest TSH content (IAK 109A) had the most balanced ratio of α/TSH-β, 1.75. The ratio was calculated by adding α subunits in TSH to free α and dividing by TSH-β in TSH plus free TSH-β. Two tumors (TtT 108D and IAK 111) maintained their α content, but had decreased TSH-β and TSH, thus yielding high α/TSH-β ratios. Another tumor (IAK 103F) grew both in euthyroid and hypothyroid animals and contained only small amounts of α, with no TSH-β or complete TSH (Table III).

TABLE III
α/β TSH Protein Ratios in Various TSH-Secreting Tumors

	IAK 109A	TtT 108D	IAK 111	IAK 103F
TSH (ng-eq/mg)	200	2.8	1	<0.05
α (ng/mg)	160	200	295	0.03
TSH-β (ng-eq/mg)	48	3	2.4	<0.05
Ratio	1.75	46	102	—[a]

[a] A ratio cannot be calculated for this tumor since no TSH or TSH-β was detected.

Total RNA was extracted from each of these individual tumors (Chen *et al.*, 1983), as well as from the pituitaries of normal euthyroid mice, mice made hypothyroid 2 months previously (early hypothyroid), and mice made hypothyroid about 1 year previously (late hypothyroid). Equal amounts of RNA were dotted onto nitrocellulose (Thomas, 1980) and hybridized with either ^{32}P-labeled α or TSH-β cDNA. The probes had essentially identical specific activities. Densitometry of the autoradiograms was used to quantitate in arbitrary units the amount of α and TSH-β mRNA/μg total RNA (Fig. 21). The calculated amounts of α and TSH-β mRNA and the ratios derived are shown in Table IV. There was an increase in both α and TSH-β mRNA with increasing hypothyroidism, but the increase in TSH-β mRNA exceeded that of α, so that the ratio of α to TSH-β reached 1. This occurred despite the fact that α mRNA in the pituitary includes α mRNA from the gonadotrophe. The tumor IAK 103F,

TABLE IV
Amounts of α and TSH-β mRNA in Pituitary Glands and TSH-Secreting Tumors

	Units α mRNA (μg RNA)	Units TSH-β mRNA (μg RNA)	Ratio α/TSH-β mRNA	Ratio α/TSH-β protein
Euthyroid pituitaries	52	16	3.2	[a]
Early hypothyroid pituitaries	149	50	3.0	[a]
Late hypothyroid pituitaries	447	438	1.0	[a]
IAK 109A tumor	309	576	0.5	1.75
TtT 108D tumor	124	91	1.4	46
IAK 111 tumor	529	80	6.6	102
IAK 103F tumor	58	86	0.7	—

[a] The α/TSH-β ratio is most unbalanced in euthyroid pituitaries and most balanced in late hypothyroid pituitaries.

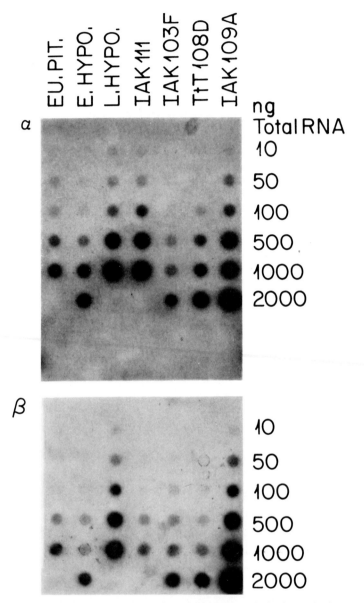

FIG. 21. Increasing concentrations of total RNA from pituitaries and TSH-secreting tumors, denatured with formaldehyde, were dotted onto nitrocellulose paper and hybridized with either ^{32}P-labeled α or TSH-β cDNA probes of the same specific activity. The amount of hybridized mRNA was detected by autoradiography and quantitated by densitometry.

which contained no detectable TSH or TSH-β, had the smallest amount of α and TSH-β mRNA. IAK 109A, which contained the most TSH, had the most α and TSH-β mRNA, with the amount of TSH-β mRNA apparently slightly exceeding that of α (Fig. 21 and Table IV). The two tumors (TtT 108D and IAK 111) that had shown striking α protein excess also showed α mRNA excess, though with imperfect correlation between message and protein levels. Since TSH and TSH-β concentrations have been quantitated in ng-eq/ml and α concentrations, in ng/mg, the protein ratios may not be completely valid. Nevertheless, our data do show a relationship between mRNA levels and protein levels. Moreover, although in the normal pituitary and certain tumors there is α mRNA excess, in tumors with high TSH content or hypothyroid pituitaries, TSH-β mRNA equals or even exceeds the amount of α mRNA. These studies suggest transcriptional control of α and TSH-β protein levels, though they do not rule out additional posttranscriptional regulation.

XIV. Conclusion

Our studies on the organization and regulation of TSH genes demonstrate the utility of molecular biologic approaches to answer important questions in endocrinology. Soon we should have the precise structure of the TSH genes elucidated. This information is necessary prior to undertaking more detailed studies of the hormonal regulation of gene transcription and RNA processing.

ACKNOWLEDGMENTS

We would like to acknowledge valuable contributions to this work by Dr. Maria E. Vrontakis, a visiting investigator in our laboratory, Mr. Edward Athanasian, a premedical student, and our technicians, Olga Agranovsky and Cynthia Wagner. We appreciate the skill and patience of Jo Ann Gili in typing this manuscript. This work has been supported by USPHS Grants CA-23185 and CA-08748 and a grant from the March of Dimes–Birth Defects Foundation (1-682). Dr. Kourides is the recipient of a USPHS Research Career Development Award AM-00679.

REFERENCES

Alexander, D. C., and Miller, W. L. (1981). *J. Biol. Chem.* **256,** 12628.
Aviv, H., and Leder, P. (1972). *Proc. Natl. Acad. Sci. U.S.A.* **69,** 1408.
Bajorunas, D. R., Rosner, W., and Kourides, I. A. (1984). *J. Clin. Endocrinol. Metab.* (in press).
Benton, W. D., and Davis, R. W. (1977). *Science* **196,** 180.
Birken, S., and Canfield, R. E. (1977). *J. Biol. Chem* **252,** 5386.
Blackman, M. R., Gershengorn, M. C., and Weintraub, B. D. (1978). *Endocrinology* **102,** 499.

Blackman, M. R., Weintraub, B. D., Rosen, S. W., Kourides, I. A., Steinwascher, K., and Gail, M. H. (1980). *J. Natl. Cancer Inst.* **65,** 81.

Blobel, G., and Dobberstein, B. D. (1975a). *J. Cell Biol.* **67,** 835.

Blobel, G., and Dobberstein, B. D. (1975b). *J. Cell Biol.* **67.** 852.

Boorstein, W. R., Vamvakopoulos, N. C., and Fiddes, J. C. (1982). *Nature (London)* **300,** 419.

Boothby, M., Ruddon, R. W., Anderson, C., McWilliams, D., and Boime, I. (1981). *J. Biol. Chem.* **256,** 5121.

Bordelon-Riser, M. R., Siciliano, M. J., and Kohler, P. O. (1979). *Somatic Cell Genet.* **5,** 597.

Cacicedo, L., Pohl, S. L., and Reichlin, S. (1981). *Endocrinology* **108,** 1012.

Canfield, R. E., Birken, S., Morse, J. H., and Morgan, F. J. (1976). *In* "Peptide Hormones" (J. A. Parsons, ed.), p. 299. Univ. Park Press, Baltimore, Maryland.

Catt, K. J., and Pierce, J. G. (1978). *In* "Reproduction Endocrinology" (S. S. C. Yen and R. B. Jaffe, eds.), p. 34. Saunders, Philadelphia, Pennsylvania.

Catt, K. J., Dufau, M. L., and Tsuruhara, T. (1973). *J. Clin. Endocrinol. Metab.* **36,** 73.

Chen, C. L. C., Dionne, F. T., and Roberts, J. L. (1983). *Proc. Natl. Acad. Sci. U.S.A.* **80,** 2211.

Chin, W. W., Habener, J. F., Kieffer, J. D., and Maloof, F. (1978). *J. Biol. Chem.* **253,** 7985.

Chin, W. W., Maloof, F., and Habener, J. F. (1981a). *J. Biol. Chem.* **256,** 3059.

Chin, W. W., Kronenberg, H. M., Dee, P. C., Maloof, F., and Habener, J. F. (1981b). *Proc. Natl. Acad. Sci. U.S.A.* **78,** 5329.

Chin, W. W., Godine, J. E., Klein, D. R., Chang, A. S., Tan, L. K., and Habener, J. F., (1983). *Proc. Natl. Acad. Sci. U.S.A.* **80,** 4649.

Choi, Y. S., Knopf, P. M., and Lennox, E. S. (1971). *Biochemistry* **10,** 659.

Counis, R., Corbani, M., Poissonier, M., and Jutisz, M. (1982). *Biochem. Biophys. Res. Commun.* **107,** 998.

D'Angelo, S. A., Paul, D. H., Wall, N. R., and Lombardi, D. M. (1976). *Endocrinology* **99,** 935.

Daniels-McQueen, S., McWilliams, S., Birken, S., Canfield, R., Landefeld, T., and Boime, I. (1978). *J. Biol. Chem.* **253,** 7109.

Davis, M. M. K., Calame, K., Early, P. W., Livant, D. L., Joho, R., Weissman, I. L., and Hood, L. (1980). *Nature (London)* **283,** 733.

Dayhoff, M. (1976). *In* "Atlas of Protein Sequence and Structure," Vol. 5. Suppl. 2, p. 122. Nat. Biomed. Research Foundation, Washington, D.C.

D'Eustachio, P., Bothwell, S. L. M., Takaro, T. K., Baltimore, D., and Ruddle, F. H. (1981a). *J. Exp. Med.* **153,** 793.

D'Eustachio, P., Ingram, S., Tilghman, S. M., and Ruddle, F. H. (1981b). *Somatic Cell Genet.* **7,** 289.

Devito, W. J., and Hedge, G. A. (1982). *Endocrinology* **111,** 1406.

Dobner, P. R., Kawasaki, E. S., Yu, L-Y, and Bancroft, F. C. (1981). *Proc. Natl. Acad. Sci. U.S.A.* **78,** 2230.

Evans, R. M., Birnberg, R. M., and Rosenfeld, M. G. (1982). *Proc. Natl. Acad. Sci. U.S.A.* **79,** 7659.

Fiddes, J. C., and Goodman, H. M. (1979). *Nature (London)* **281,** 351.

Fiddes, J. C., and Goodman, H. M. (1980). *Nature (London)* **286,** 684.

Fiddes, J. C., and Goodman, H. M. (1981). *J. Mol. Appl. Genet.* **1,** 3.

Fiddes, J. C., Talmadge, K., Boorstein, W. R., and Vamvakopoulos, N. C. (1984). *Recent Prog. Horm. Res.* **40,** 43–78.

Fontaine, Y.-A., and Burzawa-Gerard, E. (1977). *Gen. Comp. Endocrinol.* **32,** 341.

Furth, J., Moy, P., Hershman, J., and Ueda, G. (1973). *Arch. Pathol.* **96,** 217.

Gershengorn, M. C. (1978). *Endocrinology* **102,** 1122.

Giudice, L. C., and Weintraub, B. D. (1979). *J. Biol. Chem.* **254,** 12679.

Giudice, L. C., Waxdal, M. J., and Weintraub, B. D. (1979). *J. Biol. Chem.* **76,** 4798.

Godine, J. E., Chin, W. W., and Habener, J. F. (1980). *J. Biol. Chem.* **255,** 8780.

Godine, J. E., Chin, W. W., and Habener, J. F. (1981). *J. Biol. Chem.* **256,** 2475.

Godine, J. E., Chin, W. W., and Habener, J. F. (1982). *J. Biol. Chem.* **257,** 8368.

Grunstein, M., and Hogness, D. (1975). *Proc. Natl. Acad. Sci. U.S.A.* **72,** 3961.

Gurr, J. A., and Kourides, I. A. (1983). *J. Biol. Chem.* **258,** 10208.

Gurr, J. A., Catterall, J. F., and Kourides, I. A. (1983). *Proc. Natl. Acad. Sci. U.S.A.* **80,** 2122.

Harada, A., Kojima, A., and Tsukui, T. (1975). *J. Clin. Endocrinol. Metab.* **40,** 942.

Hojvat, S., Baker, G., Kirsteins, L., and Lawrence, A. M. (1982). *Neuroendocrinology* **34,** 327.

Hubbard, S. C., and Ivatt, R. J. (1981). *Annu. Rev. Biochem.* **50,** 555.

Kessler, M. J., Mise, T., Ghai, M. D., and Bahl, O. P. (1979). *J. Biol. Chem.* **254,** 7909.

Keutmann, H. T., and Williams, R. M. (1977). *J. Biol. Chem.* **252,** 5393.

Keutmann, H. T., Williams, R. M., and Ryan, R. J. (1979). *Biochem. Biophys. Res. Commun.* **90,** 842.

Kourides, I. A. (1984). *In* "The Thyroid" (S. H. Ingbar and L. E. Braverman, eds.). Harper, New York (in press).

Kourides, I. A., and Weintraub, B. D. (1979). *Proc. Natl. Acad. Sci. U.S.A.* **76,** 298.

Kourides, I. A., Weintraub, B. D., Ridgway, E. C., and Maloof, F. (1973). *J. Clin. Endocrinol. Metab.* **37,** 836.

Kourides, I. A., Weintraub, B. D., Levko, M. A., and Maloof, F. (1974). *Endocrinology* **94,** 1411.

Kourides, I. A., Weintraub, B. D., Ridgway, E. C., and Maloof, F. (1975). *J. Clin. Endocrinol. Metab.* **40,** 872.

Kourides, I. A., Weintraub, B. D., Rosen, S. W., Ridgway, E. C., Kliman, B., and Maloof, F. (1976). *J. Clin. Endocrinol. Metab.* **43,** 97.

Kourides, I. A., Re, R. N., Weintraub, B. D., Ridgway, E. C., and Maloof, F. *Clin. Endocrinol.* (1977a). *J. Clin. Invest.* **59,** 509.

Kourides, I. A., Ridgway, E. C., Weintraub, B. D., Bigos, S. T., Gershengorn, M. C., and Maloof, F. (1977b). *J. Clin. Endocrinol. Metab.* **45,** 434.

Kourides, I. A., Weintraub, B. D., Re, R. N., Ridgway, E. C., and Maloof, F. (1978). **9,** 535.

Kourides, I. A., Ridgway, E. C., and Maloof, F. (1979). *J. Clin. Endocrinol. Metab.* **49,** 700.

Kourides, I. A., Hoffman, B. J., and Landon, M. B. (1980a). *J. Clin. Endocrinol. Metab.* **51,** 1372.

Kourides, I. A., Landon, M. B., Hoffman, B. J., and Weintraub, B. D. (1980b). *Clin. Endocrinol.* **12,** 407.

Kourides, I. A., Barker, P. E., Gurr, J. A., Pravtcheva, D. D., and Ruddle, F. H. (1984). *Proc. Natl. Acad. Sci. U.S.A.* **81,** 517.

Kreil, G. (1981). *Annu. Rev. Biochem.* **50,** 317.

Krieger, D. T., and Martin, J. B. (1981). *N. Engl. J. Med.* **304,** 876.

Laemmli, U. K. (1970). *Nature (London)* **227,** 680.

Landefeld, T. D. (1979). *J. Biol. Chem.* **254,** 2685.

Landefeld, T. D., and Kepa, J. (1979). *Biochem. Biophys. Res. Commun.* **90,** 1111.

Lemarchand-Beraud, T. R., and Berthier, C. (1981). *Acta Endocrinol. (Copenhagen)* **97,** 74.

Maghuin-Rogister, G., Hennen, G., Closset, J., and Kopeyan, C. (1976). *Eur. J. Biochem.* **61,** 157.

Magner, J. A., and Weintraub, B. D. (1982). *J. Biol. Chem.* **257,** 6709.

Magner, J. A., and Weintraub, B. D. (1984). *In* "The Thyroid" (S. H. Ingbar and L. E. Braverman, eds.). Harper, New York (in press).

Marshall, M. C., Jr., Williams, D., and Weintraub, B. D. (1981). *Endocrinology* **108,** 908.

Maxam, A. M., and Gilbert, W. (1980). *Methods Enzymol.* **65,** 499.

McMaster, G. C., and Carmichael, G. C. (1977). *Proc. Natl. Acad. Sci. U.S.A.* **74,** 4835.

Miksicek, R. J., and Towle, H. C. (1983). *J. Biol. Chem.* **258,** 9575.

Moldow, R. L., and Yalow, R. S. (1978). *Life Sci.* **22,** 1859.

Morgan, F. J., Birken, S., and Canfield, R. E. (1975). *J. Biol. Chem.* **250,** 5247.

Nilson, J. H., Thomason, A. R., Cserbak, M. T., Moneman, C. L., and Woychik, R. P. (1983). *J. Biol. Chem.* **258,** 4679.

Ottenweller, J. E., and Hedge, G. A. (1982). *Endocrinology* **111,** 515.

Parnes, J. R., Velan, B., Felsenfeld, A., Ramanathan, L., Ferrini, U., Appella, E., and Seidman, J. G. (1981). *Proc. Natl. Acad. Sci. U.S.A.* **78,** 2253.

Parsons, T. F., and Pierce, J. G. (1980). *Proc. Natl. Acad. Sci. U.S.A.* **77,** 7089.

Parsons, T. F., Bloomfield, G. A., and Pierce, J. G. (1983). *J. Biol. Chem.* **258,** 240.

Pelham, H. R. B., and Jackson, R. J. (1976). *Eur. J. Biochem.* **67,** 247.

Peterson, R. E., Kourides, I. A., Horwith, M., Vaughan, E. D., Jr., Saxena, B. B., and Fraser, R. A. R. (1981). *J. Clin. Endocrinol. Metab.* **52,** 692.

Pierce, J. G. (1971). *Endocrinology* **89,** 1331.

Pierce, J. G., and Parsons, T. F. (1981). *Annu. Rev. Biochem.* **50,** 465.

Pierce, J. G., Liao, T. H., Howard, S. M., Shome, B., and Cornell, J. S. (1971). *Recent Prog. Horm. Res.* **27,** 165.

Pierce, J. G., Liao, T. H., and Carlsen, R. B. (1973). *In* "Hormonal Proteins and Peptides" (C. H. Li, ed.), Vol. 1. p. 17. Academic Press, New York.

Prentice, L. G., and Ryan, R. J. (1975). *J. Clin. Endocrinol. Metab.* **40,** 303.

Rayford, P. L., Vaitukaitis, J. L., Ross, G. T., Morgan, F. J., and Canfield, R. E. (1972). *Endocrinology* **91,** 144.

Rigby, P. W. J., Dieckmann, M., Rhodes, C., and Berg, P. (1977). *J. Mol. Biol.* **113,** 237.

Roberts, B. E., and Paterson, B. M. (1973). *Proc. Natl. Acad. Sci. U.S.A.* **70,** 2330.

Ross, D. S., Downing M. F., Chin, W. W., Kieffer, J. D., and Ridgway, E. C. (1983a). *Endocrinology* **112,** 187.

Ross, D. S., Downing, M. F., Chin, W. W., Kieffer, J. D., and Ridgway, E. C. (1983b). *Endocrinology* **112,** 2050.

Rowe, D. W., Moen, R. C., Davidson, J. M., Byers, P. H., Bornstein, P., and Palmiter, R. D. (1978). *Biochemistry* **17,** 1581.

Sairam, M. R., and Li, C-H (1977). *Can. J. Biochem.* **55,** 755.

Schorr-Toshav, N. L., Gurr, J. A., Catterall, J. F., and Kourides, I. A. (1983a). *Endocrinology* **112,** 1434.

Schorr-Toshav, N. L., Halmi, N. S., Wurzel, J. M., and Kourides, I. A. (1983b). *Horm. Metab. Res.* **15,** 485.

Shome, B., and Parlow, A. F. (1973). *J. Clin. Endocrinol. Metab.* **36,** 618.

Silva, J. E., and Larsen, P. R. (1978). *Endocrinology* **102,** 1783.

Silva, J. E., and Larsen, P. R. (1979). *Science* **198,** 502.

Southern, E. M. (1975). *J. Mol. Biol.* **98,** 503.

Spindler, S. R., Mellon, S. H., and Baxter, J. D. (1982). *J. Biol. Chem.* **257,** 11627.

Spira, O., Birkenfeld, A., Avni, A., Gross, J., and Gordon, A. (1979). *Acta Endocrinol. (Copenhagen)* **92,** 502.

Struck, D. K., and Lennarz, W. J. (1977). *J. Biol. Chem.* **252,** 1007.

Tabas, I., Schlesinger, S., and Kornfeld, S. (1978). *J. Biol. Chem.* **253,** 716.

Talmadge, K., Boorstein, W. R., and Fiddes, J. C. (1983). *DNA* **2**, 279.

Tepper, M. A., Dionne, F. T., Gee, C. E., and Roberts, J. L. (1983). *Endocrinology* **112**, 118 (Abstr.).

Thomas, P. (1980). *Proc. Natl. Acad. Sci. U.S.A.* **77**, 5201.

Vale, W., Grant, G., Amoss, M., Blackwell, R., and Guillemin, R. (1972). *Endocrinology* **91**, 562.

Vamvakopoulos, N. C., and Kourides, I. A. (1979). *Proc. Natl. Acad. Sci. U.S.A.* **76**, 3809.

Waechter, C. J., and Lennarz, W. J. (1976). *Annu. Rev. Biochem.* **49**, 95.

Wahl, G. M., Stern, M., and Stark, G. (1979). *Proc. Natl. Acad. Sci. U.S.A.* **76**, 3683.

Weintraub, B. D., Krauth, G., Rosen, S. W., and Rabson, A. S. (1975). *J. Clin. Invest.* **56**, 1043.

Weintraub, B. D., Stannard, B. S., Linnekin, D., and Marshall, M. (1980). *J. Biol. Chem.* **255**, 5715.

Weintraub, B. D., Gershengorn, M. C., Kourides, I. A., and Fein, H. (1981). *Ann. Intern. Med.* **95**, 339.

Weintraub, B. D., Stannard, B. S., and Meyers, L. (1983). *Endocrinology* **112**, 1331.

Winberry, L. K., Morris, S. M., Jr., Fisch, J. E., Glynias, M. J., Jenik, R. A., and Goodridge, A. G. (1983). *J. Biol. Chem.* **258**, 1337.

Wurzel, J. M., Curatola, L. M., Gurr, J. A., Goldschmidt, A. M., and Kourides, I. A. (1983). *Endocrinology* **113**, 1854.

DISCUSSION

J. H. Oppenheimer: That was a lovely presentation. You are assuming that the regulation of mRNA levels occurs at a transcriptional level. Have you had a chance to examine potential nuclear precursor forms of the mRNAs coding for subunits to substantiate this assumption? Moreover, have you any thoughts about the role of the protein which has been postulated by Bowers to be synthesized in response to T_3 and to function as an inhibitor of TSH secretion?

I. A. Kourides: I presume that when you say precursor forms, you mean precursor forms of messenger RNA and the processing of the messenger RNA. We have not yet done such experiments; in fact, I should be careful to point out that our studies look at a pre-translational level of regulation, but they have not directly looked at transcription. In other words, there may be direct effects on the primary message transcript, effects on message processing, or effects on messenger RNA stability.

J. H. Oppenheimer: Have you done any "runoff" experiments?

I. A. Kourides: No, but we plan to do these experiments. My personal bias is that there will be strong transcriptional control. However, we have no data now which address the question of how T_3 affects transcription.

G. D. Aurbach: Ione thank you very much for a very lucid and interesting presentation on biosynthesis of the subunits. You implied that bromocryptine inhibits messenger RNA formation for at least the α subunit and TRH stimulates production of TSH α and β subunits. What would you suppose would be the intracellular mediator of these control mechanisms, cyclic AMP, calcium? Do you have any thoughts or ideas on that question?

I. A. Kourides: I see no necessity that cyclic AMP would have to be involved, and, in fact, there are data from which it seems clear that the action of TRH does not require cyclic AMP to stimulate TSH; cAMP is not involved as an intermediary in TRH action; from the work of several investigators including Gershengorn, the "second messenger" for TRH is probably calcium. In addition, bromocryptine or other dopamine agonists do not appear to act via cyclic AMP. At this point we have no data concerning specific intracellular interme-diates in terms of TSH regulation. Our data show for bromocryptine that there is an effect on both α and TSH-β mRNA. I tried to point out that the greater effect on α mRNA that we have seen could imply an action on gonadotropin α messenger RNA. We will now study this possibility more carefully.

G. D. Aurbach: One further question. Are there any experiments using calcium ionophores to determine whether changes in intracellular calcium could influence directly mRNA formation for either subunit?

I. A. Kourides: Not in the TSH system. There are studies in GH cells looking at the effects of calcium on growth hormone and prolactin mRNA levels. Dr. Carter Bancroft is probably in the audience and has been involved in some of these studies of the effects of calcium on message levels for growth hormone and prolactin; I don't know if he would care to make any comment.

F. C. Bancroft: We have shown that calcium causes a large (10- to 20-fold) stimulation of cytoplasmic and nuclear prolactin RNA sequences in the GH$_3$ cells, while causing at most a 2-fold stimulation of growth hormone mRNA [White and Bancroft (1981). *J. Biol. Chem.* **256,** 5942]. We have also demonstrated a calcium requirement for the stimulation by thyro-tropin-releasing hormone (TRH) of prolactin mRNA in the GH$_3$ cells, implying that calcium acts as a mediator of the action of TRH on prolactin gene expression [White and Bancroft (1983). *J. Biol. Chem.* **258,** 4618]. Similar studies with epidermal growth factor (EGF) (White and Bancroft, 1983) together with recent preliminary studies examining the ability of calmo-dulin inhibitors to block the stimulation by EGF, of prolactin mRNA, suggest that calcium may also act as a mediator of the action of EGF on prolactin gene expression.

R. T. Stone: In reference to the α excess: Have you conducted experiments in which you looked at the rate of accumulation of α and β thyroid mRNA in a hypothyroid animal and stimulated with TSH?

I. A. Kourides: You asked whether we have looked at the rate of appearance of α or β message. As I stated, we haven't yet done all the time course experiments with thyroid hormone that we plan to do. We have studied different doses, but we have not done different time courses; we hope to do these experiments soon. Thus, I cannot answer what the rate of change is in the decrease of α or β message with thyroid hormone.

J. E. Rall: It seems that with T$_3$ you get more of an inhibition of β than α message, and with TRH you get some stimulation of both messages. This seem curious because you can stimulate two very different messages with the same agent. Do you think there is a common regulatory function somewhere in the 5' regions of the genes for β and α or do you think that TRH has sort of a general metabolic effect which secondarily enhances synthesis of both messages?

I. A. Kourides: We plan in the future experiments to look closely at the 5' regions of α and β TSH genes. We, too, have noted that, with certain hormones like T$_3$, there is a very discordant effect on α and β TSH gene expression. Yet it appears that other hormones which have a more modest effect on message seem to have more balanced effects. The more balanced effect of TRH and in preliminary experiments, of dexamethasone on α and β TSH mRNA is probably not just a random event. Whatever the exact interaction is between RNA polymerase and TSH genes, I suspect that there should be similarities in the 5' regions of both α and β TSH genes but also sufficient differences so that with specific hormones one could regulate α gene expression differentially from that of β TSH. I think that the level of regulation is probably going to be predominantly transcriptional; I have no data on how this transcriptional event occurs. It is possible that there could be synthesis of some inhibitory protein product that somehow interacted with the polymerases or chromatin to decrease TSH gene expression. Since this is strictly hypothetical at this point, it is perhaps not worthy of further comment.

J. Fiddes: I was very interested in your observation that there are maybe two β TSH genes because my prediction might have been that LH, FSH, and TSH might be similar in having only one gene. So I wonder how sure you are that these are two genes and what the differences are between the genes? Also is there any possibility that they may be alleles?

I. A. Kourides: I have already stated everything we know at this time about these two TSH-β genes. We have not yet subcloned them, and thus we have not done nucleotide sequencing. What we are reasonably sure of is that they have different sizes one being 1.8 kb or less and the other 1.4 kb or less. Nevertheless, their overall structure is quite similar. On the other hand, the genomic flanking regions of these genes are different so it appears that there are two genes. However, it is conceivable once the sequencing is done that the genes are actually the same and are duplicated and placed in the genome in different places. In addition, even if the mouse had two TSH-β genes, that would not necessarily imply that the human could have two as well. For example, rats have two insulin genes, whereas humans have only one insulin gene. We have not yet determined whether these two TSH-β genes could be alleles. Further work will be needed to define that.

J. Fiddes: Of course I agree it is not at all surprising that these genes were duplicated independently.

I. A. Kourides: No it is not surprising.

J. Fiddes: What about the situation in the rat? Is there a single α subunit gene and how many β subunit genes?

I. A. Kourides: We have not looked at rat genes. Originally, the implication had been from Chin's work that there might be two rat α genes; I think that he now believes there is only one rat α gene, but I am not sure of that. From Roberts' work, it is clear that there is only one rat LH-β gene, and I believe that Chin concurs on this point.

K. Sterling: This was very impressive. However, there is one thing that bothers me a little about the T_3 inhibition of the levels of messenger RNA. I believe that if T_3 is administered to a hypothyroid rat that TSH will fall within an hour and with the presumably long half-times of mRNA, I wonder if there isn't a much later effect on TSH synthesis, which doubtless is suppressed and whether there aren't other immediate mechanisms in operation.

I. A. Kourides: We have not yet done the studies to look at time points shorter than 4 days. We did the longer time points first because we were sure that we were going to see an effect then; we are now going back to look at shorter time periods in a fashion similar to the way we decreased the dose of T_3 to look at the minimum dose affecting TSH-β mRNA levels.

R. O. Greep: With great timidity I venture a question. You mentioned that the α and β genes were on different chromosomes. I wonder if you have found that awkward. Does it mean that they evolved at different times and, if they did, this would involve anticipation on the part of nature which I think doesn't exist.

I. A. Kourides: There is no definitive answer to any evolutionary question. However, there is certainly precedent for genes for various proteins being located on different chromosomes. Nature does not seem to be uncomfortable with it. In fact, α and β globin gene families are on different chromosomes, and the genes for heavy and light chains of the immunoglobulins are on multiple different chromosomes.

N. B. Schwartz: If you transplant a TSH-secreting tumor into an intact mouse, rather than one whose thyroid has been destroyed, at what level are the T_3 and the TSH regulated? Is there any regulation or does the tumor simply take over and continue to drive the thyroid?

I. A. Kourides: TSH-secreting pituitary tumors will very rarely grow in a euthyroid animal; it is only when these tumors become autonomous and do not make any TSH or TSH-β, although they may still make a little α, that they will grow in euthyroid animals. By necessity, a hypothyroid recipient is needed.

N. B. Schwartz: So then when is a tumor not a tumor? That is, should this be regarded as a tumor if it can be totally suppressed in the presence of its target gland?

I. A. Kourides: By classical pathologic criteria, these are tumors. These pituitary adenomata are quite benign and, therefore, a good model system to study TSH regulation because they are regulated by hormones in a fashion qualitatively similarly to the normal pituitary gland.

A. Means: Concerning the chromosomal localization studies, I think it should be pointed out that the use of intraspecies somatic cell genetics can be very difficult. It has been shown by Mary Riser (Baylor College of Medicine) that if you do not have as many as 50 hybrids to do a statistical analysis you can arrive at different conclusions. She recently carried out experiments where she used the α and β subunit of human chorionic gonadotropin, insulin, and adenosine deaminase all in humans and found with a statistical evaluation of 50 cells that she could feel reasonably comfortable about the chromosomal assignments of these four genes. Mary Harper from the University of California, San Diego used an *in situ* procedure that she has developed with Grady Saunders using precisely the same probes. In the four cases where Riser had reported statistically significant differences, Harper could confirm those localizations. Parenthetically, the comments about human hCG or human chorionic gonadotropin being on 10 and 18 have now been confirmed by at least two independent criteria in two different laboratories.

I. A. Kourides: That is an interesting point about α and β CG gene chromosomal localization. I would like to make a general comment about somatic cell hybrids. Somatic cell hybrids could cause confusion in chromosomal localization if one does not appreciate that a particular chromosome may only be present in a certain percentage of those hybrids and that the percentage is not always zero or 100. Thus, it is important to screen enough hybrids to have enough hybrid cells that are clear-cut positives or negatives. There is not necessarily a magic number of hybrid cells that should be studied, however.

The Mouse Mammary Tumor Virus Model in Studies of Glucocorticoid Regulation

GORDON L. HAGER, HELENE RICHARD-FOY,[1] MICHAEL KESSEL,[2] DAVID WHEELER, ALEX C. LICHTLER, AND MICHAEL C. OSTROWSKI

Laboratory of Tumor Virus Genetics, National Cancer Institute, National Institutes of Health, Bethesda, Maryland

I. The Mouse Tumor Virus Model

Steroid hormones are now thought to exert a variety of regulatory effects on their target cell's metabolism primarily through the pleiotropic modulation of gene expression. A general model incorporating currently accepted concepts in the mechanism of steroid hormone action is presented in Fig. 1. Under this model, high-affinity binding of steroid to its receptor is thought to induce a conformational change in the protein, resulting in an altered DNA (chromatin) affinity. Early subcellular fractionation studies suggested that the receptor was located primarily in the cytosol prior to hormone binding, migrating to the nucleus only after activation. This aspect of the model (cytosolic localization followed by nuclear translocation) is now questioned by some, but the general features of the model (gene activation by chromatin association of a hormone altered regulatory protein) remain intact.

Efforts to understand the mechanisms by which steroids mediate their regulatory effects have focused over the past two decades on a number of model gene systems. Experimental evidence suggesting that the expression of mouse mammary tumor virus (MMTV), a B-type retrovirus, was subject to regulation by hormones emerged more than 20 years ago (Smoller *et al.,* 1961; reviewed in Young and Hager, 1979). McGrath (1971) demonstrated that glucocorticoids were among the most potent modulators of MMTV expression. Young *et al.* (1977) and Ringold *et al.* (1977) subsequently presented evidence that the major effect on MMTV expres-

---

[1] Present address: Universite de Paris XI, Department de Chimie Biologique, Lab Hormones, 94270 Bicetre, France.

[2] Present address: Department of Mikrobiolgie, University of Heidelberg, Im Neuenheimer Feld 230, 6900 Heidelberg, Federal Republic of Germany.

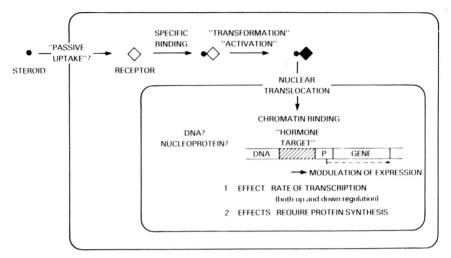

FIG. 1.   Model for steroid hormone action.

sion by glucocorticoid was at the transcriptional level. This finding focused the attention of several laboratories on the MMTV model.

The introduction of recombinant DNA technology in the 1970s, and the parallel demonstration of calcium phosphate mediated introduction of DNA into mammalian cells, permitted a direct approach to the identification of sequences involved in hormone regulation. Molecular clones of MMTV were first characterized by Donehower *et al.* (1980); the DNA sequence of the MMTV promoter and associated regulatory regions quickly became available (Hager and Donehower, 1980; Donehower *et al.*, 1981).

The life cycle (Fig. 2) of RNA tumor viruses (retroviruses) involves first the conversion of the RNA genomic information to a double-standard DNA form (unintegrated replication intermediate) by reverse transcription, then the integration of this DNA form into cellular DNA (provirus). The proviral DNA is then recognized by the normal cellular transcription apparatus (RNA polymerase II), and expression of viral messenger RNA and genomic RNA occurs. During reverse transcription of the RNA genome, sequences from the 3′ end of viral RNA (U3 sequences) are transposed to the left end of the DNA replication intermediate, and sequences from the 5′ end (U5 sequences) are copied at the right end, creating structures now referred to as the long terminal repeat (LTR). During integration, the topology of the viral genome is maintained; that is, the viral gene order is conserved, with one LTR at each end. One consequence of this process is that the sequences immediately upstream from

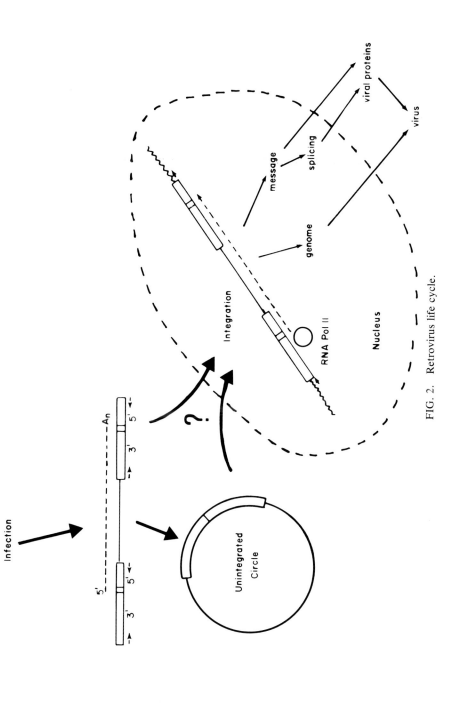

FIG. 2. Retrovirus life cycle.

the site of viral RNA transcription initiation (U3) are in fact encoded by the virus itself.

This unique structure suggests two models for the location of sequences putatively involved in the regulation of viral transcription. The sequences either would be located in the U3 region of the LTR (or possibly within other regions of viral DNA), or within cellular sequences that become juxtaposed to the viral LTR during the integration event. The availability of molecular clones of MMTV (Donehower *et al.*, 1980) immediately suggested a test of these models. Fusion of the MMTV promoter to a gene that was selectable in cultured cells, and whose expression was not normally regulated by hormone, should allow the identification of sequences containing the hormone regulatory information.

II. Identification of Glucocorticoid Regulatory Sequences

The experiment suggested above was first successfully carried out by two laboratories. We (Huang *et al.*, 1981) fused the 3' LTR from an MMTV proviral clone to the oncogene (v-ras) from Harvey murine sarcoma virus (HaMuSV; Hager *et al.*, 1979), and introduced the resulting chimeras into NIH 3T3 cells by calcium phosphate mediated transfection. We were able to show that the level of the transformation gene product (p21) was subject to regulation by dexamethasone (a synthetic glucocorticoid) in foci of transformed cells derived with these fusions. Furthermore, the appropriate fusion transcripts could be indentified in the transformants, and the steady-state concentration of this fusion transcript was induced by dexamethasone. For some of the cell lines derived in these experiments, the transformed phenotype of the cell was also subject to regulation by the presence or absence of hormone in the culture medium (Hager *et al.*, 1982). Lee *et al.* (1981) independently reported the transfer of regulation to the expression of dihydrofolate reductase. These experiments unambiguously established that the regulatory sequences must be within the viral LTR, since the normal pathway for viral integration was not operative in the transfection experiments, and a mechanism for the acquisition of specific cell sequences was therefore not available.

III. Assays for Glucocorticoid Responsiveness

The successful transfer of hormone regulation to genes normally unresponsive to hormone action provides an experimental method for further localization of sequences involved in the regulatory response. We have mapped these sequences by three independent methods.

1. We noted in our first experiments (Huang *et al.*, 1981) that the efficiency with which transformed foci could be recovered with the MMTV LTR-v-ras fusions was extremely low (approximately 1–5 foci/μg chimeric DNA). This was a surprising finding since the MMTV LTR can be a very strong promoter, at least in viral-infected cells.

We subsequently discovered (Ostrowski and Hager, 1983; Ostrowski *et al.*, 1984) that the addition of a viral enhancer element from the HaMuSV LTR to the MMTV LTR-v-ras increased the specific transformation potential (foci/μg DNA) by a factor of 50- to 100-fold. This high-efficiency focus-formation was observed, however, only when dexamethasone was present in the culture medium during the transfection protocol. The extreme sensitivity of this assay to the presence of hormone provides the basis for a rapid and simple test for hormone responsiveness of a given LTR deletion.

2. A more direct assay of transcriptional activity at a given promoter is to monitor the expression of RNA initiated at that promoter (or a gene product synthesized from that RNA) for DNA introduced into cells before it has become integrated. This kind of experiment is referred to as a transient expression assay, to distinguish it from the case where expression occurs at an integrated locus in stably transformed cell lines. Gorman *et al.* (1982) developed a sensitive transient expression system based on the chloramphenicol acetyl transferase (CAT) gene from the bacterial Tn9 transposon. We have developed vectors that contain the CAT gene under transcriptional control of the MMTV LTR (Kessel *et al.*, 1984). The expression of CAT activity in L cells transfected with these molecules is inducible by dexamethasone, providing a second assay for hormone responsiveness.

3. A third approach to the mapping of hormone responsive sequences is simply to analyze the large variety of MMTV proviruses that occur in all strains of laboratory mice, and ask if naturally occurring mutations are present in the LTRs of these strains that would serve to further localize the regions essential for regulation.

IV. Localization of the Glucocorticoid Regulatory Element by Gene Transfer

The data obtained from the first two types of assays, hormone-dependent acquisition of stable transformants, and hormone-responsive CAT activity in transient expression, are summarized from the work of Kessel *et al.* (1984). In both assay systems, the deletion of the left half of the LTR has no effect on the observed induction ratio compared to the complete LTR. In the stable transformation assay, further deletion of sequences to position approximately −350 also has little effect. Deletion of sequences between −350 and −105 results in a gradual loss of inducible transformation, until at position −105 the number of foci recovered in the presence of hormone is not significantly different than the number found in the absence of dexamethasone.

In the CAT transient expression assay, deletion of sequences between −650 and −179 also gives rise to an gradual of inducibility. In both assay systems, hormone responsiveness is lost in an incremental fashion over a considerable distance, as opposed to an abrupt change over a few nucleotides. The difference between the highly inducible complete LTR and the totally unresponsive −105 deletions must reflect the loss of sequences necessary for hormone induction. The incremental loss of induction could arise from a variety of sources. First, the position of the enhancer element in the LTR-v-ras fusions is transposed closer to the transcription initiation site as more sequences are deleted. The increase in uninduced, or constitutive, activity could therefore be due to an increased enhancer effect with decreasing distance. It is more difficult to explain the parallel rise in constitutive activity in the CAT transient expression deletions, because the enhancer element in these molecules is position invariant at the 3′ end of the CAT gene. The 5′ distance from the activator to the MMTV promoter cap site is more than 4 kb in this construction.

Alternatively, the increase in expression in the absence of hormone as sequences in the right half of the LTR are deleted might indicate a possible negative effect of these sequences. It is striking that with the complete LTR, in both the stable transformation assay and the transient expression assay, the fully induced expression is approximately equivalent to that found in each type of assay with a comparable hormone nonresponsive promoter. Thus, when the v-ras gene is driven by the HaMuSV LTR (which contains the MSV enhancer), the number of foci obtained is about the same as the induced number of foci found with the MMTV LTR-driven v-ras fusion activated with the MSV enhancer; also, the level of CAT activity found with a HaMuSV CAT fusion is approximately the same as that found with the induced MMTV LTR CAT chimera (data not shown). In both cases, the expression level for chimeras containing the complete LTR in the absence of hormone is quite low compared to the nonresponsive promoters. In other words, the presence of intact sequences containing the hormone-responsive element leads to a low activity promoter. We have speculated elsewhere on possible mechanisms for this negative effect (Hager et al., 1983). The final resolution of this issue must await the construction of point mutations that have a strong effect on induction ratios with no change in enhancer position. Such studies are underway.

We conclude at this point that the primary sequences involved in the hormone response are located between positions −350 and −105. The mutations discussed in the next section further suggest that critical sequences are located to the right of position −215. The incremental loss of regulation observed in both assays might correspond to a multiple number of hormone-receptor binding sites; such a multiplicity of sites has in fact been suggested (Payvar *et al.*, 1982; Scheidereit *et al.*, 1983).

V. Naturally Occurring Mutations in the MMTV LTR

All laboratory strains of mice and most wild mouse populations harbor several endogenous MMTV proviruses in their genomes. Some strains in addition carry vertically transmitted viruses. A total of 17 unique proviral sequences have now been characterized by restriction mapping and segregation patterns (Traina *et al.*, 1981). These various molecules provide a potential source of naturally occurring mutations in the promoter and regulatory regions of the LTR. We have molecularly cloned a number of these proviral elements (Donehower *et al.*, 1980), and have sequenced the LTR elements of the C3H-S infectious virus (Donehower *et al.*, 1981), the unit II endogenous provirus (Donehower *et al.*, 1983), and the Mtv-1 (or unit V) provirus (Johnson and Hager, 1984). In addition, the LTR sequence is available from other laboratories for the GR-P virus (Fasel *et al.*, 1982), and the GR-40 sequence endogenous to the GR genome (this provirus is apparently identical to the C3H-S unit II). The C3H-S LTR has been independently sequenced by Majors and Varmus (1983).

A sequence comparison of the four completely sequenced LTRs is presented in Fig. 3. Two striking generalization emerge from this comparison. First, although a large number of point mutations have arisen in the LTRs of these strains since their divergence, the open reading frame that covers the leftward 72% of the LTR is maintained in all four LTRs. The conservation of the reading frame strongly indicates that selection pressure must exist at the protein level, and a gene product must be expressed from this locus. Two groups have in fact recently reported the identification of a uniquely spliced MMTV messenger RNA that uniquely encode the pLTR gene product (Wheeler *et al.*, 1983; Van Ooyen *et al.*, 1983). It can be concluded that a fourth gene, whose function is currently not understood, is present in the MMTV genome. It is highly unlikely that this gene is involved in hormone regulation, since the complete reading frame can be deleted from chimeric fusions with little effect on the observed hormone response (see Section IV).

The second striking feature of the sequence comparison is the apparent mutational hot spot between positions −350 and −450 (numbering from

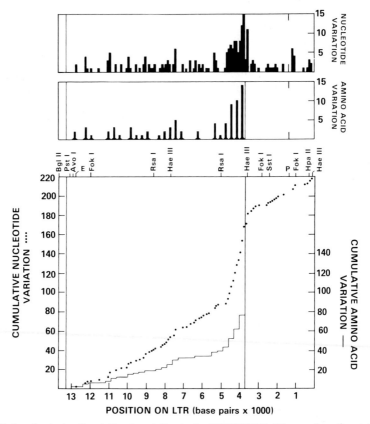

FIG. 3.   Analysis of mutational variation in the MMTV LTR. The number of mutations that have accumulated in LTRs for which the complete sequences are available have been plotted against position in the LTR. The corresponding variation for the open reading frame (or putative pLTR gene product) has also been presented. The data for this analysis include the C3H-S LTR (Donehower *et al.*, 1981; Majors and Varmus, 1983), the C3H unit II LTR (Donehower *et al.*, 1983) [identical to the GR-40 endogenous sequence (Kennedy *et al.*, 1982)], the C3H Mtv-1 provirus (Johnson and Hager, unpublished observations), and the GR-P LTR (Fasel *et al.*, 1982).

the right end of the LTR). The large variation in this region is due primarily to a large sequence rearrangement in the Mtv-1 provirus. The DNA sequences in this region for each of the molecules is presented in Fig. 4. With respect to the cap site for the initiation of transcription, there are essentially no conserved sequences between position −215 and position −325. Despite this major sequence rearrangement, however, when the Mtv-1 LTR is introduced into mouse X/C cells by transfection, Mtv-1 specific RNA in initiated at the correct cap site, and the expression of this

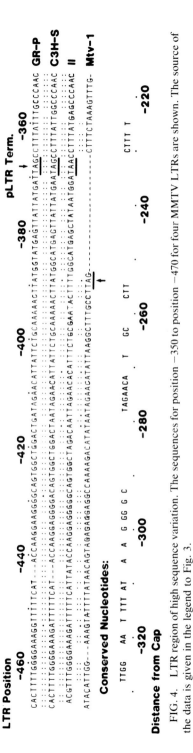

FIG. 4. LTR region of high sequence variation. The sequences for position −350 to position −470 for four MMTV LTRs are shown. The source of the data is given in the legend to Fig. 3.

RNA is subject to normal hormone regulation (10- to 15-fold induction; L. Johnson and G. Hager, unpublished observations). We therefore conclude that sequences between -325 and -215 are unessential for promoter function and hormone regulation. Coupled with the data from the gene fusion deletions discussed in Section IV, particularly the wild-type responsiveness found with the -350 LTR-v-ras fusion, these results would suggest that the critical region of the hormone response element is to the right of position -215. Further deletion to positions -179, -150, and -105 inactivates the regulatory element. The location of the hormone response element by mutational analysis is consistent with the finding of glucocorticoid receptor binding sites in the same region of the LTR DNA (Payvar *et al.*, 1982; Scheidereit *et al.*, 1983), suggesting at this level of analysis that the site functionally identified by deletion analysis is in fact a hormone receptor complex binding site. The utilization of site-directed mutagenesis of this region in the functional assays we have described should now permit a high-resolution definition of the regulatory site.

VI. Analysis of Hormone Action on Minichromosomes

The genomic DNA of mammalian cells is organized in a complex nucleoprotein structure. The basic repeating unit of this structure, the chromatosome, consists of a nucleosome and an associated length of DNA, between 140 and 220 bp. One function of this complex is to pack the very large amount of DNA present in eukaryotic cells into as small a structure as possible. Considerable evidence is now available that the local chromatin environment may also play a role in the regulation of gene expression. Genes actively involved in transcription are more sensitive to a variety of deoxynucleolytic enzymes, indicating a more open chromatin configuration (Weintraub and Groudine, 1976). In addition to this "open" structure of active genes, localized changes in chromatin structure that are detected as hypersensitive sites have been shown to occur in a variety of systems (for a review of this subject, see Elgin, 1981), and frequently (but not always) map to the 5' nontranscribed sequences, where potential regulatory sequences are expected to occur. It is now clear that these site-specific changes in nucleoprotein organization correlate well with gene activation. It is not clear whether these changes reflect an alteration in chromatin induced by the action of transcription factors that forms a nucleoprotein template structure critically required for expression of a given gene, or whether these changes simply reflect secondary perturbations of the structure accompanying the interaction of soluble regulatory molecules with sites on DNA.

Chromatin organization must also play some role in the response of target genes to hormone induction. The sequences responsive to a given hormone are frequently quite cell-specific, even though receptors for the hormone might be present in a wide variety of cell types. Indeed, Weintraub and Groudine (1983) have recently reported the activation of DNase I hypersensitive sites in sequences around the vitellogenin gene upon stimulation by estrogen.

The difficulty in dealing with the high complexity of sequence information in mammalian DNA has largely been overcome by the application of recombinant DNA technology. It is not possible, however, to study chromatin structure and its alterations with these techniques because the structures cannot be reproduced in the prokaryotic hosts used in molecular cloning. Recent efforts in our laboratory have focused on attempts to develop a system in mammalian cells for the amplification of noncomplex episomes containing hormone target promoters, with the goal of characterization and purification of these minichromosomes as nucleoprotein particles. Figure 5 is a schematic representation of this strategy. The establishment of plasmids containing the regulated MMTV promoter would permit a direct examination of the role of chromatin structure in hormone action.

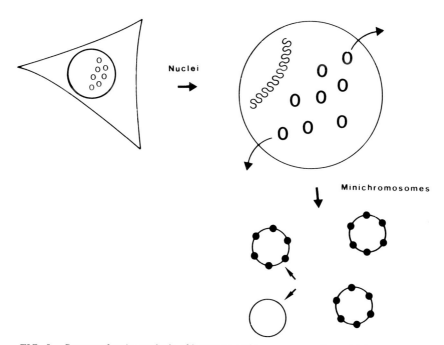

FIG. 5.   Strategy for the analysis of hormone action on noncomplex minichromosomes.

The vector we have utilized in these experiments is the bovine papilloma virus (BPV). It has been demonstrated that a fragment of this virus DNA (69% transforming fragment) can support stable replication in the episomal state of foreign pieces of DNA ligated to the fragment (see Law *et al.*, 1982, for a description of the BPV vector system). We have accordingly inserted a variety of MMTV-LTR fusions into the BPV vector, and generated clonal mouse cell lines transformed with these chimeric fusions (Ostrowski *et al.*, 1983).

VII. BPV-LTR Fusions Replicate Episomally

Figure 6 presents the structure of a typical BPV LTR construction, pm19. This molecule contains the MMTV LTR-v-ras fusion (Huang *et al.*, 1981) and the *Bam*HI–*Hin*dIII fragment of BPV. Plasmid pBR322 sequences for replication of the chimera in bacteria have been removed before introducing the vector into mouse cells.

Figure 7 presents a Southern blot analysis of total DNA from a cell line developed after transfection with pm19 DNA. The blot has been hybrid-

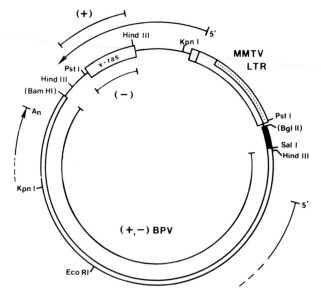

FIG. 6.   Map of the minichromosome present in clone 935.1. The structure of the episome replicating in clone 935.1 is presented. This clone was generated by transforming mouse C127 cells with DNA from plasmid pM19 (Ostrowski *et al.*, 1983), from which the pBR322 sequences had been deleted. The concentric blocks represent the regions of the chimeric DNA subcloned in M13 single-stranded phage for use as hybridization probes in the transcription extension experiments (see Fig. 9).

ized with probes specific for the LTR, v-ras, and BPV segments of the chimera. A comparison of the fragment sizes observed with each probe (shown at the right of each panel, Fig. 7) with the predictions for a circular molecule (legend to Fig. 7) indicates that the structure of sequences detected with these probes is consistent with an amplified circular molecule. Furthermore, unrestricted chimeric DNA isolated from this cell line migrates in gels as form I and form II circular DNA (data not shown). Finally, the episomal DNA can be isolated in a highly enriched fraction from these cells, and can be shown by electron microscopic visualization to contain monomeric, circular molecules of the predicted size (A. Beyers, personal communication).

The copy number control included in lane 1 (Fig. 7c) indicates that the episomes are replicating to high copy number in this cell line (approximately 200 copies/cell). Since the mouse cells carrying these episomes contain endogenous MMTV proviruses in their genomic DNA, we can address the question of whether one or more integrated copies of the fusion DNA are present in the cell. If the blots with MMTV LTR probe are overexposed to detect the endogenous proviral sequences, no additional bands are detected, indicating that the fusion DNA is uniquely episomal in these cells.

VIII. The LTR Promoter Is Regulated in the Episomal State

The amplified minichromosomes would be of little use if the LTR promoter were not subject to hormone regulation in the episomal state. To address this issue rigorously, we have carried out transcription extension experiments with minichromosomes isolated from induced and uninduced cells. The protocol for this experiment is presented in Fig. 8. Nuclei are isolated from cells harboring high-copy episomes. Minichromosomes are extracted from the nuclei under conditions (Ostrowski et al., 1983) that leave the nuclei intact, giving rise to an episomal fraction highly enriched in plasmid sequences. This fraction is estimated to be approximately 10% pure in terms of DNA mass. Approximately 50% of the transcription extension activity, however, is specific for the episome. This fraction is added to a transcription extension cocktail, and RNA polymerase molecules that were initiated in vivo are allowed to extend in the presence of ^{32}P-labeled nucleotide triphosphates. This labeled RNA is then hybridized to filters to which DNA fragments from specific strands and specific regions of the episomal DNA have been attached. The amount of hybridization to each region is thus a direct measure of the number of polymerase molecules initiated at specific promoters. The BPV 60% transforming fragment promoter (at approximately 4 o'clock on the map in Fig. 6)

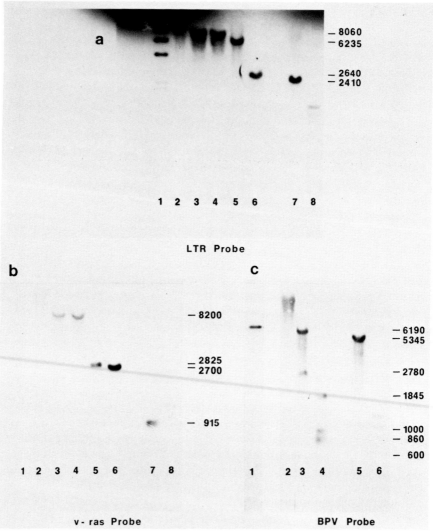

FIG. 7. Structure of BPV-MMTV plasmic replicating in a transformed mouse cell clone. Autoradiograms are shown of Southern blots made with total DNA from clone 935.1, a cell transformed by pM19, a chimeric construction containing MMTV LTR, v-ras, and BPV sequences (see Ostrowski *et al.*, 1983). The blot in a was hybridized to nick-translated LTR probe, b to v-ras probe, and c to BPV probe. Identity of restriction digest performed on DNA samples prior to electrophoresis and blotting is as follows; for each digest, the predicted fragments hybridizing with the probe utilized in that blot are given in brackets (see Ostrowski *et al.*, 1983). (a) Lane 2, *Sal*I [8794]; lane 3, *Eco*RI [8794]; lane 4, *Bam*HI [8794]; lane 5, *Kpn*I [5780]; lane 6, *Pst*I [2673]; lane 7, *Hind*III [2299]; (b) lane 2, *Sal*I [8794]; lane 3, *Eco*RI [8794]; lane 4, *Bam*HI [8794]; lane 5, *Kpn*I [2800]; lane 6, *Pst*I [2673]; lane 7, *Hind*III [893]; (c) lane 2, *Sal*I [8794]; lane 3, *Kpn*I [5780, 2800]; lane 4, *Pst*I [1770, 914, 821-771-723 triplet, 500]; lane 5, *Hind*III [5574]. Ten micrograms of restriction-digested DNA were

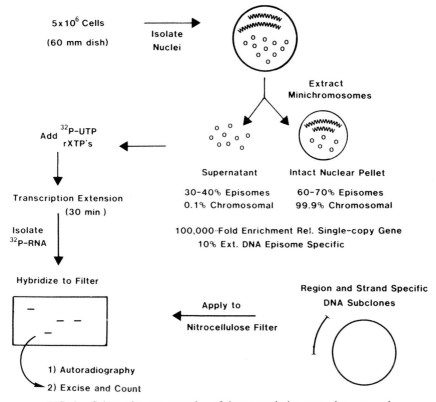

FIG. 8.   Schematic representation of the transcription extension protocol.

serves as a very useful internal control in these experiments, since this promoter would not be expected to be responsive to glucocorticoid regulation.

The results of such an experiment are presented in Fig. 9. It can be seen that a much larger number of RNA polymerase molecules (25-fold increase) extend through the sense strand of the v-ras gene (initiated at the LTR promoter) when the minichromosomes are isolated from cells grown in the presence of hormone, whereas the number of molecules extending

loaded in each gel lane. Land 1 in a and b contain λ-HindIII digested size-markers, while lane 8 in both a and b and lane 6 in c contain φX-HaeIII digested size-markers. Lane 1 in c contains a BPV-MMTV recombinant plasmid that was restricted with EcoRI. The amount of this plasmid loaded on the gel was calculated to be equivalent to 125 copies of episome per cell. The numbers to the right of the figure panels are the sizes of the fragments (in base pairs) hybridizing to the different probes.

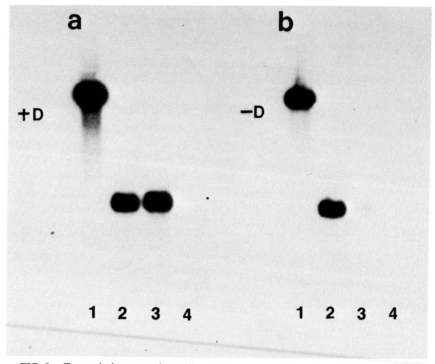

FIG. 9.   Transcription extension with minichromosomes from clone 935.1. Minichromosomes were isolated from 935.1 cells grown in the presence (a) and the absence (b) of
dexamethasone. RNA synthesis was carried out *in vitro* in the presence of ^{32}P-labeled
ribonucleotide triphosphates with endogenous RNA polymerase as described in Ostrowski
et al. (1983). In each panel, lane 1 contains unlabeled DNA from the BPV portion of the
chimera (see Fig. 6), lane 2 contains (−) strand DNA from the v-ras region, lane 3 contains
(+) strand DNA from the v-ras region, and lane 4 contains control M13 DNA. This figure is
reproduced from Ostrowski *et al.* (1983).

through the antisense strand of the v-ras gene, or through the BPV sequences (initiated at the BPV promoter), is unaffected by glucocorticoid
treatment. This constitutes direct evidence that the LTR promoter remains highly inducible when mobilized in the episomal state.

IX. Chromatin Modifications in Response to Hormone Action

We have analyzed chromatin structure of the BPV-LTR minichromosomes for structural alterations that would correlate with activation of
gene expression. First, we have probed for evidence of DNase I hypersensitive sites. These experiments were carried out using the indirect end-
labeling technique pioneered independently by Wu (1980) and by Nedos-

pasov and Georgiev (1980). To detect the presence of sites in the DNA that are unusually sensitive to DNase, chromatin or nulcei are first treated briefly with the enzyme. The DNA is then isolated, and cleaved with restriction enzymes that flank the region of interest. Labeled probes are prepared from short stretches of sequence immediately adjacent to the restriction sites. The DNA is then fractionated by gel electrophoresis and subjected to Southern transfer analysis with these probes. If random nicks have been introduced into the chromatin during the brief DNase digestion, the result from the Southern transfer analysis will be a dispersed pattern of hybridization. If nicks have been introduced into the chromatin at specific sites, then unique fragments will be detected, and the size of these fragments will locate the site of DNase hypersensitivity.

This analysis has been performed with minichromosome chromatin from hormone-treated and untreated cells (Richard-Foy et al., 1984). We detect a DNase I-hypersensitive site in the LTR of the episomal DNA that is present only in chromatin from hormone-induced cells. At the current level of resolution, this site is located approximately between positions -120 and -190 with respect to the cap site. It is unclear at this time whether the size of the hormone-induced hypersensitive site represents an increased sensitivity over a long stretch of sequence, or whether it is simply due to the relatively low resolution gel analysis utilized thus far. Nevertheless, it is quite clear that a change in chromatin structure leading to an increased nucleolytic sensitivity occurs with activation of the LTR promoter by glucocorticoid stimulation. At current levels of resolution, this hypersensitive site overlaps precisely the region that is required in the experiments described in Section IV to transfer hormone regulation. The most likely synthesis of these results is that the hormone-receptor complex binds to the chromatin in this region and induces a structural alteration that is detected as a hypersensitive site. The critical question now becomes whether this change in chromatin structure simply reflects a secondary alteration that results from the interaction of soluble regulatory factors and transcription proteins with DNA, or whether the altered nucleoprotein structure actually serves as a necessary native template for the increased level of gene transcription. The ability to fractionate the minichromosomes, and utilize them as in vitro templates should permit a direct approach to this important issue.

It would seem probable that the finding of this hypersensitive site will have implications for the mechanism of gene activation events other than the special case of hormone induction. Two advantages exist for the functional analysis of this chromatin alteration. The site has been defined on episomal elements that in principle are subject to purification, and the site can be induced at will with a known regulatory molecule.

We have also used the indirect end-labeling technique to ask whether nucleosomes in the region of the LTR promoter on the minichromosomes are nonrandomnly positioned. Early experimental results suggest that nucleosomes are located at specific positions on LTR DNA upstream from the cap site; that is, they are "phased" 5' to the site of transcription initiation. This type of experimental analysis is subject to a variety of artifacts, however; a convincing demonstration of nonrandom nucleosome positioning awaits further experimentation.

X. Summary

Experimental analysis of glucocorticoid regulation of mouse mammary tumor virus expression has proven a productive model for understanding the mechanism of hormone action. In this system the transfer of hormone regulation to genes not normally subject to regulation was first convincingly demonstrated using DNA transfection technology. These powerful tools have permitted the rapid localization of sequences critically involved in the hormone response.

We have shown that regulation of the MMTV promoter can be established for chimeras replicating as small episomal elements. The development of this system enables us to examine the mechanism of hormone activation of gene expression with noncomplex chromatin templates. Normal induction of expression can be demonstrated at the MMTV promoter mobilized in the episomal state, and changes in chromatin structure associated with promoter activation have been characterized. We are encouraged that the very difficult issue of the role of chromatin organization in gene activation can now be addressed in this system.

ACKNOWLEDGMENTS

We wish to acknowledge the important contribution to the experiments discussed here by Mr. Ronald Wolford and Ms. Diana Berard. Without their excellent technical assistance, this work could not have been completed.

REFERENCES

Donehower, L., Andre, J., Berard, D. S., Wolford, R., and Hager, G. L. (1980). *CSH Symp. Quant. Biol.* **44,** 1153.
Donehower, L., Huang, A., and Hager, G. L. (1981). *J. Virol.* **37,** 226.
Donehower, L., Fleurdelys, B., and Hager, G. L. (1983). *J. Virol.* **45,** 941.
Elgin, S. C. R. (1981). *Cell* **27,** 413.
Fasel, N., Pearson, K., Buetti, E.. and Diggelmann, H. (1982). *EMBO J.* **1,** 3.

Gorman, C. M., Moffat, L. F., and Howard, B. H. (1982). *Mol. Cell. Biol.* **2**, 1044.
Hager, G. L. (1983). *Prog. Nucleic Acid Res. Mol. Biol.* **28**, 193.
Hager, G. L., and Donehower, L. A. (1980). *ICN-UCLA Symp. Mol. Cell. Biol.* **18**, 241.
Hager, G. L., Chang, E. H., Chan, H. W., Garon, C. F., Israel, M. A., Martin, M. A., Scolnick, E. M., and Lowy, D. R. (1979). *J. Virol.* **31**, 795.
Hager, G. L., Huang, A. L., Bassin, R. H., and Ostrowski, M. C. (1982). *In* "Eukaryotic Viral Vectors" (Y. Gluzman, ed.), p. 165. Cold Spring Harbor Laboratory, Cold Spring Harbor, New York.
Hager, G. L., Lichtler, A. C., and Ostrowski, M. C. (1983). *In* "Enhancers and Eukaryotic Gene Expression" (Y. Gluzman and T. Shenk, eds.), pp. 161–164. Cold Spring Harbor Laboratory, Cold Spring Harbor, New York.
Huang, A. L., Ostrowski, M. C., Berard, D. S., and Hager, G. L. (1981). *Cell* **27**, 245.
Johnson, L., and Hager, G. L. (1984). *J. Virol.* (submitted).
Kennedy, N., Knedltschek, G., Groner, B., Hynes, N. E., Herrlich, P., Michalides, R., and Van Ooyen, A. J. J. (1982). *Nature (London)* **295**, 622.
Kessel, M., Khoury, G., Lichtler, A. C., Ostrowski, M. C., and Hager, G. L. (1984). *Nucleic Acids Res.* (submitted).
Law, M.-F., Howard, B., Sarver, N., and Howley, P. M. (1982). *In* "Eukaryotic Viral Vectors" (Y. Glusman, ed.), pp. 79–85. Cold Spring Harbor Laboratory, Cold Spring Harbor, New York.
Lee, F., Mulligan, R., Berg, P., and Ringold, G. (1981). *Nature (London)* **294**, 228.
Majors, J. E., and Varmus, H. E. (1983). *J. Virol.* **47**, 495.
McGrath, C. M. (1971). *J. Natl. Cancer Inst.* **47**, 455.
Nedospasov, A., and Georgiev, S. (1980). *Biochem. Biophys. Res. Commun.* **92**, 532.
Ostrowski, M. C., and Hager, G. L. (1983a). *In* "Workshop on Gene Transfer and Cancer." Raven, New York (in press).
Ostrowski, M. C., Richard-Foy, H., Wolford, R. G., Berard, D. S., and Hager, G. L. (1983b). *J. Cell. Mol. Biol.* **11**, 2045.
Ostrowski, M. C., Huang, A. L., Kessel, M., Wolford, R. G., and Hager, G. L. (1984). *EMBO J.* (submitted).
Payvar, F., Firestone, G. L., Ross, S. R., Chandler, V. L., Wrange, O., Carlstedt-Duke, J., Gustafsson, J.-A., and Yamamoto, K. (1982). *J. Cell. Biochem.* **19**, 241.
Richard-Foy, H., Ostrowski, M. C., and Hager, G. L. (1984). *Cell* (submitted).
Ringold, G. M., Yamamoto, K. R., Bishop, J. M., and Varmus, H. E. (1977). *Proc. Natl. Acad. Sci. U.S.A.* **74**, 2879.
Scheidereit, C., Geisse, S., Westphal, H. M., and Beato, M. (1983). *Nature (London)* **304**, 749.
Smoller, C. G., Pitka, D. R., and Bern, H. A. (1961). *J. Biophys. Biochem. Cytol.* **9**, 915.
Traina, V. L., Taylor, B. A., and Cohen, J. C. (1981). *J. Virol.* **40**, 735.
Van Ooyen, A. J. J., Michalides, R. J. A. M., and Nusse, R. (1983). *J. Virol.* **46**, 362.
Weintraub, H., and Groudine, M. (1976). *Science* **193**, 848.
Weintraub, H., and Groudine, M. (1983). *Cell* **33**, 65.
Wheeler, D. A., Butel, J. S., Medina, D., Cardiff, R. D., and Hager, G. L. (1983). *J. Virol.* **46**, 42.
Wu, C. (1980). *Nature (London)* **286**, 854.
Young, H. A., and Hager, G. L. (1979). *In* "Steroid Receptors and the Management of Cancer" (E. B. Thompson and M. Lippman, eds.), p. 45. CRC Press, Cleveland, Ohio.
Young, H. A., Shih, T. Y., Scolnick, E. M., and Parks, W. P. (1977). *J. Virol.* **21**, 139.

DISCUSSION

F. C. Bancroft: In the gene transfer experiments you showed in the first section of your talk it was necessary to employ heterologous enhancer elements to enhance the activity of the MMTV promoter. Could the presence of an enhancer element in your constructions have introduced artifacts into your deletion studies?

G. Hager: I attempted to address that point in discussing the various mechanisms by which the receptor locus could act. We have, of course, created an artificial chimera. There is no evidence that the MMTV provirus contains any kind of enhancer element. It remains an enigma as to why the MMTV LTR is such a weak promoter in gene transfer experiments. This is a uniform finding, essentially in everybody's hands. If you look at the strength of this promoter in a cell line isolated from a mammary tumor induced by MMTV, in that particular cell type, the MMTV LTR can be an extraordinarily powerful promoter. We really don't understand why the promoter is so weak in these gene fusion experiments. In order to do what I call statistically quantitative experiments, that is where you average a large number of events, it is necessary to put enhancers into the construction to get enough activity. It is of course possible that the enhancer introduces a potential artifact.

A. R. Means: Do deletion mutants in the LTR alter the nuclease periodicity or nucleosome phasing effect when such mutants are introduced into the BPV system?

G. Hager: We haven't look at that yet.

A. R. Means: It would be interesting.

G. Hager: This is a major question, which should be prefaced by reminding you that there is still an assumption that the micrococcal periodicity is a result of nucleosome phasing; that certainly needs to be substantiated with a variety of approaches, including the recently developed chemical agents that will attach nucleosome linker regions in a much less sequence specific way. If that holds up, then the question we are immediately faced with is what determines the phase. Of course, people have been grappling with this question for some years now. Are there sequences in the LTR that interact specifically with nucleosome structure? The more currently accepted idea is that phasing is simply a result of a regulatory protein binding to DNA, thereby setting up a phase which would then hold over a certain distance from the location of the DNA binding protein. Our experiments would suggest that if a regulatory protein is responsible for setting the phase, it would not be the receptor protein because the phase is present both in the presence and absence of hormone. That of course includes the additional assumption that receptor is not bound to the DNA in the absence of hormone, a concept which some people are now questioning.

J. E. Rall: You presented so much data that there are many questions one would like to ask. Did I miss the control experiment using bovine papilloma virus by itself to see if you get nucleosome phasing? I note that two-thirds of the DNA in your plasmid construct is just normal bovine papilloma virus.

G. Hager: No, the control was the LTR in both orientations; the phase was orientation independent.

J. E. Rall: Yes, but suppose that may not matter either, and the bovine papilloma virus without any LTR at all, will cause nucleosome phasing.

G. Hager: We have not analyzed BPV by itself.

J. E. Rall: Two-thirds of your DNA is BPV?

G. Hager: That is correct. We have also analyzed fusions between the LTR and a different tester gene, replacing v-ras with a chloramphenicol transferase gene; again we see the same phase. Phasing is usually considered to be localized over a limited region of DNA. I think we have proven that the DNA 3' distal to the LTR can be changed either from BPV to v-ras, or it can be changed to CAT with no effect on the phase. We have changed DNA 5' to the LTR in the sense that two completely different regions of the BPV genome can be placed immediately proximal to those sequences with no detectable effect on the phase. So I think that the controls are really pretty good.

J. E. Rall: The second question is, what kind of nonhistone nuclear proteins are present on the minichromosomes?

G. Hager: That is a question we are just beginning to ask. Our efforts in the past year have been devoted to developing cell lines where we can convince ourselves that regulation is occurring, and that minichromosomes are homogeneous, at least at the DNA level. We are just beginning to get to the biochemical approach of purifying minichromosomes and looking at the proteins. To look at the cell lines with 200 to 300 copies per cell was going to be extremely difficult, given the various aspects of the technology. I think that now that we have developed all lines with up to 1500 copies per cell, it will be feasible to look at the protein composition of the episomes.

P. Chambon: Just a remark concerning the last point you mentioned. It is not clear that when increasing the number of minichromosome copies, you will not lose the homogeneity of the population. It is known that there is not much more transcription from a strong promoter whether it is present in a recombinant which can or cannot replicate after transfection in a given cell. Apparently the proportion of transcriptionally active recombinants decreases as the total number of recombinant molecules present in a cell increases. It is well known that late in SV40 infection, only a small fraction of the minichromosomes are in fact transcriptionally active.

G. Hager: Yes, that is correct. That is another fact that led us away from the SV40 base systems to the BPV system. I have already alluded to the possibility that there could be heterogeneity in minichromosome preparations. The one major point that we need to address in a rigorous fashion is what percentage of the minichromosomes are transcriptionally active; that unfortunately is a very difficult measurement to make.

P. Chambon: I agree this is difficult, but titration of RNA polymerase molecules with labeled α-amanitin may be useful, and the number of RNA polymerase molecules could also be roughly estimated from the amount of RNA synthesized in your nuclear run-on transcription experiments. It seems to me that the fact that you do observe a regular nucleosomal pattern after micrococcal nuclease digestion argues against the presence of densely packed RNA polymerase molecules on your minichromosomes. Indeed, M. Bellard in our lab has reported that no nucleosomal repeat can be seen in the ovalbumin gene when it is transcribed at a high rate *in vivo*. [M. Bellard *et al., EMBO J.* (1980). **1**, 223–230]. Similar observations have been made by others looking, for instance, at the actively transcribed *Drosophila* genes.

G. Hager: I would reply to that by making two points. First of all, again assuming that this is the result of nucleosome phasing, the region over which that array is most pronounced is not the transcribed region. Second, I did not comment on it when I went over the data, but if you look there are some specific cutting sites downstream in the transcribed region as well. If you look at those sites in the hormone treated cells, they tend to be depressed; that would agree with your point that when there is strong transcription the nonrandom order disappears. We do see some evidence of that in the region that is actually being transcribed whereas in the region upstream from the capsite, the apparent intensity of the bands remains constant.

P. Chambon: Do you have any evidence that micrococcal nuclease may cut specifically naked DNA at about a 170 bp interval in the upstream region of the MMTV promoter where you do see evidence for phasing?

G. Hager: No, there is no evidence for this. Also, the AT composition in the linker regions is almost exactly the same as in the nucleosome region.

P. Chambon: Do you think that the presence of a "repressor" molecule may set up the phasing in the upstream region of the MMTV promoter?

G. Hager: I suspect we are a little bit like an ant crawling on an elephant in terms of knowing what all the proteins are that are involved here.

F. S. French: When you showed the slide on the sedimentation of receptor, I take it the receptor was bound to the minichromosome. I just wondered if you have extracted receptor from the chromosome and shown that it has the same sedimentation as the receptor in the host cell.

G. Hager: No, the only experiment that was done so far is to show that a cell line harboring a minichromosome of almost exactly the same size without the LTR element does not bind the labeled hormone. That is the only experiment which has been done as a control. Many chromosomes can be extracted themselves with receptors in place. This raises the interesting possibility that we may not have to purify receptor in order to use these molecules as transcription substrates since the receptor is already there and we simply could use cells with an unoccupied receptor as a control. I also want to reemphasize that with these minichromosomes we have a very nice internal control. There is no effect whatsoever of hormone on the BPV promoter itself.

P. Chambon: Do you know what happens to the DNase I hypersensitive site which is induced by glucocorticoid if you remove the hormone from the medium?

G. Hager: Not yet. We also would like to look at the kinetics of the appearance of the site.

Role of the Circadian System in Reproductive Phenomena

FRED W. TUREK, JENNIFER SWANN, AND DAVID J. EARNEST

Department of Neurobiology and Physiology, Northwestern University, Evanston, Illinois

I. Introduction

Successful reproduction in mammals involves a variety of carefully timed events. From the initiation of gamete production through pregnancy and parturition, various endocrine and neural events occur within a well-defined temporal program. Therefore, it is not surprising to find a great deal of interaction between the reproductive system and the major component of the temporal organization of animals: the circadian system.

The circadian system interfaces with the reproductive process at many different levels, but the precise relationship can vary greatly from species to species. The objective of this article is to review the different ways in which reproductive phenomena depend upon circadian information in mammals. In particular this article will examine the role of the circadian system in (1) regulating the daily pattern of release of reproductive hormones from the pituitary gland and the gonads, (2) synchronizing various events associated with ovulation to specific times of the day, (3) timing various events associated with pregnancy and parturition, and (4) measuring the length of the day in seasonal breeders—information that is used to time reproductive activity to the appropriate season of the year.

Although this paper focuses entirely on those aspects of reproduction that involve a cycling 24-hour component, it should be noted that many reproductive events also involve rhythms that have higher and lower frequencies. For example many reproductive hormones appear to be released in regularly timed bursts; these episodic pulses usually recur at intervals ranging between 1 and 4 hours (Van Cauter and Copinschi, 1981). Rhythms with periods longer than 24 hours include the ovulatory cycle, which can extend from a few days to months and annual rhythms in reproduction (see Campbell and Turek, 1981; Hoffmann, 1981b, for reviews). As discussed below, the circadian system often plays a critical role in the timing of some long-term reproductive rhythms including the 4–5 day estrous cycles in rodents and seasonal reproductive cycles. Few studies have attempted to ascertain whether or not the circadian system may be important in the timing of the high-frequency pulsatile hormonal release.

143

II. Circadian Rhythmicity

Numerous biochemical, physiological, and behavioral events in plants and animals are expressed rhythmically with a 24-hour period that matches the daily solar cycle. These diurnal rhythms continue to persist under laboratory conditions devoid of any external environmental signals, and therefore are believed to be driven by an endogenous biological clock. Such rhythms are referred to as being "circadian" because in constant environmental conditions the expressed periods are about 24 hours. The primary cue that synchronizes or entrains circadian rhythms with the 24-hour rotation of the earth is the light–dark cycle. Strictly speaking, a diurnal rhythm should not be referred to as "circadian" until it has been demonstrated that such a rhythm persists under constant environmental conditions. However, in properly controlled experiments, diurnal rhythms are usually found to persist with a circadian period. Consequently, the term circadian is often used to refer to diurnal rhythms that are observed under either artificial or natural 24-hour lighting conditions.

Over the last 30 years extensive phenomenological studies have elucidated many of the fundamental properties of diurnal rhythms. However, it has only been fairly recently that investigators have been able to find an anatomical location for the circadian clock(s) in mammals and to elucidate physiological mechanisms that underlie the generation of circadian rhythms. Such studies have also led to a better understanding of how the circadian system interacts with many other physiological processes including the reproductive system. For a more complete description of the basic properties of circadian rhythms and of ways that they control the timing of a variety of physiological events, the reader is directed to recent books (Aschoff, 1981; Aschoff *et al.,* 1982; Moore-Ede *et al.,* 1982; Brady, 1982) and review articles (Takahashi and Zatz, 1982; Moore-Ede *et al.,* 1983a,b; Turek, 1983).

III. Diurnal Variations in Gonadotropins and Gonadal Steroids

A number of studies have been carried out in humans and in animals to characterize diurnal patterns in circulating levels of LH, FSH, testosterone, and estradiol. It is not uncommon to find data in the literature supporting either of the following opposing hypotheses: (1) hormone X does not show a diurnal rhythm, or (2) hormone X does show a diurnal rhythm (Judd, 1979; Krieger and Aschoff, 1979). These discrepancies are probably primarily due to genetic differences in the populations studied as well as differences in sampling procedures and statistical analyses (Poland *et al.,* 1980; Van Cauter and Copinschi, 1981). The discovery that most hormones are released episodically at intervals ranging from 1 to 4 hours complicates any attempt to elucidate the circadian nature of hormonal patterns. Early studies of 24-hour hormonal profiles were based on blood samples collected at infrequent intervals (e.g., 1–4 hours) from single animals or on data pooled from many animals sampled at different times. Such procedures do not allow the accurate determination of the overall profile of a hormone that can increase 2- to 3-fold in 30 minutes. The superimposition of pulsatile variations upon a diurnal rhythm often results in complex profiles for which quantitative methods of analysis have only recently been developed (Van Cauter, 1979; Merriam and Wachter, 1982).

A. CHARACTERIZATION OF HORMONAL RHYTHMS

Although there is some suggestion that circulating LH and FSH levels in male rats (Kalra and Kalra, 1977; Dunn and Johnson, 1978; McLean *et al.*, 1977) and LH levels in male rams (Ortavant *et al.*, 1982) show diurnal fluctuations, most animal studies have not determined individual gonadotropin levels at frequent enough intervals (e.g., 10–30 minutes) over a 24-hour period to adequately characterize the diurnal pattern. An exception to this are 24-hour studies in male rhesus monkeys which showed a clear increase in serum LH levels at night when blood was collected at 20-minute intervals (Plant, 1981).

Studies with repeated blood sampling in adult human males have in general not revealed any marked diurnal fluctuation in serum LH and FSH levels (Boyar *et al.*, 1972; Rubin *et al.*, 1975; Judd, 1979; Miyatake *et al.*, 1980) (Fig. 1). However, following an extensive examination of the literature, Krieger and Aschoff (1979) found that in general, reported values for serum LH levels tended to be higher during late sleep and before noon, and lower during early sleep and in the afternoon. A more rigorous statistical analysis of LH profiles is necessary before any definitive statement about the circadian nature of the release of this hormone in men can be made. In women sampled during their early follicular phase, a decline in serum LH levels has been observed shortly after sleep onset with a return to normal or a rebound above normal levels during the later stages of sleep (Kapen *et al.*, 1973, 1980). As for other pituitary hormones (Rubin and Poland, 1976; Van Cauter and Copinschi, 1981; Moore-Ede *et al.*, 1982), the various stages of sleep can influence gonadotropin release.

In contrast to the weak or absent circadian variation in serum LH and FSH levels seen in adult humans, there are pronounced changes in late prepubertal and pubertal boys and girls (Kapen *et al.*, 1974; Judd *et al.*, 1977; Judd, 1979; Rebar and Yen, 1979; Beck and Wuttke, 1980). In both sexes elevations in LH and FSH occur during sleep. As puberty pro-

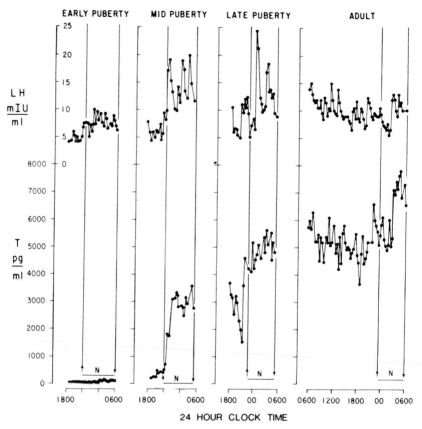

FIG. 1. Serum luteinizing hormone (LH) and testosterone (T) in pubertal and adult human males. While there is a clear nighttime (N) elevation in both LH and T during puberty, only serum T levels show a clear nighttime elevation in adults. (From Judd, 1979.)

gresses, there is a gradual increase in daytime gonadotropin release such that by the end of puberty serum gonadotropin levels are similar during day and night (Fig. 1) (Judd, 1979; Rebar and Yen, 1979).

Diurnal fluctuations in serum testosterone levels in males have been observed in a wide variety of animal species including voles, rats, sheep, and monkeys (Goodman *et al.*, 1974; Van Horn *et al.*, 1976; Perachio *et al.*, 1977; Keating and Tcholakian, 1979; Plant, 1981; Bremner *et al.*, 1983). Most investigations in human males reveal a marked diurnal rhythm in circulating testosterone levels in young adults with serum T levels being elevated during the night (Rubin *et al.*, 1975; Judd, 1979; Guignard *et al.*, 1980). Since there is little, if any increase in serum LH at night, the sleep related increase in circulating T levels may be due to other factors such as testicular blood flow, Leydig cell response to T, and/or circadian fluctuations in other hormones. In studies involving female animals, there are clear circadian changes in serum estradiol and progesterone levels near the time of ovulation (see Section IV). Few studies have examined the diurnal profile of gonadal steroid hormones during other stages of the cycle. A report by Aedo *et al.* (1981) suggests that neither progesterone nor estradiol shows circadian variation during the follicular periovulatory luteal phases of the human menstrual cycle. However, since blood samples were only taken at 3-hour intervals, more extensive studies are required before any definitive statements can be made.

At the time of puberty in humans there are pronounced diurnal rhythms in serum estradiol in females and testosterone in males (Boyar *et al.*, 1976; Rebar and Yen, 1979; Judd, 1979). While serum testosterone levels rise in phase with the nocturnal increase in serum LH levels in boys (Fig. 1), the diurnal increase in serum estradiol in females occurs during the day, after circulating LH and FSH levels have declined. It has been suggested that the paradoxical rise in serum estradiol levels may be due to a delayed ovarian response to the preceding rise in gonadotropins (Boyar *et al.*, 1976; Rebar and Yen, 1979).

A recent report by Bremner and colleagues (1983) indicates that the diurnal fluctuation in circulating testosterone is a function of age, since the nocturnal rise in serum testosterone levels observed in young men (mean age, 25.2 years) is absent in healthy elderly men (mean age 71 years) (Fig. 2). Previous reports in the literature were inconsistent with respect to the effects of aging on circulating testosterone levels since sampling regimes were often inadequate to accurately characterize the circadian hormonal profile. This study points out the importance of taking into account the time of day of sampling in order to adequately characterize circulating hormonal levels.

B. PHYSIOLOGICAL SIGNIFICANCE OF CIRCADIAN RHYTHMICITY IN REPRODUCTIVE HORMONES

While the importance of intermittent, rather than continuous, release of LHRH for normal pituitary gonadotropin secretion has been elegantly demonstrated in human and nonhuman studies (Knobil, 1980: Pohl *et al.*, 1983), the significance of diurnal variations in hypothalamic, pituitary, and/or gonadal hormones remains unknown. Indeed, it is not at all clear at what level the search for a significance in the circadian hormonal release should be carried out. Circadian variation in reproductive hormone levels may be necessary for normal response of target tissues. This could result from interactions with other hormonal rhythms and/or correspond to an

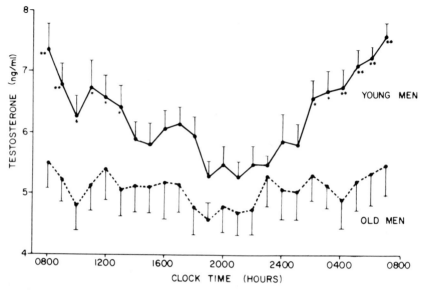

FIG. 2.   Hourly serum testosterone levels (mean ± SEM) in normal young ($N = 17$; mean age = 25.2 years) and old ($N = 12$; mean age = 71 years) men. Significant levels of the differences between young and old men at each time point are indicated by * ($p < 0.05$) or ** ($p < 0.01$). The absence of an asterisk indicates no significant differences at that time point (From Bremner *et al.*, 1983.)

altered circadian response of the target tissues. The circadian variation in hormone concentrations may enable the same hormone to act differently at various times of the day. Hormonal rhythms may also be important in the feedback control system between the central nervous system and the endocrine organs. Finally, the significance of circadian hormonal rhythms may be related to the necessity to synchronize a variety of endocrine and neural events for maximum efficiency.

There is a close correlation between diurnal hormone patterns and the sleep–wake cycle, which also shows circadian variation (Weitzman, 1980). There is good evidence to suggest that at least for some hormones, there is a direct action of sleep on hormone secretion that is superimposed on a sleep-independent endogenous circadian rhythm of hormone release (Weitzman *et al.*, 1983). The close correlation between hormonal release and sleep suggests a functional link between the two in the synchronization of various physiological events.

The clinical significance of circadian rhythmicity in reproductive hormones is not known. A major difficulty in addressing this question is the fact that changes in the circadian profile are often associated with changes in the pulsatile release of the hormone. For example, in patients with anorexia nervosa, the diurnal pattern of pituitary LH release is usually either infantile (serum LH levels constantly low) or pubertal (serum LH levels rise during the night). However, it is not clear if the disruption of normal reproductive physiology that is associated with anorexia nervosa is due to a loss in the normal episodic release of pituitary LH or to a change in the circadian profile (Boyar *et al.*, 1976; Katz *et al.*, 1977; Pirke *et al.*, 1979; Roulier *et al.*, 1981). Only in the past few years has it been recognized that disorders in the circadian organization of hormonal secretions may be involved in the etiology of some endocrine diseases. Whether disruptions of the normal diurnal pattern of reproductive hormones plays a role in the etiology of certain dysfunctions of the reproductive system still needs to be determined.

IV. Role for the Circadian System in the Timing of Ovulation

In mammals specific events in the ovarian cycle occur at intervals much longer than 24 hours. Nevertheless, data from different rodent species demonstrate that estrous-related events, such as the timing of the surge in pituitary LH release, ovulation, the increase in progesterone secretion, and the onset of sexual receptivity, are linked to the circadian system and occur at specific times of day on the days when they occur (Schwartz, 1969; Rusak and Zucker, 1979; Campbell and Turek, 1981). Although there is little evidence to indicate that the timing of the LH surge in nonrodent species is regulated by the circadian system, it should be noted that few comprehensive studies have actually addressed this question. Recent studies in humans (Edwards, 1981; Testart *et al.*, 1982; Seibel *et al.*, 1982) indicate that the preovulatory LH surge occurs in the majority of women in the early morning, and suggest that the circadian involvement in timing events in the ovarian cycle may be more widespread than previously thought.

A. CIRCADIAN TIMED EVENTS OF THE ESTROUS CYCLE

In rats, hamsters, and mice held under standard laboratory lighting conditions (e.g., LD 14 : 10) it has been clearly established that ovulation occurs at a fixed time relative to the light–dark cycle (Alleva *et al.*, 1968; Schwartz, 1969; Bingel and Schwartz, 1969). A phase-shift in the LD cycle results in a subsequent phase shift in the timing of ovulation (Alleva *et al.*, 1968). The circadian nature of the timing of ovulation is supported by the fact that ovulation continues to occur near the expected time of day after an acute exposure to constant light (LL) or constant darkness (DD) (McCormack and Sridaran, 1978).

The hormonal events inducing ovulation in rodents are well understood (Campbell and Turek, 1981). On a background of high circulating estrogen levels, a surge of LH occurs on proestrus resulting in ovulation on the morning of estrus. Numerous studies have now clearly demonstrated that the proestrus LH surge is tightly controlled by a neural circadian clock. When rats and hamsters are entrained to a light–dark (LD) cycle, the LH surge occurs with a fixed phase relationship to the LD cycle (Bast and Greenwald, 1974; Stetson and Gibson, 1977; Carrillo and Sawyer, 1978; Gallo, 1981). In hamsters exposed to constant darkness, preovulatory LH and FSH release occurs at specific times of the day indicating that an endogenous circadian pacemaker is regulating the timing of preovulatory gonadotropin release (Stetson and Anderson, 1980). Recent studies by Levine and Ramirez (1982) show increased release of LHRH from the medial basal hypothalamus at the time of the preovulatory gonadotropin surge, implying its role in triggering the surge.

The hormonal events accompanying the ovarian cycle, particularly rising estrogen and progesterone levels, induce sexual receptivity in female rodents (Campbell and Turek, 1981). In regularly cycling female hamsters exposed to a LD 16 : 8 cycle the onset of lordosis behavior occurs near the time of lights off (Alleva *et al.,* 1971; Swann and Turek, 1982) once every 4 days. During exposure to constant light, the occurrence of lordosis continues to show cyclicity with a period slightly greater than 96 hours (Alleva *et al.,* 1971; Fitzgerald and Zucker, 1976; Swann and Turek, 1982) and shows a free-running rhythm that bears a fixed phase relationship to the circadian rhythm of locomotor activity (see below).

Further support for the concept that the circadian system regulates the timing of events associated with the ovarian cycle is the observation that if the LH surge is blocked by an injection of pentobarbital prior to the expected preovulatory increase in pituitary LH release, the LH surge occurs 24 hours later and ovulation is also delayed by 24 hours (Everett and Sawyer, 1950; Norman and Spies, 1974; Terranova, 1980; Van der Schoot, 1980). Using a variety of drugs that block the LH surge and ovulation when administered during the "critical period," Everett and Tyrey (1982) found that electrical stimulation of the medial preoptic area following drug treatment induced normal ovulatory amounts of LH. Thus the suppressive action of these drugs does not appear to be due to an effect on the availability or release of LHRH, or on the responsiveness of the pituitary or ovary. Instead, these drugs probably act by preventing the circadian neural signal from reaching LHRH neurons.

Even though the circadian-timed LH surge occurs only once every 4 or 5 days, there is strong evidence indicating that the neural signal is generated daily. Indeed, ovariectomized estrogen-primed (OVX-E_2) rats show a daily release in LH at a time of day similar to that observed on proestrous in intact animals (Legan and Karsch, 1975; Legan *et al.*, 1975). As with the normal preovulatory surge in LH, the daily surges seen in OVX-E_2 animals are coupled to the light–dark cycle (Chazal *et al.*, 1977). Further support for a daily neural signal for LH release is that an LH surge can be induced on diestrus in intact rats by the administration of exogenous estrogen and that this induced surge can be blocked by an injection of pentobarbital (Geiger *et al.*, 1981).

Estrogen treatment of ovariectomized hamsters can also trigger daily LH surges (Norman and Spies, 1974; Stetson *et al.*, 1978), and this daily surge can be delayed 24 hours by barbiturate blockade (Stetson *et al.*, 1981). Unlike rats however, daily surges in acutely ovariectomized hamsters have been observed even without estrogen treatment (Stetson *et al.*, 1978; Shander and Goldman, 1978) indicating that the circadian neural signal can induce LH surges even in the absence of estrogens. Daily afternoon surges in LH have also been observed in intact and OVX lactating hamsters as well as in intact and OVX hamsters exposing to nonstimulatory short days that induce acyclicity in this species (Bridges and Goldman, 1975). Thus, in cycling hamsters exposed to photostimulatory long days, LH surges occur only once every 4 days while surges occur daily in noncycling hamsters. The physiological mechanisms governing the transition between LH surges once every 4 days to surges every day as well as the events leading to ovarian dysfunction associated with daily surges of LH remain unknown.

B. RELATIONSHIP BETWEEN CIRCADIAN RHYTHM OF LOCOMOTOR ACTIVITY AND OVARIAN CYCLES

A variety of experimental findings indicate that the same circadian clock (or clock system) that regulates the activity rhythm in rodents also controls the timing of events associated with the ovarian cycle. There is especially strong support for this hypothesis in the golden hamster. Under a standard light–dark cycle, such as LD 14:10 or LD 16:8, the onset of activity in hamsters occurs at about the time of lights off every day whereas the onset of lordosis occurs a few hours prior to activity onset every 4 days (Fig. 3). Furthermore, during exposure to constant light the activity rhythm free-runs with a period that is usually greater than 24 hours, and the onset of lordosis behavior continues to occur near the onset of activity once every four complete activity cycles (Fitzgerald and Zucker, 1976; Swann and Turek, 1982). Carmichael *et al.* (1981) have also demonstrated that the onset of behavioral estrus is a quadruple multiple of the period of the activity rhythm during entrainment to light–dark cycles

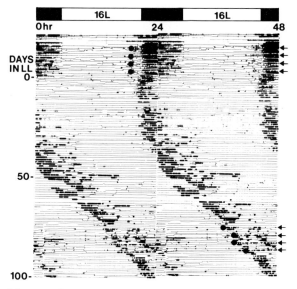

FIG. 3. Activity record over 121-day period of a female hamster exposed to LD 16:8 cycle (diagrammed at top) for 3 weeks before being transferred into constant light (LL). Activity data in this and Fig. 4 have been double plotted over a 48-hour time scale to aid in visual examination of data. During exposure to LD 16:8 locomotor activity was confined mainly to the 8-hour period of darkness. During exposure to LL, the activity rhythm free-ran with a period greater than 24 hours. On days 7–19 of LD 16:8 and again on days 75–87 of LL, the female was exposed briefly to a male hamster at 2-hour intervals to determine time of onset of lordosis behavior. Black dots (indicated by arrows) represent time on that day when lordosis behavior was first observed. (From Swann and Turek, 1982.)

with periods of 21.5–23.5 hours. Thus, in hamsters entrained to cycles of 21.5–22.0 hours, behavioral estrous cycles of 86–88 hours are observed. Changing the period of the LD cycle also modifies the phase relationship between activity onset and the onset of lordosis (Carmichael *et al.*, 1981). Changes in the phase relationship between two or more circadian rhythms are commonly observed when the period of the entraining agent is altered (Aschoff, 1979). Such changes could reflect the fact that separate, but coupled, circadian oscillators underlie the activity and lordosis onsets, or that there is an alteration in the coupling strength between a single circadian pacemaker and its target tissues under different entraining conditions.

The proestrous surges in LH and FSH also have a fixed phase relationship to the circadian rhythm of activity (Stetson and Gibson, 1977). In photorefractory cycling female hamsters exposed to LD 6:18, the preovulatory release of LH and FSH was found to occur 2–3 hours before the onset of activity even though the phase relationship between the onset of activity and light off varied between 0 and 6 hours (Stetson and Gibson, 1977). In hamsters exposed to different light–dark cycles (i.e., 6–22 hours of light/24 hours), it was found that a precise temporal relationship was maintained between the LH surge and activity onset, whereas the phase relationship between the LH surge and the light–dark cycle was variable (Moline *et al.*, 1981). In photorefractory hamsters free-running in constant darkness, the preovulatory release of LH and FSH continued to occur at a specific time of the animal's circadian day, 2–3 hours before the onset of activity (Stetson and Anderson, 1980).

Three additional observations in hamsters support the hypothesis that the onset of activity and the daily timed events of the estrous cycle are regulated by the same circadian oscillator(s). First, occasionally a simultaneous induction of arrhythmicity of the locomotor activity rhythm and constant behavioral estrus has been observed in hamsters exposed to continuous light (Stetson *et al.*, 1977). Second, the addition of deuterium oxide to the drinking water lengthens the period of both the activity rhythm and the period of lordosis onsets such that a stable phase relationship between these two rhythms is maintained (Fitzgerald and Zucker, 1976). Third, lesions of the suprachiasmatic nuclei, a region of the hypothalamus known to be involved in the generation of circadian rhythms, disrupt both the activity rhythm and the estrous cycle resulting in random irregular bouts of activity and a concurrent state of constant estrus (Stetson and Watson-Whitmyre, 1976).

Recent evidence in hamsters suggests that more than one circadian oscillator controls the timing of both the activity rhythm and the circadian-based events of the estrous cycle. In about 50% of hamsters exposed to constant light (LL) for a prolonged period of time, the activity rhythm dissociates or "splits" into two distinct components (Pittendrigh and Daan, 1976; Turek *et al.*, 1982). Initially, these two components may free-run with different periods for several days until they reach a 180° antiphase relationship with respect to each other (Fig. 4). At this point, the two activity bouts recouple and in the "split condition" free-run with the same period. According to the convention established by Pittendrigh and Daan (1976), the components are labeled either evening (E) or morning (M) on the basis of their extrapolated position in the active phase prior to the occurrence of splitting. This "splitting" phenomenon strongly suggests that at least two mutually coupled circadian pacemakers underlie the rhythm of activity.

In view of the close relationship between the timing of estrous events and the circadian rhythm of locomotor activity, we recently sought to determine if one or both of the circadian oscillators underlying the rhythm

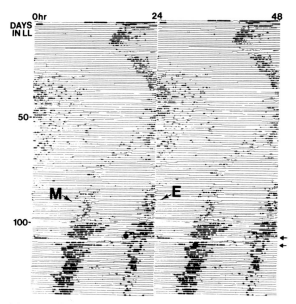

FIG. 4. Activity record over 136-day period of a female hamster maintained in constant light (LL). On about day 65, the activity rhythm split into two components designed as M (morning) and E (evening). On days 103–111, the female was briefly exposed to a male hamster at 2-hour intervals to determine time of onset of lordosis behavior. Black dots (indicated by arrows) represent time on that day when lordosis behavior was first observed. (From Swann and Turek, 1982.)

of activity was responsible for timing the onset of lordosis behavior by monitoring lordosis behavior in female hamsters with a split rhythm of activity (Swann and Turek, 1982). Regular (i.e., 4-day) or irregular (i.e., non-4-day) cycles in lordosis behavior continued to occur in about 90% of the animals with a split activity rhythm. In about one-third of females with a split activity rhythm, the onset of lordosis occurred near the onset of the E component while in a second third of the animals lordosis behavior began near the onset of the M component. Importantly, the onset of lordosis was associated on different days with either the E or M component in the remaining animals (Fig. 4). Thus, in the majority of hamsters with a split rhythm of activity, estrous cyclicity is maintained and the onset of lordosis can be associated with either of the two oscillators underlying the circadian rhythm of activity. Similarly, Carmichael et al. (1981) observed that estrous onset could be associated with either the entrained or free-running component of the activity rhythm in a single female hamster whose rhythm of activity had split into two components during entrainment to an LD cycle with a period less than 24 hours.

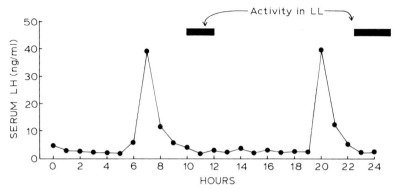

FIG. 5.   Twenty-four hour serum LH profile in a single ovariectomized estrogen-treated hamster bled once an hour via an indwelling atrial cannula. The animal had previously been exposed to constant light (LL) for many weeks during which the circadian rhythm of activity had split into two components. The timing of the two activity bouts relative to the time of the two LH surges is indicated by the horizontal black bars.

One question that arises from the observation that the onset of lordosis can be associated with either of the two circadian oscillators underlying the rhythm of activity is whether two LH surges would occur in a single day in an animal with a split rhythm of activity. This would be a surprising result since in a cycling animal with an intact rhythm of activity only a single LH surge is observed. Alternatively, the LH surge may always be associated with only one of the circadian oscillators underlying the activity rhythm, but the onset of lordosis behavior may be associated with either oscillator because the onset of lordosis may not be a precise marker for the state of the circadian system underlying estrous cyclicity (Swann and Turek, 1982).

In order to probe in more detail the relationship between the estrous cycle and the circadian rhythm of activity in split animals, we recently monitored serum LH levels in ovariectomized estrogen-treated hamsters with an intact or a split rhythm of activity during exposure to LL (Swann and Turek, 1983). In all animals with an intact activity rhythm ($N = 6$), a single LH surge occurred about 1–4 hours before the onset of activity. Surprisingly, in all females showing a split activity rhythm, two LH surges per 24 hours were observed. The LH surges occurred 0–4 hours before the onset of the nearest bout of activity (Fig. 5). Taken together, these results suggest that the LH surge and the onset of locomotor activity are regulated by the same circadian oscillators, and when these oscillators are expressed independently in the split state, each is equally capable of triggering a bout of activity and an LH surge.

The results summarized in this section suggest that either (1) a single set of circadian oscillators underlies both the circadian activity rhythm and the estrous rhythm or (2) two separate sets of circadian oscillators that are normally coupled to each other drive the two rhythms. Adler (1978) has suggested that it might be possible to distinguish between these two hypotheses by determining if the estrous and circadian oscillators could be experimentally separated from one another. Indeed, such separation has been observed. For example, Weber and Adler (1978) found no correlation between the induction of persistent estrus (the occurrence of which indicates the absence of preovulatory LH surges) and a free-running activity rhythm in rats exposed to unusual LD cycles, and that persistent estrus could be induced in rats whose activity rhythm remained entrained. Similarly, unlike in hamsters (Stetson et al., 1978), there is a time-lag in LL-induced arrhythmicity of locomotor activity and the onset of persistent estrus in rats (Shimizu et al., 1983). Persistent estrus has also been observed in rats whose activity rhythm is entrained to an LD 21 : 3 cycle (Shimizu et al., 1983). Further support for the separability of estrous-related events from the rhythm of activity is the finding that the circadian activity rhythm reentrains at a slower rate following reversal of the photoperiod than do circadian-based estrous cycle rhythms (Campbell and Finkelstein, 1978), and that during initial exposure to LL there is a temporal dissociation between activity onset and the hormonal events of estrus (Campbell and Schwartz, 1980). However, such dissociations between estrous events and activity may simply be due to differences in coupling strength between a common set of central circadian pacemakers and the driven rhythms of activity and estrus. More conclusive evidence that the activity rhythm and the estrous cycle are driven by separate sets of circadian oscillators would require that the two rhythms show different periods under either free-running or entrained conditions.

C. NEURAL EVENTS UNDERLYING CIRCADIAN CONTROL OF OVARIAN CYCLES

Investigations on the neurochemical events mediating the neural control of proestrous changes in LHRH activity have focused on the catecholamines. Barraclough and Wise (1982) have recently reviewed the complex and often conflicting literature on this subject. Many of the discrepancies are due to the variety of experimental paradigms that have been employed to address the role of catecholamines in the preovulatory release of gonadotropins. Based on measurements of catecholamine turnover rates (an index of secretion) and changes in LHRH concentrations in discrete hypothalamic nuclei, Barraclough and Wise (1982) conclude that norepinephrine initiates the preovulatory surge in gonadotropins by evoking the release of newly accumulated LHRH from axonal terminals in the median eminence. However, there is also substantial evidence suggesting the involvement of a variety of other neurotransmitters in the control of the gonadotropin surge, particularly serotonin and dopamine (Weiner and Ganong, 1978; Barraclough and Wise, 1982). In addition, acetylcholine and endorphins have also been implicated in the regulation of LHRH and possibly the release of gonadotropins on proestrus (Cicero, 1980; Egozi *et al.*, 1982; Sylvester *et al.*, 1982). As Barraclough and Wise (1982) have pointed out, the LHRH neuronal system has a number of higher order inputs which may either inhibit or stimulate LHRH release. Thus, it is not known which neurotransmitters directly control the circadian preovulatory gonadotropin release and which neurotransmitters simply modify this response. Undoubtedly various neurochemicals are involved in (1) the generation of circadian signals by a neural clock, (2) the relaying of information to the neural clock (e.g., positive feedback effects of estrogens on gonadotropin surge), and (3) the interaction between the neural clock and the LHRH neuronal system.

Attempts to localize the biological clock responsible for generating and transmitting the neural signal triggering gonadotropin release on proestrous have centered around the bilaterally paired suprachiasmatic nucleus (SCN) of the hypothalamus. There is now substantial evidence from lesion studies implicating the SCN in the control of a variety of circadian rhythms including eating, sleeping, drinking, pineal *N*-acetyltransferase activity, locomotor behavior, and heart rate (Rusak and Zucker, 1979; Turek, 1983). Both *in vivo* and *in vitro* studies on the metabolism and electrical activity of the SCN also demonstrate the intrinsic ability of this area of the hypothalamus to generate circadian signals (Inouye and Kawamura, 1979; Schwartz *et al.*, 1980; Green and Gilette, 1982; Shibata *et al.*, 1982).

Lesions in the SCN region in rats and hamsters have been found to induce constant behavioral estrus, to block ovulation, and to abolish the LH surge in either intact or ovariectomized steroid-treated animals (Fig. 6) (Stetson and Watson-Whitmyre, 1976; Brown-Grant and Raisman, 1977; Gray *et al.*, 1978; Samson and McCann, 1979b; Coen and MacKinnon, 1980; Kawakami *et al.*, 1980; Wiegand *et al.*, 1980; Wiegand and Terasawa, 1982). Ablation of areas near the SCN, including the organum vasculosum lamina terminalis (OVLT) (Samson and McCann, 1979b) or the medial preoptic nucleus (MPN), a small periventricular structure immediately caudal to the OVLT (Terasawa *et al.*, 1980; Wiegand *et al.*, 1980), have also been found to produce the constant estrous syndrome and to block the LH surge in ovariectomized rats treated with steroids. It

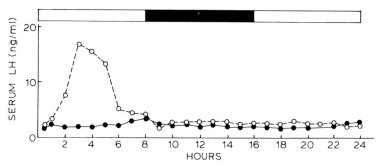

FIG. 6.   Twenty-four hour serum LH profile in two representative ovariectomized estrogen-treated hamsters bled once an hour while maintained on a LD 16:8 light–dark cycle
(horizontal black bar at top depicts time of lights off). Prior to the collection of blood, the
animals had either sustained a Sham-SCN lesion (O---O) or a lesion that totally destroyed
the SCN (●—●).

has been suggested that lesions in the SCN area may induce persistent
estrus and/or interfere with the daily surge of gonadotropins via two different mechanisms (Gray *et al.*, 1978; Wiegand and Terasawa, 1982).
First, lesions of the SCN itself may disrupt the circadian neural signal that
determines the occurrence and timing of preovulatory gonadotropin release. Second, lesions of the MPN may disrupt the steroid-sensitive and/
or GnRH-containing neurons that are necessary for the gonadotropin
surge. Further studies are required in order to identify more precisely the
neural events generating and transmitting circadian signals from LHRH
cell bodies to axonal terminals in the median eminence.

Despite the diversity of neurochemical events and neuroanatomical
pathways that have been associated with the proestrous release of gonadotropins, two general assumptions appear valid at this time. First, neurons within the SCN probably comprise the neural clock responsible for
generating the circadian signal that triggers the proestrous release of gonadotropic hormones. Second, norepinephrine plays an important role in
the release of LHRH from axon terminals in the median eminence at the
time of the preovulatory LH surge. However, how the SCN is coupled to
norepinephrine containing fibers is not known. Circadian signals from the
SCN may directly or indirectly influence norepinephrine release at dendritic terminals synapsing with LHRH cell bodies. Alternatively, circadian signals from the SCN may initiate changes in norepinephrine release
by acting on noradrenergic cell bodies in the lower brain stem that give
rise to axonal terminals in the anterior hypothalamic and preoptic areas.

V. Involvement of Circadian System during Pregnancy

The time of birth for many mammalian species (including humans) shows a diurnal variation for which the light–dark cycle is an important environmental synchronizer (Kaiser and Halberg, 1962; Lincoln and Porter, 1976; Bosc and Nicolle, 1980). In rats, parturition takes place mainly during the light phase and a shift in the light–dark cycle during mid-pregnancy can shift the time of birth by a few fours (Lincoln and Porter, 1976; Sherwood et al., 1983). Maximum serum relaxin levels and basal serum progesterone levels both occur during the light phase approximately 24 hours before birth and these two photic-regulated hormonal events may be indicative of an increasingly effective endogenous circadian luteolytic process that is involved with the termination of pregnancy (Sherwood et al., 1983).

The duration of pregnancy is a precisely timed event with little intraspecies variation. Because of the important role played by the circadian system in regulating various reproductive processes, studies have been carried out in both mice and hamsters to determine if gestation length is governed by the number of light–dark cycles or by the passage of absolute time (Lanman and Seidman, 1977; Davis and Menaker, 1981; Carmichael and Zucker, 1982). Exposure of pregnant mice to 21 hour days or hamsters to 20, 23, or 28 hour days did not have any effect on the absolute duration of gestation when compared to control animals maintained on 24 hour photoperiods. Thus, the duration of pregnancy is not based on the counting of circadian days, but rather is of a fixed length after insemination or fertilization (Davis and Menaker, 1981; Carmichael and Zucker, 1982).

A clear role for the circadian system in the maintenance of pregnancy has been demonstrated in rodents. Gunnet and Freeman (1983) have recently reviewed the literature indicating that diurnal surges in prolactin are responsible for maintaining the first half of pregnancy in rats. Stimulation of the uterine cervix, which normally occurs during mating, induces two large surges of prolactin per day: one during the day and the other at night. These prolactin surges maintain corpora lutea function and the production of progesterone by the corpora lutea maintains pregnancy until a placenta luteotropin takes over during the second half of pregnancy. Following a fertile mating, the two prolactin surges continue for 10 days while the surges last for 12–13 days during pseudopregnancy.

These two daily surges in prolactin following coital stimulation have been referred to as a "unique neuroendocrine response" because a brief cue provided by cervical stimulation results in a twice-daily surge in

prolactin that continues for many days in the absence of any reinforce-
ment or reapplication of the stimulus (Gunnet and Freeman, 1983). Both
prolactin surges are entrained by the LD cycle and a phase shift in the LD
cycle leads to a phase shift in both surges. In constant darkness, or
following enucleation, the rhythm in prolactin surges free-runs with a
circadian period.

Gunnet and Freeman (1983) have suggested that a master circadian
pacemaker (entrained by the LD cycle) may be coupled to two secondary
oscillators regulating the diurnal or nocturnal prolactin surges. The stimulus provided by mating serves to couple the master clock to the prolactin
secretory oscillators. As with other circadian rhythms regulated by the
light–dark cycle, the suprachiasmatic nucleus (SCN) appears to act as, or
be an important component of, the master oscillator responsible for the
circadian rhythm in prolactin surges. Lesioning of the SCN, or of its
posterior efferents, results in the termination of both the nocturnal and
diurnal surges of prolactin (Bethea and Neill, 1980; Yogev and Terkel,
1980). Interestingly, lesions of the medial preoptic area (MPOA) in intact
and ovariectomized rats induce a nocturnal but not a diurnal surge in
prolactin (Freeman and Banks, 1980). Lesioning of the MPOA after induction of the diurnal and nocturnal surges by cervical stimulation abolishes the diurnal but not the nocturnal prolactin surge. These results have
led to the hypothesis that the MPOA contains neurons that are inhibitory
to nocturnal but stimulatory to diurnal surges of PRL (Freeman and
Banks, 1980). Additionally, electrical stimulation of the dorsomedial–
ventromedial areas (DMN–VMH) of the hypothalamus induces diurnal
and nocturnal surges in intact and ovariectomized rats suggesting an involvement of this area in the control of the circadian release of prolactin
(Freeman and Banks, 1980). How cervical stimulation acts to couple the
SCN circadian pacemaker to neurons responsible for the twice-daily
surges of PRL in the MPOA and DMN–VMH areas is not known.

VI. Role of the Circadian System in the Timing of Photoperiodically Controlled Seasonal Reproductive Cycles

In the majority of vertebrate species inhabiting the temperate zones of
the world, the young are born during specific times of the year when the
probability of survival for both the parents and their offspring is maximum. The primary environmental cue synchronizing the time of mating
with the appropriate time of the year is the seasonal change in daylength
(Turek and Campbell, 1979; Hoffmann, 1981b; Follett and Follett, 1981).
The strong reliance on daylength for the timing of the reproductive season
is undoubtedly due to the noise-free nature of this variable and therefore

its reliability as a marker of the phase of the seasonal environmental cycle. It should be noted that in addition to reproductive activity, a variety of other physiological and behavioral annual cycles (e.g., milk production, growth, pelage color) are also regulated by the seasonal change in daylength (Hoffmann; 1981b; Tucker and Ringer, 1982).

The importance of daylength in the regulation of the annual reproductive cycle has been demonstrated in a variety of mammalian species including hamsters, voles, ferrets, sheep, deer, horses, mink, as well as a number of subhuman primates (Turek and Campbell, 1979; Van Horn and Eaton, 1979; Hoffmann, 1981b). Photoinhibitory daylengths can lead to testicular regression and the cessation of mature sperm production in the male, anovulation in the female, and the termination of sexual behavior in both sexes. Much of our understanding of the endocrine events involved in photic-induced changes in hypothalamic–pituitary–gonadal activity in mammals is derived from studies on two model species: golden hamsters (a long-day breeder) and sheep (a short-day breeder). Changes in daylength induce changes in hypothalamic LHRH release and gonadal steroid production. There is now good evidence suggesting the photoperiod alters pituitary gonadotropin release by two processes (Turek and Ellis, 1981; Goodman and Karsch, 1981). First, the fact that changes in daylength alter the negative feedback effects of gonadal steroids on pituitary gonadotropin release suggests the existence of a "steroid-dependent" process. Second, pituitary gonadotropin release can also be altered by the photoperiod in the absence of gonadal (and adrenal) steroids, indicating a "steroid-independent" process is also involved.

In order for seasonal changes in daylength to alter hypothalamic–pituitary–gonadal function, two events must take place. First, a system must be involved in the measurement of daylength, and second, information from the daylength-measuring system must be relayed to the hypothalamic–pituitary axis responsible for gonadotropin release. As discussed below, the circadian system is used to measure the length of the day, the suprachiasmatic nucleus (SCN) is probably the location of the circadian clock(s), and the pineal gland is involved in the transfer of information from the circadian clock measuring photoperiodic time to the hypothalamic–pituitary–gonadal axis.

A. PHOTOPERIODIC TIME MEASUREMENT

Since it was first discovered that seasonal change in daylength was a primary environmental signal for the regulation of annual reproductive cycles, a great deal of attention has been directed at answering the question, "How do living organisms measure the length of the day?" Although early work in this field focused on the idea that animals measured the total duration of the light or dark period by some sort of hourglass mechanism, it is now clear that in both birds and mammals, photoperiodic time measurement is based on a circadian rhythm of responsiveness to light (for reviews see Turek and Campbell, 1979; Hoffmann, 1981b; Follett and Follett, 1981).

Two general models have been advanced to account for the role of the circadian system in photoperiodic time measurement (Pittendrigh, 1972). In the "external coincidence" model, light serves a dual role. First, light entrains a circadian rhythm of responsiveness to itself, and second, when external light is coincident, or not coincident, with a photosensitive phase of that rhythm, the organism will interpret the photoperiod as a long, or short day, respectively. In the "internal coincidence" model, light serves only to entrain two or more circadian oscillators that underlie the photoperiodic response. This model suggests that since the phase relationships between internal circadian oscillators may vary under different photoperiodic conditions (e.g., a change in the ratio of light to dark), an inductive configuration between internal oscillators mediating photoperiodic time measurement will only occur under certain light–dark cycles (Pittendrigh, 1981). A common feature of both the internal and external coincidence models is that the critical factor determining whether a particular light–dark cycle will stimulate or inhibit reproductive function depends upon the phase relationship between light and the circadian oscillator(s) involved in the transmission of information about daylength to the hypothalamic–pituitary–gonadal axis.

The hypothesis that the circadian system is involved in photoperiodic time measurement is supported by the results of two different experimental approaches. One approach has been to elucidate the neural and endocrine events mediating the effects of light on reproduction; these physiological approaches will be discussed in Parts B and C of this section. A second approach has involved the exposure of animals to a variety of unusual light–dark cycles and the subsequent determination of whether the animal interpreted the light–dark cycle as a long or short day. A common feature of these light–dark cycles is that light is only present for a short period of time relative to the total amount of darkness. The most common experimental paradigms that are used to test for the involvement of the circadian system in photoperiodic-time measurement are referred to as "resonance," "T," and "night interruption" experiments.

1. Resonance Experiments

"Resonance" experiments refer to studies in which groups of animals are exposed to one of a series of light–dark cycles where a fixed photoperiod of short duration is coupled to varying durations of darkness such that the period (T) of the light dark cycle is lengthened systematically by 12-hour increments. In a typical resonance experiment, groups of animals will be exposed to one of the following light–dark cycles LD 6 : 18, LD 6 : 30, LD 6 : 42, LD 6 : 54. Such studies have now been carried out in four mammalian species, golden hamsters, laboratory rats, voles, and sheep (Elliott *et al.*, 1972; Grocock and Clarke, 1974; Nelson *et al.*, 1982; Almeida and Lincoln, 1982). The response of the reproductive system to resonance light cycles has been similar in all mammalian species tested to date; when the period of the LD cycle is 24 or 48 hours (e.g., LD 6 : 18 or LD 6 : 42) the photoperiod is interpreted as a short day, while periods of 36 or 60 hours (e.g., LD 6 : 30 or LD 6 : 54) are read as a long day. This is true whether the species examined is a long-day breeder, such as the hamster or a short-day breeder, such as the sheep. Thus, testicular function is maintained or induced in hamsters exposed to LD 6 : 30 (Elliott *et al.*, 1972) while testicular regression occurs in sheep transferred from stimulatory short days to LD 6 : 30 (Almeida and Lincoln, 1982).

The results of resonance studies indicate that neither the duration of light nor the duration of dark, nor a ratio between the two is the determining factor for inducing a photoperiodic response. Instead, the results indicate that time measurement involves a response to light that varies on a circadian basis. Thus, under an LD 6 : 18 or LD 6 : 42 photoperiod, the phase relationship between light and the underlying circadian rhythm(s) involved in photoperiodic time measurement is such that the photoperiod is interpreted as a short day, while under LD 6 : 30 or LD 6 : 54 the phase relationship induces a long day response. A direct test of this hypothesis would be to monitor the phase of the circadian rhythm(s) responsible for the measurement of day length. However, at the present time this rhythm has not been identified (but see Section C below). Instead, a directly measurable circadian rhythm such as the rhythm of locomotor activity has been used to track the state of the circadian system under the assumption that the photoperiodic rhythm(s) of sensitivity to light is regulated by the same circadian clock or that at least the two rhythms are regulated by two tightly coupled circadian clocks. Elliott and his colleagues (1972, 1976) demonstrated in the hamster that the phase relationship between the circadian activity rhythm and the LD cycle does indeed vary systematically under resonance photoperiods, and that the effect of light on the hamster's reproductive system depends primarily on the coincidence of the light period with specific phases of the activity rhythm. In the case of the hamster, when light is only coincident with the inactive phase of the hamster's activity rest cycle (i.e., subjective day for this nocturnal species) the photoperiod is interpreted as a short day and testicular regression occurs (i.e., under LD 6 : 18 or LD 6 : 42 cycles). In contrast, when light is coincident occasionally with the active phase (i.e., subjective night), the photoperiod is interpreted as a long day and testicular function is maintained (i.e., under LD 6 : 30 or LD 6 : 54).

2. T Experiments

The term "T experiment" has been used to refer to studies in which groups of animals are exposed to one of a series of light–dark cycles in which a fixed photoperiod is coupled to varying durations of darkness such that the period (T) of the light–dark cycle remains close to 24 hours (e.g., T = 23 to 25 hours). The use of T cycles enables the investigator to position the time of light at different phase points of the circadian system. This is due to the fact that entrainment to a light–dark cycle involves control of both the phase and period of the circadian rhythm, and as T is varied, the phase relationship of the circadian system to the LD cycle is altered as a function of the phase shift needed each day for the period of the endogenous rhythm to equal the period of the entraining light–dark cycle (Pittendrigh, 1981). Elliott has successfully used the T experiment paradigm to map out the circadian rhythm of sensitivity of the golden hamster's reproductive response to 1-hour light pulses (Elliott, 1976, 1981; Elliott and Goldman, 1981). By changing T of the light–dark cycle from 23.34 to 24.67 hours, while maintaining the duration of light at a fixed 1-hour interval, Elliott was able to position the 1 hour of light at different phase points of the circadian rhythm of activity; a reference rhythm used to ascertain the phase relationship between the light and the circadian system. As predicted from the hypothesis that a circadian rhythm of sensitivity to light underlies photoperiodic time measurement, the testicular response of hamsters depended markedly on T. When T was close to 24 hours (e.g., T = 23.93 or 24.14 hours), testicular regression occurred indicating the animals interpreted the LD cycle as a short day. Under T cycles further from 24 hours (e.g., T = 23.34 or 24.67 hours), testicular regression was blocked. An analysis of the phase relationship between the time of the light pulse and the circadian rhythm of activity revealed that the photoperiodic response to the different T cycles was strongly correlated with the circadian time at which light was presented (Fig. 7). In the case of the hamster, the time of sensitivity to the photostimulatory effects of light on the circadian system corresponds closely to the subjective night phase of the hamster's activity rhythm.

The results from both T and resonance experiments in hamsters emphasize the importance of the phase relationship between light and the circadian system in determining whether or not photic stimulation of the reproductive system will occur. Both sets of experiments utilize the fact that by

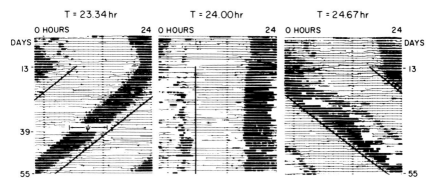

FIG. 7. Entrainment of the activity rhythm of three representative hamsters initially exposed to constant darkness before being transferred to one of three light cycles with different periods (T) on day 13. Each T cycle was made up of a 1-hour period of light coupled to dark periods of varying duration. The heavy lines connect the midpoints of the 1-hour pulses. The phase relationship (ψ) between the onset of activity and the light pulse is a function of T. Testicular growth was stimulated in hamsters exposed to T cycles of 23.34 and 24.67 hours and inhibited in animals exposed to a T of 24.00 hours. (From Elliott, 1981.)

changing the period of the LD cycle, normally noninductive light intervals (e.g., 1–6 hours of duration) would be read as a long day. Eskes and Zucker (1978) have used a different experimental approach to demonstrate the same point. They were able to alter the phase relationship between a normally noninductive photoperiodic light–dark cycle (LD 10 : 14) and the circadian system by changing the endogenous period of the system. This was accomplished by administering deuterium oxide (D_2O) in the water, a treatment known to lengthen the free-running circadian rhythm of activity. Treatment of hamsters with D_2O altered the phase relationship of hamsters exposed to LD 10 : 14 in such a manner that the 10-hour period of light was now coincident with the photosensitive phase of the hamster's rhythm of sensitivity to light. As a result, testicular regression which normally occurs during exposure to LD 10 : 14 in the hamster was blocked.

3. Night Interruption Experiment

Night interruption experiments refer to studies in which animals are exposed to short days with the night being interrupted by a short pulse of light. A typical night-interruption paradigm may involve exposure of animals to an LD 6 : 18 light cycle with a daily 15–60 minute light pulse interrupting the dark phase at various time points. Night interruption experiments have been carried out on a variety of different mammalian species including golden hamsters, Djungarian hamsters, voles, sheep, and mink (Ravault and Ortavant, 1977; Lincoln, 1978; Hoffmann, 1979;

Rudeen and Reiter, 1980; Grocock, 1981; Boissin-Agasse *et al.*, 1982; Earnest and Turek, 1983a; Ellis and Follett, 1983). Night interruption lighting schedules are often referred to as skeleton photoperiods since they are designed to simulate the time of "lights-on" and "lights-off" of complete photoperiods. In all cases it has been found that the interruption of the night at certain circadian phases with a brief pulse of light can lead to a long-day response of the reproductive system.

Caution should be taken in interpreting the results of night interruption experiments. First, positive results from a night interruption experiment (i.e., a long-day response is induced by the pulse of light during the night of an otherwise short day), although being consistent with the hypothesis that a circadian rhythm of sensitivity to light underlies photoperiodic time measurement, do not demonstrate the validity of such a hypothesis. Indeed, such results are equally compatible with an hourglass hypothesis for photoperiodic time measurement where the critical factor is the total duration of an uninterrupted night. To conclusively demonstrate circadian involvement in photoperiodic time measurement, it is necessary to carry out resonance and/or T experiments. Once these studies have been carried out for a given species, then the night interruption paradigm can be useful in mapping out the circadian rhythm of sensitivity to light. However, defining the circadian phases at which the coincidence of light will lead to a long-day response is not as straightforward as at first it may appear. Unless there is some independent measure of how the circadian system is entraining to the night interruption lighting schedule, it is not known which of the two periods of light is being interpreted as dawn and which as dusk. Using the activity rhythm as a marker of the phase relationship between the circadian system and the LD cycle, we have found that a single 1-second pulse of light interrupting the dark period of an LD 6:18 lighting schedule can be interpreted as a "lights-off" signal in some animals and a "lights-on" signal in others (Earnest and Turek, 1983a).

Night interruption experiments in golden hamsters have demonstrated that very short pulses of light can influence the neuroendocrine–gonadal axis in this species. As little as 1 to 6 seconds of light interrupting the night of an otherwise short nonstimulatory light cycle can mimic the effects of long days and maintain testis function and/or induce testicular growth (Earnest and Turek, 1983a; Ellis and Follett, 1983). Indeed, 10-second pulses of light during the night, when delivered only once every 2, 4, or 7 days, can also partially or totally prevent the inhibitory effects of short days on neuroendocrine–gonadal activity in hamsters (Earnest and Turek, 1984).

It is even possible to mimic the photostimulatory effects of an LD 14:10 light cycle on testicular function in hamsters with only two 1-

second pulses of light separated by dark intervals of 14 and 10 hours (Earnest and Turek, 1983a). It is important to note that in this study the activity rhythm of all of the animals entrained such that their active period occurred during the 10 hours of darkness. Thus the circadian system entrained in an identical fashion to the two 1-second pulses of light as they would have to a complete LD 14 : 10 light cycle. If the animals had entrained such that the active phase occurred during the 14-hour dark period, then it is anticipated that testicular regression would have occurred because in this case, the skeleton photoperiod is being "read" as a short day (i.e., LD 10 : 14). Indeed, Elliott and Goldman (1981) have shown that the same LD cycle can be photostimulatory or nonstimulatory with respect to testicular activity depending on the way the circadian system entrains to a skeleton photoperiod. After free-running in constant darkness for 34 days, 18 hamsters were exposed to a skeleton photoperiod for 63 days consisting of two 15-minute pulses separated by intervals of darkness lasting 13.5 and 10 hours. Because the pulses of light were first introduced at different circadian phase points, some of the animals ($N = 10$) entrained such that locomotor activity occurred during the 10-hour dark interval. Thus, these animals were interpreting the skeleton photoperiod as an LD 14 : 10 light cycle, and in all cases, testicular function was maintained. In contrast, the remaining animals ($N = 8$) entrained such that locomotor activity occurred during the 13.5 hour dark interval. Thus, these animals interpreted the skeleton photoperiod as an LD 10.5 : 13.5 light cycle, and testicular regression was observed in all these animals. These results again point to the importance of the phase relationship between the LD cycle and the circadian cycle in determining whether a given photoperiod will be interpreted as a long or short day.

The fact that short pulses of light in either a night interruption or a T experiment paradigm can stimulate neuroendocrine–gonadal activity raises the possibility that attempts to mimic the effects of light with pharmacological agents may yield insight on the neurochemical events that mediate the effects of light on the circadian system involved in photoperiodic time measurement. In a recent experiment (Earnest and Turek, 1983b), we attempted to mimic the effects of a 1-second night interruption on reproductive function with an intraventricular injection of carbachol, a cholinergic agonist. This experiment was inspired by the work of Zatz who had previously demonstrated that carbachol could mimic the phase shifting effects of light on circadian rhythmicity in mice and rats (Zatz, 1979; Zatz and Herkenham, 1981). We were able to show that the inhibitory effects of a short day photoperiod (LD 6 : 18) on testicular function were prevented by nighttime, but not daytime, intraventricular injections of carbachol. Importantly, carbachol injections were found to stimulate testicular function only in those animals in which the injection also altered the entrainment of the circadian rhythm of activity. We have also recently demonstrated that while daily injections of saline have no effect on the free-running rhythm of activity in DD, injection of carbachol once every 23.33 or once every 24 hours to hamsters maintained in DD could entrain the circadian rhythm of activity (Earnest and Turek, unpublished results). Importantly, testicular function was maintained in animals injected with carbachol once every 23.33 hours, while testicular regression occurred in animals injected with carbachol once every 24 hours (Fig. 8). Thus in both a night interruption and a T experiment paradigm carbachol injections mimic the effects of light on both the circadian rhythm of activity and testicular function. These results suggest that acetylcholine may play an important role in mediating the effect of light on the circadian clock(s) responsible for regulating the circadian rhythm of activity and photoperiodic time measurement. At the present time, the site at which acetylcholine exerts its action is unknown; acetylcholine may be released by neurons that carry information from the retina to the circadian system, or it may be a neurotransmitter within the circadian system itself.

Taken together, the results obtained from "resonance," "T," and "night interruption" experiments demonstrate that the circadian system is involved in photoperiodic time measurement. It appears that the coinci-

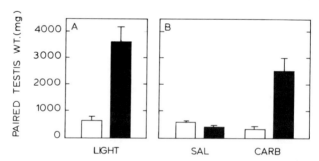

FIG. 8.   (A) mean (±SEM) paired testis weights of hamsters after a 9-week exposure to a T cycle of 24 hours (LD 1 : 23: open bar) or 23.33 hours (LD 1 : 22.33: black bar). This differential gonadal response to the 1-hour light pulses is due to different phase relationships between the 1-hour light pulses and the circadian system (see Fig. 7). (B) Mean paired testis weights of hamsters receiving intraventricular injections of either saline or carbachol while being exposed to constant darkness for 9 weeks. The open bars represent animals that were injected once every 24 hours while the black bars represent animals injected once every 23.33 hours. Injections of carbachol entrained the circadian rhythm of locomotor activity and mimicked the effects of light on gonadal function. Testicular function was only stimulated when the injections of carbachol were coincident with that portion of the circadian locomotor activity rhythm known to be sensitive to the stimulatory effects of light, i.e., when T of the injection was 23.33 hours.

dence, or lack of coincidence, of light with certain phases of a circadian oscillator(s) involved in the photoperiodic response will determine whether the light cycle is interpreted as a long or short day. Whether some form of the internal and/or external coincidence model is involved in the photoperiodic response is not known. Once the circadian system has interpreted the photoperiod as being a long or a short day, this information is relayed to the hypothalamic–pituitary–gonadal axis and changes in reproductive activity occur. In the last decade a good deal of progress has been made in elucidating the neural and endocrine events involved in photoperiodic time measurement and the coupling between the circadian and reproductive systems. As described below, the suprachiasmatic nuclei and the pineal gland play a central role in this response.

B. SUPRACHIASMATIC NUCLEI

In view of the fact that (1) a circadian clock(s) is involved in photoperiodic time measurement (Elliott and Goldman, 1981) and (2) the suprachiasmatic nucleus (SCN) of the hypothalamus appears to contain a circadian clock that is involved in the generation of a variety of different circadian rhythms (Rusak and Zucker, 1979; Turek, 1983; Moore, 1983), an obvious place to look for the clock involved in photoperiodic time measurement is the SCN. Indeed, early studies in the golden hamster demonstrated that destruction of the SCN abolishes the photoperiodic gonadal response, and lesioned animals remain reproductively competent irrespective of photoperiodic treatment (Rusak and Morin, 1976; Stetson and Watson-Whitmyre, 1976). In addition, lesions of the SCN in hamsters abolish both (1) short-day induced changes in the negative feedback effects of testosterone on pituitary gonadotropin release (Turek et al., 1980) and (2) the attenuated castration response that occurs during exposure to short days (Turek et al., 1983). Thus, the inhibitory effects of short days on hypothalamic–pituitary–gonadal activity are abolished by SCN lesions in this species. The SCN also appears to play a role in the timing of photoperiodically controlled seasonal cycles in ewes. SCN-lesioned ewes often continue to show estrus cycles and ovulation during the normally quiescent nonbreeding period (Domański et al., 1980; Przekop and Domański, 1980). Unfortunately, the role of the SCN in the photoperiodic control of seasonal reproductive cycles has only been examined in these two mammalian species. Why an impairment of the circadian organization leads to the maintenance of reproductive competence during exposure to nonstimulatory lighting conditions in both hamsters and sheep is not known. There is no a priori reason to expect that disruption of the circadian system involved in photoperiodic time measurement would result in the maintenance of gonadal function regardless of daylength. It is of great interest to determine what effect lesioning of the SCN has on the gonadal response of other photoperiodic species.

While total destruction of both SCN completely disrupts short-day induced testicular regression in the hamster, partial destruction of SCN tissue can lead to a partial inhibition as demonstrated by either a delay in the onset of regression and/or the prevention of complete gonadal atrophy (Turek and Pickard, 1981). Since the SCN appears to be functioning as a biological clock involved in photoperiodic time measurement, these results suggest that information about daylength is conveyed from the circadian system to the neuroendocrine–gonadal axis in a graded rather than an all-or-none fashion.

The mechanism by which partial or complete destruction of SCN tissue renders the hamster totally, or partially, unresponsive to the inhibitory effects of short days is not completely understood. Although there may be a direct neural input from the SCN to the pituitary gonadotropin control centers that are responsive to manipulations of daylength, it appears that at least part of the effects of the SCN on reproductive function are mediated by a multisynaptic pathway from the SCN to the pineal gland.

C. PINEAL GLAND

The photoperiodic control of seasonal reproductive activity has been found to be disrupted by pinealectomy in a variety of different mammalian species including golden hamsters, Djungarian hamsters, ferrets, voles, white-footed mice, and sheep (Turek and Campbell, 1979; Hoffmann, 1981a). Indeed, we know of no photoperiodic mammalian species that has been adequately investigated in which pinealectomy does not somehow alter the normal response of the neuroendocrine–gonadal axis to photoperiodic manipulations. The type of effect that pinealectomy has on the photoperiodic response can vary widely from species to species as exemplified by the fact that pinealectomy prevents short-day induced testicular regression in the golden hamster but induces testicular regression in Turkish hamsters exposed to photostimulatory long days (Carter et al., 1982).

There is now substantial evidence suggesting that the photoperiodic control of the release of the pineal hormone melatonin plays a critical role in regulating hypothalamic–pituitary–gonadal activity. The synthesis and release of melatonin is tightly coupled to the light–dark cycle such that melatonin levels in both the pineal gland and the blood are high at night and low during the day (Reiter, 1982). The administration of melatonin has been shown to inhibit as well as stimulate neuroendocrine gonadal activity in a variety of mammalian species (Turek and Campbell, 1979; Reiter, 1980, 1982; Hoffmann, 1981b). Recent studies on both Djungarian hamsters and sheep indicate that the duration of nighttime melatonin release determines whether the photoperiod will be interpreted as a long or a short day (Carter and Goldman, 1983; Bittman, 1983).

The diurnal rhythm in melatonin production is regulated by the SCN. Bilateral lesioning of the SCN leads to the abolishment of the diurnal rhythm in pineal N-acetyltransferase (NAT) activity; NAT is an enzyme involved in the synthesis of melatonin (Moore, 1981). It has been known for a number of years that pineal melatonin synthesis is under the direct control of a β-adrenergic input from the superior cervical ganglion (SCG) (Binkley, 1983). The preganglionic neurons that innervate the SCG in turn derive from the intermediolateral nucleus (IMLN) of the spinal cord (Rando et al., 1981). Anatomical and physiological studies suggest that the neural pathway from the SCN to the IMLN involves the paraventricular nucleus (PVN) of the hypothalamus (Swanson and Cowan, 1975; Swanson and Kuypers, 1980; Swanson and Sawchenko, 1980; Pickard and Turek, 1983a). SCN efferents project monosynaptically to regions of the PVN that project monosynaptically to the IMLN (Swanson and Kuypers, 1980). Recent studies have demonstrated that PVN lesions disrupt the normal diurnal fluctuations in pineal melatonin and NAT levels in rats and hamsters (Bittman, 1983; Klein et al., 1983) and block short day induced testicular regression in the hamster (Pickard and Turek, 1983a,b; Bittman, 1983) in a manner similar to that observed following either SCN

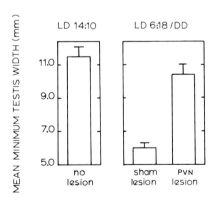

FIG. 9.   Mean (±SEM) minimum testis width observed in control animals maintained on a photostimulatory LD 14 : 10 light cycle for 13 weeks (left) and in sham-lesioned and PVN-lesioned animals maintained on a nonstimulatory LD 6 : 18 light cycle for 10 weeks followed by 3 weeks of constant darkness (DD). PVN lesions prevented short-day induced testicular regression, but did not disrupt the circadian rhythm of locomotor activity during exposure to LD 6 : 18 or DD. (From Pickard and Turek, 1983b.)

lesions or pinealectomy (Fig. 9). Importantly, PVN lesions that block short-day induced testicular regression do not affect the circadian rhythm of activity suggesting that different efferent pathways connect the SCN to the pineal gland and centers in the brain responsible for locomotor activity (Pickard and Turek, 1983b).

Although many of the details are missing, the general outline of how the circadian system is involved in photoperiodic time measurement, and ultimately the photic-control of neuroendocrine–gonadal function, is emerging. The results from studies involving unusual light–dark cycles (i.e., resonance, T, and night-interruption experiments) have demonstrated that a circadian oscillator is involved in measuring day length, and that the key feature of photoperiodic time measurement involves the phase relationship between the photoperiod and the circadian system. The location of the photoperiodic circadian clock(s) is probably in the SCN which directly receives photic information from the eye via a retinohypothalamic tract. The SCN in turn regulates pineal melatonin synthesis via a neural pathway involving the PVN, IMLN, and SCG. The rhythm in pineal melatonin release then influences hypothalamic–pituitary–gonadal activity.

VII. Conclusions

Many of the neural, endocrine, morphological, and behavioral events associated with reproduction in mammals receive temporal information from the circadian system. This information serves to coordinate events involved in the reproductive process as well as to synchronize this process with the internal and external environment of the organism. Over the past decade, a great deal of progress has been made in describing the relationships between the reproductive and circadian systems. In addition, some of the physiological events that link the two systems have recently been discovered. However, many of the neurochemical and neurophysiological events that mediate the interactions between the two systems remain to be discovered. Over the next decade, many advances will be made by both circadian and reproductive biologists in elucidating the neural events that underlie circadian rhythmicity and reproductive physiology. At present there is little communication between these two groups of investigators. Both communities would profit greatly by the establishment of greater interactions with one another.

REFERENCES

Adler, N. T. (1978). *In* "Sex and Behavior: Status and Prospectus" (T. E. McGill, D. A. Dewsbury, and B. O. Sachs, eds.), p. 115. Plenum, New York.
Aedo, A. R., Landgren, B. M., and Diczfalusy, E. (1981). *Contraception* **23,** 407.

Alleva, J. J., Waleski, M. V., Alleva, F. R., and Umberger, E. J. (1968). *Endocrinology* **82,** 1227.

Alleva, J. J., Waleski, M. V., and Alleva, F. R. (1971). *Endocrinology* **88,** 1368.

Almeida, O. F. X., and Lincoln, G. A. (1982). *Biol. Reprod.* **27,** 1062.

Aschoff, J. (1979). *Z. Tierpsychol.* **49,** 225.

Aschoff, J. (1981). "Handbook of Behavioral Neurobiology: Biological Rhythms," pp. 1–563. Plenum, New York.

Aschoff, J., Dann, S., and Groos, G. A. (1982). "Vertebrate Circadian Systems: Structure and Physiology," pp. 1–363. Springer-Verlag, Berlin and New York.

Barraclough, C. A., and Wise, P. M. (1982). *Endocrine Rev.* **3,** 91.

Bast, J. D., and Greenwald, G. S. (1974). *Endocrinology* **94,** 1295.

Beck, W., and Wuttke, W. (1980). *J. Clin. Endocrinol. Metab.* **50,** 635.

Bethea, C. L., and Neill, J. D. (1980). *Endocrinology* **107,** 1.

Bingel, A. S., and Schwartz, N. B. (1969). *J. Reprod. Fertil.* **19,** 223.

Binkley, S. (1983). *Endocrine Rev.* **4,** 255.

Bittman, E. L. (1983). *Biol. Reprod.* **28** (Suppl. 1), 122.

Bittman, E. L., Lehman, M. N., and Winans, S. S. (1983). *Neurosci. Abstr.* **9,** 318.

Boissin-Agasse, L., Boissin, J., and Ortavant, R. (1982). *Biol. Reprod.* **26,** 110.

Bosc, M. J., and Nicolle, A. (1980). *Reprod. Nutr. Dev.* **20,** 735.

Boyar, R., Perlow, M., Hellman, L., Kapen, S., and Weitzman, E. (1972). *J. Clin. Endocrinol. Metab.* **35,** 73.

Boyar, R. M., Wu, R. H. K., Roffwarg, H., Kapen, S., Weitzman, E. D., Hellman, L., and Finkelstein, J. W. (1976). *J. Clin. Endocrinol. Metab.* **43,** 1418.

Brady, J. (1982). "Biological Timekeeping," pp. 1–197. Cambridge Univ. Press, London and New York.

Bremner, W. J., Vitiello, M. V., and Prinz, P. N. (1983). *J. Clin. Endocrinol. Metab.* **56,** 1278.

Bridges, R. S., and Goldman, B. D. (1975). *Biol. Reprod.* **13,** 617.

Brown-Grant, K., and Raisman, G. (1977). *Proc. R. Soc. London Ser. B* **198,** 279.

Campbell, C. J., and Finkelstein, J. S. (1978). *In* "Environmental Endocrinology" (I. Assenmacher and D. S. Farner, eds.), pp. 196. Springer-Verlag, Berlin and New York.

Campbell, C. S., and Schwartz, N. B. (1980). *Endocrinology* **106,** 1230.

Campbell, C. S., and Turek, F. W. (1981). *In* "Biological Rhythms" (J. A. Aschoff, ed.), p. 523. Plenum, New York.

Carmichael, M. S., and Zucker, I. (1982). *J. Reprod. Fertil.* **66,** 691.

Carmichael, M. S., Nelson, R. J., and Zucker, I. (1981). *Proc. Natl. Acad. Sci. U.S.A.* **78,** 7830.

Carrillo, A. J., and Sawyer, C. H. (1978). *Acta Endocrinol.* **88,** 274.

Carter, D. S., and Goldman, B. D. (1983). *Endocrinology* **113,** 1261.

Carter, D. S., Hall, V. D., Tamarkin, L., and Goldman, B. D. (1982). *Endocrinology* **111,** 863.

Chazal, G., Faudon, M., Gogan, F., Hery, M., Kordon, C., and Laplante, E. (1977). *J. Endocrinol.* **75,** 251.

Cicero, T. J. (1980). *Fed. Proc. Fed. Am. Soc. Exp. Biol.* **39,** 2551.

Coen, C. W., and MacKinnon, P. C. B. (1980). *J. Endocrinol.* **84,** 231.

Davis, F. C., and Menaker, M. (1981). *J. Comp. Physiol.* **143,** 527.

Domanski, E., Przekop, F., and Polkowska, J. (1980). *J. Reprod. Fertil.* **58,** 493.

Dunn, J. D., and Johnson, D. C. (1978). *Neuroendocrinology* **27,** 126.

Earnest, D. J., and Turek, F. W. (1983a). *Biol. Reprod.* **28,** 557.

Earnest, D. J., and Turek, F. W. (1983b). *Science* **219,** 77.

Earnest, D. J., and Turek, F. W. (1984). *J. Androl.* (in press).

Edwards, R. G. (1981). *Nature (London)* **293**, 253.

Egozi, Y., Avissar, S., and Sokolvsky, M. (1982). *Neuroendocrinology* **35**, 93.

Elliott, J. A. (1976). *Fed. Proc. Fed. Am. Soc. Exp. Biol.* **35**, 2339.

Elliott, J. A. (1981). *In* "Biological Clocks in Seasonal Reproductive Cycles" (B. K. Follett and D. E. Follett, eds.), p. 203. Wright Press, Bristol.

Elliott, J. A., and Goldman, B. D. (1981). *In* "Neuroendocrinology of Reproduction" (N. T. Adler, ed.), p. 377. Plenum, New York.

Elliott, J. A., Stetson, M. H., and Menaker, M. (1972). *Science* **178**, 771.

Ellis, D. H., and Follett, B. K. (1983). *Biol. Reprod.* **29**, 805.

Eskes, G. A., and Zucker, I. (1978). *Proc. Natl. Acad. Sci. U.S.A.* **75**, 1034.

Everett, J. W., and Sawyer, C. H. (1950). *Endocrinology* **47**, 198.

Everett, J. W., and Tyrey, L. (1982). *Endocrinology* **111**, 1979.

Fitzgerald, K. M., and Zucker, I. (1976). *Proc. Natl. Acad. Sci. U.S.A.* **73**, 2923.

Follett, B. K., and Follett, D. E. (1981). "Biological Clocks in Seasonal Reproductive Cycles," pp. 1–292. Wright Press, Bristol.

Freeman, M. E., and Banks, J. A. (1980). *Endocrinology* **106**, 668.

Gallo, R. V. (1981). *Biol. Reprod.* **24**, 100.

Geiger, J. M., Plas-Roser, S., and Aron, Cl. (1981). *J. Interdiscip. Cycle Res.* **12**, 109.

Goodman, R. L., and Karsch, F. J. (1981). *In* "Biological Clocks in Seasonal Reproductive Cycles" (B. K. Follett and D. E. Follett, eds.), p. 223. Wright Press, Bristol.

Goodman, R. L., Hotchkiss, J., Karsch, F. J., and Knobil, E. (1974). *Biol. Reprod.* **11**, 624.

Gray, G. D., Sodersten, P., Tallentire, D., and Davidson, J. M. (1978). *Neuroendocrinology* **25**, 174.

Green, D. J., and Gillette, R. (1982). *Brain Res.* **245**, 198.

Grocock, C. A. (1981). *J. Reprod. Fertil.* **62**, 25.

Grocock, C., and Clarke, J. (1974). *J. Reprod. Fertil.* **39**, 337.

Guignard, M. M., Pesquies, P. C., Serrurier, B. D., Merino, D. B., and Reinberg, A. E. (1980). *Acta Endocrinol.* **94**, 536.

Gunnet, J. W., and Freeman, M. E. (1983). *Endocrine Rev.* **4**, 44.

Hoffmann, K. (1979). *Experientia* **35**, 1529.

Hoffmann, K. (1981a). *In* "The Pineal Organ: Photobiology-Biochemistry-Endocrinology" (A. Oksche and P. Pevet, eds.), p. 123. North-Holland Publ., Amsterdam.

Hoffmann, K. (1981b). *In* "Handbook of Behavioral Neurobiology: Biological Rhythms" (J. Aschoff, ed.), Vol. 4, p. 449. Plenum, New York.

Hoffmann, K., Illnerova, H., and Vanecek, J. (1981). *Biol. Reprod.* **24**, 551.

Inouye, S. T., and Kawamura, H. (1979). *Proc. Natl. Acad. Sci. U.S.A.* **76**, 5962.

Judd, H. L. (1979). *In* "Endocrine Rhythms" (D. T. Krieger, ed.), p. 299. Raven, New York.

Judd, H. L., Parker, D. C., and Yen, S. C. (1977). *J. Clin. Endocrinol. Metab.* **44**, 865.

Kaiser, I. H., and Halberg, F. (1962). *Ann. N.Y. Acad. Sci.* **98**, 1042.

Kalra, P. S., and Kalra, S. P. (1977). *Endocrinology* **101**, 1821.

Kapen, S., Boyar, R., Perlow, M., Hellman, L., and Weitzman, E. D. (1973). *Life Sci.* **13**, 693.

Kapen, S., Boyar, R. M., Finkelstein, J. W., Hellman, L., and Weitzman, E. D. (1974). *J. Clin. Endocrinol. Metab.* **39**, 293.

Kapen, S., Vagenakis, A., and Braverman, L. (1980). *J. Clin. Endocrinol. Metab.* **51**, 302.

Katz, J. L., Boyar, R. M., Roffwarg, H., Hellman, L., and Weiner, H. (1977). *Psychosoma. Med.* **39**, 241.

Kawakami, M., Arita, J., and Yoshioka, E. (1980). *Endocrinology* **106**, 1087.

Keating, R. J., and Tcholakian, R. K. (1979). *Endocrinology* **104**, 184.
Klein, D. C., Smoot, R., Weller, J. L., Higa, S., Markey, S. P., Creed, G. J., and Jacobwitz, D. M. (1983). *Brain Res. Bull.* **10**, 647.
Knobil, E. (1980). *Recent Prog. Horm. Res.* **36**, 53.
Krieger, D. T., and Aschoff, J. (1979). *In* "Endocrinology" (L. J. DeGroot, ed.), Vol. 3, p. 2079. Greene & Stratton, New York.
Lanman, T. J., and Seidman, L. (1977). *Biol. Reprod.* **17**, 224.
Legan, S. J., and Karsch, F. J. (1975). *Endocrinology* **96**, 57.
Legan, S. J., Coon, G. A., and Karsch, F. J. (1975). *Endocrinology* **96**, 50.
Levine, J. E., and Ramirez, V. D. (1982). *Endocrinology* **111**, 1439.
Lincoln, D. W., and Porter, D. G. (1976). *Nature (London)* **260**, 780.
Lincoln, G. A. (1978). *J. Reprod. Fertil.* **52**, 179.
McCormack, C. E., and Sridaran, R. (1978). *J. Endocrinol.* **76**, 135.
McLean, B. K., Rubel, A., and Nikitovitch-Winer, M. B. (1977). *Neuroendocrinology* **23**, 23.
Merriam, G. R., and Wachter, K. W. (1982). *Am. J. Physiol.* **243**, E310.
Miyatake, A., Morimoto, Y., Oisho, T., Hanasaki, N., Sugita, Y., Iijima, S., Teshima, Y., Hishikawa, Y., and Yamamura, Y. (1980). *J. Clin. Endocrinol. Metab.* **51**, 1365.
Moline, M. L., Albers, H. E., Todd, R. B., and Moore-Ede, M. C. (1981). *Horm. Behav.* **15**, 451.
Moore, R. Y. (1981). *In* "Neurosecretion and Brain Peptides" (J. B. Martin, S. Reichlin, and K. L. Bick, eds.), p. 449. Raven, New York.
Moore, R. Y. (1983). *Fed. Proc. Fed. Am. Soc. Exp. Biol.* **42**, 2783.
Moore-Ede, M. C., Sulzman, F. M., and Fuller, C. A. (1982). "The Clocks that Time Us: Physiology of the Circadian Timing System," pp. 1–448. Harvard Univ. Press, Cambridge, Massachusetts.
Moore-Ede, M. C., Czeisler, C. A., and Richardson, G. S. (1983a). *N. Engl. J. Med.* **309**, 530.
Moore-Ede, M. C., Czeisler, C. A., and Richardson, G. S. (1983b). *N. Engl. J. Med.* **309**, 469.
Nelson, R. J., Bamat, M. K., and Zucker, I. (1982). *Biol. Reprod.* **26**, 329.
Norman, R. L., and Spies, H. G. (1974). *Endocrinology* **95**, 1367.
Ortavant, R., Daveau, A., Garnier, D. H., Pelletier, J., de Reviers, M. M., and Terqui, M. (1982). *J. Reprod. Fertil.* **64**, 347.
Perachio, A. A., Alexander, M., Marr, L. D., and Collins, D. C. (1977). *Steroids* **29**, 21.
Pickard, G. E., and Turek, F. W. (1983a). *Neurosci. Lett.* **43**, 67.
Pickard, G. E., and Turek, F. W. (1983b). *Neurosci. Abstr.* **9**, 626.
Pirke, K. M., Fichter, M. M., Lund, R., and Doerr, P. (1979). *Acta Endocrinol.* **92**, 193.
Pittendrigh, C. S. (1972). *Proc. Natl. Acad. Sci. U.S.A.* **69**, 2734.
Pittendrigh, C. S. (1981). *In* "Handbook of Behavioral Neurobiology: Biological Rhythms" (J. Aschoff, ed.), Vol. 4, p. 95. Plenum, New York.
Pittendrigh, C. S., and Dann, S. (1976). *J. Comp Physiol.* **106**, 333.
Plant, T. M. (1981). *Biol. Reprod.* **25**, 244.
Pohl, C. R., Richardson, D. W., Hutchinson, J. S., Germak, J. A., and Knobil, E. (1983). *Endocrinology* **112**, 2076.
Poland, R. E., Rubin, R. T., and Weischsel, M. E., Jr. (1980). *Psychoneuroendocrinology* **5**, 209.
Przekop, F., and Domański, E. (1980). *J. Endocrinol.* **85**, 481.
Rando, T. A., Bowers, C. W., and Zigmond, R. E. (1981). *J. Comp. Neurol.* **196**, 73.
Ravault, J. P., and Ortavant, R. (1977). *Ann. Biol. Anim. Biochem. Biophys.* **17**, 459.

Rebar, R. W., and Yen, S. S. C. (1979). *In* "Endocrine Rhythms" (D. T. Krieger, ed.), p. 259. Raven, New York.

Reiter, R. J. (1980). *Endocrine Rev.* **1**, 109.

Reiter, R. J. (1982). *In* "Frontiers in Neuroendocrinology" (W. F. Ganong and L. Martini, eds.), p. 287. Raven, New York.

Roulier, R., Conte-Devolx, B., Castanas, E., Bert, J., and Codaccioni, J. L. (1981). *In* "Human Pituitary Hormones: Circadian and Episodic Variations" (E. van Cauter, ed.), p. 310. Nyhoff, The Hague.

Rubin, R. T., and Poland, R. E. (1976). *Psychoneuroendocrinology* **1**, 281.

Rubin, R. T., Gouin, P. R., Lubin, A., Poland, R. E., and Pirke, K. M. (1975). *J. Clin. Endocrinol. Metab.* **40**, 1027.

Rudeen, P. K., and Reiter, R. J. (1980). *J. Reprod. Fertil.* **60**, 279.

Rusak, B., and Morin, L. P. (1976). *Biol. Reprod.* **15**, 366.

Rusak, B., and Zucker, I. (1979). *Physiol. Rev.* **59**, 449.

Samson, W. K., and McCann, S. M. (1979a). *Endocrinology* **105**, 939.

Samson, W. K., and McCann, S. M. (1979b). *Brain Res. Bull.* **4**, 783.

Schwartz, N. B. (1969). *Recent Prog. Horm. Res.* p. 1.

Schwartz, W., Davidsen, L. C., and Smith, C. B. (1980). *J. Comp. Neurol.* **189**, 157.

Seibel, M. M., Shine, W., Smith, D. M., and Taymor, M. L. (1982). *Fertil. Steril.* **37**, 709.

Shander, D., and Goldman, B. (1978). *Endocrinology* **103**, 1383.

Sherwood, O. D., Downing, S. J., Golog, T. G., Gordon, W. L., and Tarbell, M. K. (1983). *Endocrinology* **113**, 997.

Shibata, S., Oomura, Y., Kita, H., and Hattori, K. (1982). *Brain Res.* **247**, 154.

Shimizu, K., Furuya, T., Takeo, Y., Shirama, K., and Maekawa, K. (1983). *Experientia* **39**, 104.

Stetson, M. H., and Anderson, P. J. (1980). *Am. J. Physiol.* **238**, R23.

Stetson, M. H., and Gibson, J. T. (1977). *J. Exp. Zool.* **201**, 289.

Stetson, M. H., and Watson-Whitmyre, M. (1976). *Science* **191**, 197.

Stetson, M. H., Watson-Whitmyre, M., and Matt, K. S. (1977). *J. Interdiscip. Cycle Res.* **8**, 350.

Stetson, M. H., Watson-Whitmyre, M., and Matt, K. S. (1978). *Biol. Reprod.* **19**, 40.

Stetson, M. H., Watson-Whitmyre, M., Dipinto, M. N., and Smith, S. G. (1981). *Biol. Reprod.* **24**, 139.

Swann, J., and Turek, F. W. (1982). *Am. J. Physiol.* **243**, R112.

Swann, J. M., and Turek, F. W. (1983). *Biol. Reprod.* **28**, (Suppl. 1), 50.

Swanson, L. W., and Cowan, W. M. (1975). *J. Comp. Neurol.* **160**, 1.

Swanson, L. W., and Kuypers, H. G. J. M. (1980). *J. Comp. Neurol.* **194**, 555.

Swanson, L. W., and Sawchenko, P. E. (1980). *Neuroendocrinology* **31**, 410.

Sylvester, P. W., Van Vugt, D. A., Aylsworth, C. A., Hanson, E. A., and Meites, J. (1982). *Neuroendocrinology* **34**, 269.

Takahashi, J. S., and Zatz, M. (1982). *Science* **217**, 1104.

Terasawa, E., Wiegand, S. J., and Bridson, W. E. (1980). *Am. J. Physiol.* **238**, E533.

Terranova, P. F. (1980). *Biol. Reprod.* **23**, 92.

Testart, J., Frydman, R., and Roger, M. (1982). *J. Clin. Endocrinol. Metab.* **55**, 374.

Tucker, H. A., and Ringer, R. K. (1982). *Science* **216**, 1381.

Turek, F. W. (1983). *BioScience* **33**, 439.

Turek, F. W., and Campbell, C. S. (1979). *Biol. Reprod.* **20**, 32.

Turek, F. W., and Ellis, G. B. (1981). *In* "Biological Clocks in Seasonal Reproductive Cycles" (B. K. Follett and D. E. Follett, eds.), p. 251. Wright Press, Bristol.

Turek, F. W., and Pickard, G. E. (1981). *In* "Photoperiodism and Reproduction" (R.

Ortavant, J. Pelletier, and J.-P. Rovault, eds.), p. 175. Institute National De La Recherche Agronomique, Paris.

Turek, F. W., Jacobson, C. D., and Gorski, R. A. (1980). *Endocrinology* **107**, 942.

Turek, F. W., Earnest, D. J., and Swann, J. (1982). In "Vertebrate Circadian Systems" (J. Aschoff, S. Dann, and G. Groos, eds.), p. 203. Springer-Verlag, Berlin and New York.

Turek, F. W., Losee-Olson, S. H., and Ellis, G. B. (1983). *Neuroendocrinology* **36**, 335.

Van Cauter, E. (1979). *Am. J. Physiol.* **237**, E255.

Van Cauter, E., and Copinschi, G. (1981). "Human Pituitary Hormones: Circadian and Episodic Variations." Nyhoff, The Hague.

Van der Schoot, P. (1980). *J. Endocrinol.* **86**, 451.

Van Horn, R. N., Beamer, N. B., and Dixson, A. F. (1976). *Biol. Reprod.* **15**, 523.

Van Horn, R. N., and Eaton, G. G. (1979). In "The Study of Prosimian Behavior" (G. A. Doyle, ed.), p. 79. Academic Press, New York.

Vomachka, A. J., and Greenwald, G. S. (1980). *Biol. Reprod.* **22**, 1127.

Weber, A. L., and Adler, N. T. (1978). *Biol. Reprod.* **19**, 425.

Weiner, R. I., and Ganong, W. F. (1978). *Physiol. Rev.* **58**, 905.

Weitzman, E. D. (1980). In "Neuroendocrinology" (D. T. Krieger and J. C. Hughes, eds.), p. 85. Sinauer, Sunderland, Massachusetts.

Weitzman, E. D., Zimmerman, J. C., Czeisler, C. A., and Ronda, J. (1983). *J. Clin. Endocrinol. Metab.* **56**, 352.

Wiegand, S. J., and Terasawa, E. (1982). *Neuroendocrinology* **34**, 395.

Wiegand, S. J., Terasawa, E., Bridson, W. E., and Goy, R. W. (1980). *Neuroendocrinology* **31**, 147.

Yogev, L., and Terkel, J. (1980). *Neuroendocrinology* **31**, 26.

Zatz, M. (1979). *Fed. Proc. Fed. Am. Soc. Exp. Biol.* **38**, 2596.

Zatz, M., and Herkenham, M. A. (1981). *Brain Res.* **212**, 234.

DISCUSSION

G. Slaughter: In your animals exposed to the 1-second light pulse where you may be at the threshold of the stimulus, it appeared that you had two groups of animals with varying responses. Do you think those groups are genetically different in their ability to respond to a stimulus of that duration?

F. W. Turek: I don't know, for example we did not try to breed those animals to see if we could select for threshold differences.

H. L. Bradlow: Two questions: first, do you need two spaced 1-second light pulses to entrain the animals. If you shifted from a 14 light 10 dark cycle to a 24 dark regime and at the appropriate clock time put in a single 1-second pulse will they hold in phase or do you need two to position them in the proper cycle?

F. W. Turek: It would depend upon the period of the light–dark cycles. If a 1-second light pulse was presented once every 24 hours, the animals would entrain so that the light pulse would not fall in the photosensitive phase. However, if the 1-second light pulse was presented once every 23.3 hours then entrainment would occur such that light would fall on the sensitive phase. In that case, my guess is that the pulse of light would indeed be sufficient to maintain testicular function.

H. L. Bradlow: And how would a single pulse work in a 25 hour cycle?

F. W. Turek: If the period of the cycle was 25 hours, then a 1-second pulse of light would also probably be sufficient to maintain testicular function since the light pulse would be coincident with the sensitive phase.

H. L. Bradlow: You have clearly shown that a SCN lesion will block the regression of the testes. If the testes were already regressed and the lesioning was then carried out, will they grow back? In other words, will you abolish the inhibition?

F. W. Turek: Yes, bilateral destruction of the SCN will induce testicular recrudescence in animals with regressed testes in a similar manner as occurs when hamsters are transferred from short to long days.

H. L. Bradlow: So essentially, on a short-day regime you get testicular regression and it is maintained as long as you don't have a specific lesion.

F. W. Turek: It appears that the testes remain enlarged in the absence of short-day information being relayed from the SCN to the pineal gland. In the absence of the SCN, such information cannot reach the pineal gland.

D. L. Foster: As an extension of Dr. Bradlow's question, would you comment on the effects of lesioning the suprachiasmatic nucleus or effects of pinealectomy on testis growth in sexually immature hamsters. Do such males attain puberty at the normal time?

F. W. Turek: In the golden hamster, the photoperiod does not influence the timing of the onset of puberty. Thus in hamsters born and raised on short days, the reproductive system develops normally for the first 5–8 weeks of life, and then the inhibitory effects of short days become apparent. We have not been able to alter the time course of puberty by pinealectomy, and I don't think lesions of the SCN would alter pubertal events which are not dependent on photic information.

D. L. Foster: It is important to point out that there are species differences with respect to the role of the pineal in the pubertal process. In contrast to the hamster, disruption of pineal function in the female sheep has profound effects on the timing of puberty. Dr. Steven Yellon, a postdoctoral fellow in my laboratory, has recently demonstrated that bilateral removal of the superior cervical ganglia in 6-week-old lambs reared in natural photoperiod abolishes the nocturnal rise in circulating melatonin and prevents onset of puberty at the normal age of 30 weeks. In the absence of normal pineal function, the prepubertal period is extended by twofold, and first ovulation occurs at approximately 60 weeks of age.

F. W. Turek: The key here is that the lamb is sensitive to the effects of daylength early in life while the golden hamster is not. I think pinealectomy will only have a major effect on hypothalamic–pituitary–gonadal function when the reproductive system is sensitive to daylength. For example, pinealectomy can influence the timing of puberty in Siberian hamsters raised on short days; this species unlike the golden hamster, but like the lamb, is responsive to daylength early in life.

S. Y. Ying: In your 1-second light pulse studies, would the light intensity also be important?

F. W. Turek: We have not carried out experiments involving different light intensities. Michael Menaker has been looking at questions related to the threshold and quality of light necessary for entrainment and photic-induced changes in reproductive functions. The threshold for both functions is quite low (around 1 lux) and we work well above threshold light intensities.

S. Y. Ying: Have you also turned off the lights for 1 second in a constant regimen?

F. W. Turek: Yes, if you turn off the lights for a short time period there will not be an inhibition of the reproductive system because light will still be coincident with the photosensitive phase.

S. Y. Ying: Would other environmental factors such as noise act as the pacemaker?

F. W. Turek: We have not been able to entrain hamsters to nonphotic signals. We have tried daily disturbances, saline and melatonin injections, as well as exposure to a receptive female. None of these agents influence the rhythm of activity. We have never been able to affect the reproductive system with other environmental factors in terms of stimulating reproduction while hamsters are exposed to nonstimulatory short days. However, it is possible to inhibit the reproductive system by exposing the animals to very cold temperature or food deprivation, even though they are exposed to stimulatory long days.

W. Wehrenberg: Fred, that was a very illuminating presentation you just gave us. I have a couple of questions which I hope you can shed some light on. During constant light you observed a splitting of the activity rhythm. When you follow plasma LH concentrations in these animals, you observed two surges, one associated with each activity rhythm. In contrast, in animals with only one activity rhythm you observed only one LH surge. My question is, was the total LH released in animals with the two LH surges equivalent to the total LH released in animals with just one surge?

F. W. Turek: We do not see any differences in terms of the total LH released, but I want to qualify that statement. In some animals LH levels reach values above the maximum amount detectable. So I can't really say what the maximum amount is in some animals.

W. Wehrenberg: A second question, when the animals are without photic influences, i.e., free-running, the activity rhythm was about 25 hours. Yet I noticed that when you made lesions of the SCN the activity rhythm was less than 24 hours. What explained this shift?

F. W. Turek: If we lesion a single SCN in animals exposed to LL, we see a decrease in the period of the free-running rhythm about 90% of the time. This is observed in animals with either an intact or a split activity rhythm. Interestingly, this also occurs in cockroaches in which a circadian pacemaker is thought to reside in each optic lobe; removal of one optic lobe decreases the free-running period. We think this is telling us something about the way circadian pacemakers interact with each other to generate a single rhythm. However, what this means at any sort of anatomical or neurochemical level is not known. It definitely is a characteristic of circadian systems; once you start removing pieces of the pacemaker(s), the period of the expressed rhythm shortens.

R. Goodman: I think you have to be a bit careful about how you interpret the carbachol data. You clearly showed that a cholinergic agonist mimics the effects of light, but it doesn't necessarily follow that light is acting via acetylcholine. A more definitive test would be to determine if a cholinergic antagonist will block the effects of that 1-second light pulse. Have you done that experiment?

F. W. Turek: Yes, that is what David Earnest is doing now. At the present time he is trying to do two things. He is trying to determine if the SCN is the site of action of carbachol by applying carbachol directly to the SCN. Second, he is using cholinergic antagonists to see if he can block the effects of short light pulses.

R. Goodman: I assume that each individual animal has its own free-running period. Is there any information available on whether that's genetically determined or that something occurring during pregnancy determines an individual animal's free-running period.

F. W. Turek: Very few studies have been done to look at the genetic basis of biological rhythms in mammals. Studies in invertebrates have demonstrated that it is possible to select for specific circadian characteristics, such as period and phase. Fred Davis has found that mice raised from birth in either a short LD cycle (i.e., 20 hours) or a long LD cycle (i.e., 28 hours), show similar free-running periods when exposed to constant conditions as adults. Thus learning probably plays little, if any, role in determining the period of endogenous circadian rhythms. Interestingly, we have very preliminary evidence which indicates that young hamsters born to and raised by a female hamster with a split rhythm of activity are more likely to have a split activity rhythm as an adult, than an animal born to and raised by a mother with an intact activity rhythm. Whether this has a genetic basis, or is due to the exposure either *in utero* and/or during development to a mother with a split circadian system is not known.

R. E. Peter: With Alice Hontela in my laboratory, we have studied the daily cycles of gonadotropin release in the goldfish. Goldfish that are actively undergoing ovarian recrudescence or that are holding in a preovulatory condition have a regular daily cycle of gonadotropin release, whereas fish that are undergoing ovarian regression or that are sexually regressed do not have such daily cycles. When goldfish are exposed to stimulatory environmental conditions, such as a long photoperiod and warm water temperatures (20°C), the daily cycle is accentuated. If we continue the exposure to these conditions for an extended period, the daily cycle disappears by having the nadir serum GTH levels increase to the apogee levels, resulting in an overall increase in serum gonadotropin levels coincident with the onset of ovarian regression.

F. W. Turek: You get an overall increase in gonadotropins when the gonads are regressed?

R. E. Peter: That's right. In other experiments we've done daily injections of low dosages of gonadotropin, and found that female goldfish are responsive, in terms of ovarian growth, to a daily injection only at certain times of the day. Interestingly, this coincides reasonably well with the time of day when the fish would normally have a surge of gonadotropin release. With Mr. Louis Garcia, we found most recently that if we incubate ovarian follicles from female goldfish *in vitro* and test their steroid release response to gonadotropin, the follicles that respond best to gonadotropin are ones taken from fish at the time of the daily surge of gonadotropin release. If we take follicles from goldfish some hours later, when the fish are at the nadir levels of the daily cycle in serum gonadotropin, these follicles have very little responsiveness to gonadotropin *in vitro,* and in fact don't show a clear dose-dependent response in steroid release. What this indicates, I think, is that coincident with the daily cycle of gonadotropin release, there is also a daily variation in receptors for gonadotropin in the ovary. What synchronizes this change in receptors with the gonadotropin cycle is an interesting question; whether gonadotropin can synchronize its own responsiveness is hard to say. The question is whether in the mammals, where you have elegantly demonstrated a daily variation in responsiveness within the brain, do you have evidence for variations in responsiveness at the pituitary and gonadal levels?

F. W. Turek: No, we do not have any evidence for that, however, I should add that I do not know of very many experiments that have addressed that question. We do know that the response of the reproductive system to melatonin injections varies during the day. It would not surprise me at all that there's a circadian change in either the gonadal or the pituitary response to specific hormones. Along these lines, may I show another slide? This is an important finding which indicates that increased LH and FSH levels are not always correlated with an active reproductive state. This is a slide I borrowed from Kay Jorgenson and Nenna Schwartz in which they summarize LH and FSH levels as well as progesterone and estrogen levels in female hamsters that are either exposed to long days, and thus are showing normal estrous cycles, or to short days, which have induced anestrous. Notice that in the female hamster exposed to long days there is a surge in serum LH and FSH levels on proestrous. However, during exposure to short days, ovulation has ceased, then daily surges of LH, FSH, and progesterone are observed. Now this raises all sorts of question. If you get daily surges in LH and FSH why isn't ovulation occurring? How do you go from an animal that's showing a surge once every 4 days to one that's showing a surge every day?

H. Robertson: You have drawn our attention to the effect of the circadian rhythm on the time of day of the LH surge in the rat, the hamster, and the human. Some 25 years ago we studied this in the ewe and found that the time of onset of estrus in the ewe is biphasic. One group having a peak between 0500 and 0700 hours and another with a peak 12 hours later. We subsequently showed that LH was discharged from the pituitary 2–6 hours after the onset of estrus. The biphasic distribution of the time of LH release in the ewe is of interest since the mean duration of the estrus cycle is 16.5 days, and it is tempting to speculate whether this may be related to the 12 hour difference between the two peaks of LH rather than to the presence of two populations of sheep, one with a 16 day cycle length and another with a cycle length of 17 days.

P. M. Wise: I have a question relative to the animals which exhibit "split" running behavior patterns. In the hamsters which you ovariectomize and treated with estradiol, you demonstrated two LH surges a day. Do you think that multiple LH surges on 1 day occur in the "split" animals that are not ovariectomized and estrogen-treated where you demonstrated periodic lordotic behavior?

F. W. Turek: I do not predict that ovary-intact animals with a split activity rhythm will have multiple LH surges. However, I also did not predict that the ovariectomized estrogen-treated animals with a split activity rhythm would have 2 LH surges—so much for my prediction. My prediction is based on the idea that once you get an LH surge in an animal with an intact ovary, increased progesterone levels will block the next LH surge. Jennifer Swann is working on this question right now.

G. Gibori: How do your data apply to humans? You have shown, in your animal model, that exposure to only 6 hours of light per day causes a dramatic decrease in testosterone levels and testis weight. Is it possible that exposure to short day affects man similarly?

F. W. Turek: To start with, the reason the hamster responds to seasonal changes in day length is so mating takes place at a specific time of the year. The human is a very unusual species; we are ready to mate at any time of the year, any time of the month, week , day, or hour! On the other hand, perhaps primitive man was a seasonal breeder and there are still vestiges of seasonality. Certainly, seasonality is seen in other primate species. Epidemiological studies have been carried out showing that in the human male serum testosterone levels are high during the late summer–early fall. There are old reports which indicate that before the advent of electricity, amenorrhea was highest during the short days of winter in Scandinavian countries. The difficulty here is trying to separate out the effects of depression which may set in during the long nights of winter from any direct effect of daylength on reproduction. In any case, the human reproductive system is certainly not regulated to any large extent by the seasonal changes in daylength. Whether these is a loose relationship, I don't know. It is interesting to note that there are manic depressive people who get depressed in the winter. Now I know I get depressed in the winter in Chicago too, but in these people it is a very clear syndrome. Investigators at the NIMH are now treating these people with extra light during the night and they are getting some positive results. It is of course difficult to separate out the placebo effect from the effects of the light, but the idea that humans still are influenced by the seasonal change in the light–dark cycle is very likely. Indeed, while reproduction may only be marginally influenced by daylength in humans, other physiological systems may be affected. For example, the incidence of heart attack is higher at one time of year than at others; there may be a number of endocrine changes which occur in response to the seasonal change in day length.

G. J. MacDonald: I would like to ask if you envision a role for the adrenal gland in the circadian system.

F. W. Turek: I don't see the adrenal gland as playing a major role in regulating neural oscillators in the brain. Removal of the adrenal glands has little, if any effect on measurable circadian rhythms. With respect to the seasonal reproductive cycle, I don't see the adrenals as playing a major role there either. We and others have shown that photic-induced changes in neuroendocrine–gonadal functions still occur in the absence of the adrenal glands.

R. B. Billiar: We have some autoradiographic data that would support the suggestion that the suprachiasmatic nucleus does have a nicotinic cholinergic receptor. Namely, if we use the antagonist α-bungarotoxin which is a well established antagonist for the peripheral niconitic cholinergic receptor then we do get labeling of the SCN in the rat. If we ovariectomize a rat the SCN labeling will selectively disappear and estrogen administration will restore the labeling. Interestingly, if we neonatally androgenize the female the SCN α-BTX binding will still disappear after we ovariectomize the adult. Whereas if we castrate an adult male rat we still get α-bungaratoxin labeling of the SCN just as in the intact male. This leads me to my question, also concerned with the LH surge and locomotor activity. If you neonatally androgenize the female and then as an adult ovariectomize her and then give her estrogen do you or do you not get these LH surges and do they correlate with locomotor activity?

F. W. Turek: We haven't done that.

R. B. Billair: The reason I asked is that the neonatally androgenized female rats still maintain their circadian rhythms but I assume they would not have the LH surges in response to the estrogen.

F. W. Turek: That would be my prediction. Only a few studies have been done with neonatally androgenized animals with respect to looking at circadian rhythmicity. There is some indication that the circadian system is sexually dimorphic, and following the treatment of young females with androgen, the circadian system during the adult stage has male characteristics.

I. Callard: The circuitous route of the nerve pathway from the central nervous system to the pineal has always fascinated me and I wondered that now you have included the paraventricular nucleus in the picture whether you have the evidence of a direct dorsal route from the paraventricular nucleus?

F. W. Turek: No, we don't.

I. Callard: In your hypothalamic islands does your cut go above the PVN?

F. W. Turek: I believe that in the studies of Inouye the hypothalamic islands did not include the PVN.

I. Callard: You might be interested to know that there is at least one reptile with a tract that runs from the paraventricular dorsal to terminate in the region of the pineal/paraphyseal area. This is a neurosecretory tract which might be worth looking into with regard to the integration of information of the pineal into the circadian system.

F. W. Turek: We are very interested in the effects of CRF on rhythmicity. Because of the relationship between the PVN and the SCN, David Keefe in my laboratory has injected CRF into the lateral ventrical to look for effects on the circadian system. We are finding major shifts in the circadian rhythm of activity following an injection of CRF. This is not a trivial statement to make since at the present time only a few pharmacological manipulations have been found to directly affect the circadian system.

R. E. Frisch: In regard to seasonality and human reproduction, I would like to comment that data from the Bush people of the Kalahari desert, where nutrition is suboptimal, show a rise in the birth rate 9 months after the seasonal increase in the food supply.

F. W. Turek: It's also true 9 months after Lent ends!

N. B. Schwartz: I would like to go back to the question that was raised about the ovarian cycle in the goldfish. There is some evidence in the mouse suggesting that there is a circadian rhythm in the responsiveness of intact mice on regular light–dark cycles to injected gonado-tropin, a study which Don Lamond did many years ago. With respect to the hamster following these daily surges of LH, we think that what is happening in the ovary is that the follicles are not ever maturing. We see a lot of interstitial tissue from which, presumably, the progesterone is coming. There are no mature antral follicles in the ovary. What one sees is medium-sized follicles undergoing atresia. We think that these daily light surges are killing the follicles before they mature.

E. L. Marut: In regard to the loose association of the light–dark cycle in human female reproduction, there was a report about 15 years ago (unfortunately I cannot remember the citation) where a clinical trial was carried out on women with irregular but ovulatory menstrual cycles. They were told to sleep with the lights on at night from day 10 to day 13 of each menstrual cycle and an unusually high number of those women consistently ovulated on the fourteenth day, where they had not before. Do you see an analogy between that sort of study and that entraining the hamsters with light pulses at specific sensitive times?

F. W. Turek: The difficulty is in trying to separate a seasonal from a circadian effect. We know that a variety of mental and physical disorders may be associated with a disorganized circadian system. So one of the things light could have done in the studies to which you referred is to synchronize rhythms associated with reproduction. The extra light may not be mimicking the effects of long days by triggering the long day response. Instead it may be synchronizing some rhythms which are out of synchrony with each other and now ovulation occurs. In terms of what is important for reinitiating ovulation, it can be tricky to separate out the synchronous effect of light from the inductive effect of light.

E. L. Marut: That's right. As you mentioned, it is difficult to separate the long nights–short days effect from the depression that ensues, just as with women who work night shifts who very often will have abnormalities of their menstrual cycles. Is it simply because they hate to work the night shift or because they have their light–dark exposure disrupted? One more quick question. Have you noted any differences in the effects of either SCN or PVN lesions that are dependent on the light–dark cycle the animal was exposed to either prior to the time of the lesioning or at the time of the lesioning?

F. W. Turek: I don't think I would predict differences but we haven't looked.

K. V. Werder: Do you have any evidence that the response you are observing following a shift in day–light cycles is mediated by the prolactin secretion?

F. W. Turek: Andy Bartke and Bruce Goldman have shown very strong correlations between prolactin levels and the gonadal response. Prolactin levels decrease in conjunction with short-day induced testicular regression. At first I tended to disregard prolactin as a major hormone in the seasonal response, particularly since in sheep prolactin levels are inversely correlated with the testis response. On the other hand the data are now quite convincing that prolactin can affect the reproductive system in hamsters.

R. O. Greep: I noticed that you said that you slapped yourself on the head to remind you of a particular incident and I wonder if everybody in the audience realizes the background of that piece of human behavior! In the fourth century B.C. Herophilus of Alexandria studying the pineal proposed that the pineal was a valve between the rear of the brain and the front of the cortex and that you could improve your memory by slapping the side of the head. That idea persisted despite Galen in the second century who objected strongly to it, but it persisted through the seventeenth century so it lasted for almost 2000 years and it has become such an established part of human behavior that very often you'll see people slap their head like that when they're trying to think of something.

RECENT PROGRESS IN HORMONE RESEARCH, VOL. 40

Neuroendocrine Basis of Seasonal Reproduction

FRED J. KARSCH, ERIC L. BITTMAN, DOUGLAS L. FOSTER,
ROBERT L. GOODMAN, SANDRA J. LEGAN, AND JANE E. ROBINSON

*Reproductive Endocrinology Program, Departments of Physiology and Obstetrics and
Gynecology, The University of Michigan, Ann Arbor, Michigan*

I. Strategy of Seasonal Breeding

It comes as no surprise that the vast majority of animals give birth to their young at a specific time of the year. This is so because not all seasons are equally well suited for survival. As a result, selection pressures have favored the propagation of those genes which couple the time of birth to the most appropriate phase of the annual cycle of climate and food availability. In temperate climates, the young of many species are born in the early springtime. This enables them to take advantage of the abundant food resource and be maximally developed and competitive before encountering the environmental hardships of winter. Springtime, however, is not the optimal season of birth for all regions. In hot arid climates, for example, the most severe environmental challenges occur during the droughts of summer, so the birth season is shifted accordingly (Zucker *et al.*, 1980).

Regardless of when the birth season occurs, it results from a number of biological processes, one of which is a recurring alternation between periods of fertility and infertility. Unlike births, however, which are clustered in one season, the time of the fertile period in this annual reproductive cycle varies markedly depending on the interval from conception to birth (Fig. 1). Among those species which are born in the spring, for example, the horse has a gestation period of nearly 1 year; the fertile period thus occurs in the springtime. Sheep, deer, and rhesus monkeys have gestation periods of about 5–6 months; they enter their breeding season in late summer or autumn, thus allowing birth in the spring. Finally, many rodents and birds, which have a very short interval from conception to birth, begin their breeding season in the spring of the same year that they bear their young.

To synchronize their fertile period to the most suitable time of the year, seasonal breeders rely on environmental cues which enable them to antic-

185

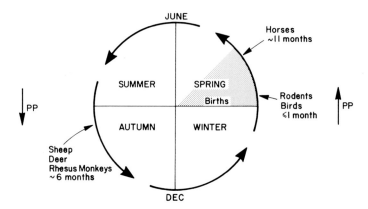

FIG. 1.   Timing of annual reproductive cycle of exemplary seasonal breeders. Approximate onset of breeding period shown by arrows pointing toward circle. Months are approximate intervals from insemination to birth. Note time of breeding depends on interval to birth. Shaded area, usual birth period. PP, photoperiod.

ipate the "season of plenty." Of the many environmental variables available, photoperiod is perhaps the most commonly used synchronizing agent. Unlike some of the other climatic variables such as temperature and rainfall, the seasonal cycle of daylength is constant from one year to the next, and thus it has especially good predictive value. Species that use photoperiod as a synchronizing agent can be separated into two general groups, long-day breeders which enter their breeding season as daylength increases in the springtime and short-day breeders that become fertile as daylength decreases in the autumn.

Regardless of whether an animal is a long- or short-day breeder, the regulation of the annual reproductive cycle by daylength is a classic instance of the interplay between the brain and the endocrine system in coordinating the normal reproductive process. The thrust of this article is to develop our current concepts of the neuroendocrine mechanisms whereby an external cue, photoperiod, regulates the annual reproductive cycle in one seasonal breeder, the female sheep. We have selected as our experimental model the Suffolk ewe, a breed which displays a marked seasonality to its pattern of estrous cyclicity.

It is important to stress at the outset that seasonal reproduction is so vital to the propagation of a species that many different strategies have evolved among animals to accommodate the climatic challenges specific to their differing environments. The system to be described, therefore, is but one example of how nature accomplishes this remarkable process of reversible fertility, a process described as "Nature's Contraceptive" by Drs. Lincoln and Short (1980) in their contribution to this publication several years ago.

II. Role of Photoperiod in Timing the Annual Reproductive Cycle

Being a short-day breeder, the Suffolk ewe becomes sexually active in the late summer to early autumn. Unless she becomes pregnant, repeated 16-day estrous cycles persist until late winter when the 6-month anestrous season begins. Two types of experiments have demonstrated that photoperiod is the primary synchronizing agent for the annual reproductive cycle of the ewe, and that daylength sets both the timing and the duration of the breeding season.

The first type of experiment deals with photoperiodic reversals. Nearly 50 years ago, Marshall (1937) described the consequences of transferring the ewe across the equator, such that the seasonal swings in photoperiod and other environmental variables were shifted by 6 months. After a period of adjustment, the annual reproductive cycle was found to shift in accordance with the environment in the new locale. Over the course of the next 30 years, a number of experiments which employed reversed artificial photoperiods clearly demonstrated that light is the environmental cue which caused this response (Yeates, 1949; Thwaites, 1965; Wodzicka-Tomaszewska et al., 1967). Results of one such study, illustrated in Fig. 2, indicate that regardless of whether the photoperiod is natural or reversed, decreasing daylength is associated with reproductive induction and increasing daylength with reproductive arrest. In contrast, an attempt to reverse the timing of the annual reproductive cycle with shifts in an-

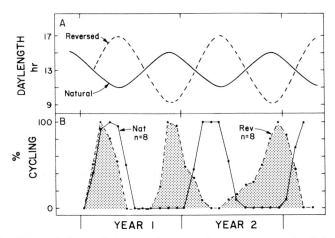

FIG. 2.   Effect of photoperiod reversal on annual reproductive cycle of the ewe. (A) Solid line, natural photoperiod; dashed line, reversed, accentuated, artificial photoperiod. (B) Solid line, incidence of estrous cycles under natural (Nat) light. Shaded area, estrous cycles in ewes transferred to reversed (Rev) photoperiod at beginning of year 1. Note photoperiod reversal causes a shift in the annual reproductive cycle. n, Number of ewes. Redrawn from Thwaites (1965).

other environmental variable, temperature, was not successful (Wodzicka-Tomaszewska *et al.*, 1967).

The second type of experiment produces an acceleration of the seasonal reproductive cycle with artificial photoperiods. One such study,
illustrated in Fig. 3, has compared the timing of the breeding season in our
flock of Suffolk ewes maintained outdoors under natural Michigan environmental conditions (top panel) to that of ewes housed indoors in an
artificial photoperiod alternated between long and short days every 90 or
120 days (bottom panels). Each shift to artificial long days caused termination of estrous cycles; each shift to short days reinstated cyclicity after

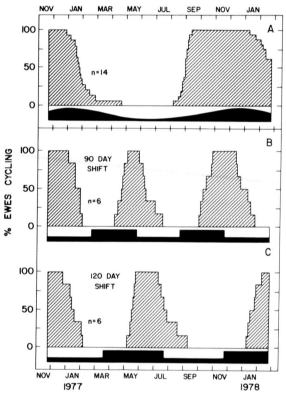

FIG. 3.   Photoperiodic acceleration of seasonal reproductive cycle of the ewe. Incidence
of estrous cycles in ewes maintained outdoors in natural photoperiods (A) or indoors in
artificial photoperiods alternated every 90 (B) or 120 (C) days between long (16L : 8D) and
short (8L : 16D) daylengths. Horizontal bars at bottom of each histogram are relative amount
of light (open area) and dark (closed area) each day. Note 90-day light shifts cause two
breeding and anestrous seasons each year. n, Number of ewes. Redrawn from Legan and
Karsch (1980).

a lag of about 50 days. As a consequence, the annual reproductive cycle was shortened, and in ewes subjected to the 90-day alternations in photoperiod, two breeding and anestrous seasons occurred over the course of 1 year. Further, by the end of the study, the reproductive condition of ewes exposed to the 90-day light shift was completely out of phase with that of ewes housed in an adjacent room and treated with the 120-day shift (February 1978). Importantly, the two groups were exposed to the same seasonal changes in all other environmental variables.

The results from both types of experiments lend strong support to the view that daylength is the primary synchronizing agent for the annual reproductive cycle of the Suffolk ewe. Not only does this cue serve to align the onset of breeding activity to the most appropriate time of year, it also sets the duration of the breeding season. Further, should other environmental variables contribute to this timekeeping process, their influence would seem to be subordinate to that of photoperiod. Given the deterministic role of daylength in this seasonal breeder, we may turn our attention to the question of how photic signals are perceived, processed neurally, and transmitted to the ovaries to regulate estrous cyclicity.

III. Hypothalamo-Pituitary Mechanisms Which Mediate Photoperiodic Regulation of Estrous Cyclicity

One central mechanism which processes both external and internal environmental signals is the ''LH pulse generator.'' This neuroendocrine mechanism gives rise to the pulsatile mode of gonadotropin secretion and serves to mediate the reproductive response to daylength. In this section, we will focus on the functional interplay between the LH pulse generator and the ovaries during both breeding and anestrous seasons. We will then turn our attention to the pathway which carries photoperiodic information from the external environment to this pulse generating system.

Recent studies of Levine *et al.* (1982) and Clarke and Cummins (1982) have demonstrated that, in the ewe, the LH pulse generator produces bursts of GnRH release from hypothalamic nerve terminals. These bursts are coupled with, and are presumably the cause of, the pulses of LH discharged from the anterior lobe of the pituitary (Fig. 4). It is also known that the nature of the LH pulse pattern changes dramatically throughout the course of both the estrous and the seasonal reproductive cycles of the ewe, and that these changes control the time of ovulation. Let us now examine how the LH pulse generator determines the time of ovulation during the estrous cycle, the nature of the changes produced by photoperiod, and how these changes lead to the seasonal onset and cessation of ovarian cyclicity.

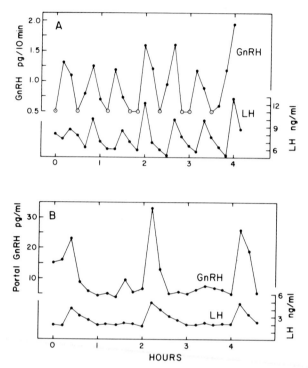

FIG. 4. Temporal relationship between pulses of LH and GnRH release in ovariecto-mized ewes. (A) Coincident patterns of LH in peripheral blood (obtained every 10 minutes) and GnRH in perfusate (obtained over 10-minute period) from push-pull cannula with tip positioned in median eminence. Open circles, undetectable. Redrawn from Levine *et al.* (1982). (B) Coincident patterns of LH in peripheral blood and GnRH in hypothalamo-hypophyseal portal blood (both obtained every 12 minutes). Redrawn from Clarke and Cummins (1982). Note each LH pulse is associated with a simultaneous pulse of GnRH.

A. LH PULSE GENERATOR AND THE ESTROUS CYCLE

To understand how photic input to the LH pulse generator leads to seasonal changes in gonadal activity, it is first necessary to consider the sequence of endocrine events which normally leads to ovulation during the estrous cycle of the ewe. These preovulatory events occur during a 2–3 day follicular phase and include a precipitous drop in progesterone, a progressive rise in tonic LH secretion, a sustained increase in estradiol secretion, and the LH surge (Fig. 5, left). The pivotal step in this sequence is the sustained increase in tonic LH secretion. This LH rise is initiated at luteolysis by the acute withdrawal of progesterone, a potent negative feedback hormone in the ewe (Baird and Scaramuzzi, 1976;

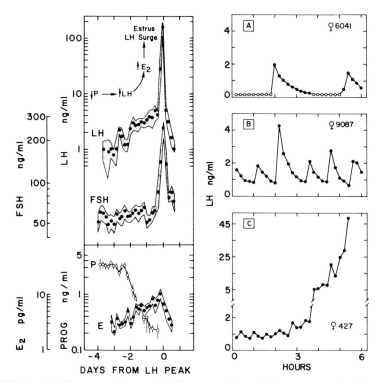

FIG. 5. *Left.* Sequence of events leading to ovulation in the estrous cycle of the ewe. Concentrations (mean ± SEM) of LH, FSH, progesterone (P), and estradiol (E) in serum obtained from 6 ewes every 4 hours for 4 days immediately prior to LH peak. *Right.* Patterns of LH pulses in representative ewes during estrous cycle: (A) late luteal phase (open circles, undetectable); (B) 24–48 hours before preovulatory LH peak; (C) just before and during onset of LH surge (note break in scale for LH). Samples obtained every 12 minutes. Note, an increase in LH pulse frequency underlies the rise in serum LH between P drop and onset of LH surge. From Goodman and Karsch (1981).

Karsch *et al.,* 1977, 1979, 1980). The resultant increase in serum LH permits the final stages of follicular maturation and drives the progressive increase in estradiol secretion needed to trigger the preovulatory LH surge (Goodman *et al.,* 1981a; McNatty *et al.,* 1981; McNeilly *et al.,* 1982). This rise in tonic LH secretion is the critical event because it is susceptible to control by factors in the external and internal environments, and it is the means by which these factors govern ovarian cyclicity. Thus, if there is a sustained increase in tonic LH secretion, ovulation can occur; if there is not, the remaining steps in the preovulatory sequence are prevented and ovulation is blocked (Legan and Karsch, 1979; Goodman and Karsch, 1980b).

The pulse generator enters this picture because changes in the pulsatile pattern of LH release underlie the sustained rise in tonic LH secretion during the follicular phase. At this time, LH pulse frequency increases from a luteal phase nadir of one pulse every 3–4 hours to a maximum of about one pulse every 30 minutes just prior to the onset of the preovulatory LH surge (Fig. 5, right). In fact, the frequency of LH pulses just prior to the surge is so great that a clear pulse pattern is obscured when samples are obtained every 12 minutes, the interval we routinely employ to characterize LH secretory dynamics at other times of the cycle (Fig. 5C). By reducing the sampling interval to 4 minutes, however, a well-organized pattern of high-frequency pulses of LH is disclosed (up to one pulse every 30 minutes, Fig. 6, insets).

The importance of this increase in frequency to the estrous cycle has been demonstrated in experiments in which LH, or GnRH, was "pulse" injected into anovulatory sheep. Repeated injection of LH, switching from a luteal to a follicular phase frequency, drives a normal estradiol rise which leads to the LH surge and ovulation in both prepubertal and anestrous sheep (Ryan and Foster, 1980; McNeilly *et al.*, 1982). Further, when such high-frequency pulses of LH were generated experimentally, by a

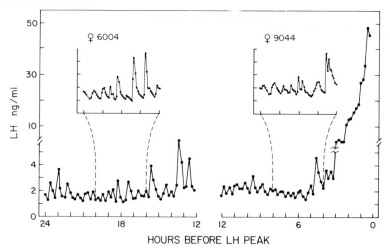

FIG. 6.   LH pulse pattern leading up to preovulatory LH surge in representative ewes. Samples were obtained every 12 minutes during first and last 4 hours, and every 4 minutes during middle 4 hours of each 12-hour period of observation. Lower tracing plots only 12-minute samples from middle 4-hour period. Upper tracing includes each 4-minute sample during that same 4-hour period (expanded time scale). Note sawtooth patterns of 12 minute samples reflects highly organized pattern of frequent pulses revealed by 4-minute samples. Modified from Karsch *et al.* (1983).

sequence of pulsed injections of GnRH designed to approximate the normal frequency changes, ovulation was induced during the anestrous season (Legan, 1982; McLeod *et al.*, 1982). Therefore, it is through this acceleration of LH, and presumably GnRH discharge, that the LH pulse generator provides the signal for the ovaries to produce the next step in the preovulatory sequence, the sustained estradiol rise.

The primary factors controlling the time of ovulation during the estrous cycle are the ovarian steroids, and this control is exerted by modulation of the output of the LH pulse generator. As illustrated in Fig. 7, removal of these steroids by ovariectomy during the luteal phase leads to a marked increase in both frequency and amplitude of LH pulses (Fig. 7A; compare to luteal phase pattern in Fig. 5A). Immediate replacement of a luteal phase level of progesterone, provided by a constant-release Silastic im-

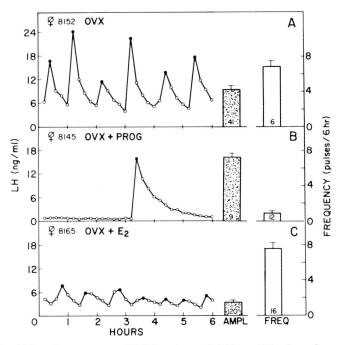

FIG. 7. Effect of progesterone (PROG) and estradiol (E$_2$) on LH pulses of ewes ovariectomized (OVX) 12 days previously during luteal phase of an estrous cycle in mid-breeding season. *Left*, data from representative ewes. *Right*, mean + SEM amplitude and frequency of pulses for all ewes. Numbers in bars are number of pulses (amplitude) and number of 6-hour observation periods (frequency). Closed circles indicate peaks of LH pulses. (A) No steroid treatment. (B) Silastic PROG implant to produce serum PROG level 3–4 ng/ml. (C) E$_2$ implant to produce E$_2$ level of 3–5 pg/ml serum. Note, PROG decreases only frequency (FREQ). E$_2$ decreases only amplitude (AMPL). From Goodman and Karsch (1980a).

plant, prevented this increase in frequency but did not decrease the amplitude (Fig. 7B). Replacement with a physiological level of estradiol, however, was found to have the opposite effect, a marked reduction in LH pulse amplitude but no decrease in frequency (Fig. 7C). This effect of estradiol on amplitude may be accounted for by an action on the pituitary to decrease its responsiveness to GnRH (Goodman and Karsch, 1980a). Progesterone, in contrast, was found not to reduce the response of the pituitary to an exogenous pulse of GnRH (Goodman and Karsch, 1980a).

These findings lead to the conclusion that the frequency of LH pulses during the estrous cycle is modulated primarily by progesterone, which acts in the brain to prolong the interval between bouts of GnRH discharge. In contrast, the amplitude of LH pulses is limited by estradiol which acts, at least in part, upon the pituitary gland to diminish its response to each pulse of GnRH. Further, it seemed reasonable to postulate that the marked increase in frequency of LH pulses during the follicular phase of the cycle is solely a consequence of the withdrawal of progesterone at luteolysis. Additional experiments to test this hypothesis, however, revealed convincingly that a second hormone is required for the extremely high-frequency pulses during the follicular phase. Specifically, it was found that estradiol contributes to the acceleration of pulse frequency following the withdrawal of progesterone (Karsch et al., 1983).

The foregoing actions of steroids on the LH pulse generator have led to a working model for the steroidal control of ovulation during the estrous cycle of the ewe (Fig. 8). According to this model, the elevated secretion of progesterone in the luteal phase holds the pulse generator in check, thus causing a low frequency of GnRH and, consequently, LH pulses. At this time of the cycle, the basal level of estradiol serves to limit the amplitude of LH pulses by acting, at least in part, upon the anterior pituitary to decrease its response to GnRH, and perhaps also to reduce the rate of gonadotropin biosynthesis (Landefeld et al., 1983). The characteristic low-frequency pulses of LH do not provide a sufficient sustained gonadotropic stimulus to support the final stages of follicular maturation and to drive the preovulatory estradiol rise. As a result, the normal preovulatory sequence cannot be completed. Thus, by virtue of its ability to limit the frequency of the LH pulse generator, progesterone prevents ovulation during the luteal phase of the cycle (Fig. 8A).

When this progesterone blockade is lifted at luteolysis, the activity of the LH pulse generator is permitted to increase, so GnRH and LH pulse frequency begin to accelerate. Without progesterone to oppose its action, estradiol further enhances frequency, possibly by directly addressing the neural component of the LH pulse generating mechanism. In addition,

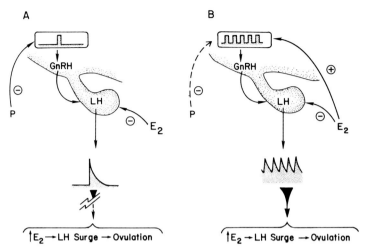

FIG. 8.   Model for control of ovulation during estrous cycle of ewe. (A) Luteal phase: preovulatory sequence (bottom) is blocked (broken arrow) by elevated progesterone (P) which reduces the frequency of LH pulse generator. (B) Follicular phase: frequency of LH pulse generator increases due to combined effect of P withdrawal (broken line) and estradiol (E_2) stimulation. This permits the preovulatory sequence. At both cycle stages, estradiol decreases amplitude of LH pulses by acting, at least in part, on the anterior pituitary. Modified from Goodman and Karsch (1981).

LH pulse amplitude remains low due to the continued presence of estradiol, and perhaps also because the frequency becomes so great that LH or GnRH synthesis cannot keep pace with the increased rate of their own release. The resulting high-frequency, low-amplitude pulses of LH produce the sustained elevation in circulating LH needed to promote follicular maturation and the preovulatory estradiol rise. The latter induces the LH surge which causes ovulation (Fig. 8B).

The keystone of this model is that the *frequency* of LH pulses is deterministic to ovulation. Progesterone is an organizer of the estrous cycle by virtue of its capacity to hold the LH pulse generator in check. Importantly, estradiol by itself cannot inhibit LH pulse frequency. Although the role of FSH has not been clarified in this model, it is tempting to view it as a permissive hormone because circulating concentrations of FSH are sufficient for follicular maturation to occur at any time during the normal estrous cycle (Smeaton and Robertson, 1971). Further, FSH secretion either does not change (Fig. 5), or decreases slightly (Salamonsen et al., 1973; Baird et al., 1981), between luteal regression and onset of the preovulatory gonadotropin surge.

B. PHOTOPERIODIC REGULATION OF LH PULSE GENERATOR

In addition to its control by steroids, the LH pulse generator of the ewe is highly susceptible to regulation by variables in the external environment. Two external variables which have received particular attention are olfactory and photic cues. The immediate induction of a volley of hourly LH pulses in anestrous ewes following exposure to pheromones from an unfamiliar ram exquisitely illustrates the activation of the LH pulse generator by olfactory cues (Poindron *et al.*, 1980; Martin *et al.*, 1983a). Concerning photic cues, regulation of the pulse generator by daylength is evident throughout the course of the annual reproductive cycle. Two types of effects have been described, both in ewes in which seasonal variations in gonadal steroids were eliminated by ovariectomy.

1. Direct Photoperiodic Drive

The first effect of daylength can be observed by monitoring LH pulse patterns in long-term ovariectomized ewes during the course of the annual cycle of natural photoperiod (Goodman *et al.*, 1982). Under such conditions, LH pulses are relatively infrequent, but large during the long days of summer. They gradually shift to high-frequency, low-amplitude pulses during the short days of winter, and then revert to the low-frequency pattern the next summer. One such example is illustrated in Fig. 9 in

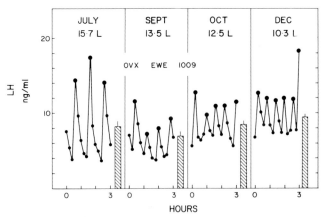

FIG. 9. Example of direct photoperiodic drive to LH pulse generator. Representative LH pulse patterns in the same ovariectomized (OVX) ewe at various times during exposure to decreasing natural daylengths (July–December). Samples were obtained every 12 minutes; peak of LH pulse identified by large points. Bars indicate serum LH concentration (mean + SE) for each observation period. Photoperiod (in hours light/day) is indicated below month in each panel. Note pulse frequency increases as daylength decreases. From J. E. Robinson, H. M. Radford, and F. J. Karsch (unpublished).

which the LH pulse frequency in a typical ovariectomized ewe is shown
to shift from 3 pulses/3 hours in July, to 4 in September, 5 in October, 6 in
December, and although not illustrated, back to about 3 pulses/3 hours the
following July. Additional experiments have demonstrated that such
changes in the LH pulse generator of the ovariectomized ewe can be
driven experimentally by artificial photoperiods (Bittman *et al.*, 1982;
Robinson, 1983). Since this effect of light is evident in the absence of
gonadal steroids, we have come to call it "direct photoperiodic drive" to
the LH pulse generator.

2. Steroid Negative Feedback

The second effect of daylength, which is much more dramatic, is observed in the ovariectomized ewe treated with a constant release Silastic
implant of estradiol to maintain a fixed basal level of the steroid in the
circulation (Goodman *et al.*, 1982; Martin *et al.*, 1983b). An example from
one such experiment is illustrated in Fig. 10, which depicts the serum LH
profile 3 days after insertion of the implant into the same ovariectomized
ewe, first during anestrus and then during the breeding season. In anestrus, estradiol obliterated LH pulses during the 8-hour observation period
in the example illustrated (a single LH pulse/8 hours was observed in each
of a few ewes in this study). Nevertheless, these ewes remained highly
responsive to a small pulse of exogenous GnRH (Fig. 10A, inset, note

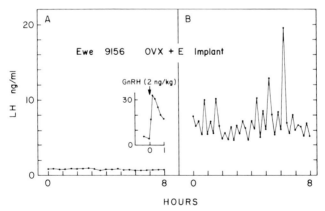

FIG. 10. Demonstration that season dramatically alters effect of estradiol (E) on
pulsatile LH secretion in ovariectomized (OVX) ewe. LH pulse patterns on day 3 after
inserting identical Silastic E implant (producing 3–5 pg E/ml serum) into the same OVX ewe
(maintained in natural environment) during anestrus (A) and breeding season (B). Inset in A
shows LH before and after iv bolus (arrow) of synthetic GnRH on day 4 (note scale change
for LH). Note, in anestrus, estradiol blocks LH pulses but not pituitary response to small
dose of GnRH. Redrawn from Goodman *et al.* (1982).

scale change). Quite a different picture emerged during the breeding season (Fig. 10B). High-frequency pulses of LH persisted despite the presence of the estradiol implant, a result which was obtained even when the implant was left in place for a longer period (e.g., see Fig. 7C). The only suppressive effect of estradiol in the breeding season was on LH pulse amplitude, indicating that estradiol had lost its ability to slow the pulse generator.

Other studies have shown that this seasonal change in the effect of estradiol can be reproduced indoors under artificial photoperiods (Bittman et al., 1982). These observations lead to the conclusion that the inhibitory photoperiods of anestrus enable estradiol to act within the brain to depress LH pulse frequency; this action is totally abolished by the inductive photoperiods of the breeding season.

The foregoing change in the effectiveness of estradiol in suppressing the LH pulse generator constitutes the basis of the well-documented seasonal shift in the negative feedback action of this steroid on gonadotropin secretion (Legan et al., 1977; Martin et al., 1983b). This change can be monitored indirectly throughout the year simply by measuring serum LH concentrations in samples obtained every few days from ovariectomized ewes in which the estradiol implant is left in place (Fig. 11B). When estradiol can inhibit pulse frequency during the anestrous period of spring

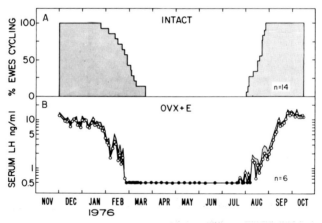

FIG. 11. Seasonal change in potency of estradiol negative feedback on LH secretion in sheep. (A) Incidence of estrous cycles in intact ewes maintained outdoors. (B) Mean + SEM (shaded area) serum LH concentration throughout the year in ovariectomized ewes treated with sc Silastic estradiol implant (OVX + E) which maintained serum estradiol levels of 3–5 pg/ml. n, Number of ewes; solid circles, undetectable LH values. Note, suppressive effect of estradiol is much greater during the spring/summer anestrous period than in the breeding season. From Legan and Karsch (1979).

and summer, serum LH concentrations are undetectable (high response to estradiol). When estradiol cannot inhibit frequency during the breeding season of autumn and winter, LH levels are elevated (low response to estradiol). Importantly, the waxing and waning of this response to estradiol negative feedback are temporally associated with the transitions between breeding and anestrous seasons in ewes with intact ovaries (Fig. 11A).

It remains to be determined whether the changes in direct photoperiodic drive and steroid negative feedback are mechanistically coupled or distinct. For example, the potency of estradiol feedback may be secondary to the level of direct photoperiodic drive, such that the greater the drive, the weaker the feedback effect. Alternatively, the seasonal swings in potency of estradiol may reflect a shift in estradiol metabolism, or a change in the steroid response apparatus in those neurons which mediate estradiol negative feedback (a change which is independent of direct photoperiodic drive). A recent observation which is germaine to this issue is that pentobarbital anesthesia can reverse both steroid-dependent and steroid-independent suppression of LH pulses during anestrus. Thus, treatment with pentobarbital was found to cause an acute increase in LH pulse frequency in anestrus; this effect was not observed in the breeding season (Goodman and Meyer, 1984). This has led to the intriguing hypothesis that inhibitory neurons, which are activated under long days and blocked by pentobarbital, mediate both direct photoperiodic drive and estradiol negative feedback to the LH pulse generator in anestrus (see comment by R. L. Goodman in Discussion).

C. MODEL FOR PHOTOPERIODIC CONTROL OF OVARIAN CYCLICITY

The foregoing observations have led to a conceptual model for photoperiodic determination of estrous cyclicity in the ewe. Under the inductive influence of the short days of the breeding season, there is a high drive to the LH pulse generator which gives it the potential to elicit frequent bursts of GnRH discharge from hypothalamic neurons (Fig. 12A). In addition, the concentrations of estradiol which normally circulate cannot feed back to slow the LH pulse generator (if anything, estradiol seems to enhance frequency at this time). Therefore, LH pulse frequency can increase to a rate sufficient for completion of the preovulatory sequence, provided progesterone is not present to hold the LH pulse generator in check. Ovulation thus follows within 3 to 4 days of luteolysis and repeated estrous cycles can occur.

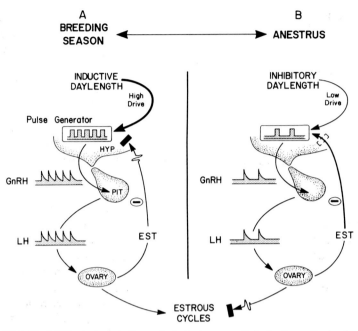

FIG. 12.   Model for photoperiodic control of estrous cyclicity in sheep. Basis of model is that interaction between changing photoperiodic drive and potency of estradiol (EST) negative feedback to pulse generator determines transitions between breeding season (A) and anestrus (B). Solid rectangles depict blockade; open one removal of blockade. Relative frequencies of LH and GnRH pulses are indicated. See text for details.

Under the inhibitory daylengths of anestrus, there is a low photoperiodic drive to the LH pulse generator (Fig. 12B). Furthermore, the pulse generator becomes exquisitely sensitive to inhibition by estradiol, such that the basal level of estradiol which is secreted is sufficient to evoke a profound suppressive effect. As a consequence, the frequency of hypothalamic GnRH discharge is greatly diminished. The resulting low-frequency pulses of LH do not provide sufficient gonadotropic support for a sustained estradiol rise. The preovulatory sequence is thus blocked and estrous cycles cannot occur. The ovarian follicle, therefore, delimits its own destiny in anestrus via a highly effective negative feedback loop between estradiol and the LH pulse generator.

The central feature of this model is that the transitions between the breeding season and anestrus are a direct and inevitable consequence of shifts in frequency of the LH pulse generator. In a sense, therefore, this is much the same as our working model for the control of ovulation during the estrous cycle (Fig. 8). The main difference is that progesterone organizes the time of ovulation during the estrous cycle by virtue of its being above or below a threshold level; estradiol may be viewed as organizing the time of ovulation in the seasonal reproductive cycle by virtue of whether or not the pulse generator is susceptible to its inhibitory effect.

Although not tested in its entirety, this model has received extensive experimental support. Representative lines of evidence are now listed (except where cited, documentation is provided in earlier reviews of Legan and Karsch, 1979; Goodman and Karsch, 1980b; Karsch, 1980; and in McNeilly *et al.*, 1982). First, the LH pulse generating system is clearly compromised in anestrus because pulse frequency in intact ewes is extremely low, and sustained increases in tonic LH secretion are not normally observed. Second, the ovary is not limiting in anestrus because it can respond normally to LH pulses; it can generate a preovulatory estradiol rise in response to a sustained tonic LH rise; and ovulation and corpus luteum formation can occur following an experimentally produced LH surge (although there is some evidence to suggest the follicle may become less responsive to LH at the transition into anestrus, S. J. Legan, unpublished). Third, the LH surge system is not limiting in anestrus because a preovulatory LH surge can be induced by a rise in estradiol which mimics that of the normal follicular phase (but there is some disagreement as to whether sensitivity of the surge system to estradiol changes with season, see Land *et al.*, 1976; Howland *et al.*, 1978; Goodman *et al.*, 1981b). Fourth, the capacity of the pituitary to respond to high-frequency pulses of GnRH is not limiting in anestrus (McLeod *et al.*, 1982; Legan, 1982, 1983). Fifth, the spontaneous transition into the breeding season is heralded by an increase in frequency of LH pulses (I'Anson, 1983), a finding which is consistent with the view that the onset of cyclicity is promoted by an acceleration of the LH pulse generator. Such an increase in frequency has also been suggested to promote onset of the breeding season of the ram (Lincoln and Short, 1980) and the onset of reproductive function at puberty in both sexes of sheep (Ryan and Foster, 1980; Olster and Foster, 1983).

This completes our consideration of the hypothalamo-hypophyseal mechanisms which mediate the seasonal occurrence of estrous cyclicity. The most crucial point of control seems to rest within the system which governs the tonic mode of LH secretion, specifically whether or not estradiol can suppress the neural processes which lead to the pulsatile pattern of LH release. There is thus a solid experimental basis for the concept that photoperiod regulates the timing of the annual reproductive cycle by directing the activity of this LH pulse generator. Let us now turn our attention to the pathway whereby the photic cues are received and relayed to the pulse generating system.

IV. Photoperiodic Pathway to LH Pulse Generator

The pathway which is believed to transmit photic information to the hypothalamo-hypophyseal axis of photoperiodic rodents is presented in Fig. 13. According to this scheme, which is derived largely from work in the golden hamster (Reiter, 1980; Bittman *et al.*, 1983c; Turek *et al.*, 1984), light cues activate photoreceptors in the retina and are transmitted via a monosynaptic tract to the suprachiasmatic nuclei of the hypothalamus. From there, the photic signal is relayed to the paraventricular nuclei, eventually to the superior cervical ganglia, and then to the pineal gland. The pineal transduces the neural input into hormonal output in the form of a circadian rhythm of melatonin secretion. This melatonin rhythm serves to modulate hypothalamo-hypophyseal activity and, in turn, the seasonal changes in reproductive function. Each step of this postulated photoneuroendocrine pathway will now be examined for the ewe. In addition, evidence will be advanced to suggest that specific characteristics of the melatonin pattern produce the alterations in the LH pulse generator which determine whether or not estrous cycles occur.

A. LOCATION OF THE PHOTORECEPTOR

While it might seem obvious that the eyes should contain the photoreceptor, evidence from birds, reptiles, and fish demonstrates convincingly that most classes of vertebrates do not use their eyes for the reproductive response to daylength (Benoit, 1964; Menaker and Keatts, 1968; Underwood, 1975; Day and Taylor, 1983). Rather, light penetrates the skull and impinges upon extraretinal photoreceptors located deep in the brain (Follett, 1978). When we became interested in this issue in the ewe, only three photoperiodic mammals had been studied (ferret, golden hamster, Mongolian gerbil). Although each was found to require retinal photoreceptors, each was a long-day breeder (Thomson, 1954; Hoffman and Reiter, 1965; Dixit *et al.*, 1977; Herbert *et al.*, 1978). In addition, evidence for the existence of extraretinal photoreceptors in neonatal rats suggests that at least one mammal has retained the potential to respond to light independent of the eyes (Zweig *et al.*, 1966; Wetterberg *et al.*, 1970).

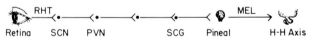

Retina   SCN   PVN   SCG   Pineal   H-H Axis

FIG. 13. Postulated neuroendocrine pathway for transmission of photic cues from the retina to the hypothalamo-hypophyseal (H-H) axis of the golden hamster. RHT, retinohypothalamic tract. SCN and PVN, suprachiasmatic and paraventricular nuclei of hypothalamus, respectively. MEL, melatonin. See text for details.

With regard to the ewe, our initial leaning was that sheep cannot possibly employ extraretinal photoreceptors to control seasonal reproduction because the thick skull and overlying skin would provide a formidable barrier to the penetration of light. Two early observations, however, forced us to abandon this assumption, making it necessary to obtain empirical evidence for the locus of the photoreceptor in the ewe. First, normal daylight has been found to traverse the skull of the living sheep, and to activate photosensitive probes implanted surgically in various parts of the brain including the hypothalamus (Van Brunt *et al.*, 1964). Second, appropriately timed breeding seasons have been found to persist in ewes following blinding by section of the optic nerve (Clegg *et al.*, 1965). The latter observation, while consistent with extraretinal photoreception, is inconclusive because it was not established that the changes in reproductive condition were driven by photoperiod after blinding. The authors themselves offered another explanation: "If the receptor for light is destroyed, the animal reverts to an inherent biological rhythm which, in the case of the sheep, coincides with the seasonal variations in reproductive activity."

A crucial point thus emerges: Any valid test of the importance of each putative component of the photoneuroendocrine pathway must employ an experimental model in which changes in reproductive state are unambiguously demonstrated to be driven by photoperiod.

1. Experimental Model

Our approach for developing a suitable model was to exploit the finding that the seasonal changes in estrous cyclicity can be driven artificially by 90-day alternations between short and long days (8 hours light/day and 16 hours light/day, respectively; Fig. 14). A similar photoperiodic drive is evident when the measured variable is not the occurrence of estrous cycles, but the response to estradiol negative feedback, monitored by serum LH concentrations in ovariectomized ewes bearing constant-release estradiol implants (Fig. 14B). Exposure to long days leads to a potentiation of estradiol negative feedback in ovariectomized ewes (fall in LH). Transfer to short days reverses this effect. The response to estradiol negative feedback has proven to be an easily measured and extremely useful indicator of reproductive induction. We have selected it as the measured variable in our experiments to test various components of the photoneuroendocrine pathway (occasionally monitoring estrous cycles of intact ewes as a check). There are several distinct benefits to this index of reproductive induction, one being that it is an accurate reflection of the activity of the LH pulse generator under conditions in which ovarian steroids do not change.

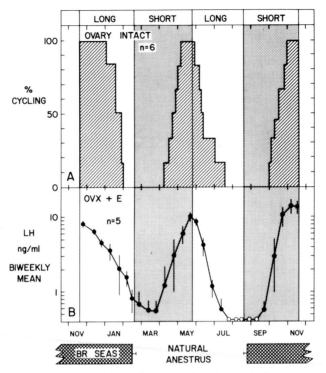

FIG. 14. Experimental model used to test the photoperiodic response. Artificial photoperiod alternated every 90 days between long days (16L : 8D, open areas) and short days (8L : 16D, shaded areas). (A) Estrous cycles in 6 ewes with intact ovaries. (B) Response to estradiol negative feedback on LH secretion, measured as serum LH in 5 ovariectomized (OVX) ewes treated with sc Silastic estradiol (E) implants which produced 3–5 pg E/ml serum. Samples were obtained 3 times each week and LH levels were pooled to obtain a mean (±SEM) value for each 2-week period. Open circles, undetectable values. Bar at bottom shows average (and SEM) date of onset and cessation of breeding season in control flock of ewes maintained outdoors. Note, definitive test of response to daylength is reproductive induction in short days during natural anestrus. Redrawn from Legan and Karsch (1980).

An especially important feature of this model pertains to *timing* of the experimentally produced shifts in estradiol negative feedback in relation to the natural transitions between breeding and anestrous seasons outdoors (illustrated by bar at bottom of Fig. 14). One particular light shift, the transfer to short days in late February, produces reproductive induction in the middle of the natural anestrous season. Since this particular response is totally out of phase with the natural seasonal reproductive cycle, it is unquestionably driven by light. It thus becomes our definitive test of the photoperiodic response.

2. Effect of Blinding

One of a series of studies which utilized this model to locate the photoreceptor is illustrated in Fig. 15. In this study, potency of estradiol negative feedback and estrous cyclicity was monitored in the same groups of ewes for nearly 5 years, during which time they were subjected to alternations between the long and short photoperiods every 90 days. After displaying the definitive photoperiodic response in 2 successive years (LH rise in ovariectomized ewes during natural anestrus, April and May of years 1 and 2), each ewe was blinded by bilateral orbital enucleation. Surprisingly, the ewes again responded to this test, although not as robustly, during the following year (see LH rise in short days beginning February of year 3). Up to this point, a sighted ram had been housed in the same room for the purpose of checking estrus in the group of blind ewes with intact ovaries. When the LH rise in anestrus of year 3 became evident, however, the sighted ram was removed. Thereafter, all blind ewes failed to respond to the definitive test of the photoperiodic response (April and May of years 4 and 5). Nevertheless, the seasonal swings in LH persisted. The first of these swings was synchronous with the onset of the natural breeding season (see LH rise in September of year 3 with reference to bar at bottom of Fig. 15). Subsequent LH shifts, however, tended to occur progressively later than the natural transitions outdoors, and when the study was terminated during the mid-anestrous season of year 5, LH had not plunged to a low level.

These observations, in conjunction with complementary findings in four other groups of blind ewes in this series of experiments (Legan and Karsch, 1983), lead to the conclusion that *retinal* photoreceptors are required for timing of the annual reproductive cycle of the ewe. In the absence of these receptors, the ewe may receive photoperiodic information indirectly via the ram, possibly by means of olfactory cues. When deprived of both the photoreceptor and the ram, the ewe remains seasonally reproductive, although the transitions may occur at a slightly different time from one year to the next.

The latter conclusion raises the important question of why seasonality persists in the absence of photoperiodic input. There are two possible explanations. Either another meteorological or geophysical cue can take over in the absence of photoperiodic input or, as suggested by Clegg *et al.* (1965), there is an endogenous circannual rhythm of reproduction which is normally synchronized by light, but which "free runs" in its absence. Although neither of the two explanations can be eliminated, several lines of evidence favor the endogenous rhythm. First, no other cueing agent (with the possible exception of the ram) has yet been found to drive

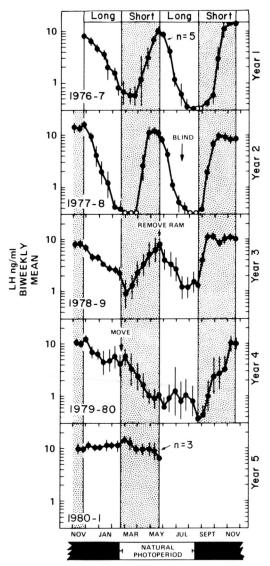

FIG. 15. Effect of blinding on photoperiodic response. Biweekly mean (±SEM, see legend Fig. 13) serum LH concentration in the same ovariectomized ewes treated sc with Silastic estradiol implants during 4.5-year period. Photoperiod was alternated every 90 days between long days (16L : 8D, open areas) and short days (8L : 16D, shaded areas). All ewes were blinded in July of year 2 (arrow); the sighted ram removed from room in May of year 3 (arrow); ewes moved to adjacent room in February of year 4 (arrow). Data for each year are plotted in successive vertical panels. n, Number of ewes. Two ewes died after 4 years; data in year 5 are for the 3 remaining ewes. Horizontal bar at bottom shows date of onset and termination of breeding season (mean and SEM) in control flock maintained outdoors (closed area is breeding season; open area is anestrus). Note absence of response to photoperiod in years 4 and 5. Modified from Legan and Karsch (1983).

seasonal reproduction in the ewe. Even if such a cue were to exist and were relatively stable from year to year, the reproductive transitions in our blind ewes should have remained reasonably well synchronized from 1 year to the next, and certainly among individual blind ewes within a given year. The seasonal transitions, however, tended to drift out of phase with the natural breeding cycle. Further, although obscured by our pooling of data for presentation in Fig. 15, the reproductive transitions among individual blind ewes tended to become asynchronous within a given year (see Legan and Karsch, 1983). Also consistent with the existence of a circannual rhythm is the finding that alternations between breeding and anestrous conditions have been found to persist in sighted ewes held on a fixed daylength for a prolonged period, but the reproductive shifts were neither synchronized among ewes nor in phase with the natural breeding cycle (Ducker et al., 1973). Finally, endogenous circannual rhythms in a variety of physiological and behavioral functions have been well documented in a host of different species (Pengellay, 1974; Gwinner, 1981). Available evidence, therefore, favors an endogenous circannual rhythm of reproduction in the ewe, a rhythm which is normally synchronized by light acting via retinal photoreceptors.

B. EXISTENCE OF A RETINOHYPOTHALAMIC TRACT

A monosynaptic tract, which links the retina to the suprachiasmatic nuclei of the hypothalamus, has been identified in a number of species (Moore and Lenn, 1972; Moore, 1973; Eichler and Moore, 1974). This tract, which is distinct from the primary optic system used for visual image perception, is a good candidate for the first connection in the photoneuroendocrine pathway because it links the photoreceptor with that region of the brain believed to have a major timekeeping function in mammals (Stetson and Watson-Whitmyre, 1976; Rusak and Zucker, 1979; Turek et al., 1984).

In conjunction with Dr. S. S. Winans, we have identified a retinohypothalamic tract in the ewe. This was accomplished by autoradiographic localization of tritiated proline which had been injected into the vitreous chamber of the eye. When deposited there, the radioactive amino acid is taken up by retinal ganglion cells, incorporated into proteins, and transported by axoplasmic flow to terminals. Detectable radioactivity does not accumulate beyond the terminals, because once released into a synapse, it disperses rapidly. One week after the injection, the brain was removed and the hypothalamus serially sectioned for autoradiographic localization of terminal fields. Significant radioactivity was found to accumulate in hypothalamic terminals, exclusively in the region of the paired suprachiasmatic nuclei (Legan and Winans, 1981). Thus the ewe, like other mammals, has a monosynaptic tract from the retina to the suprachiasmatic nuclei.

It remains to be determined whether the role of the suprachiasmatic nuclei in biological timekeeping and seasonal breeding, which has been described in rodents, can be extended to sheep. Nevertheless, there is evidence that destruction or denervation in the area of this important region of the brain disrupts the annual reproductive cycle of the ewe (Domanski *et al.*, 1972; Przekop, 1978; Przekop and Domanski, 1980; Pau *et al.*, 1982). Further, it is not known whether suprachiasmatic neurons of the sheep project to the paraventricular nuclei and whether, as in the hamster, the latter region serves to transmit photic information to the superior cervical ganglia which innervate the pineal (Bittman *et al.*, 1983c; Turek *et al.*, 1984). It is known, however, that the superior cervical ganglia of sheep relay photic cues to the pineal (Lincoln, 1979; Yellon and Clayton, 1983). As will now be shown, a great deal of information is available concerning the role of the pineal and its hormone, melatonin, in mediating the reproductive response to photoperiod in the ewe.

C. ROLE OF THE PINEAL GLAND

There can be little doubt that the pineal is required for the reproductive response to photoperiod in several species of long-day breeders (Thorpe and Herbert, 1976; Farrar and Clarke, 1976; Reiter, 1980; Hoffmann, 1981). Our early work in the ewe, however, led to the unwarranted conclusion that the pineal was not necessary in this short-day breeder (Roche *et al.*, 1970). Importantly, the design of those experiments, and a number of others conducted since then in the ewe, failed to account for the fact that the male may influence the reproductive state of the female and that the ewe remains seasonal when deprived of all photoperiodic input. Several more recent studies clearly favor a role for the pineal in sheep, the most compelling of these being performed on the ram (Lincoln, 1979; Barrell and Lapwood, 1979). It became necessary, therefore, to reevaluate the role of the pineal gland, and its hormone melatonin, in mediating the reproductive response to daylength in the ewe. After mastering the arduous procedure of removing the pineal, which in sheep is a deep brain structure embedded in blood vessels, we tested whether the pineal is needed for 90-day alternations between artificial long and short days to drive appropriate changes in ovarian cyclicity and response to the negative feedback action of estradiol. (In this and subsequent studies to be described, rams were excluded from the rooms and ovarian cycles were monitored by serum progesterone concentrations.)

1. Ovarian Cyclicity

A group of ewes with intact ovaries was pinealectomized in early spring and after entering the breeding season in early autumn, the ewes were moved indoors along with unoperated controls. Thereafter, both groups were subjected to 90-day shifts between artificial long and short days for 1.5 years. Control ewes showed unambiguous responses to photoperiod, including onset of cycles under short days during the natural anestrous season of 2 successive years (Fig. 16A). The reproductive pattern of pinealectomized ewes, however, was entirely different. As in the blind ewes, seasonality persisted but it was not photoperiodically controlled.

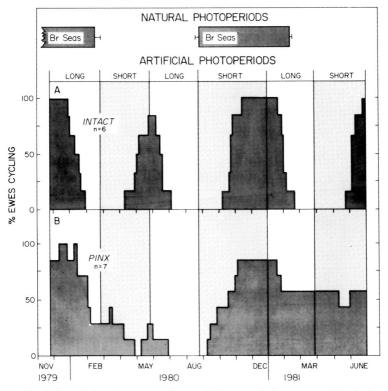

FIG. 16.   Effect of pinealectomy on photoperiodic control of estrous cyclicity in the ewe. Top bar. Mean (and SEM) date of onset and termination of breeding season (BrSeas) in control flock of intact ewes maintained outdoors. Histograms indicate incidence of repeated estrous cycles in 6 intact ewes (A) and 7 pinealectomized ewes (PINX, B) subjected to alternations between long days (16L : 8D, open areas) and short days (8L : 16D, shaded areas) approximately every 90 days. Ewes were PINX in spring of 1979. Note PINX ewes fail to respond to *both* long and short days. From Bittman *et al.* (1983a).

Thus, exposure to short days during natural anestrus was ineffective in driving onset of cycles (Fig. 16B, February–May 1980). Similarly, long days failed to cause reproductive arrest (January–March 1981). The shifts which did occur between breeding and anestrous conditions tended to become asynchronous among pinealectomized ewes and out of phase with the natural seasonal transitions (compare histogram at bottom to bar at top of Fig. 16).

2. Response to Estradiol-Negative Feedback

Pinealectomy of estradiol treated ovariectomized ewes also abolished the reproductive response to photoperiod (Fig. 17). Unlike sham-operated controls, which responded reliably to the light shifts with robust swings in circulating LH, most pinealectomized ewes failed to respond to short days with a typical LH rise during the natural anestrous season of two successive years (February–May 1980 and March–June 1981). Further, pinealectomy eliminated the suppressive effect of long days (e.g., December–March 1981). Again, seasonal swings in LH persisted, but these became asynchronous among ewes and damped over time (note large standard errors in Fig. 17 bottom panel at end of study). Two putatively pinealectomized ewes, however, seemed to remain reproductively responsive to photoperiod (dashed lines in Fig. 17). One of these was found to have a small nighttime rise of serum melatonin and was thus judged to be incompletely pinealectomized; the other unfortunately died before a melatonin profile was obtained.

The preceding results lead to the inescapable conclusion that the pineal gland must be present to mediate the effect of photoperiod on ovarian cyclicity in the ewe, and that this function is likely to be effected through changes in potency of estradiol in the feedback inhibition of tonic LH secretion. Importantly, the pineal is not merely progonadal or antigonadal; rather, it is needed for the response to *both* inductive and inhibitory daylengths. This raises the intriguing question of how the pineal can mediate opposite reproductive responses. The most attractive hypothesis is that the pineal participates in the measurement of daylength. How the pineal serves this timekeeping function leads to a consideration of the secretion of its hormone, melatonin, the last step in the photoneuroendocrine pathway to be considered here.

D. MELATONIN—A TIMEKEEPING HORMONE

Being one of the few seasonal breeders in which a radioimmunoassay for *circulating* melatonin is available, the sheep is an ideal model for studying the role played by this hormone in the reproductive response to

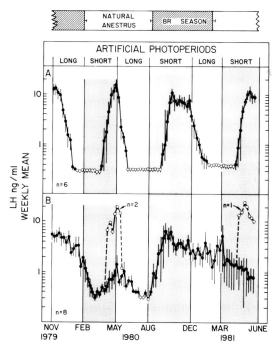

FIG. 17. Effect of pinealectomy on photoperiodic regulation of response to estradiol negative feedback, monitored as serum LH concentrations in ovariectomized ewes treated with sc Silastic estradiol implants (producing 3 pg/ml serum estradiol). Top bar. Mean (and SEM) dates of onset and termination of breeding season in a control flock of intact ewes maintained outdoors. LH values depict weekly mean (±SEM) for twice weekly samples in 6 pineal intact ewes (A) and 8 pinealectomized ewes (B) housed in artificial photoperiods alternated between long days (16L : 8D, open areas) and short days (8L : 16D, shaded areas) approximately every 90 days. Dashed lines show data from ewes judged to be incompletely pinealectomized where they markedly diverged from the rest of the group (see text). Note pinealectomy eliminated response to both long and short photoperiod. Modified from Bittman *et al.* (1983a).

daylength. Using such an assay, Rollag and Niswender (1976) first determined that the secretion of melatonin in sheep is rhythmic, and that the properties of this rhythm generally conform to those inferred from earlier studies of pineal melatonin content and enzyme activities in rodents (Rudeen *et al.*, 1975; Klein, 1978; Tamarkin *et al.*, 1979; Goldman *et al.*, 1981). Specifically, they reported that significant secretion of melatonin in the ewe occurs only at night, that its secretion is effectively suppressed by light, and that it is a circadian rhythm which persists in constant darkness but is normally entrained by the light/dark cycle. Further, photoperiod shapes the melatonin rhythm in the ewe, so that its secretory pattern

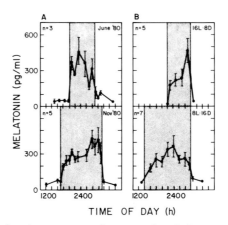

FIG. 18. Twenty-four hour patterns of serum melatonin in ewes (ovariectomized and treated with estradiol implant) exposed to either natural (A, June and November) or artificial (B, long and short) photoperiods. Shading indicates dark period. Values are mean ± SEM. n, Number of ewes. Note, duration of nocturnal melatonin rise is proportional to length of night. Modified from Bittman *et al.* (1983b).

changes during the course of the year (Rollag *et al.*, 1978; Arendt *et al.*, 1981). The latter point is illustrated in Fig. 18 which describes 24-hour profiles of circulating melatonin in Suffolk ewes maintained in contrasting natural conditions (June vs November) and in corresponding artificial photoperiods (16 vs 8 hours light/day). Regardless of whether light is natural or artificial, we find the *duration* of the nighttime melatonin rise to be the feature of the rhythm which is most affected by photoperiod, the duration being directly proportional to the length of the night.

Another property of the melatonin rhythm is its rapid adjustment in response to a change in daylength. For example, following an abrupt decrease from 16 to 8 hours of light each day, the melatonin rise begins to lengthen during the first long night. By the second long night, the duration is almost completely reset (Fig. 19). A further aspect of the melatonin rhythm in the ewe is that it is abolished by removal of the pineal (Fig. 20A and B). Regardless of whether the day is long or short, we find serum melatonin concentrations to be extremely low and arrhythmic following complete pinealectomy.

Melatonin, therefore, would seem to have all the properties expected of a timekeeping hormone. Its secretion is sensitive to light and changes under different photoperiods; it originates from a structure known to mediate the photoperiod response; it has the characteristics of a circadian rhythm. With regard to the latter property, there is now compelling evidence that circadian rhythms are used to measure the length of the day in

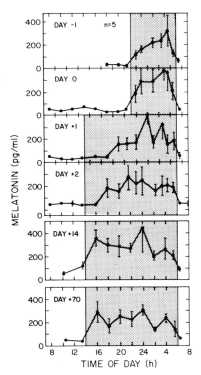

FIG. 19.   Resetting of melatonin pattern after a light shift. Mean (±SEM) serum melatonin concentration in the same 5 ewes on last 2 days (day −1, day 0) of 90-day period of
exposure to long days (16L : 8D) and on days 1, 2, 14, and 70 after shift to short days
(8L : 16D) by advancing time of lights off. Shaded areas depict dark period. Ewes were
ovariectomized and treated with estradiol implants producing 3–5 pg/ml serum estradiol.
Note rapid adjustment of melatonin pattern. From Bittman et al. (1983b).

a wide variety of birds and mammals, including sheep (Hamner, 1964;
Follett and Sharp, 1969; Elliott, 1976; Lincoln et al., 1981; Almeida and
Lincoln, 1982; Turek, 1984). Finally, melatonin can have profound effects
on the reproductive state when administered to long-day breeding hamsters and ferrets, and short-day breeding sheep (Thorpe and Herbert,
1976; Tamarkin et al., 1976; Bittman, 1978; Reiter, 1980; Nett and
Niswender, 1982; Kennaway et al., 1982).

Despite the foregoing implications of a timekeeping function for melatonin, it remained to be determined for any species, whether restoration
of consecutive, *physiological* nighttime rises in circulating melatonin
could reinstate the reproductive response to daylength in the absence of
the pineal. To make such a determination, we devised a portable back-
pack infusion system which permitted patterned intravenous delivery of

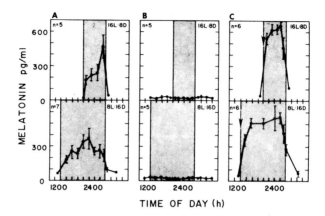

FIG. 20.   Effect of pinealectomy and infusion of melatonin on 24-hour pattern of serum
melatonin (mean ± SEM) in ewes exposed to artificial long (16L:8D) or short (8L:16D)
photoperiods. (A) Pineal intact ewes (repeated from Fig. 18). (B) Pinealectomized (PINX)
ewes. (C) PINX ewes infused with melatonin (see text, arrow shows time pumps turned on).
Shading indicates period of darkness. n, Number of ewes (ovariectomized and treated with
estradiol implant). Note pinealectomy abolishes, and infusion restores, the nighttime rise in
melatonin. (Mean level at night in PINX ewes infused with melatonin approximated highest
nighttime peaks in individual PINX ewes.) Modified from Bittman et al. (1983b).

melatonin into unrestrained pinealectomized ewes for periods of 1 year or
more. By simple adjustment of settings on the battery-powered infusion
pump, the duration and amplitude of the experimentally produced rise in
circulating melatonin could be set to approximate the duration and amplitude of the rise produced endogenously in pineal intact ewes (Fig. 20C).
Two experiments were then performed. The first assessed whether melatonin could account for the inductive effect of short days; the other determined whether melatonin could reinstate the suppressive effect of long
days.

1. Melatonin Mediates Reproductive Induction

Ovariectomized ewes bearing estradiol implants were pinealectomized
in the mid-breeding season, the completeness of surgery being verified by
abolition of the nighttime rise in melatonin. Approximately 1 month before onset of the natural anestrous season (and 1–2 months after surgery),
experimental ewes were equipped with the melatonin delivery system.
Controls were pinealectomized but not infused. During the next 90 days
(late December–late March), both groups were exposed to long days.
Each night, the experimental ewes were infused with a long-day pattern of
melatonin. During the next 90 days (March–June), both groups were ex-

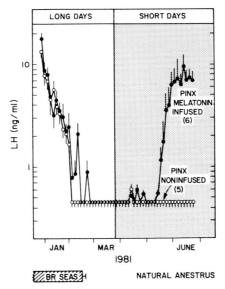

FIG. 21. Melatonin mediates reproductive response to short days. Mean (±SEM) serum LH concentration in two groups of pinealectomized (PINX) ewes that were ovariectomized and treated with estradiol implants. Closed circles, 6 ewes infused with melatonin each night (see text for details of treatment). Open circles, 5 noninfused controls. Open area is initial period of exposure to 90 long days (16L : 8D); shaded area represents subsequent 90 short days (8L : 16D). Serum melatonin values presented in Fig. 20B and C. Bar at bottom shows date (mean + SEM) of transition into anestrus in flock of intact ewes maintained outdoors. Note marked LH rise during anestrus in melatonin-infused ewes. Redrawn from Bittman *et al.* (1983b).

posed to short days, and the infusion pattern of melatonin into experimental ewes was switched to one corresponding to short days. The strategy for this study was to conduct a definitive test for melatonin action by attempting to provoke reproductive induction during the natural anestrous season.

During the initial 90 long days, LH fell precipitously to an undetectable level around the onset of natural anestrus, regardless of whether or not melatonin was infused (Fig. 21). This similarity between LH patterns of the experimental and control groups was expected because seasonality persists in pinealectomized ewes (Fig. 17), and this experiment was initiated just prior to the natural transition into anestrus. Furthermore, both groups had been pinealectomized for just a few months, and this is not sufficient time for a clear reproductive asynchrony to develop among ewes (see previous section on effect of pinealectomy, see also Bittman *et al.*, 1983a).

In marked contrast to the similar patterns during the initial 90-day period of long days, the LH profiles were totally different during the subsequent 90-day period of short days. LH remained undetectable in the noninfused controls, verifying that pinealectomy abolishes the reproductive response to short days. In contrast, a robust LH rise occurred in the pinealectomized ewes receiving the short day pattern of melatonin (Fig. 21, March–June). Importantly, the amplitude of this LH response (more than 20-fold) was just as great as that in a concurrent group of pineal intact controls similarly transferred from long to short days (not illustrated, see Bittman et al., 1983b). Moreover, the mean latency to onset of the LH rise (67 days) did not differ from that of the pineal intact controls.

These findings provide compelling evidence that the pineal drives reproductive induction in short days through its nocturnal secretion of melatonin. Since the melatonin rhythm of pineal intact ewes is reset within days after transfer from a long to a short photoperiod (see Fig. 19), these observations also indicate that the long latency from stimulus to response (about 2 months) arises at a level beyond the pineal in the photoneuroendocrine pathway to the LH pulse generator.

2. Melatonin Mediates Reproductive Arrest

Since the pineal was also found to mediate the suppressive effect of long days in the ewe, a second study was performed to assess whether melatonin also drives the photoinhibitory response. The experimental approach was similar to that of the preceding study, except the sequence of treatments was reversed. During an initial priming period, pinealectomized ewes were infused nightly with the short-day pattern of melatonin in short days to synchronize reproductive induction. Treatment was then switched to nightly infusion of the long-day pattern of melatonin in long days.

A precipitous drop in circulating LH occurred in all pinealectomized ewes which received the long-day pattern of melatonin, but not in a separate group of noninfused pinealectomized controls (Fig. 22). The melatonin-induced decline in LH was identical, in magnitude and time course, to that which occurred in a concurrent group of pineal intact ewes (not illustrated). Furthermore, the LH drop did not occur in an additional control group of pinealectomized ewes which received the short-day melatonin pattern in short days for the entire study (thus verifying that the LH fall in experimental ewes was driven by the switch in treatment rather than by a development of refractoriness to melatonin—data not shown, see Bittman and Karsch, 1984).

The foregoing results lead to the conclusion that the nocturnal rise of melatonin mediates the suppressive effect of long days, as well as the

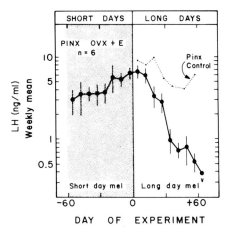

FIG. 22.   Melatonin mediates reproductive response to long days. Mean (±SEM) serum LH concentration in 6 pinealectomized (PINX) ewes that were ovariectomized and treated with Silastic estradiol implants (OVX + E). Prior to day 0, the ewes were housed in short days (8L : 16D, shaded area) and infused with a short-day pattern of melatonin (mel). After day 0, the ewes were exposed to long days (16L : 8D, open area) and treated with a long-day pattern of melatonin. Small points and dotted line illustrate mean serum LH concentration in 2 control noninfused, PINX, OVX + E ewes. v, Undetectable. Note, LH plummets during exposure to long-day melatonin pattern in long days. Redrawn from Bittman and Karsch (1984).

inductive effect of short days. This conclusion is in keeping with the concept that melatonin participates in the measurement of photoperiod, and in addition, it prompts the intriguing question: how does melatonin code for daylength?

3. How Melatonin Codes Daylength

Our initial approach to answering this question has been to distinguish between two alternative conceptual models, the permissive and the deterministic models illustrated in Fig. 23. According to the former, the melatonin rhythm permits the discrimination of daylength by some other neural timekeeping device (Elliott and Goldman, 1981). Light entrains the melatonin rhythm but the characteristics of this rhythm are inconsequential; all that is needed is for some melatonin rhythm to be present. According to the deterministic model, light shapes the melatonin rhythm and a particular characteristic of this rhythm, in turn, dictates the reproductive state. Thus, short-day melatonin causes photoinduction; the long-day pattern drives reproductive arrest.

The experimental strategy to distinguish between these models has been to mismatch photoperiod and the melatonin rhythm. Two such mis-

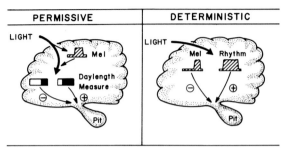

FIG. 23. Hypothetical models for how melatonin codes daylength. Mel, melatonin. Pit, anterior lobe of pituitary gland. +, Stimulatory; −, inhibitory. Open and closed areas of rectangles on left indicate relative lengths of daily light and dark periods, and represent discrimination of long and short days by some daylength measuring system. See text for details.

matches are possible, long-day melatonin infused under short days and short-day melatonin provided under long days. If the permissive model holds, the response should be appropriate to the prevailing photoperiod. Conversely, if melatonin is deterministic, the response should conform to the melatonin pattern.

In one mismatch experiment, two groups of pinealectomized ewes which had been reproductively suppressed with long-day melatonin in long days were transferred to the inductive short photoperiod. At the same time, the melatonin infusion in the control was switched to a short-day pattern (match), and as expected, serum LH concentrations increased as typically occurs in an inductive photoperiod (Fig. 24A). The other group continued to receive the long-day melatonin pattern after being transferred to short days (mismatch). Without exception, the response to the mismatch was appropriate to the long-day melatonin pattern, not to the inductive photoperiod. Thus, LH remained suppressed (Fig. 24B).

In the second such study, pinealectomized ewes displaying elevated serum LH concentrations were infused with a long-day pattern of melatonin and exposed either to long days (match) or short days (mismatch). Again the response was appropriate to the long-day melatonin pattern. LH fell precipitously regardless of whether the photoperiod was inductive or inhibitory (Fig. 25). Results from a third experiment using the converse mismatch (short-day melatonin in long days) are equally conclusive; the response conformed to the inductive melatonin pattern, not to the inhibitory photoperiod (S. M. Yellon, unpublished).

Results from our mismatch experiments, therefore, lend compelling support to the conclusion that the circadian rhythm of melatonin secretion

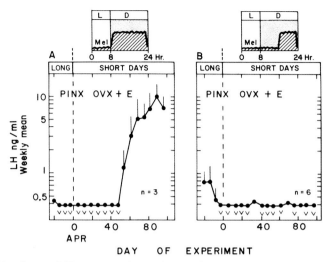

FIG. 24. Serum LH concentrations when melatonin (Mel) and photoperiod were matched (A, short-day Mel in short days, 8L : 16D) or mismatched (B, long-day Mel in short days) beginning on day 0. Prior to day 0, ewes were treated with long-day Mel pattern in long days (16L : 8D). Ewes were pinealectomized (PINX), ovariectomized (OVX), and treated with Silastic estradiol (E) implants which produced 3 pg E/ml serum. LH values are weekly mean (±SEM), samples obtained twice weekly. n, Number of ewes. v, Undetectable values. The specific light (L)/dark (D) cycle and Mel pattern infused each night after day 0 are shown schematically at top (see text for details). Note, LH response after day 0 in mismatch (B) conformed to the long-day melatonin pattern, not the inductive photoperiod. From Bittman and Karsch (1984).

is not merely permissive to the reproductive response to photoperiod. Rather, melatonin determines it. This conclusion leads to the question of which particular feature of the nightly melatonin rise might code for daylength in the ewe. Those characteristics which have been considered include: amplitude, duration, phase relative to the 24-hour light/dark transitions, and the specific shape of the elevation at night (*amplitude:* Lincoln *et al.,* 1981; *duration:* Carter and Goldman, 1983; Bittman *et al.,* 1983b; Bittman and Karsch, 1984; *phase:* Tamarkin *et al.,* 1976; Panke *et al.,* 1980; Almeida and Lincoln, 1982; Watson-Whitmyre and Stetson, 1983; *shape:* Arendt *et al.,* 1981). Recent observations in the Djungarian hamster indicate that duration is the property which is critical to the discrimination of daylength in that long-day breeder (Carter and Goldman, 1983). Although information available for the sheep does not categorically eliminate any of the four characteristics mentioned above, our studies in the ewe are certainly consistent with the hypothesis that the critical feature is duration, the property we find to be most obviously affected by photoperiod (see Fig. 18).

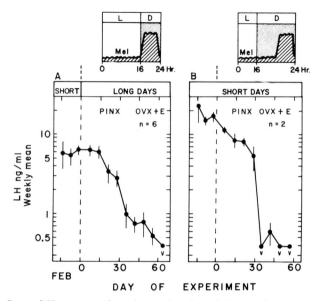

FIG. 25.   Serum LH concentration when melatonin and photoperiod were matched (A, long-day melatonin in long days) or mismatched (B, long-day melatonin in short days). Top illustrates specific light treatments and schematic patterns of melatonin infusion. See text and legend to Fig. 24 for further details. Note LH response after day 0 for mismatch (B) was appropriate to the inhibitory melatonin pattern, not to photoperiod. From Bittman and Karsch (1984).

V. Melatonin and the LH Pulse Generator

It is now time to return to the LH pulse generator and to question how the melatonin signal modulates the activity of this neuroendocrine determinant of estrous cyclicity. Although the answer to this question is largely a mystery, the frequency of the pulse generator is known to be susceptible to regulation by the pineal, both in the presence and absence of ovarian steroids (Bittman et al., 1982). Further, prolonged exposure of the ewe to a short-day pattern of melatonin has been found to drive an increase in frequency of LH pulses in the presence of estradiol (Bittman et al., 1982). It also seems clear that the reproductive transitions, which can be generated in the pinealectomized ewe by a physiologic pattern of melatonin, do not result from a direct action of the hormone on the anterior pituitary and a modulation of its response to GnRH (E. L. Bittman, unpublished). It thus seems reasonable to postulate that the primary actions of melatonin in this system are directed toward the neural elements of the LH pulse generator.

Such information, however, merely scratches the surface of this important area of neuroendocrine integration, and many compelling questions remain. How does the pulse generator, which can oscillate as rapidly as once or twice each hour, decode the signal provided by a 24-hour rhythm of melatonin? Does melatonin act directly upon the pulse generator, or must melatonin interact with another system which then addresses the pulse generator? Why is such a long period of time required for the effects of melatonin on the pulse generator to become evident?

VI. Conclusion

Despite the many unanswered questions, a great deal of insight has been gained into the complex interplay between the neural and endocrine response systems which underlie the seasonal reproductive process in the short-day breeding ewe. Evidence has been presented which supports the scheme presented in Fig. 26. Specifically, light cues activate retinal photoreceptors and are transmitted via a monosynaptic tract to the supra-

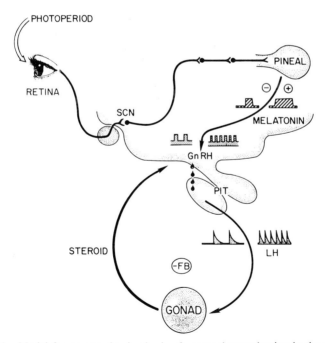

FIG. 26. Model for neuroendocrine basis of seasonal reproduction in the ewe. SCN, suprachiasmatic nuclei. +, Inductive. −, Inhibitory. PIT, pituitary gland. −FB, negative feedback between ovaries and LH pulse generator.

222   FRED J. KARSCH ET AL.

chiasmatic nuclei of the hypothalamus. After interacting with the circadian system, the photic information is relayed to the pineal gland which transduces the neural message into a hormonal signal in the form of a circadian rhythm of melatonin secretion. The pattern of this melatonin signal, which is interpreted as inductive or suppressive, sets the frequency of the LH pulse generator and determines the capacity of this neural oscillator to respond to the negative feedback action of estradiol. The resulting changes in the episodic pattern of gonadotropin secretion, in turn, dictate whether or not estrous cycles can occur.

Without a doubt, nature has chosen to employ a most intriguing hierarchy of temporal organization to ensure the newborn lamb begins its life at the time of year most suitable to its survival. What a truly remarkable system it is that enables a *circannual* rhythm of reproduction to be timed by a *circadian* rhythm of melatonin, which acts via a *circhoral* rhythm of hypothalamo-hypophyseal activity to regulate the *16-day* estrous cycle of the ewe.

ACKNOWLEDGMENTS

We are indebted to a great many people who have contributed to this work. We thank Douglas Doop who cares for our animals, helps perform our experiments, and maintains our Sheep Research Facility. Barbara Glover has helped perform the assays, and Marjorie Hepburn and Mark Byrne have prepared our analytical reagents. Drs. Gordon D. Niswender, Mark D. Rollag, and Leo E. Reichert, Jr. has supplied antibodies and purified hormones for radioimmunoassays. We acknowledge Ann Betz, Ruth Lum, and Sue Bareis for help in preparing the manuscript and general administrative assistance. Finally, special thanks are extended to Dr. A. Rees Midgley, Jr., whose enthusiasm and unyielding efforts to the Reproductive Endocrinology Program have created an atmosphere of excitement and excellence. This work was supported by research and training grants from the National Institute of Child Health and Human Development, The Ford Foundation, and the Michigan Society of Fellows.

REFERENCES

Almeida, O. F. X., and Lincoln, G. A. (1982). *Biol. Reprod.* **27**, 1062.
Arendt, J., Symons, A. M., and Laud, C. (1981). *In* "Photoperiodism and Reproduction in Vertebrates" (R. Ortavant, J. Pelletier, and J-P. Revault, eds.), p. 219. INRA, Versailles.
Baird, D. T., and Scaramuzzi, R. J. (1976). *J. Endocrinol.* **70**, 237.
Baird, D. T., Swanston, I. A., and McNeilly, A. S. (1981). *Biol. Reprod.* **24**, 1013.
Barrell, G. K., and Lapwood, K. R. (1979). *J. Endocrinol.* **80**, 397.
Benoit, J. (1964). *Ann. N.Y. Acad. Sci.* **117**, 204.
Bittman, E. L. (1978). *Science* **202**, 648.
Bittman, E. L., and Karsch, F. J. (1984). *Biol. Reprod.* **30**, 585.
Bittman, E. L., Karsch, F. J., and Dempsey, R. J. (1982). *Annu. Meet., 64th, Endocrine Soc. Abstr.* No. 983.

Bittman, E. L., Karsch, F. J., and Hopkins, J. W. (1983a). *Endocrinology* **113**, 329.

Bittman, E. L., Dempsey, R. J., and Karsch, F. J. (1983b). *Endocrinology* **113**, 2276.

Bittman, E. L., Lehman, M. N., and Winans, S. S. (1983c). *Soc. Neurosci. Abstr.* **9**, Part 1, 318.

Carter, D. S., and Goldman, B. D. (1983). *Endocrinology,* **113**, 1261.

Clarke, I. J., and Cummins, J. T. (1982). *Endocrinology,* **111**, 1737.

Clegg, M. T., Cole, H. H., and Ganong, W. F. (1965). USDA Miscellaneous Publication No. 1005, p. 96.

Day, J. R., and Taylor, M. H. (1983). *J. Exp. Zool.* **227**, 453.

Dixit, V. P., Sharma, O. P., and Agrawal, M. (1977). *Endokrinologie* **70**, 13.

Domanski, E., Przekop, F., and Skubiszewski, B. (1972). *Acta Neurobiol. Exp.* **32**, 753.

Ducker, M. J., Bowman, J. C., and Temple, A. (1973). *J. Reprod. Fertil. Suppl.* **19**, 143.

Eichler, V. B., and Moore, R. Y. (1974). *Acta Anat.* **89**, 359.

Elliott, J. A. (1976). *Fed. Proc. Fed. Am. Soc. Exp. Biol.* **35**, 2339.

Elliott, J. A., and Goldman, B. D. (1981). *In* "Neuroendocrinology of Reproduction: Physiology and Behavior" (N. T. Adler, ed.), p. 377. Plenum, New York.

Farrar, G. M., and Clarke, J. R. (1976). *Neuroendocrinology* **22**, 134.

Follett, B. K. (1978). *In* "Control of Ovulation" (D. B. Crighton, G. R. Foxcroft, N. B. Haynes, and G. E. Lamming, eds.), pp. 267–293. Butterworths, London.

Follett, B. K., and Sharp, P. J. (1969). *Nature (London)* **223**, 968.

Goldman, B., Hall, V., Hollister, C., Reppert, S., Roychoudhury, P., Yellon, S., and Tamarkin, L. (1981). *Biol. Reprod.* **24**, 778.

Goodman, R. L., and Karsch, F. J. (1980a). *Endocrinology* **107**, 1286.

Goodman, R. L., and Karsch, F. J. (1980b). *In* "Progress in Reproductive Biology, 5. Seasonal Reproduction in Higher Vertebrates" (R. J. Reiter and B. K. Follett, eds.), p. 134. Karger, Basel.

Goodman, R. L., and Karsch, F. J. (1981). *In* "Biological Clocks in Seasonal Reproductive Cycles" (B. K. Follett and D. E. Follett, eds.), p. 223. Wright, Bristol.

Goodman, R. L., and Meyer, S. L. (1984). *Biol. Reprod.* **30**, 374.

Goodman, R. L., Reichert, L. E., Jr., Legan, S. J., Ryan, K. D., Foster, D. L., and Karsch, F. J. (1981a). *Biol. Reprod.* **25**, 134.

Goodman, R. L., Legan, S. J., Ryan, K. D., Foster, D. L., and Karsch, F. J. (1981b). *J. Endocrinol.* **89**, 229.

Goodman, R. L., Bittman, E. L., Foster, D. L., and Karsch, F. J. (1982). *Biol. Reprod.* **27**, 580.

Gwinner, E. (1981). *In* "Handbook of Behavioral Neurobiology, Vol. 4. Biological Rhythms" (J. Aschoff, ed.), p. 391. Plenum, New York.

Hamner, W. M. (1964). *Nature (London)* **203**, 1400.

Herbert, J., Stacey, P. M., and Thorpe, D. H. (1978). *J. Endocrinol.* **78**, 389.

Hoffmann, K. (1981). *In* "Handbook of Behavioral Neurobiology, Vol. 4, Biological Rhythms" (J. Aschoff, ed.), p. 449. Plenum, New York.

Hoffman, R. A., and Reiter, R. J. (1965). *Science* **148**, 1609.

Howland, B. E., Palmer, W. M., Sanford, L. M., and Beaton, D. B. (1978). *Can. J. Anim. Sci.* **58**, 547.

I'Anson, H. (1983). *Biol. Reprod.* **28** (Suppl. 1), Abstr. 64.

Karsch, F. J. (1980). *Physiologist* **23** (No. 6), 29.

Karsch, F. J., Legan, S. J., Hauger, R. L., and Foster, D. L. (1977). *Endocrinology* **101**, 800.

Karsch, F. J., Foster, D. L., Legan, S. J., Ryan, K. D., and Peter, G. K. (1979). *Endocrinology* **105**, 421.

Karsch, F. J., Legan, S. J., Ryan, K. D., and Foster, D. L. (1980). *Biol. Reprod.* **23**, 404.

Karsch, F. J., Foster, D. L., Bittman, E. L., and Goodman, R. L. (1983). *Endocrinology* **113,** 1333.

Kennaway, D. J., Gilmore, T. A., and Seamark, R. F. (1982). *Endocrinology* **110,** 1766.

Klein, D. C. (1978). *In* "The Hypothalamus" (S. Reichlin, R. J. Baldessarini, and J. B. Martin, eds.), p. 303. Raven, New York.

Land, R. B., Wheeler, A. G., and Carr, W. R. (1976). *Ann. Biol. Anim. Biochim. Biophys.* **16,** 521.

Landefeld, T. D., Kepa, J., and Karsch, F. J. (1983). *J. Biol. Chem.* **258,** 2390.

Legan, S. J. (1982). *Biol. Reprod.* **26** (Suppl. 1), Abstr. 31.

Legan, S. J. (1983). *Biol. Reprod.* **28** (Suppl. 1), Abstr. 63.

Legan, S. J., and Karsch, F. J. (1979). *Biol. Reprod.* **20,** 74.

Legan, S. J., and Karsch, F. J. (1980). *Biol. Reprod.* **23,** 1061.

Legan, S. J., and Karsch, F. J. (1983). *Biol. Reprod.* **29,** 316.

Legan, S. J., and Winans, S. S. (1981). *Gen. Comp. Endocrinol.* **45,** 317.

Legan, S. J., Karsch, F. J., and Foster, D. L. (1977). *Endocrinology* **101,** 818.

Levine, J. E., Pau K-Y. F., Ramirez, V. D., and Jackson, G. L. (1982). *Endocrinology* **111,** 1449.

Lincoln, G. A. (1979). *J. Endocrinol.* **82,** 135.

Lincoln, G. A., and Short, R. V. (1980). *Recent Prog. Horm. Res.* **36,** 1.

Lincoln, G. A., Almeida, O. F. X., and Arendt, J. (1981). *J. Reprod. Fertil. Suppl.* **30,** 23.

Marshall, F. H. A. (1937). *Proc. R. Soc. London Ser. B* **122,** 413.

Martin, G. B., Scaramuzzi, R. J., and Lindsay, D. R. (1983a). *J. Reprod. Fertil.* **67,** 47.

Martin, G. B., Scaramuzzi, R. J., and Henstridge, J. D. (1983b). *J. Endocrinol.* **96,** 181.

McLeod, B. J., Haresign, W., and Lamming, G. E. (1982). *J. Reprod. Fertil.* **65,** 215.

McNatty, K. P., Gibb, M., Dobson, C., and Thurley, D. C. (1981). *J. Endocrinol.* **90,** 375.

McNeilly, A. S., O'Connell, M., and Baird, D. T. (1982). *Endocrinology* **110,** 1292.

Menaker, M., and Keatts, H. (1968). *Proc. Natl. Acad. Sci. U.S.A.* **60,** 146.

Moore, R. Y. (1973). *Brain Res.* **49,** 403.

Moore, R. Y., and Lenn, N. J. (1972). *J. Comp. Neurol.* **146,** 1.

Nett, T. M., and Niswender, G. D. (1982). *Theriogenology* **17,** 645.

Olster, D. H., and Foster, D. L. (1983). *Biol. Reprod.* **28** (Suppl. 1), Abstr. 25.

Panke, E. S., Rollag, M. D., and Reiter, R. J. (1980). *Comp. Biochem. Physiol.* **66A,** 691.

Pau, K-Y. F., Kuehl, D. E., and Jackson, G. L. (1982). *Biol. Reprod.* **27,** 999.

Pengelley, E. T. (ed.). (1974). "Circannual Clocks." Academic Press, New York.

Poindron, P., Cognie, Y., Gayerie, F., Orgeur, P., Oldham, C. M., and Ravault, J-P. (1980). *Physiol. Behav.* **25,** 227.

Przekop, F. (1978). *Acta Physiol. Pol.* **29,** 393.

Przekop, F., and Domanski, E. (1980). *J. Endocrinol.* **85,** 481.

Reiter, R. J. (1980). *Endocrine Rev.* **1,** 109.

Robinson, J. E. (1983). *Biol. Reprod.* **28** (Suppl. 1), Abstr. 62.

Roche, J. F., Karsch, F. J., Foster, D. L., Takagi, S., and Dziuk, P. J. (1970). *Biol. Reprod.* **2,** 251.

Rollag, M. D., and Niswender, G. D. (1976). *Endocrinology* **98,** 482.

Rollag, M. D., O'Callaghan, P. L., and Niswender, G. D. (1978). *Biol. Reprod.* **18,** 279.

Rudeen, P. K., Reiter, R. J., and Vaughan, M. K. (1975). *Neurosci. Lett.* **1,** 225.

Rusak, B., and Zucker, I. (1979). *Physiol. Rev.* **59,** 449.

Ryan, K. D., and Foster, D. L. (1980). *Fed. Proc. Fed. Am. Soc. Exp. Biol.* **39,** 2372.

Salamonsen, L. A., Jonas, H. A., Burger, H. G., Buckmaster, J. M., Chamley, W. A., Cumming, I. A., Findlay, J. K., and Goding, J. R. (1973). *Endocrinology* **93,** 610.

Scaramuzzi, R. J., and Baird, D. T. (1977). *Endocrinology* **101,** 1801.

Smeaton, T. C., and Robertson, H. A. (1971). *J. Reprod. Fertil.* **25**, 243.

Stetson, M. H., and Watson-Whitmyre, M. (1976). *Science* **191**, 197.

Tamarkin, L., Westrom, W. K., Hamill, A. I., and Goldman, B. D. (1976). *Endocrinology* **99**, 1534.

Tamarkin, L., Reppert, S. M., and Klein, D. C. (1979). *Endocrinology* **104**, 385.

Thomson, A. P. D. (1954). *Proc. R. Soc. London Ser. B* **142**, 126.

Thorpe, P. A., and Herbert, J. (1976). *J. Endocrinol.* **70**, 255.

Thwaites, C. J. (1965). *J. Agric. Sci.* **65**, 57.

Turek, F., Swann, J., and Earnest, D. J. (1984). *Recent Prog. Horm. Res.* **40**, 143.

Underwood, H. (1975). *J. Comp. Physiol.* **99**, 71.

Van Brunt, E. E., Shepherd, M. D., Wall, J. R., Gonong, W. F., and Clegg, M. T. (1964). *Ann. N.Y. Acad. Sci.* **117**, 217.

Watson-Whitmyre, M., and Stetson, M. H. (1983). *Endocrinology* **112**, 763.

Wetterberg, L., Geller, E., and Yuwilder, A. (1970). *Science* **167**, 884.

Wodzicka-Tomaszewska, M., Hutchinson, J. C. D., and Bennett, J. W. (1967). *J. Agric. Sci.* **68**, 61.

Yeates, N. T. M. (1949). *J. Agric. Sci.* **39**, 1.

Yellon, S. M., and Clayton, J. A. (1983). *Biol. Reprod.* **28** (Suppl. 1), Abstr. 27.

Zucker, I., Johnston, P. G., and Frost, D. (1980). *In* "Progress in Reproductive Biology, 5. Seasonal Reproduction in Higher Vertebrates" (R. J. Reiter and B. K. Follett, eds.), p. 102. Karger, Basel.

Zweig, M., Snyder, S. H., and Axelrod, J. (1966). *Proc. Natl. Acad. Sci. U.S.A.* **56**, 515.

DISCUSSION

D. Pomerantz: I would like to pose questions in two areas. First, I noted that the time that elapsed between either changing the photoperiod or applying the infusions of melatonin until you observed altered LH secretion seemed to be at least 30 days. I am wondering if you have any explanation as to why it takes the neural and secretory mechanisms so long to respond to the change in melatonin?

F. J. Karsch: This is an extremely interesting question which we have asked ourselves for years. While I do not know the answer, I can reject a few possibilities and then speculate as to what the general nature of the change may be. First, the lag does not seem to reflect time for development of pituitary mechanisms needed to respond appropriately to high frequency pulses of GnRH. A number of workers have found that repeated hourly bolus injections of GnRH into anestrous ewes immediately produces appropriate gonadotropin responses and eventual ovulation. Second, the lag does not seem to be based on the time required for GnRH neurons to develop the capacity to produce high-frequency discharges of the releasing hormone. The anestrous ewe can respond to other external signals, such as introduction of the ram after a period of isolation, with hourly pulses of LH (and presumably GnRH) (Martin *et al.*, 1983). Third, the lag cannot be explained by the time needed for the pattern of the circadian rhythm of melatonin to adjust following a light shift. This requires only a few days as I described in my presentation. By exclusion, then, the 50-day latency most likely results from a process after the level of the pineal gland and before the level of the GnRH neuron—perhaps in the link between the melatonin receptor and the LH pulse generator.

In speculating about the basis for the lag, I might point to examples of structural changes in the brain with season. Structural changes have been seen in hypothalamic neurons in certain bats and in neurons controlling vocalizations in birds (Nottebohm, *Science* **214**, 1368, 1981). The explanation which I find most attractive for the 50-day lag is that the response to melatonin includes morphological changes in neurons which control the activity of the pulse generator, or perhaps in the pulse generator itself. These changes may take quite some time.

Further, it should be pointed out that much shorter lags have been observed in other species. In the Japanese quail, for example, a pronounced increase of gonadotropin is seen on the first day of photoinduction, although this is probably not mediated by the pineal (Follett *et al., J. Endocrinol.* **74**, 449, 1977).

D. Pomerantz: For the second area, I would like to ask you to guess once again. I was really intrigued about the effect of the presence of a male and that he was a really good supplier of time cues. How do you envision the presence of the male interacting in the system, is it simply his motor activity, is he a provider of pheromones, if he is a pheromone supplier what is the neural pathway, is there melatonin involvement at all in the ability of the male to change the patterns of LH secretion in the blinded ewes?

F. J. Karsch: I suspect there are at least two types of effects which the ram may have. One is a relatively long-term seasonal effect due to chronic exposure to the male, such as I described in our blind ewes. The other is a much more acute effect observed following introduction of the ram to seasonally anestrous ewes previously isolated from the male. A great deal more is known of the acute effect (e.g., Poindron *et al.,* 1980; Martin *et al.,* 1983). The acute influence of ram introduction, which is called the "ram effect," is now known to be an olfactory response triggered by a pheromone which is discharged on the wool of the ram. Within minutes of exposure to this pheromone, the negative feedback effect of estradiol is disrupted, the LH pulse generator is activated, and an hourly rhythm of LH pulses is established. This, in turn, produces a preovulatory estradiol rise which induces the LH surge and ovulation. Tactile or motor activity of the ram is not needed for the "ram effect"; in fact the presence of the ram is not even required. All that is needed is the wool of the ram, or a wool extract which contains the active substance. With regard to the more long-term seasonal effect of the ram which may have influenced our blind ewes, there is no information as to the nature of the cue or its mode of action, other than it would appear to alter the response to the negative feedback action of estradiol on gonadotropin secretion. The neural pathways which mediate either of these influences of the ram are not known.

D. Pomerantz: Do you think that in the normal situation where the ewe is exposed to the ram, that the pineal mechanisms are in fact all that important?

F. J. Karsch: With regard to the acute "ram effect" I have just described, it is evident only if the ewe has been isolated from the male. In the normal situation on a farm, males and females are not totally isolated. I expect, therefore, that this effect would not be a driving influence. As concerns the postulated long-term seasonal effect of the ram, it is important to point out that the ram was sighted and the ewes were not. We do not know whether such an effect of the ram would be evident if the females could sense daylength. Further, the response in blind ewes housed with a ram was not as robust as that in sighted ewes (animals shown were estradiol-treated castrates), and although not described in my presentation, an influence of the ram on estrous cycles was not observed in blind ewes which had intact ovaries (Legan and Karsch, 1983). Thus, I expect that photoperiod is normally the primary external cue for the seasonal reproductive cycle of the ewe and that the presence of the ram may modify the response to the light cue. Further, it should be noted that the reproductive activity of the ram is also seasonally modulated by photoperiod through pineal mediated mechanisms, so again the light cycle is the primary synchronizing agent.

R. Osathanondh: I have a question in regard to the blinding experiment. What happens if an animal has been blinded since birth, in other words, her brain has never been triggered by photic stimuli via the retina, what would happen in regards to the reproductive seasonality and melatonin rhythm?

F. J. Karsch: I cannot answer your question; we have not studied the effect of blinding at the time of birth. Moreover, information in other species may be difficult to interpret in terms of the system we describe here for the ewe, because the ewe remains reproductively seasonal in the absence of photoperiodic drive. This is not the case for a number of the other seasonal breeders which have been studied. It may be helpful to have Hamish Robertson comment on this point. He mentioned to me just before my presentation that he monitored the occurrence of estrous cycles in a lamb that was found to be born blind.

H. Robertson: Perhaps I could comment on the question of what happens if you're lucky enough to find a lamb that is born blind. We found one and followed it and, much to our surprise, in the presence of a ram it started ovulating at the normal time of year.

R. Osathanondh: May I just point out one thing that has been reported in the journal *Fertility and Sterility* (S. Lehrer, *Fertil. Steril.* **38**, 751, 1982) in which the investigator has studied congenitally blind women in the school for the blind. The blind women do not seem to have any problems with ovulation or reproduction but, as Dr. Turek has pointed out, the human is probably much different from animals with regard to reproductive activity.

F. J. Karsch: I do not really think the human and sheep are as different as you suggest. Blind individuals of both species have perfectly normal ovarian cycles. What blinding does in sheep is abolish photoperiodic drive of the annual reproductive cycle. Since humans are not obviously reproductively seasonal, nor photoperiodic, I would expect that blinding would have little effect on reproduction. Thus, it is the seasonality component which is different, not necessarily the mechanisms which operate during each estrous or menstrual cycle.

W. Wehrenberg: Fred, you raised the question of how melatonin codes for daylight. The evidence you presented argues rather conclusively that the deterministic model is the correct model. I agree with this conclusion for your series of experiments. The question I would like to raise concerns data reported by Fred Stormshack at Corvalis, Oregon. He has shown that the subcutaneous implantation of Silastic capsules containing melatonin in mink can advance the furring out process in these animals. This event takes place during the long-day photoperiod even though these animals are short-day breeders. His experiments argue that the pattern of delivery of melatonin is not critical for this physiological event and thus led me to suggest that the permissive role is also a viable model by which melatonin might code for daylight.

F. J. Karsch: It is entirely possible that the melatonin message is processed in different ways among the species which utilize this hormone to synchronize seasonal changes in physiological processes. Nevertheless, I think we must be extremely careful in interpreting experiments in which melatonin is delivered constantly, when its normal pattern of secretion is rhythmic. On the one hand, it is quite possible that a sustained elevation of the hormone may not yield meaningful information concerning the length of the day, and that any response which does occur may do so for reasons unrelated to photoperiod. On the other hand, a normal type of melatonin pattern may persist following placement of a constant release implant, with the endogenous nighttime rise being superimposed upon an elevated baseline.

C. S. Nicoll: With regard to the persistence of the seasonal reproductive cycle in the blinded ewes, have you considered the possibility that lunar cycles could be involved in this phenomenon? The reason I ask is based on work done by some of my colleagues in Berkeley and in Seattle at the University of Washington (Grau *et al., Science* **211**, 607, 1981). They have been studying the seaward migration of salmon and found that it is triggered by surges in thyroid hormone levels in plasma. These surges are initiated by the new moon each month. Once the surges are big enough, the animals are induced to migrate downstream to the sea. It is interesting that the animals can detect the phase of the new moon even when they are indoors and they cannot see the moon. Clearly, these animals are responding to changes in the lunar cycle even though they cannot see it. If salmon can do this, maybe sheep can also do it. One would expect that it is the gravitational effect since it occurs indoors where they cannot see the light of the moon. I think that these results in salmon illustrate that people working on seasonal breeders should consider the possible influence of lunar cycles.

F. J. Karsch: We cannot really exclude an influence of lunar cycles. I would be very surprised if they act to synchronize the annual reproductive cycle of the ewe. To my knowledge, lunar cycles are not seasonal. Also, if lunar cycles could synchronize seasonal breeding, one would expect that seasonal reproductive changes in blind or pinealectomized ewes would remain synchronized among individuals. Although it is not evident from the data I presented which described group means, the reproductive changes in individual blind and pinealectomized ewes drift over time and become asynchronous among animals. As a result, some animals are turned on while others are turned off. Thus, with the possible exception of the ram, I doubt that the reproductive changes in our blind or pinealectomized ewes were under the influence of any synchronizing agent, lunar or otherwise.

G. D. Niswender: I might just add that there are species of plenaria with fission only at night, and that the fissioning appears to be a melatonin-mediated event. These animals cue on lunar cycles even when they are housed in the interior rooms of large buildings where there is no light from outside.

F. Turek: I would just like to comment on how I think we are beginning to link some theoretical explanations for photoperiodic time measurement with physiological mechanisms. In one of my slides I showed a hypothetical rhythm of sensitivity to light which was driven or entrained by some circadian clock and the phase relationship between the light and the rhythm of sensitivity determined if the light would be stimulatory or not. I think what you have found in the sheep and what Bruce Goldman has found in the Siberian hamster suggests that the hypothetical rhythm of sensitivity may be the melatonin rhythm which is driven by the suprachiasmatic nucleus and that when light is coincident with a certain phase of the melatonin rhythm, one can alter the pattern of that rhythm. Some very nice studies by Klaus Hoffman in the Siberian hamster have shown that a 1-minute pulse of light in the middle of the night of an otherwise short LD cycle will mimic the effects of long days on both the reproductive system and the pattern of pineal NAT levels.

F. J. Karsch: Yes, that is a very good point. I feel that our studies regarding the way melatonin codes for daylength forces us to think along the line that photoperiod, and the circadian system, may exert their primary influence above the level of the pineal gland. Perhaps the role of light and the circadian system is limited to shaping an entraining the rhythm of pineal melatonin secretion, and beyond the pineal, these factors are no longer involved.

H. Robertson: The question has been raised as to whether, under certain conditions, the ewe can become an induced ovulator. I have held the view for a long time that the difference between a spontaneous and an induced ovulating species is not so clear cut as we tend to think and there is now considerable evidence to support the view that ovarian activity in the ewe can be induced by the presence of the ram and this is not dependent upon coital stimulation. I have always been critical of data reported on the effect of changing the photoperiodicity to which sheep have been exposed, since the exposure is generally of short duration and superimposed on animals entrained to natural daylight. It may be of interest that over a period of 7 years I raised three generations of sheep in continuous 24 hour light. These sheep were, therefore, never exposed to any circadian photoperiodicity and, presumably, not to circadian changes in melatonin secretion. Nevertheless in the presence of rams they appeared, as judged by sexual receptivity, to have periods of several ovarian cycles interspersed with short anovulatory periods. Unfortunately this work was carried out before it became possible to monitor ovarian activity in the absence of the ram by sequential plasma progesterone determinations.

F. J. Karsch: Our results in blind ewes certainly complement your views of the influence of the ram on the reproductive condition of the ewe. Also, our studies show that the ram is not needed for persistence of seasonality in ewes rendered nonphotoperiodic.

D. C. Collins: In a series of studies carried out in collaboration with Drs. Gordon, Wilson, and Walker of the Yerkes Primate Research Center, we have demonstrated the occurrence of seasonally restricted ovulations in the rhesus monkey housed in an outdoor environment that exposes them to natural light. We have monitored the ovulatory and menstrual history of 12 female rhesus monkeys during a 20-month period encompassing two reproductive periods. At the beginning of the study, all of the females were nursing infants of 1–4 months of age. Pregnancy was prevented by vasectomy of the males in this group. The resumption of ovulation occurred in November and December for all 12 animals in the first year. The timing of the resumption of ovulation appeared to be related to the age of the infant. All females exhibited multiple ovulations, although the absolute number varied. No ovulations occurred after March and the summer months were characterized by anovulatory cycles and amenorrhea. The ovulations resumed in September in these nonlactating subjects, a significantly earlier time than that seen following parturition and lactation.

Our results clearly show that ovulations are restricted to the fall and winter months followed by anovulation in the spring and summer. The anovulatory period is characterized by low levels of LH, FSH, estradiol-17β, and progesterone. The seasonal onset of ovulation is preceded by a change in the pattern of gonadotropin secretion. The onset of the anovulatory period is characterized by significant decreases in FSH and LH. The timing of the endocrine events associated with seasonal ovulations in the rhesus monkey suggests that the light–dark cycle is important since the changes occur at about the autumal and vernal equinox.

In conclusion, female rhesus monkeys living in an outdoor environment exhibit a seasonal period of ovulation in the fall and winter. Our data are consistent with the hypothesis that the seasonal ovulatory pattern is controlled by an environmental factor, such as photoperiod, mediated through changes in the neuroendocrine system controlling gonadotropin secretion.

R. E. Peter: In goldfish, Alice Hontela and I have found that a single daily injection of melatonin, or three daily injections of melatonin, given approximately 4 hours before the normal time for the daily pulse of gonadotropin release acutely suppresses the daily pulse. We think this is an indication that melatonin may serve in some way as a means of suppressing pulses of gonadotropin in fish exposed to environmental conditions unfavorable for gonadal development, specifically short photoperiods. The pineal is known to have an antigonadal effect in goldfish under short photoperiods. In the sheep, you had relatively long time periods before you detected an effect to melatonin. Do you have any information that demonstrates effects on pulses of LH within a few days after beginning infusion of melatonin in pinealectomized sheep?

F. J. Karsch: No, we have not examined LH pulse patterns directly during the first few days after beginning melatonin infusions into pinealectomized ewes. We have, however, monitored mean serum LH concentrations in estradiol-treated ovariectomized ewes. These values provide an indirect monitor of the activity of the LH pulse generator, and we have not observed a change until several weeks after the switch in the melatonin pattern.

R. E. Peter: If I can add another item of information relative to the input of olfactory information. Another candidate for this input is the nervus terminalis. Its cell bodies are located on the olfactory bulbs. Fibers follow the olfactory tracts and the optic nerves out to the retina to end among bilpolar retinal cells. Some endings also occur in the ventral-basal preoptic region, perhaps in the suprachiasmatic nucleus. Interestingly the cell bodies and fibers of the nervus terminalis in fishes and other lower vertebrates contain LH-RH or GnRH. This provides a means for transfer of LH-RH or GnRH to the retina where it can influence activity of bipolar cells and, of course, it raises the possibility that the nervus terminalis could also influence activity of the suprachiasmatic nucleus or other preoptic nuclei.

S. Cohen: I have one comment. The comment is—you use the term gonad and steroids. I do not think you meant any gonads or any steroids. Is there any special reason you did not specifically say ovary or estradiol?

F. J. Karsch: I am speaking of a rather generalized phenomenon. The gonads may be either the testes or the ovaries. The same type of control system seems to operate in the male, with the active steroids being secreted by the testes. Further, the seasonal change is not specific to estradiol. A seasonal shift in potency of steroid negative feedback has been described for other steroids. It is quite possible that such changes would be evident for all steroids which exert their suppressive effects by acting within the brain. Thus, I suspect that we are dealing with a rather widespread phenomenon which pertains to both sexes and which operates in a variety of seasonal breeders.

D. Schulster: Relevant to the regulation of LH secretion by melatonin: what is known of the direct effect of melatonin on the characteristics of the receptors for GnRH at the level of the pituitary membrane?

F. J. Karsch: I do not know of any evidence for effects of melatonin on receptors for GnRH in the pituitary. Melatonin has been found to alter the response to GnRH in pituitaries of immature rats incubated *in vitro* (Martin and Klein, *Science* **191,** 301, 1976). We need to remember, however, that the albino rat is not normally a photoperiodic species. Further, it is not known whether the patterns and amounts of melatonin which are normally secreted by the rat pineal can affect the pituitary directly. As concerns a pituitary site for melatonin action in our seasonally breeding sheep, unpublished studies by Eric Bittman have examined the response to low dose pulses of GnRH under conditions of differing photoperiods and melatonin patterns. He found no evidence for an action of melatonin upon the pituitary gland. Thus, I would suspect the major action of melatonin is exerted within the brain. Also, I should stress, the most important effect of photoperiod seems to be on *frequency* of gonadotropin pulses, and this type of change would seem to favor a neural site of action. Nevertheless, the available evidence does not permit us to exclude an effect on the pituitary as well.

D. Keefe: Could there be an indirect effect of melatonin on the reproductive system? The light–dark cycle entrains the hormonal rhythms of a variety of hormones, such as corticosterone and prolactin, that affect the reproductive system. Could it be that melatonin affects the reproductive system by changing these hormonal rhythms? I wonder, in your experiments where you mismatched the light–dark cycle with the melatonin infusions, did you look into the rhythms of reproductively active hormones such as prolactin and cortico-steroids? Would they follow the melatonin rhythm or the photoperiod?

F. J. Karsch: This is an interesting question. As of yet, we have not monitored rhythms of other hormones in our studies in which photoperiod and melatonin were mismatched. Are you aware of information which would suggest that other hormones might mediate the effects of melatonin on GnRH?

D. Keefe: No I am not. Is an intact hypothalamic–pituitary–adrenal axis necessary for photoperiodism in reproduction? Is intact prolactin secretion required for a photoperiodic response in reproduction?

F. J. Karsch: We have not studied the importance of the adrenal in mediating the reproductive response to photoperiod in the ewe. In the golden hamster, however, the adrenal gland is not needed for these responses to occur in either the male or the female (Bittman and Goldman, *J. Endocrinol.* **83**, 113, 1979; Ellis and Turek, *Endocrinology* **106**, 1338, 1980). A possible role for prolactin has attracted considerable interest because seasonal changes in gonadal function are temporally associated with changes in prolactin secretion (Walton *et al., J. Endocrinol.* **75**, 127, 1977). It also seems that an increase in prolactin secretion may heighten the effectiveness of steroids in suppressing gonadotropin secretion in the albino rat and, in the human, certain types of amenorrhea are marked by elevated secretion of prolactin (McNeilly, *J. Reprod. Fertil.* **58**, 537, 1980). Nevertheless, we do not yet know whether the annual cycle of prolactin plays a role in mediating the effect of the melatonin rhythm on gonadotropin secretion which we see in the ewe. I would guess that the variations in prolactin might be associated with one of the many other changes in physiological functions known to occur with season.

C. Irvine: The very striking changes that you showed in melatonin in response to different photoperiods were either in intact ewes or in ovariectomized estrogen-replaced ewes. There is some evidence for an effect of sex steroids at the pineal, based on demonstration of receptors for gonadal steroids and on the influence of steroids on pineal enzymes including HIOMT. In view of these effects, I was wondering if you had looked at the changes in melatonin in ovariectomized ewes without steroid replacement?

F. J. Karsch: No studies of others dealing with the effects of sex steroids on melatonin secretion in sheep have indicated that ovariectomy leads to an increase in the amplitude of the nighttime melatonin rise but does not alter its duration. Since there are profound quantitative differences in the secretion of ovarian steroids from one season to the next, a seasonal change in amplitude of the nightly melatonin rise might be a reasonable expectation. Data in the ewe are somewhat difficult to interpret due to large variation in nighttime melatonin levels (see Rollag *et al.,* 1978 and Arendt *et al.,* 1981). There is evidence in the ram, however, to suggest that changes in the light cycle, which produce alterations in testicular function, are associated with rather marked changes in the amplitude of the nightly melatonin rise (see Lincoln *et al.,* 1981). In our own studies which I described here, however, no effect of photoperiod on the amplitude of the melatonin rise was apparent, possibly because our ewes were ovariectomized and treated with constant release estradiol implants.

G. R. Merriam: You have carefully shown us how important melatonin is for distributing photoperiodic information to the LH-RH pulse generator. In your pinealectomized animals, have you determined if melatonin plays a role in distributing information to other hormones like prolactin which show both seasonal changes and also a pronounced circadian rhythm, or to hormones like cortisol that have a pronounced circadian component but little seasonal variation?

F. J. Karsch: No.

R. Goodman: I would like to turn to the SCN. You suggested that this nucleus is where the interaction of photoperiod with the endogenous circadian rhythm in photosensitivity occurs. The hypothesis that the biological clock resides in the SCN is based mainly on data in rodents. There are data in monkeys, for instance, that SCN lesions do not abolish the diurnal rhythm in cortisol. So I think we have to be a bit careful about concluding that the SCN contains the biological clock in species other than rodents.

F. J. Karsch: Your comment is very well taken. The role of the suprachiasmatic nucleus in biological timekeeping in the sheep remains to be determined. As I mentioned in my talk, there is information to suggest that the normal seasonal reproductive cycle is disrupted when the area in or around the suprachiasmatic nucleus is destroyed by electrolytic lesions or when its fiber tracts are interrupted by knife cuts. This is in keeping with a role for the suprachiasmatic nucleus as a component of the biological clock in the ewe, but it does not prove it.

F. Turek: In SCN lesion studies that have been carried out in primates, some but not all circadian rhythms were abolished. So, even in primates the SCN is a focus for studies on the location of the biological clock. In addition, studies have been carried out in birds in which lesions of the SCN also abolished circadian rhythmicity. Although studies on the role of the SCN in the generation of circadian rhythms have only been carried out in a few species, it does appear to play a critical role in the circadian organization in species as diverse as birds, rodents, and primates.

G. Callard: Fred, in your talk you alluded to the work that some of your colleagues were doing on the neural mechanisms which underlie changes in estrogen feedback sensitivity. I wonder if you or they would care to tell us what their findings are.

F. J. Karsch: You are referring to experiments which Bob Goodman has performed since leaving our laboratory in Michigan. Perhaps he would comment on those studies.

R. Goodman: We have examined the effects of pentobarbital anesthesia on LH pulses in intact ewes. Pentobarbital administration to intact anestrous ewes produced a dramatic increase in LH secretion primarily by increasing pulse frequency. In contrast, during the breeding season pentobarbital suppressed LH secretion. In interpreting these data, we have assumed that pentobarbital acts to suppress neuronal activity. Thus our working hypothesis is that in anestrus a set of neurons, activated by the inhibitory photoperiod, actively inhibits GnRH pulses; pentobarbital suppresses these inhibitory neurons to allow an increase in LH during anestrus. We also postulate that these neurons are not active in the breeding season to account for the seasonal difference we see in the effects of pentobarbital.

G. Callard: That addresses the direct drive question, I think, but how about estrogen feedback sensitivity?

R. Goodman: To put estrogen feedback into the model, we postulate that the neurons that are active in anestrus but not the breeding season are estradiol sensitive. Thus, in anestrus estradiol inhibits LH pulse frequency by increasing the activity of these hypothetical inhibitory neurons. Since these neurons are not functional in the breeding season, estradiol loses its ability to strongly suppress LH secretion at this time of year.

G. Callard: So you do not envision any changes, for example, in estrogen receptors?

R. Goodman: The data on estrogen receptors are inconclusive at this time. We certainly cannot rule out a role for seasonal changes in estrogen receptors.

G. MacDonald: There is evidence the pineal gland may provide some control over the primate menstrual cycle. Some years ago Dr. Virginia Fiske and I (*Fertil. Steril.* **26,** 609, 1975) administered melatonin (10 mg/day) from day 7 or 9 to day 17 following the start of menstruation to regularly cycling *Macaca fascicularis* that were housed in a room with a controlled light : dark (12 : 12) schedule. We found that the expected progesterone increase associated with corpus luteum formation was delayed or prevented during the cycle that melatonin was administered. In the cycle following treatment the expected preovulatory estrogen increase was more variable in time and the occurrence of a second estrogen peak increased. These findings suggest melatonin delayed the release of LH and provides the possibility of a pineal influence over the primate menstrual cycle.

R. Guillemin: Is there an effect of the long-term exposure to the ram in the pinealectomized animal?

F. J. Karsch: We have not looked at this. The influence of long-term exposure to the ram was suggested in our studies in blind ewes. These animals had intact pineals and a free-running circadian rhythm of melatonin secretion. We do not know, therefore, whether ram pheromones utilize a pathway which includes the pineal. I would not think so because the ram can effect the LH pulse generator within minutes, but with photoperiod, the response takes about 2 months.

Somatocrinin, the Growth Hormone Releasing Factor

Roger Guillemin, Paul Brazeau, Peter Böhlen,
Frederick Esch, Nicholas Ling, William B. Wehrenberg,
Bertrand Bloch, Christiane Mougin, Fusun Zeytin,
and Andrew Baird

*Laboratories for Neuroendocrinology, The Salk Institute for Biological Studies,
La Jolla, California*

I. Introduction[1]

In their proposal of a humoral hypothalamic control of adenohypophysial secretions, Green and Harris had left open two possibilities: (1) that the hypothalamic humoral mediator would be a single substance—the pituitary secretion being thus either of all hormones simultaneously, or, if eventually shown to be solitary for one hormone or another, that the specificity would be due to a modulation of peripheral origin (steroids, thyroid hormones, etc.); or (2) that there would be several hypothalamic neurohumors, each one being particularly involved in the secretion of one pituitary hormone. Subsequent physiological studies yielded results best explained by a multiplicity of hypothalamic hypophysiotropic factors. This became an inescapable conclusion when TRF (thyrotropin releasing factor) was characterized: TRF would stimulate exclusively the secretion of thyrotropin (TSH), not of ACTH (adrenocorticotropin), or GH (growth hormone) or the gonadotropins (LH and FSH). This remains true even though it was shown later that TRF can stimulate the secretion of prolactin (PRL) along with that of TSH. Indeed the ensuing years saw the characterization of LRF, that stimulates the secretion of both gonadotropins LH and FSH, and of CRF, that specifically stimulates the secretion of ACTH and β-endorphin. It only remained to characterize a growth hormone releasing factor, GRF. There were many efforts to this end for almost 20 years. Based on questionable bioassays, they yielded results that ultimately had to be recognized as artifacts (a fragment of the β-chain of hemoglobin, Schally *et al.*, 1971; Veber *et al.*, 1971; an inactive decapeptide, Yudaev *et al.*, 1972; never fully characterized peptides, Wilber *et al.*, 1971; Nair *et al.*, 1978, etc.). These efforts also led to the recognition and eventual characterization, in extracts of the hypothalamus, of somatostatin, a powerful inhibitor of the secretion of GH (Krulich *et al.*, 1968; Brazeau *et al.*, 1973).

---

[1] Historical and narrative by R. G.

233

With knowledge of the pitfalls of the bioassays and efficient ways of removing the interfering somatostatin from the crude hypothalamic extracts (affinity chromatography, gel filtration) we started anew to look for GRF in 1978. Rapidly we showed that it was possible by gel filtration on Sephadex G-75 or G-50 to separate all forms of bioactive somatostatin (SS-14, SS-28) from a single zone of the effluent containing GRF activity, based on an *in vitro* assay system measuring by RIA the secretion of ir-GH by rat pituitary cells grown as a monolayer. Almost as rapidly it became obvious that we had, in each hypothalamic fragment, only minute amounts of GRF, probably no more than 10–50 fmol, assuming a potency for GRF to be of the order of that of the already characterized hypothalamic releasing factors.

I then decided that we should investigate in parallel another possible source of GRF, namely those tumors, mostly islet cells adenomas, or carcinomas known in patients to accompany a full-blown syndrome of acromegaly in the absence of a pituitary adenoma (see Leveston *et al.*, 1981, for a review of such cases). Indeed, from early studies by Frohman *et al.* (1980) the GRF activity recognized by these authors in the extract of one such tumor appeared to have chromatographic behavior very similar, if not identical, to those of the material we were purifying from hypothalamic extracts.

At first, clinician colleagues holding such GRF-secreting tumors were not anxious to part with aliquots of the GRF-secreting tissues for us to attempt to isolate GRF from them. Then, in 1981, a 200-mg fragment of a lung tumor which had caused acromegaly was obtained from B. Scheithauer at the Mayo Clinic. The amount of tissue obtained was so small that we decided to keep it frozen for use at some later date when we would have more refined technology for isolation and sequencing than what was available at that time; attempts to grow GRF-secreting cells out of that tissue were unsuccessful (2 years later we received 57 g of the same tumor which unfortunately had been kept in formalin; we could not find GRF activity in it). In August 1981 Fusun Zeytin joined us from the laboratories of Armen Tashjian at Harvard, bringing with her about 400 mg of an islet cell tumor which had caused acromegaly in a patient (Ms. B. G.) of Michael Thorner, University of Virginia. The tissue had been sent by Michael Thorner to Armen Tashjian in the hope of growing GRF-secreting cells out of it, in parallel with similar efforts conducted by Michael Cronin at the University of Virginia (no group succeeded in that task). With the generous agreement of both Armen Tashjian and Michael Thorner, we extracted what remained of that tumor aliquot and isolated ca. 100 pmol of a single GRF entity for which we obtained an amino acid composition on October 24, 1981. No sequence data were attempted, since our then available sequencing equipment would not have had the necessary sensitivity. At that time, Michael Thorner agreed to provide us with an additional 5 g of that tumor. Again that tissue was kept in liquid nitrogen, untouched, until we would have high-resolution sequencing capability, which was now expected for February–March 1982 through the delivery of one of the prototypes of the gas-phase sequencer instrument developed by Hood, Hunkapiller, and collaborators (Hewick *et al.*, 1981) and to be manufactured by Applied Biosystems, Foster City, CA.

In September 1981, I gave a lecture at the old Faculté de Médecine in Paris, in one of the plenary sessions of the annual meeting of the French Société d'Endocrinologie. The title of the lecture was "Evidence for a central nervous system control of the secretion of growth hormone" and discussed primarily physiological and pharmacological data and also some clinical studies particularly relating sleep and GH secretion. In that lecture I mentioned the existence of the tumors as ectopic sources of GRF, a possibility, though rare, not be overlooked in the diagnosis of the etiology and surgical treatment of acromegaly without any obvious pituitary adenoma, quoting the recent case of Thorner. I also explained my interest in obtaining tissues of any such tumor as a possible source of GRF. A couple of months later I received a letter from Dr. Geneviève Sassolas of the Alexis Carrel University in Lyons, France, describing a patient (Mr. T. W.) whose history and case report fitted the clinical picture of an ectopic GRF-secreting tumor. I wrote back with a couple of questions and suggestions and on March 31, 1983, a second letter from Geneviève Sassolas describing new clinical findings confirmed the presence of a tumor of the pancreas in that patient. I immediately contacted her in Lyons by telephone. The patient was scheduled for surgery on April 16. On April 13 Fusun Zeytin left for Lyons equipped to collect tumor tissue so as to grow GRF-secreting cells out of it (another unsuccessful attempt, as it turned out) and to organize things with the surgical team of Dr. Christian Partensky to obtain the bulk of the pancreas tumor in optimal conditions, the tumor to be diced in liquid nitrogen within minutes of surgical removal. Fusun returned to the laboratories on April 18 with the bulk (ca. 200 g) of two separate tumors both found in the pancreas of the patient. By April 21 small aliquots of both tumors had been extracted and filtered on G-75 by Peter Böhlen and we knew from the assays of Paul Brazeau that both tumors contained large quantities of bioactive somatostatins, with minute amounts of GRF activity in one, but large amounts in the other (5–10,000 times more GRF activity than that found in an equivalent weight of hypothalamic extracts). Two aliquots of 7 g each of that GRF-rich tumor were processed; three peptides with GRF activity were obtained in homogeneous forms on May 10 and May 17; on May 22 Fred

Esch completed the first amino acid sequence of a GRF. On May 28 Nicholas Ling had reproduced that sequence by solid-phase synthesis and purified it to homogeneity on June 1. On June 4 Paul Brazeau showed that the synthetic replicate had, *in vitro*, the full biological activity of the native material. We now knew that we had isolated and characterized GRF and reproduced it by synthesis; the sequence of events had taken less than a month and a half. *In vivo* activity was shown on June 6 by Bill Wehrenberg by iv injection into rats anaesthetized with pentobarbital. These results were announced at a poster session at the meeting of the Endocrine Society on June 16, though the primary structure was not shown. The primary structures of the tumor-derived GRF (hpGRF-44) and of two biologically active fragments (hpGRF-37, hpGRF-40) were reported in *Science* (Guillemin *et al.*, 1982); by the end of the year we had published a series of papers describing the results of *in vitro* studies on the mechanism of action of GRF, *in vivo* studies including the use of a monoclonal antibody against rat hypothalamic GRF, localization of GRF neurons in the brain of primates, synthesis of fragments and analogs, etc. Indeed a great deal of what was presented at the Laurentian meeting had been concluded by December 1982.

From the amino acid composition obtained in October 1981, we knew that the GRF peptide isolated from the first 400-mg sample of the tumor obtained from Michael Thorner was closely related to one of the molecules isolated from the Lyons tumor. Processing of the 5-g fragment of that tumor revealed a single molecule with GRF activity. Fred Esch determined the primary structure of that material to be identical to that of the hpGRF-40 characterized earlier from the other tumor. This was reported in *Biochem. Biophys. Res Commun.* (Esch *et al.*, 1982). Rivier *et al.* (1982), in *Nature (London)*, reported the structure of the GRF peptide they had isolated and characterized independently of our own efforts from another fragment of the Thorner tumor, also as that of hpGRF-40. The same group (Spiess *et al.*, 1983) reported a structure for hypothalamic rat GRF as that of a 43-residue peptide with a free carboxy terminus. At the writing of this review we have isolated and characterized hypothalamic GRF from porcine, bovine, and ovine origins (Böhlen *et al.*, 1983c; Esch *et al.*, 1984). They are all 44-residue peptides with an amidated carboxyl terminus, closely related to the sequence of the human tumor-derived GRF. Human hypothalamic GRF was isolated by us and shown to correspond to hpGRF-44-NH$_2$, along with a minor component corresponding to hpGRF-40 (Böhlen *et al.*, 1983a). Since we had only 8 human hypothalami for that study, sequencing was out of the question and the preceding conclusions are based on chromatographic and immunological results.

The complete structure of the precursor molecule of human GRF was obtained in the Spring of 1983 by molecular cloning (Gubler *et al.*, 1983); it confirmed the complete sequence 1–44, with evidence of a Leu[44]-Gly-Arg sequence (in the precursor) recognized as the substrate for amidation of the C-terminal residue (Leu[44]).

Clinical studies were initiated as soon as we got clearance from the FDA early in January 1983. At the writing of this review more than 1500 individuals have received GRF, synthesized in our laboratories by Nicholas Ling. Judging from the literature, probably several hundred other subjects have received synthetic GRF of various sources, as well as the fragment GRF-40. The pharmaceutical industry has already announced large-scale production of GRF (*Le Monde*, 21 September, 1983). Somatocrinin (a word I have proposed to replace the initials GRF, and an obvious mirror image of the name of its physiological counterpart, somatostatin) had as spectacular a beginning as its earlier search had been slow and elusive. The remarkable series of events I have recounted was made possible only by the generosity and scientific awareness of a keen physician, passing to a group of well-prepared laboratory colleagues that rare pathology specimen that could not have been exploited otherwise. Galen had praised and advocated that intellectual approach two thousand years ago.

II. Isolation of Tumor-Derived and Hypothalamic GRFs

The existence of peptides with the biological activity of GRF, produced ectopically in rare cases of pancreatic islet tumors and variously located carcinoids, is well documented (Frohman *et al.*, 1980; Beck *et al.*, 1973; Caplan *et al.*, 1978; UzZafar *et al.*, 1979; Leveston *et al.*, 1981; Thorner *et al.*, 1982; Böhlen *et al.*, 1982). Several GRF peptides have now been isolated from two separate pancreatic tumors that caused acromegaly. From one tumor (tumor I) provided by G. Sassolas (Sassolas *et al.*, 1983) three GRF peptides were first isolated by our group and their structures determined: hpGRF-44, hpGRF-40, and hpGRF-37, consisting of 44, 40, and 37 amino acids, respectively (Böhlen *et al.*, 1983b). Isolation was accomplished by means of a rapid and efficient 4-step procedure, including (1) tissue extraction in 0.3 M hydrochloric acid, (2) gel filtration, and (3,4) two steps of reverse-phase HPLC using systems of different solute selectivities (Fig. 1). Peptide purification was monitored with a highly sensitive *in vitro* bioassay that tests the ability of column fractions to stimulate the release of growth hormone from rat anterior pituitary cells in serum-free monolayer culture (Brazeau *et al.*, 1982a). The second tumor

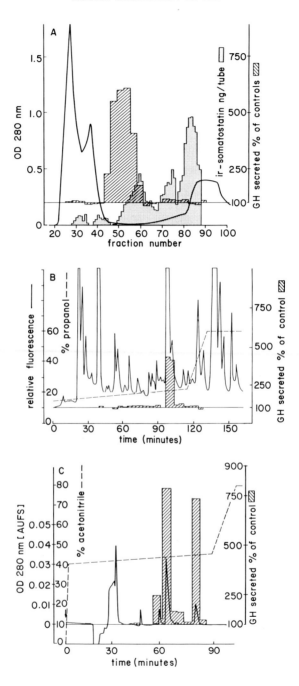

(tumor II), provided by M. Thorner, University of Virginia (Thorner *et al.*, 1982), contained only one GRF form, identical to hpGRF-40 isolated from tumor I. It was isolated independently by our group (Böhlen *et al.*, 1982, 1983b), using the methodology outlined above, and by Rivier *et al.* (1982), using a similar microanalytical approach.

The isolation of GRFs from these two pancreatic tumors reveals a considerable degree of dissimilarity among GRF-producing neoplastic tissues. Tumor I contained three forms of GRF, with the 44-residue COOH-terminal amidated peptide (the "mature" peptide) possessing the highest potency in our *in vitro* assay. The carboxyl terminally shortened peptides hpGRF-40 and hpGRF-37, with a free COOH-terminal, which possess reduced *in vitro* bioactivity, may represent products arising from multiple parallel processing of the GRF precursor protein, or alternatively may be (still active) proteolytic degradation products of hpGRF-44. The contrasting finding that tumor II only contains hpGRF-40 but not the parent peptide hpGRF-44 suggests that pro-GRF is processed differently in different tumor tissues. This view is also supported by our finding of two major forms of GRF in a human lung carcinoid (Böhlen *et al.*, 1982). The two islet cell tumors differed also with respect to their GRF concentration. While tumor I yielded 7.5 nmol total GRF/g of tissue, only 0.45 nmol GRF/g was isolated from tumor II. Finally, dissimilarity exists with regard to expression of the somatostatin gene. Tumor I, but not tumor II, was found to contain significant quantities of both somatostatin-14 and somatostatin-28 (Böhlen *et al.*, 1983b).

FIG. 1.   Isolation of GRF peptides from a pancreatic islet cell tumor (provided by G. Sassolas, Lyons, France). [This tumor also contained several forms of immunoreactive somatostatin (A), two of which were isolated and characterized as somatostatin-14 (fractions 78–88) and somatostatin-28 (fractions 52–65) by amino acid sequence.] (A) Gel filtration of acidic tissue extract (50 ml) of 7 g tumor on Sephadex G-75 (120 × 4.5 cm). Eluent 5*M* acetic acid, flow rate 60 ml/hour, fraction volume 15 ml. The first and last absorbance peaks correspond to exclusion and salt volumes of the column respectively. (B) Semipreparative reverse-phase HPLC of pool of bioactive gel filtration fractions 43–58 on C18 column using pyridine formate/*n*-propanol as mobile phase. Flow rate 0.8 ml/minute. Bioassay was performed with pooled or individual aliquots (5–10 μl) of column fractions. To avoid losses due to lyophilization, pooled gel filtration fractions were applied directly to the reverse-phase column by pumping the sample onto the column prior to starting the elution gradient. (C) Reverse-phase HPLC of bioactive fractions from semipreparative chromatography (B) using analytical C18 column in conjunction with 0.2% (v/v) heptafluorobutyric acid/acetonitrile. Flow rate 0.6 ml/minute. The sample was loaded (after 3-fold dilution) as described above. AUFS, Absorbance units full scale. Bioassay was performed with aliquots of individual or pooled column fractions that had been dried in the presence of 100 μg serum albumin.

A. ISOLATION OF HYPOTHALAMIC GRFs

Is hpGRF identical in structure to the physiological growth hormone releasing factor in the human hypothalamus? In an attempt to answer this question, we obtained 8 human hypothalamic fragments and processed them by gel filtration and reverse-phase HPLC, as in the above methodology for the pancreatic tumors. Bioassay and two radioimmunoassays of different epitope specificity revealed the presence of two major forms of GRF activity which coelute with human pancreas GRFs, hpGRF-44-NH$_2$ and hpGRF-40 under highly resolutive conditions (Böhlen *et al.*, 1983a). The bioactive material coeluting with hpGRF-44-NH$_2$ is recognized by two antibodies which are directed against the amidated carboxyl terminal sequence and the central portion of the GRF-44 peptide. The bioactive GRF which coelutes with hpGRF-40 reacts only with the antibody recognizing the central portion of hpGRF. These data provide compelling evidence that the human hypothalamus contains the same major molecular forms of GRF that were identified in the pancreas tumors. A similar conclusion was reached by Spiess *et al.* (1983), who stated further that clostripain digestion fragments of the purified native human hypothalamic GRFs gave identical mappings to those obtained with synthetic hpGRF-44 and hpGRF-40. Obviously final proof of identity between human hypothalamic and ectopically produced GRF remains in establishing the primary structures of the hypothalamic peptide, an undertaking that simply requires a larger number of human hypothalami than was available to us.

Several groups have, in the past, reported or claimed purification and/ or characterization of hypothalamic GRF from various species (Dhariwal *et al.*, 1965; Schally *et al.*, 1969, 1971; Veber *et al.*, 1971; Wilber *et al.*, 1971; Malacara *et al.*, 1972; Stachura *et al.*, 1972; Wilson *et al.*, 1974; Johansson *et al.*, 1974; Boyd *et al.*, 1978; Nair *et al.*, 1978; Brazeau *et al.*, 1981b; Arimura *et al.*, 1983; Sykes and Lowry, 1983). None of these attempts resulted in the determination of the chemical structure of an unquestionable hypothalamic growth hormone releasing factor. This was due primarily to the nonspecificity of the bioassays used to follow the presumed GRF in the purification procedures. It was not until 1983 that several hypothalamic GRFs from various animal species were isolated, chemically characterized, and shown to have true GH-releasing activity using acceptable criteria *in vitro* and *in vivo*. By the batch-processing of 80,000 rat hypothalami through acid extraction, gel filtration, and several steps of preparative, semipreparative and analytical reverse-phase HPLC, Spiess *et al.* (1983) isolated 3.4 nmol of a GRF characterized as a 43-amino acid peptide with a free C-terminus. This structure shows major homology with human GRF, with 15 substitutions or deletions from that of human GRF-44. Recently our group isolated and characterized porcine hypothalamic GRF (Böhlen *et al.*, 1983c). The antibody raised against hpGRF-40 which recognizes the central portion of the GRF sequence was found to bind with porcine GRF to the same degree as hpGRF-44 or hpGRF-40 (parallel displacement curves in the RIA). The RIA established for human GRF (Brazeau *et al.*, 1984) was therefore used for monitoring peptide purification. A carboxyl terminal amidated 44-residue peptide with only 3 substitutions from the sequence of human GRF (see Table VI) was isolated from 2500 porcine hypothalami, using an approach that included immunoaffinity chromatography besides gel filtration and two reverse-phase HPLC steps. Immunoaffinity chromatography with Affi-gel-bound purified IgG antibodies, as designed by Nicholas Ling, provided a powerful tool for the purification of pGRF from crude tissue extracts. Owing to the high efficiency of this step it was possible to isolate quantities of GRF sufficient for full structural characterization from relatively small amounts of tissue (6 nmol pGRF-44 from 2500 hypothalami). Other isolation procedures which omit the immunoaffinity step yielded pure pGRF as well but with substantially lower yield.

Using the same purification scheme, including the immunoaffinity chromatography step, we have also isolated and characterized bovine hypothalamic GRF (see Table VI). We have also isolated hypothalamic ovine GRF and hypothalamic caprine (goat) GRF, again using the purification scheme described above. The primary structures are being established by Fred Esch at the writing of this review.

B. STRUCTURE OF prepro-GRF

The primary structures of two precursors for human pancreas GRF were established by molecular cloning and DNA sequence analysis of cDNA coding for preproGRF-mRNA (Gubler *et al.*, 1983). The two forms of mRNA code for preproGRF-107 and -108. The two polypeptides contain the sequence of hpGRF-44 flanked by basic processing sites. The precursors include a putative signal sequence and a COOH-terminal amidation signal for hpGRF-44, the latter in keeping with our demonstration that the carboxyl terminus of hpGRF-44 is amidated. PreproGRF-108 differs from prepro-GRF-107 by the insertion of serine in the COOH-terminal portion of the precursor (in position 104). The molecular weight of prepro-GRF as determined by *in vitro* translation of tumor poly(A)$^+$-RNA, followed by immunoprecipitation with hpGRF-specific antiserum and sodium dodecyl sulfate–polyacrylamide gel electrophoresis was shown to be approximately 13,000, which agrees with the size of a 107 or 108 amino acid peptide (Fig. 2).

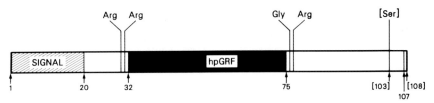

FIG. 2. Schematic representation of preproGRF-107 and -108. The sequence of hpGRF-44 (in black) is flanked by processing sites consisting of basic amino acids. A glycine residue immediately adjacent to the carboxyl terminus of GRF mediates the amidation of hpGRF-44. A hydrophobic sequence at the amino terminus (probably 20 amino acids in length) represents the signal sequence. Two cryptic sequences of 9 (amino terminal) and 31 (carboxyl terminal) amino acids comprise the rest of the precursor protein. Prepro-GRF-107 lacks the residue serine-103.

III. Determination of the Primary Structure of Tumor-Derived and Hypothalamic GRFs

The strategy and methodology employed in each instance are identical; thus only the structural elucidation of hpGRF-44, considered as a representative study, will be discussed in detail.

Amino Acid Analysis. Peptides were hydrolyzed in sealed evacuated ignition tubes containing 5 μl 6 N HCl and 7% thioglycollic acid for 24 hours at 110°C (Böhlen and Schroeder, 1982). Amino acid analyses of 10–100 pmol of peptide hydrolyzates were performed with a Liquimat III amino acid analyzer (Kontron, Zurich, Switzerland) equipped with a proline conversion fluorescence detection system (Böhlen and Mellet, 1979).

Edman Degradation. The sequential degradation of peptides was performed with an Applied Biosystems Model 470A gas phase sequencer as described (Hunkapiller *et al.*, 1983) with several modifications. The dipeptide, Phe-Leu, was used instead of Gly-Gly to precycle the Polybrene (Aldrich). Longer coupling (1200 seconds) times in all cycles and a longer cleavage time (1665 seconds) in the first cycle were used to enhance the repetitive and initial yields, respectively. Finally, an extensive methanol wash (180 seconds, 3.8 ml) was used to clean the conversion flask after each cycle and thus reduce cycle to cycle carryover. The phenylthiohydantoin amino acid derivatives were unambiguously identified by high-pressure liquid chromatography as described (Hunkapiller and Hood, 1983).

Cyanogen Bromide Digestions. Six nanomoles of peptide in 1 ml of (0.5% heptafluorobutyric acid, 48% acetonitrile) was rapidly dried in a 17 × 100-mm polypropylene tube using a Savant vacuum centrifuge. Upon dissolution of the peptide with 100 μl 70% formic acid, a small crystal of

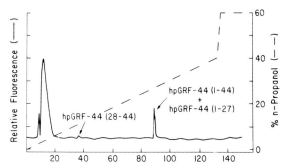

FIG. 3. Reverse-phase liquid chromatography of a cyanogen bromide digest of hpGRF-44 (6 nmol). Digestion and chromatography protocols were as described in the text. Gradient elutions were at 0.6 ml/minute and room temperature with pyridine formate/n-propanol. The column effluents were collected in 1.1-ml fractions and monitored with an automatic fluorescamine detection system (Böhlen et al., 1975).

cyanogen bromide was added and the reaction mixture capped and vortexed. After incubation for 12 hours in the dark, the cyanogen bromide-generated peptide fragments were purified with an Altex Model 322 high-pressure liquid chromatography system equipped with a Brownlee RP-18 guard column (10 μm; 4.6 × 30 mm), a Brownlee RP-18 analytical column (5 μm; 4.6 × 250 mm), and a modified pyridine formate/n-propanol system (Rubinstein et al., 1977) consisting of 1% pyridine, 1.5% formate in solvents A and B, with B also containing 60% n-propanol. The isolation of a homogeneous preparation of the cyanogen bromide digestion fragment, hpGRF-44(1–27), required rechromatography of the material in the peak (Fig. 3) containing this fragment and the undigested hpGRF-44.

A. HIGH-PRESSURE LIQUID CHROMATOGRAPHY COMPARISON OF NATIVE hpGRF-44 AND SYNTHETIC REPLICATES

The synthetic replicates of hpGRF-44 were synthesized in two forms, i.e., with a free acid and an amidated carboxyl terminus. Two different high-pressure liquid chromatography systems were employed to effect separation between the free acid and amidated forms of synthetic replicates and, in turn, to ascertain with which form the native peptide would coelute. An Altex Model 322 high-pressure liquid chromatography system with a Brownlee RP-18 (10 μm; 4.6 × 30 mm) guard column, an Altex Ultrasphere ODS (5 μm; 4.6 × 250 mm) analytical column, and triethylammonium phosphate/acetonitrile buffers (Rivier, 1978) were used to separate the free acid and amidated carboxy terminal forms of the peptide

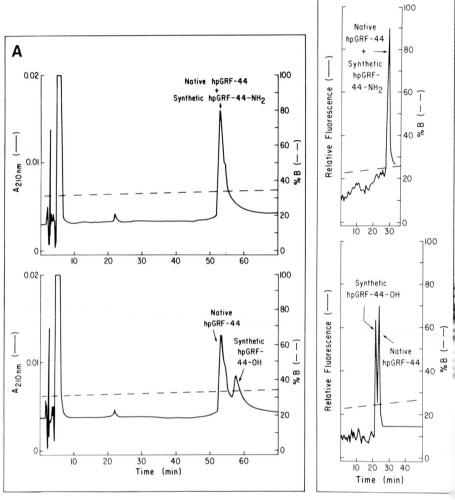

FIG. 4. Reverse-phase and ion-exchange liquid chromatography of native hpGRF-44 with its synthetic replicates containing either a free acid or an amidated carboxy terminus; 250–500 pmol quantities of each peptide were chromatographed at room temperature. (A) Reverse-phase gradient elutions of the peptide at 1.5 ml/minute employed an 80-minute linear gradient from 31 to 35%B, where solvent A was 0.25 N triethylammonium phosphate, pH 3.0 and solvent B was 20% 0.25 N triethylammonium phosphate, pH 3.0, and 80% acetonitrile. (B) Ion-exchange gradient elutions of the peptide at 0.6 ml/minute employed a 60-minute linear gradient from 22.5 to 27.5%B, where solvent A was 0.045 N sodium acetate, pH 6.01 and solvent B was 0.91 N sodium acetate, pH 6.01. Additionally, both solvents contained 30% n-propanol.

by reverse-phase methodology. Chromatography conditions are described in Fig. 4.

An Altex Model 332 high-pressure liquid chromatography system with a TSK IEX-535K (10 μm; 4.6 × 150 mm) carboxymethyl ion-exchange analytical column, 0.045 and 0.91 M sodium acetate, pH 6.0 buffers, each containing 30% n-propanol, were used in the second system to achieve a normal-phase separation of the peptide derivatives. Chromatography conditions are described in Fig. 4.

The primary structure of hpGRF-44 was established by sequence analyses of the intact peptides and their cyanogen bromide digestion fragments. The structure of hpGRF-44 (1–40) was established by Edman degradation of the intact peptide. Confirmation of these data and determination of the remaining carboxy terminal sequence were accomplished by cyanogen bromide digestion of the hpGRF-44, high-pressure liquid chromatographic isolation of the digestion fragments (Fig. 3), and subsequent structural characterization of these fragments by amino acid analyses (Table I) and Edman degradations (Tables II, III, and IV). These results were obtained with a total of 7.5 nmol peptide and are summarized in Table V.

TABLE I

Amino Acid Compositions of hpGRF-44 and Its Cyanogen Bromide Digestion Fragments

Amino acid	hpGRF-44 ($n = 8$)	hpGRF-44(1–27) ($n = 1$)	hpGRF-44(28–44) ($n = 2$)
Asx	4.05 ± 0.27 (4)[a]	2.85 (3)[a]	1.02 (1)[a]
Thr	0.93 ± 0.09 (1)	0.75 (1)	0
Ser	3.76 ± 0.20 (4)	1.95 (2)	1.91 (2)
Glx + Hse	6.87 ± 0.29 (7)	2.90 (3)	4.71 (5)
Gly	3.43 ± 0.48 (3)	1.30 (1)	2.37 (2)
Ala	4.93 ± 0.19 (5)	3.15 (3)	1.94 (2)
Val	0.89 ± 0.06 (1)	0.87 (1)	0
Met	1.04 ± 0.16 (1)	0	0
Ile	1.84 ± 0.15 (2)	1.67 (2)	0
Leu	4.99 ± 0.22 (5)	4.00 (4)	1.05 (1)
Tyr	2.10 ± 0.36 (2)	2.15 (2)	0
Phe	0.96 ± 0.37 (1)	1.20 (1)	0
His	0	0	0
Trp	0	0	0
Lys	2.02 ± 0.37 (2)	2.37 (2)	0
Arg	6.09 ± 0.61 (6)	2.35 (2)	4.00 (4)
Cya	0	0	0
Pro	0	0	0

[a] Values in parentheses were deduced from sequence analyses.

TABLE II
Sequence Analysis of hpGRF-44[a]

Cycle number (N)	Residue number	>PhNCS-AA	Yield (pmol)	Carryover from (N − 1) (pmol)
1	1	Tyr	719	—
2	2	Ala	531	29.0
3	3	Asp	281	21.4
4	4	Ala	551	19.7
5	5	Ile	322	21.3
6	6	Phe	341	14.8
7	7	Thr	86.3	11.9
8	8	Asn	237	0
9	9	Ser	44.2	15.0
10	10	Tyr	200	2.7
11	11	Arg	163	20.2
12	12	Lys	178	30.6
13	13	Val	200	20.4
14	14	Leu	153	26.5
15	15	Gly	89.3	28.4
16	16	Gln	106	43.0
17	17	Leu	105	57.3
18	18	Ser	8.9	70.8
19	19	Ala	84.7	3.0
20	20	Arg	50.0	37.3
21	21	Lys	54.4	41.9
22	22	Leu	91.0	28.1
23	23	Leu	73.0	—
24	24	Gln	33.8	32.1
25	25	Asp	28.7	29.7
26	26	Ile	21.5	10.6
27	27	Met	34.6	22.1
28	28	Ser	5.3	4.0
29	29	Arg	20.9	2.7
30	30	Gln	17.1	12.9
31	31	Gln	58.4	—
32	32	Gly	22.0	15.7
33	33	Glu	17.2	12.5
34	34	Ser	3.4	12.8
35	35	Asn	14.0	0.8
36	36	Gln	8.4	8.4
37	37	Glu	11.7	0
38	38	Arg	5.3	4.1
39	39	Gly	13.0	4.0
40	40	Ala	7.5	9.2
41	41	X	—	—
42	42	X	—	—
43	43	X	—	—
44	44	X	—	—

[a] Amount applied, 1500 pmol; initial yield, 37.3%; average repetitive yield, 89.7%. In all degradations the initial yield estimates were obtained by extrapolation of all phenylthiohydantoin amino acid yields back to cycle number one using the average repetitive yield.

TABLE III

Sequence Analysis of the CNBr Fragment: hpGRF-44(1–27)[a]

Cycle number (N)	Residue number	>PhNCS-AA	Yield (pmol)	Carryover from (N − 1) (pmol)
1	1	Tyr	221	—
2	2	Ala	239	7.4
3	3	Asp	150	11.9
4	4	Ala	219	17.3
5	5	Ile	194	28.3
6	6	Phe	178	18.8
7	7	Thr	62.4	11.0
8	8	Asn	176	10.4
9	9	Ser	33.1	14.2
10	10	Tyr	106	0
11	11	Arg	158	20.6
12	12	Lys	217	0
13	13	Val	77.8	22.5
14	14	Leu	92.3	15.1
15	15	Gly	32.9	14.4
16	16	Gln	49.9	13.7
17	17	Leu	54.7	9.7
18	18	Ser	5.8	14.2
19	19	Ala	25.9	0
20	20	Arg	34.3	2.5
21	21	Lys	29.6	0
22	22	Leu	26.0	13.7
23	23	Leu	27.3	—
24	24	Gln	27.0	10.8
25	25	Asp	17.4	19.9
26	26	X	—	5.9
27	27	X	—	—

[a] Amount applied, 540 pmol; initial yield, 57.4%; average repetitive yield, 88.9%.

B. DETERMINATION OF THE NATURE OF THE CARBOXYL TERMINUS OF hpGRF-44

Evidence for the nature of the carboxyl terminus of each of the hpGRF peptides was obtained from high-pressure liquid chromatography studies in which hpGRF-44 was cochromatographed with synthetic replicates possessing a free carboxyl or an amidated carboxyl terminus. These studies were carried out with both reverse-phase and ion-exchange high-pressure liquid chromatography systems, and the results are illustrated in Fig. 4 and clearly show the peptide possessing an amidated carboxyl terminus.

TABLE IV
Sequence Analysis of the CNBr Fragment: hpGRF-44(28–44)[a]

Cycle number (N)	Residue number	>PhNCS-AA	Yield (pmol)	Carryover from (N − 1) (pmol)
1	28	Ser	27.6	—
2	29	Arg	274	0
3	30	Gln	188	5.4
4	31	Gln	260	—
5	32	Gly	200	0
6	33	Glu	110	37.0
7	34	Ser	30.2	20.9
8	35	Asn	127	0
9	36	Gln	114	43.1
10	37	Glu	99.7	15.2
11	38	Arg	107	22.1
12	39	Gly	115	18.5
13	40	Ala	98.6	21.8
14	41	Arg	80.6	27.3
15	42	Ala	95.1	20.1
16	43	Arg	55.4	23.4
17	44	Leu	1.5	23.5

[a] Amount applied, 490 pmol; initial yield, 64.3%; average repetitive yield, 89.1%.

At the time of this review the structures of hypothalamic growth hormone releasing peptides from porcine (Böhlen et al., 1983c), bovine (Esch et al., 1984), and rat (Spiess et al., 1983) sources have also been elucidated; they are compared with the sequences of various homologous intestinal peptides in Table VI. Porcine and bovine hypothalamic GRFs are, like human GRF, 44 residues, C-terminus amidated peptides. Porcine GRF has only 3 substitutions and bovine GRF 5 substitutions from the amino acid sequence of human GRF. Rat GRF shows 14 amino acid substitutions from the sequence of human GRF.

IV. Synthetic Replicates of GRFs: Structure–Activity Relationships

Total synthesis of hpGRF-44, hpGRF-40, hpGRF-37, and fragments thereof, as well as of pGRF, bGRF, and rGRF, was achieved by solid-phase peptide synthesis methodology (Ling et al., 1980). The synthetic peptides were tested in the normal rat anterior pituitary cell monolayer culture system (Brazeau et al., 1982a). Of the hpGRF peptides tested, hpGRF-44 was found to be the most potent (ED_{50} = 15 pM; ED_{max} = 100

TABLE V

Sequence Analyses of hpGRF-44 and Its Cyanogen Bromide Fragments

Peptide	Amount analyzed (nmol)	Primary structure
Intact hpGRF-44	1.5	Y-A-D-A-I-F-T-N-S-Y-R-K-V-L-G-Q-L-S-A-R-K-L-L-Q-D-I-M-S-R-Q-Q-G-E-S-N-Q-E-R-G-A-X-X-X-X
CNBr fragment hpGRF-44(1–27)	0.54	Y-A-D-A-I-F-T-N-S-Y-R-K-V-L-G-Q-L-S-A-R-K-L-L-Q-D-X-X
CNBr fragment hpGRF-44(28–44)	0.49	S-R-Q-Q-G-E-S-N-Q-E-R-G-A-R-A-R-L

TABLE VI

Sequence Analyses of GRF Peptides and Various Intestinal Peptides

	5	10	15	20	25	30	35	40
hpGRF	YADA I FTN S YRKVLGQL S ARK L LQ D I M S RQQGES NQERGARARL - NH$_2$
pGRF	YADA I FTN S YRKVLGQL S ARK L LQ D I M S RQQGERNQEQGARVRL - NH$_2$
rGRF	HADA I FTS S YRR I LGQL YARK L LH E I MNRQQGERNQEQR SRFN - OH
PHI-27$_{porcine}$	HADGVFTS S YRR I LGQL S AKK Y LE S L I - NH$_2$
VIP$_{porcine}$	H S DAVFTDNYTRLRKQMAVKK WLN S I LN - NH$_2$
Glucagon	H S QGTFTS DY SKYLDS R RAQD F VQWLMNT - OH
Secretin$_{porcine}$	H S DGTFTS ELSRLRDS ARLKR L LQGLV - NH$_2$

p*M*). Based on a potency ranking of 100 for hpGRF-44 progressive deletion of the COOH-terminal residues of hpGRF-44 resulted in a gradual
loss of activity until hpGRF-(1–28)-OH as shown in Table VII. Fragments
shorter than (1–28) possess very little activity. These studies indicate that
the biologically active core of the molecule probably resides in the NH$_2$-
terminal part of the molecule. Furthermore, amidation of the COOH-
terminal residue increases the potency of the hpGRF peptides approximately 1.5-fold over that of the free acid forms. Met-27 is not an exclusive
requirement for biological activity as it can be replaced by norvaline (see
Table VIII). Similarly, Tyr-1 has been replaced by other amino acids
shown in Table VIII. Except for His-1 substitution all other modifications
yielded less potent analogs. Interestingly, rat GRF is equipotent to
hpGRF-44, whereas pig GRF is ca. 75% the potency of hpGRF-44, with

TABLE VII

Relative Potencies of COOH-Terminal Deletion Analogs of
hpGRF-44-NH$_2$

Analogs	Potency	(95% confidence limits)
hpGRF-44-NH$_2$	100	
hpGRF(1–44)OH	61	(50–75)
hpGRF(1–40)NH$_2$	49	(38–62)
hpGRF(1–40)OH	30	(25–37)
hpGRF(1–37)NH$_2$	28	(23–33)
hpGRF(1–37)OH	12	(9–16)
hpGRF(1–34)OH	17	(12–25)
hpGRF(1–31)OH	9	(6–12)
hpGRF(1–28)OH	6	(4–9)
hpGRF(1–24)OH	0.014	—
hpGRF(1–21)OH	<0.002[a]	—
hpGRF(1–19)OH	<0.001[a]	—

[a] Dose–response curve not parallel to standard.

TABLE VIII

Relative Potencies of Position 27 or 1 Substituted Analogs of hpGRF-40-OH

Analog	Potency	(95% confidence limits)
hpGRF-44-NH$_2$	100	
[Norval^{27}]hpGRF-40-OH	91	(74–112)
[Ala-Tyr^1]hpGRF-40-OH	4.2	(2.4–6.5)
[Arg-Tyr^1]hpGRF-40-OH	0.4	(0.1–1.1)
[Ac-Tyr^1]hpGRF-40-OH	10	(7–14)
[D-Tyr^1]hpGRF-40-OH	0.006[a]	—
[Ala^1]hpGRF-40-OH	0.84	(0.7–1.0)
[Phe^1]hpGRF-40-OH	3.1	(2.5–3.9)
[His^1]hpGRF-40-OH	54	(46.5–63.2)
[Trp^1]hpGRF-40-OH	0.006[a]	—
Rat GRF	93.7	(82.6–106.3)
Pig GRF	75	(69–81)

[a] Dose–response curve not parallel to standard.

overlapping confidence limits and bGRF may be somewhat less potent than pGRF, all the assays being done with the rat pituitary cells *in vitro*.

In early studies we have obtained evidence that N-terminally deleted analogs of hpGRF (such as [desTyr^1]GRF or [desTyr^1-Ala^2]-GRF) can be considered as partial agonists-antagonists of GRF, the antagonism being of the competitive type (Ling and Brazeau, 1983). There is considerable interest both fundamental and clinical in potent competitive antagonists of GRF.

V. *In Vitro* Studies on the Mechanism of Action of GRF

In the early stages of these studies we systematically assayed in parallel the effects of a purified preparation of rat hypothalamic GRF along with the synthetic replicates of hpGRF. As we became convinced, from data obtained in multiple approaches, the most important being the characterization of hypothalamic GRFs, that the tumor-derived material (hpGRF) was identical structurally and functionally to the GRF of hypothalamic origin, we stopped the practice of using a hypothalamic GRF reference standard in all experiments. Results of some of the early studies with the hypothalamic GRF reference standard will be presented here since historically they were important data leading to the proposal of the identity of the hypothalamic or ectopically produced GRF.

Two types of *in vitro* pituitary cell preparations were used: the "classic" monolayer tissue culture system using rat pituitary cells, kept in culture for 4 days, then used in short-term, 3- to 4-hour studies with one treatment or another, occasionally with shorter sampling times such as 5, 10, 15, or 30 minutes. The exact description of the technique for dissociation of the cells, plating, and handling on day 4 have been described in detail earlier (Brazeau *et al.* 1982a). The second type of *in vitro* pituitary cell preparation used in some experiments is that of a perifusion system, allowing continuous sampling of the pituitary effluent as ell as very short stimulation pulses (≥ 1 minute). Preparation of cells for the perifusion system has also been described in detail (Brazeau *et al.*, 1982c).

A. RADIOIMMUNOASSAYS

RIAs for rat GH are conducted using Sinha's monkey–antimouse GH immune serum (Sinha *et al.*, 1972); RIAs for PRL, TSH, LH, FSH, are conducted using the antisera provided by the National Pituitary Agency NIADDK (Dr. A. Parlow). RIAs for β-endorphin use the antiserum RB-100 (Guillemin *et al.*, 1977) prepared in this laboratory. RIA for cAMP uses Miles-Yeda anti-cAMP immune serum; the antiserum is reconstituted 1 : 15 and we omit the succinylation reaction; the trace is obtained from New England Nuclear (NEX130). Calculation of standard curves and experimental values are done with the use of the program described in (Faden *et al.*, 1980).

B. PEPTIDES

1. Reference Standard Preparation for Rat Hypothalamic GRF

This is a purified preparation of GRF from rat hypothalamic extract. Following gel filtration on Sephadex G-75 in 30% acetic acid, a step that removes all somatostatin-14 and most of somatostatin-28, the zone of the effluent with GRF activity is further purified by two steps of HPLC. A GRF preparation so obtained from 2400 rat hypothalamic fragments was aliquoted in 1.0-ml vials in tissue culture medium and kept frozen at $-20°C$; 50 μl of this solution corresponds to the ED_{50} in a complete dose–response curve; that amount of the extract is defined as 1 unit of GRF activity, and that preparation of hypothalamic GRF is referred to as GRF reference standard (Brazeau *et al.*, 1981b).

2. Synthetic hpGRF and Fragments

All synthetic replicates of the tumor-derived GRF (GRF-44) were prepared by solid-phase synthesis methods as routinely used in this laboratory (Ling *et al.*, 1980). When we refer to synthetic hpGRF-44 we imply that the molecule is in the amidated form, as is the native material; on the other hand synthetic hpGRF-40 or hpGRF-37 refer to peptides in the free acid form, as are the native extracted peptides.

3. Somatostatin-28 and -14

Somatostatin-28 and -14 were synthesized by solid-phase methods (Ling et al., 1980).

4. Chemicals

IBMX (3-isobutyl-1-methylxanthine), 8Br.cAMP (Na salt), PGE_2, cycloheximide, and $CoCl_2$ were purchased from Sigma Chemical Co. Cholera toxin and forskolin were purchased from Calbiochem-Behring Co.

5. Statistical Analyses

Comparisons of the effects of various treatments were conducted by the multiple comparison test of Dunnett following an analysis of variance (program EXBIOL) (Sakiz, 1964). Multiple dose–response curves in the bioassays were analyzed for simultaneous fitting by the 4-parameter logistic equation of De Lean et al. (1978) (program ALLFIT). The same data were also studied by regression analysis and calculations of relative potencies with 95% confidence limits (program BIOPROG) (Rodbard, 1974).

C. SPECIFICITY OF GRF FOR THE RELEASE OF ir-GH

When tested in the in vitro assay described above, purified hypothalamic GRF, native tumor-derived GRF-40 or synthetic GRF-44, at doses ranging from 0.6 to 40 units or 3.1 to 400 fmol, respectively, which are known to reach E_{max} for stimulation of GH secretion, release only ir-GH, i.e., they have no effect on the secretion of ir-β-endorphin, FSH, LH, TSH, or PRL (Table IX). Similar results have now been obtained with the synthetic replicates of hypothalamic rat, porcine and bovine GRFs.

D. DOSE–RESPONSE RELATIONSHIPS

In a large number of experiments, purified rat hypothalamic GRF, native tumor-derived GRF-37, GRF-40, and GRF-44, as well as synthetic hpGRF-37, hpGRF-40, and hpGRF-44 all show identical dose–response curves when studied at doses ranging from 0.6 to 40 U of GRF reference standard for the hypothalamic material and 3.1 to 400 fmol/ml for the various isolated or synthetic hpGRFs. These doses are known to extend to E_{max} (see Fig. 5). Figure 5 shows the results of one such experiment in which hypothalamic GRF, native hpGRF-44, synthetic hpGRF-44, synthetic hpGRF-40, and synthetic hpGRF-37 were assayed at multiple dose

TABLE IX

Specificity of Hypothalamic GRF, Native or Synthetic Tumor-Derived GRF to Release GH, not TSH, PRL, FSH, LH, β-Endorphin (βE)[a]

Hypothalamic GRF (GRF reference std) in GRF units/ml	GH released[b] (ng/ml)	TSH released[c] (ng/ml)	PRL released[c] (ng/ml)	FSH released[c] (ng/ml)	LH released[c] (ng/ml)
0	870 ± 26	52 ± 3	384 ± 18	330 ± 19	1056 ± 102
0.63	1710 ± 60	47 ± 2	347 ± 12	291 ± 21	901 ± 42
1.25	2626 ± 24	78 ± 19	394 ± 7	315 ± 12	1012 ± 63
2.50	3923 ± 40	61 ± 11	375 ± 11	355 ± 6	1077 ± 15
5	5586 ± 52	27 ± 7	410 ± 11	276 ± 16	820 ± 90
10	6803 ± 46	40 ± 7	386 ± 20	251 ± 17	873 ± 57
20	7060 ± 75	61 ± 6	424 ± 33	283 ± 7	856 ± 52
40	7213 ± 122	63 ± 17	475 ± 10	358 ± 25	1169 ± 173
Native tumor-derived hpGRF-40 (fmol/ml)					
6.3	1903 ± 43	47 ± 6	485 ± 13	235 ± 5	761 ± 71
12.5	2163 ± 62	52 ± 13	371 ± 13	221 ± 20	679 ± 76
25	3480 ± 35	57 ± 6	388 ± 14	269 ± 11	901 ± 49
50	4820 ± 57	21 ± 4	406 ± 34	285 ± 6	947 ± 56
100	6746 ± 122	51 ± 4	369 ± 22	252 ± 24	827 ± 26
200	7070 ± 124	50 ± 3	432 ± 20	259 ± 23	844 ± 75
400	7606 ± 163	39 ± 1	405 ± 10	258 ± 4	856 ± 53

Synthetic hpGRF-44-NH$_2$ (fmol/ml)	GH released[b] (ng/ml)	TSH released[c] (ng/ml)	PRL released[c] (ng/ml)	FSH released[c] (ng/ml)	LH released[c] (ng/ml)	βE released[c] (ng/ml)
0	343 ± 12	308 ± 80	217 ± 12	125 ± 5	569 ± 35	1157 ± 159
3.1	647 ± 9	416 ± 19	258 ± 18	130 ± 19	598 ± 42	1153 ± 66
6.3	733 ± 13	382 ± 93	248 ± 3	142 ± 14	507 ± 34	1054 ± 66
12.5	1123 ± 12	297 ± 19	305 ± 42	170 ± 15	745 ± 25	1151 ± 47
25	1447 ± 7	304 ± 65	273 ± 17	140 ± 9	592 ± 47	997 ± 80
50	1720 ± 30	343 ± 26	284 ± 9	179 ± 34	629 ± 34	1001 ± 10
100	2046 ± 17	307 ± 64	302 ± 10	181 ± 5	686 ± 37	1225 ± 36
200	2133 ± 13	377 ± 48	309 ± 5	146 ± 11	625 ± 10	1226 ± 37

[a] Results of two independent experiments are shown (top and bottom). In all cases, numbers ± SEM shown come from duplicate RIA measurements for each treatment in triplicate, i.e., added to three tissue culture wells in the bioassay.

[b] Analysis of variance (EXBIOL) of all results showed a highly significant treatment effect; subsequent linear regression-analysis (BIOPROG) showed the results to be linearly distributed when relating effects and doses (see data in Fig. 1 for more evidence on this statement).

[c] Analysis of variance (EXBIOL) of all results showed no significant treatment effects.

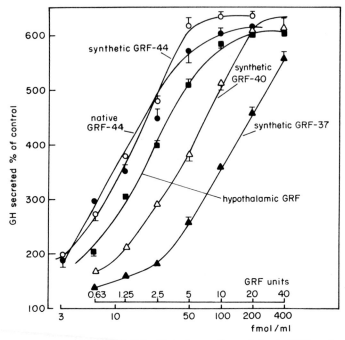

FIG. 5. Dose–response curves for multiple doses of hypothalamic GRF, native hpGRF-44, synthetic GRF-40, and synthetic GRF-37. The vertical bar on symbols represents standard error of the mean; when no such bar appears, standard error of the mean is no greater than the height of the symbol as drawn to indicate value of the mean response.

levels. Calculations (ALLFIT) of the statistical fit of these curves by the 4-parameter logistic polynomial model of DeLean *et al.* (1978) confirm that they have identical slopes (parameter b) and identical values for parameter d which represents the value of the maximal effect (E_{max}) of an agonist. In other words, in the *in vitro* assay, purified hypothalamic GRF and tumor-derived GRFs, native or synthetic, have all identical effects and intrinsic activity, i.e., they must activate the cell machinery involved in the release of growth hormone through the same mechanism (action) and to the same maximal extent (effect). The results show also that each of the 3 forms of tumor-derived GRF has a different specific activity. If the potency of native hpGRF-44 or of its synthetic replicate is taken as 100, in the assay described in Fig. 5 in which all the peptides were tested simultaneously on the same cell preparation, the potency of native or synthetic hpGRF-40 is 30 (95% confidence limits: 25 and 37); the potency of native or synthetic hpGRF-37 is 12 (95% confidence limits: 9 and 16). From calculation of the mean potency in 6 independent experiments hpGRF-44 is 2.6 times more potent than GRF-40 with 95% confidence limits of 2.3 and 3.2. These results lead to calculating that one unit of GRF activity in the purified hypothalamic extract used as the reference standard corresponds to ca. 10 fmol GRF-44. Thus the extract of one rat hypothalamic fragment contains 350–500 fmol of GRF-44. Based on extensive studies (not shown here) of various extraction methods for fresh rat hypothalamic tissues, that figure was never seen to vary more than 2-fold.

E. IS THE ACTION OF GRF ON THE RELEASE OF GH DEPENDENT ON THE PRESENCE OF EXTRACELLULAR Ca^{2+}?

Data presented in Table X shows that a blocker of calcium uptake, $CoCl_2$ at 0.2 mM, inhibits partially and at 2.0 mM abolishes completely the response to hypothalamic or synthetic hpGRF-40 or synthetic hpGRF-44.

F. IS THE ACTION OF GRF TO RELEASE GH MEDIATED BY THE ADENYLATE CYCLASE-cAMP SYSTEM?

Increasing cellular content of cAMP by adding 8Br.cAMP is doses ranging from 0.9×10^{-5} to 2.4×10^{-2} M stimulates release of GH with the same slope of the dose–response curve as that obtained for increasing doses of hypothalamic GRF, native hpGRF-44, or synthetic hpGRF-40 (Fig. 6a). The same maximal effect (E_{max}) is reached (Fig. 6a) for all forms of GRF and for 8Br.cAMP. In presence of 8Br.cAMP (4×10^{-5} to 4×10^{-3} M) the GH secretion stimulated by increasing doses of synthetic hpGRF-40 shows effect additivity of the two agonists, at the lower doses of GRF and at the higher doses of 8Br.cAMP, but in all cases the same E_{max} is reached in presence or absence of 8Br.cAMP (Fig. 6b).

The increasing availability of endogenous cAMP by adding the inhibitor of phosphodiesterases, IBMX (10^{-7} to 10^{-4} M) stimulates secretion of GH as a function of the dose of IBMX added with a slope of the dose–response curve statistically different from that obtained for hypothalamic GRF or synthetic hpGRF-40 (Fig. 6c). When synthetic hpGRF-40 is added at a maximally stimulating dose (400 fmol/ml) in the presence of IBMX in increasing concentrations (1.10^{-7} to 10^{-4} M), the value of E_{max} is never higher than that produced by the maximally stimulating dose of GRF alone (Fig. 6c).

Similarly, cholera toxin (10^{-9} to 10^{-12} M), an activator of the regulatory subunit, and forskolin (10^{-5} to 10^{-8} M), a stimulator of the catalytic subunit of adenylate cyclase, stimulate secretion of growth hormone with dose–response curves statistically different from that of synthetic

TABLE X

Effect of CoCl₂ on GH-Releasing Activity of Hypothalamic GRF or Synthetic GRF-40 and GRF-44

Hypothalamic GRF GRF reference standard (in GRF units)	CoCl₂	GH released (ng/ml)	CoCl₂ (mM)	GH released (ng/ml)
0	0	900 ± 23	2	523 ± 6
0.63	0	1856 ± 45	2	513 ± 14
1.25	0	2520 ± 46	2	520 ± 6
2.5	0	3347 ± 44	2	543 ± 14
5.0	0	4673 ± 70	2	550 ± 23
10.0	0	5410 ± 65	2	613 ± 19
20.0	0	5580 ± 51	2	563 ± 22
40.0	0	5623 ± 67	2	560 ± 15
Synthetic hpGRF-40 (fmol/ml)				
0	0	1530	0.2	1050
6.3	0	2923 ± 17	0.2	1393 ± 46
12.5	0	4166 ± 14	0.2	1627 ± 17
25	0	5397 ± 16	0.2	2033 ± 21
50	0	6867 ± 46	0.2	2546 ± 13
100	0	8690 ± 12	0.2	3503 ± 79
200	0	8973 ± 51	0.2	3677 ± 59
400	0	9097 ± 14	0.2	3667 ± 67
Synthetic hpGRF-44 (fmol/ml)				
0	0	323 ± 7	2	150 ± 6
3.1	0	637 ± 20	2	150 ± 10
6.3	0	943 ± 27	2	150 ± 10
12.5	0	1273 ± 22	2	147 ± 18
25	0	1647 ± 37	2	157 ± 7
50	0	2017 ± 20	2	166 ± 9
100	0	2343 ± 20	2	167 ± 9
200	0	2383 ± 49	2	207 ± 7

hpGRF-40 (Fig. 6d and e); when the same multiple doses of cholera toxin or forskolin are added, in the presence of a maximally effective dose of synthetic hpGRF-40, the maximal response (GH secretion) to all treatments is not different from the E_{max} observed with GRF alone (Fig. 6d and e).

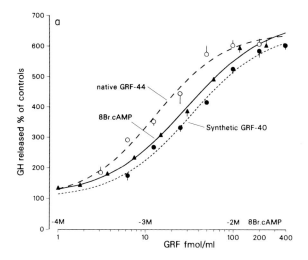

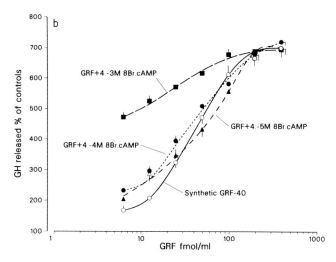

FIG. 6. (a) Parallelism and identical E_{max} for the log dose–response curves for 8Br.cAMP, native hpGRF-44, and synthetic hpGRF-40, (b) Multiple doses of synthetic hpGRF-40 alone and in the presence of three different concentrations of 8Br.cAMP: additivity at the lower dose of both agonists but identical E_{max} for all agonists alone or in combination. (c) Multiple doses of synthetic hpGRF-40, multiple doses of IBMX showing dose–response curves and identical E_{max}; multiple dose of IBMX with a maximally stimulating dose of GRF (400 fmol/ml) show no increase in the E_{max} value as obtained for GRF alone. (d) Same description and conclusion as in c, now for cholera toxin. (e) Same description and conclusion as in c, now for forskolin. In all figures, the standard error of the mean value for any treatment is indicated by a vertical bar; when no such bar is shown, the standard error of the mean is smaller than the height occupied by the sign depicting that value of the mean.

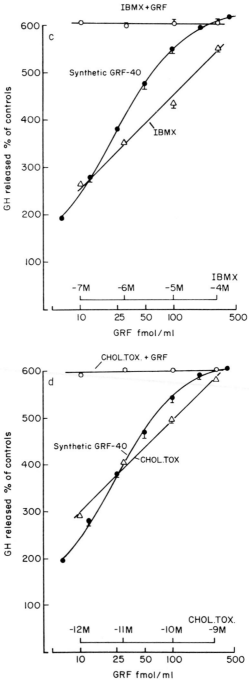

FIG. 6c and d.   See legend on p. 259.

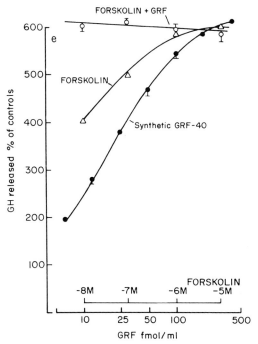

FIG. 6e.   See legend on p. 259.

Direct measurement of cAMP released in the culture fluid by the pituitary cells shows an increase as a function of the dose of GRF added to the monolayer pituitary culture. Efflux of cAMP reaches a plateau for the same doses of hpGRF-44 that also yield E_{max} for GH secretion. The increases in released cAMP parallel the increases in released GH as a function of the potency of GRF added (Fig. 7) or available [see for instance cAMP released by the same doses of hpGRF-40 in the absence or presence of $CoCl_2$ (Fig. 7) comparing with the effects, in the same experiment, of $CoCl_2$ on the release of GH, Table X).

G. GRF AND PROSTAGLANDIN PGE$_2$ STIMULATE SECRETION OF GH BY DIFFERENT PATHWAYS AND MECHANISMS

In contradistinction to the results obtained with 8Br.cAMP, IBMX, cholera toxin, and forskolin, studies of interrelationships between prostaglandin PGE$_2$ and GRF give entirely different results. The dose–response curve to PGE$_2$ is totally divergent from that observed for hypothalamic GRF or synthetic hpGRF-44 (Fig. 8a and b); moreover, PGE$_2$ E_{max}

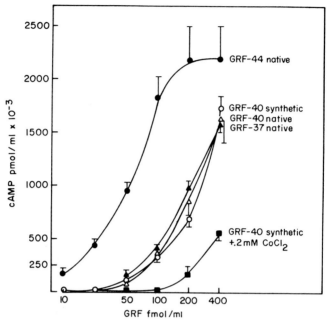

FIG. 7.   cAMP released/4 hours in incubation fluids of monolayer pituitary cultures with multiple doses of several preparations of hpGRF, also in presence of 0.2 mM CoCl$_2$ added to GRF-40.

never reaches that due to GRF (Fig. 8a and b) even at the highest tolerable doses of PGE$_2$ (10^{-2} M). When multiple doses of synthetic hpGRF-44 are studied on GH secretion in the presence of PGE$_2$ (10^{-8} to 10^{-5} M) a remarkable additivity of effects is observed at all doses, with values for E_{max} of the combined treatments far greater than those regularly observed for GRF alone (Fig. 8a and b).

H. HOW RAPID IS THE EFFECT OF GRF IN ELICITING RELEASE OF GH AND IS IT DEPENDENT ON THE SYNTHESIS OF SOME INTERMEDIATE PROTEIN?

Results presented in Fig. 9 from one perifusion experiment with dispersed pituitary cells show that the effect of hypothalamic GRF or of synthetic hpGRF-44 to stimulate release of GH is demonstrable in ca. 30 seconds following the contact of GRF with pituitary cells. In this perifusion system the effect of GRF is relatively short-lived, the duration of effect being related to the dose of GRF for identical pulse durations. Data reported in Table III show that the effect of synthetic hpGRF-40 on the release of GH is not modified by doses of cycloheximide as high as 100 μg/ ml, added 2 hours prior to GRF. These doses are well above those necessary to inhibit protein synthesis in the same *in vitro* system (Vale *et al.*, 1968).

I. ANTAGONISM BETWEEN GRF AND SOMATOSTATIN

As shown in Fig. 10a and b, somatostatin-28 or somatostatin-14 inhibits the response to hypothalamic GRF or native hpGRF-44 in a typical noncompetitive relationship. Analysis of the dose–response curves by the polynomial equation of De Lean *et al.* (1978), using the program ALLFIT,

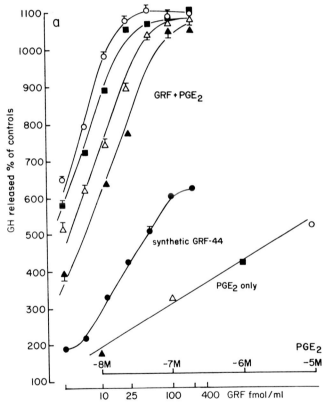

FIG. 8.   (a and b) Results from two independent experiments showing the dose–response curves to concentration of PGE$_2$ as shown, also responses to synthetic hpGRF-44 alone and in the presence of multiple concentrations of PGE$_2$. Note the additivity of the maximal effect due to each agonist. Standard error of the mean is shown by a vertical bar when that standard error is greater than the height of the sign showing the value of the mean.

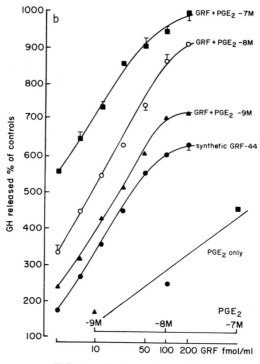

FIG. 8b.   See legend on p. 263.

shows that values for parameter *b* (slopes) are statistically identical (for
each set of curves), and so are values for parameter *c* (ED_{50}) for each set
of curves. Similarity of the ED_{50} of the agonist (GRF) in the presence or
absence of the antagonist (somatostatin) is one of the main criteria for
noncompetitive inhibition. Values for parameter *a* (response at dose 0 of
the agonist) and *d* (E_{max}) are different when comparing each set of curves;
heterogeneity of the values for *a* indicate that somatostatin also affects
the basal secretion of GH by the pituitary cells *in vitro*. Heterogeneity of
the values for *d* is another criteria of noncompetitive antagonism: the
antagonist (somatostatin) acts at some locus other than the receptor of
GRF to prevent the full activity of the agonist. The greater inhibition by
somatostatin-28 than that due to (equimolar amounts) of somatostatin-14
(Fig. 10b) reflects the greater potency of somatostatin-28 when compared
to the tetradecapeptide as originally reported by us in *in vitro* and *in vivo*
systems (Brazeau *et al.*, 1981a).

   These data show that the biological activity of hypothalamic GRF is
qualitatively indistinguishable from that of any of the three characterized

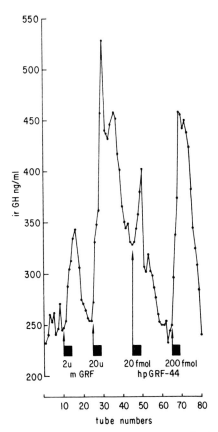

FIG. 9.   Rapidity of the pituitary response to hypothalamic GRF or synthetic GRF-44 is shown in a perifusion system using dispersed pituitary cells. Each fraction collected is 250 μl, for 33.8 seconds; total duration of each GRF pulse is 155 seconds.

forms of tumor-derived GRF or of their synthetic replicates. This conclusion has now been reinforced and extended with availability of synthetic replicates of hypothalamic porcine, bovine, and murine GRFs. The slopes of the dose–response curves are identical and so are the values for maximal stimulations (E_{max}) obtained with the hypothalamic or the tumor-derived preparations of GRF, native or synthetic. What differs are the specific activities (number of biological units/mole) of these various preparations. All evidence points to hpGRF-44 as being the primary form of human GRF: It is statistically more potent than any other form; it exists as a C-terminal amide, the form in which many neuropeptides (TRF, LRF, CRF, bombesin, substance P, vasopressin, oxytocin, etc.) and peptide hormones (α-MSH, secretin, cholecystokinin, gastrin, gastrin releas-

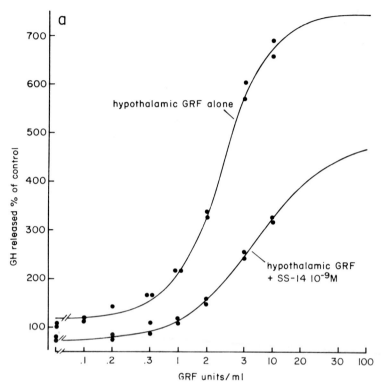

FIG. 10. (a and b) Somatostatin-14 or somatostatin-28 inhibit the response to hypotha
lamic GRF or native hpGRF-44 in typical noncompetitive antagonism. Results of two independent experiments. Symbols show actual experimental data; lines are the theoretical
curves computer calculated and drawn, from the 4-parameter logistic equations for each set
of data; curves shown here are drawn without constraints (program ALLFIT).

ing peptide, etc.) have been characterized, and have maximal activity or
are exclusively active (TRF, LRF, CRF, vasopressin, etc). Moreover, the
amino acid sequence of GRF-44 shows that GRF-37 and GRF-40 could be
generated from GRF-44, by cleavage at the NH_2-terminal side of the Arg
residues in position 38 and 41, as has been found to be the case for
dynorphin (1–8) (Minamino et al., 1980) from dynorphin and for
dynorphin B (rimorphin) from the COOH-terminal of the β-neoendorphin
precursor (Kadikani et al., 1981). Finally, and as shown above (see Section II,B), knowledge of the primary structure of the precursor of hpGRF,
preproGRF, deduced from its encoding cDNA, confirms the complete
sequence of GRF-44 with evidence of an amidating signal. The same
conclusion has just been published by Mayo et al. (1983) showing by

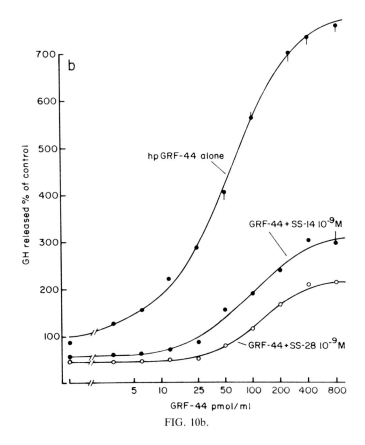

FIG. 10b.

molecular cloning the same sequence of the precursor of GRF using, as source of GRF-mRNA, tissue from the pancreatic tumor from Thorner's patient in which only GRF-40 was found and characterized (Esch *et al.*, 1982; Spiess *et al.*, 1983).

The high specific activity (number of biological units per mole) of hpGRF-44 is worthy of comment. The data reported here show hpGRF-44 to be significantly active in releasing GH in the monolayer culture assay at ≤ 3 fmol/ml or $3 \times 10^{-12} M$. In the dispersed pituitary cell perifusion assay the minimal active dose is ≤ 5 fmol/250 μl/30 seconds. The potency of hpGRF-44 is thus not only in the same range as that of TRF, LRF, CRF, but even greater, in comparable assay systems *in vitro*. Such high potency of the material, along with its specificity for influencing the secretion of only GH, speaks in favor of its physiological significance as a GH-releasing factor.

The early results reported here show that extracellular Ca^{2+} is necessary in the mechanism of action of GRF. The evidence presented here is
best explained by proposing that the adenylate cyclase-cAMP system is
involved in the mechanism of action of GRF in stimulating the secretion
of GH. The biological system used here is not a homogeneous population
of somatotrophs; therefore, the only specificity attributable to the results
obtained stems exclusively from the specificity of GRF in acting only on
somatotrophs (since there is no evidence that it stimulates secretion by
the pituitary of anything else other than GH). Cronin *et al.* (1982) have
recently reported comparable preliminary results.

Recently Lewin *et al.* (1983) reported that synthetic hpGRF-44 increases in a dose-dependent manner and with a half-maximal effect at 35
± 8 pM the activity of a cAMP-dependent protein kinase present in purified hog anterior pituitary granules. Analysis of the phosphorylation kinetics suggested that the peptide did not significantly change the reaction's V_{max} but produced a major increase in the enzyme affinity for
cAMP: the apparent K_m for the nucleotide decreasing from 700 nM in
control, unstimulated conditions to 15 pM in the presence of 100 pM
GRF-44 (see Fig. 11). Less potent analogs of GRF-44 such as GRF-37 or
[Phe^1]-GRF-40 had lower effects on the cAMP-dependent protein kinase
of the pituitary granules in relation to their lower potency in the bioassay
for GH release; an analog, GRF(2–40), inactive in stimulating the secretion of GH, had no evident effect on the phosphorylating enzyme of the
pituitary granules at doses as high as 0.1 μM. The authors conclude by
suggesting that GRF stimulates secretion (release) of growth hormone by

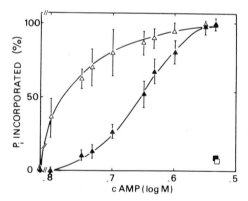

FIG. 11.   Histone phosphorylation by purified hog pituitary granules at different concen-
trations of cAMP without (closed triangle) and with (open triangle) 100 pM GRF. Mean ±
SEM from 4 different preparations. P_i values shown by the squares are in the presence of the
Walsh reagent at the concentration of cAMP shown on the *x* axis. (From Lewin *et al.*, 1983).

activating exocytosis through a phosphorylation mechanism mediated by a granular receptor coupled with a cAMP-dependent protein kinase.

Using techniques of immunocytochemistry on tissue sections prepared for electron microscopy, and with several antisera raised against hpGRF provided by our laboratory, Dubois *et al.* (1984) concluded that they could visualize immunoreactive GRF grains in normal pituitary somatotrophs of man and rhesus monkey. The immunoreactive GRF grains are located on GH-secretory granules as well as in the cell nucleus. No image is seen in rat pituitary preparations, in agreement with the fact that the hpGRF antisera prepared by us do not read rat GRF. However, when hpGRF in injected intravenously into rats (and we know that hpGRF is highly active in stimulating the secretion of growth hormone in the rat), Dubois *et al.* report that they can see immunoreactive GRF grains, again located on GH-secretory granules, as early as 3 minutes after injection of hpGRF, their number increasing at first and then decreasing as the somatotrophs become degranulated as they secrete GH, while the immunoreactive GRF grains are seen in the nucleus from 3 minutes up to 30 or 60 minutes after injection. No such images are seen with hpGRF(1–28), a biologically active fragment of GRF not recognized by the antiserum used above. Similarly, no such images are seen following injection of hpGRF(28–40), a biologically inactive fragment recognized by the antiserum provided by us and used here.

These elegant conclusions are surprisingly well in agreement with the biochemical results of Lewin *et al.* (see above) on the modus and locus of action of GRF at the level of the GH-secretory granules; they also are in accord with results of the effect of GRF on GH-mRNA levels (see below). In view of the complexity and unusual methodology involved in these studies, the conclusions of Dubois *et al.* would gain weight and acceptance if they could be confirmed by others and/or by the use of other methods such as the colloidal gold labeling of antibodies.

The striking additivity at all dose levels, including maximally stimulating doses of GRF and PGE_2 demonstrated above, implies that PGE_2 stimulates secretion of GH *in vitro* by a mechanism different from that of GRF. Since the maximum effect (E_{max}) of either agonist can be additive it also implies that PGE_2 and GRF release two independent pools of available GH.

The rapidity of action of GRF either of hypothalamic origin or as hpGRF-44 showing activation of the somatotrophs in seconds is in keeping with similar characteristics for the other hypothalamic releasing factors, TRF, LRF, CRF. Frohman *et al.* (1980), using perifusion of whole rat pituitaries, had reported that the GRF material they had purified from a human carcinoid that had caused acromegaly also elicited rapid release of GH. The frequency of sample collection, however, was far slower than the one used here (5 minutes vs 30 seconds) for a 15-minute GRF-pulse, vs 120-second GRF pulse in our own experiments. In that same report Frohman *et al.* (1980) elaborated on various characteristics of the material with GRF activity they had purified from several human tumors which had caused acromegaly. Many of their proposals regarding molecular size, significance of the NH_2- and COOH-terminals, discrepancies with activity of hypothalamic extract, conclusions as to existence of precursor forms, etc, of their active material are at variance with our present knowledge of the fully characterized hpGRF. It is always difficult to draw such conclusions when dealing with nonhomogeneous material. The merit of Frohman *et al.* in that report (1980), as well as that of other reports (UzZafar *et al.*, 1979; Beck *et al.*, 1973; Leveston *et al.*, 1981; Caplan *et al.*, 1978), is in having brought forth early evidence for GRF activity in extracts of peripheral tumors accompanying acromegaly, thus leading to the then novel concept of ectopic production of GRF-like substances.

The noncompetitive nature of the inhibition of the activity of hypothalamic GRF or hpGRF-44 by somatostatin, though never reported as such by others (Cronin *et al.*, 1982; Frohman *et al.*, 1980), was not an unexpected finding. There is no evidence that somatostatin or any of its many analogs ever behaved as a partial agonist (on the release of growth hormone); indeed, the latest proposal (Reyl and Lewin, 1981) for the subcellular mechanism of action of somatostatin would lead one to expect results and conclusions as to a noncompetitive mode for the antagonism between somatostatin and GRF.

With the availability of highly purified preparations of somatomedin C and IGF-I and IGF-II, we have recently demonstrated that these peripheral GH-induced polypeptides can inhibit directly at the pituitary level the GH-releasing activity of GRF (Brazeau *et al.*, 1982c). The inhibitory activity is seen at concentrations of 0.5–10 ng/ml (1×10^{-10} to 1.3×10^{-9} M) in either short-term (3–4 hours) or long-term (24 hours) incubation. These results are in agreement with Berelowitz *et al.* (1981), who proposed a direct negative pituitary feedback effect of somatomedin-C, but at variance with their data showing, under their experimental conditions, that a long-term ($\geq$24 hours) contact with somatomedin-C would be necessary. In our experiments, IGF-II was also active as an inhibitor of GRF, though less potent than IGF-I. The effect of the somatomedins is specific for the secretion of growth hormone and is not duplicated by other growth factors such as epidermal growth factor (EGF) or fibroblast growth factor (FGF).

The effect of hpGRF-44 was studied concomitantly on GH release and GH-mRNA levels in normal pituitary cells in monolayer culture as above and in GH$_3$ cells, a cell line known to secrete GH and PRL spontaneously, and extensively used by others to study the mechanism of the secretion of GH or of PRL with various secretagogues (TRF) or inhibitors (somato-statin). The cytoplasmic dot hybridization technique (White and Bancroft, 1983) was used to examine the effect of GRF. Pituitary cells incubated for 24 hours with 25 to 44 fmol GRF had significant increase in GH-mRNA levels. Maximal GH-mRNA levels (2.5-fold increases over controls) were noted following a 72-hour incubation of normal pituitary cells with 10^{-9} M GRF. In a similar experimental paradigm GRF did not stimulate PRL release or relative PRL-mRNA levels. GRF does not elevate GH-mRNA or PRL-mRNA levels in GH$_3$ cells; GRF does not stimulate either the secretion of GH by GH$_3$ cells (Gick *et al.*, 1983). These observations and conclusions have recently been confirmed by Barinaga *et al.* (1983) study-ing the transcriptional regulation of the GH gene by GRF.

In closing this section on *in vitro* studies with GRF, it is intriguing to mention the first, and so far only, evidence of a secretory activity of GRF not at pituitary level. Zeytinoglu *et al.* (1983) have shown that high doses of hpGRF-44 ($1-10 \times 10^{-6}$ M) increase in a dose-dependent manner the secretion of neurotensin as well as cAMP content and release by a cell line originating from a medullary thyroid carcinoma (MTC). Because of the homogeneity of such a cell line, and because the various parameters studied so far on the GRF-stimulated secretion of neurotensin parallel remarkably similar effects on the GRF-induced secretion of GH by pitui-tary cells, the MTC cell line may be an elegant model to use or consider.

VI. *In Vivo* Studies with Synthetic Replicates of GRF in Laboratory Animals

With the availability of the synthetic replicates of GRF, extensive *in vivo* studies could be initiated. Initially it was necessary to establish the dose–response relationship between GRF and plasma GH levels, as well as the specificity of GRF. Figure 12 illustrates the dose–response relation-ship between hpGRF-44 and plasma GH levels in anesthetized male rats. More detailed investigations of the time course as well as the minimum and maximum effective dose of GRF necessary to stimulate GH secretion (Wehrenberg *et al.*, 1982a, 1983a) have been reported. These results have shown that in rats the pituitary GH response to GRF is very rapid and of short duration, that is, the pituitary GH response is maximal at 3–5 min-utes and plasma GH concentrations are returning to baseline within 15 minutes. The minimum effective dose is approximately 100 ng/kg and the lowest dose producing a maximal effect approximately 10 μg/kg (4).

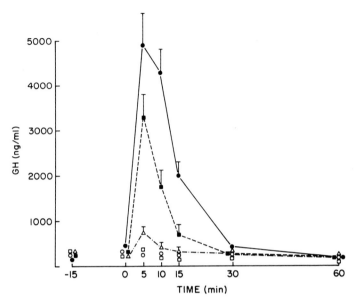

FIG. 12.   Plasma growth hormone levels in response to the intravenous administration of
saline (□) and of synthetic hpGRF-44 at 0.01 μg (○), 0.1 μg (△), 1.0 μg (■), and 10.0 μg (●).
Male Sprague–Dawley rats weighting 280 to 320 g were anesthetized with sodium pentobarbital (50 mg/kg) intraperitoneally at time −30 minutes. Samples (0.2 ml) were drawn by
venipuncture at times indicated; saline or hpGRF-44 was administered immediately after
time 0. Four animals were used for each treatment. Results are shown as the mean of
responses, with the vertical line representing the standard error of the mean.

Synthetic hpGRF-44 is a potent secretagogue of GH in the dog (Guillemin *et al.*, 1982). In complete agreement with *in vitro* observations (see
Table XI), GRF administration produced no changes in the plasma concentrations of LH, FSH, TSH, PRL, and corticosterone (Wehrenberg *et
al.*, 1982a).

For obvious reasons, animals anesthestized with sodium pentobarbital
are not the best model for studies designed to investigate mechanisms
regulating GH secretion. Therefore studies were initiated in conscious,
freely moving rats outfitted with chronic indwelling venous catheters and
maintained in isolation chambers. In animals so prepared the administration of GRF during the interval between spontaneous GH pulses (Tannenbaum and Martin, 1976) failed to elicit a consistent increase in plasma GH
concentrations (Wehrenberg *et al.*, 1982c). Of the 15 rats so treated, only
5 demonstrated an increase in GH comparable to what we had observed in
anesthetized rats. Figure 13 illustrates 4 individual examples of the incon-
sistency observed in the response. In contrast, GRF consistently elicited

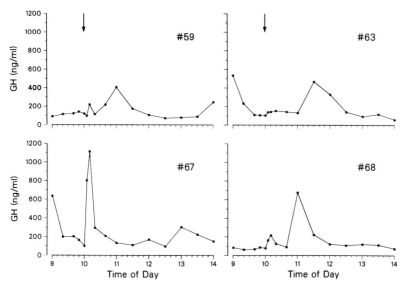

FIG. 13. The effect of 10 μg hpGRF-44 or −40 (iv) on GH secretion in 4 individual, conscious, freely moving male rats. Injections (indicated by arrows) were made at a time known to be between spontaneous GH pulses. Note the absence of response in rat 63 and the partial response in rats 59 and 68 as compared to the response in rat 67.

a dramatic and immediate increase in plasma GH when these animals were pretreated with antibodies raised against somatostatin, the hypothalamic inhibitor of GH release (Fig. 14).

To establish further the dynamic role of somatostatin in modulating the GH response to GRF, rats were subjected to a 72-hour fast, a procedure which increases endogenous somatostatin (Tannenbaum et al., 1978). In such animals GRF iv administration fails to increase plasma GH concentrations; however, a response could regularly be elicited with GRF in these fasting rats if they were first pretreated with somatostatin antibodies (Wehrenberg et al., 1982b).

As evidenced by Figs. 13 and 14, the concentration of plasma GH during spontaneous pulses can approach the concentrations obtained following exogenous administration of GRF. A possible criticism of studies involving the exogenous administration of GRF is that one cannot be certain whether the increase in plasma GH would be caused by GRF injection or a spontaneous GH pulse. During the course of the isolation and purification of GRF, Richard Luben developed several monoclonal antibodies against rat hypothalamic GRF using in vitro techniques (Luben et al., 1982). Passive immunization of rats with these antibodies has been shown specifically to inhibit the pulsatile secretion of GH presumably by

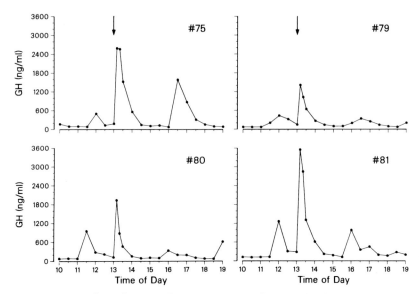

FIG. 14.   The effect of 1 μg hpGRF-44 or −40 on GH secretion in 4 individual, conscious, freely moving male rats pretreated with 5.8 mg protein of antibodies against somatostatin. Injections (indicated by arrows) were made at a time known to be between spontaneous GH pulses. Note the change in dose of hpGRF administered and scale of GH concentrations as compared to Fig. 13.

neutralizing hypothalamic GRF (Wehrenberg *et al.*, 1982c). One of these monoclonal antibodies against rat hypothalamic GRF does not recognize the GRF isolated from the human sources and thus permits an answer to the criticism of spontaneous versus stimulated increases in plasma GH. Indeed, combining the passive immunization treatment of the monoclonal antibodies with treatment with somatostatin antiserum results in a unique animal model. This model is ideal in that it represents an immediate, noninvasive, yet reversible, functional lesion of the hypothalamo-pituitary axis which is specific for only endogenous somatostatin and rat GRF. Using this model, the pituitary GH response to human GRF follows a dose–response relationship (Wehrenberg and Ling, 1983); this response is virtually unchanged over time to either a low (0.25 μg) or a high (5 μg) dose when administered at hourly intervals (Fig. 15).

GRF is active in stimulating GH secretion in rats with functional or anatomical lesions of the central nervous system that have been shown to inhibit endogenous growth hormone secretion (Wehrenberg *et al.*, 1983b). These animal models include electrolytic lesions of the ventromedial hypothalamus, a chemical lesion of the arcuate nucleus induced by neonatal treatment with monosodium glutamate, a functional lesion of catechol-

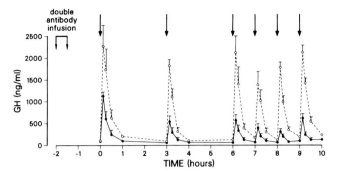

FIG. 15. The capacity of the pituitary in conscious, free moving male rats ($n = 6$) to secrete GH response to repeated intravenous injections of a moderate (0.25 μg; ●) and maximal (5 μg; ○) dose of hpGRF-40. Two hours before the first injection rats were treated with antiserum against somatostatin and monoclonal antibody against rat hypothalamic growth hormone releasing factor. Arrows indicate the injection of synthetic hpGRF-40. Data points represent the mean GH concentration; the vertical bars represent the SEM.

amine synthesis by pretreatment with α-methyl-*p*-tyrosine, and a functional lesion of catecholamine storage with reserpine. These results further demonstrate that GRF is indeed a secretagogue of GH by acting directly on the pituitary and not at some proximal locus within the central nervous system.

In 1946 Hans Selye stated that "while the pituitary is actively engaged in increased corticotropin hormone production it is apparently less capable of elaborating growth hormone, prolactin and gonadotropic hormones". This "shift in hormone production," as described by Selye, is now well recognized. Two examples include the stress-induced changes in gonadal and thyroid function (Ducommun *et al.,* 1967; Sachar, 1975). One possible mechanism that might account for this "pituitary shift" is an interaction of the pertinent releasing factors at the pituitary level. With the synthetic replicates of luteinizing hormone releasing factor (LRF), corticotropin releasing factor (CRF), thyrotropin releasing factor (TRF), and growth hormone releasing factor (GRF) now available, we decided to examine that hypothesis.

This was tested *in vitro* and *in vivo* using a 2^4 factorial experimental design (Table XI). This experimental design allows for the evaluation of both the main treatment effects of the hypothalamic releasing factors as well as all of the possible interactions between them. Significant main treatment effects both *in vitro* and *in vivo* were LRF on LH and FSH, CRF on ACTH and β-endorphin, TRF on TSH, and GRF on GH. These results confirm the specificity of the four releasing factors on their respective target cells. There were no significant interactions between any of the

TABLE XI

Experimental Design of a 2^4 Factorial Experiment to Study Interactions between Releasing Factors[a]

LRF	CRF	TRF	GRF
0	0	0	0
0	0	0	1
0	0	1	0
0	0	1	1
0	1	0	0
0	1	0	1
0	1	1	0
0	1	1	1
1	0	0	0
1	0	0	1
1	0	1	0
1	0	1	1
1	1	0	0
1	1	0	1
1	1	1	0
1	1	1	1

[a] 0, No; 1, Yes.

releasing factors on anterior pituitary hormone secretions (Wehrenberg *et al.*, 1984). These results suggest that the changes in pituitary secretion that are observed in health and disease are not due to interactions between the hypothalamic releasing factors at the level of the pituitary, but rather to the secondary interactions that modify pituitary activation or response. These results also indicate that the clinical pituitary reserve test can be expanded to include, as a single bolus mixture, all four hypothalamic releasing factors, since any lack of response will reflect a pituitary problem and not an interaction of the secretagogues administered.

IN VIVO EFFECTS OF GRF OTHER THAN HYPOPHYSIOTROPIC

In acute toxicity studies conducted to satisfy requirements of the FDA for ultimate clinical applications of GRF, we have found GRF to be an unusually innocuous substance. Intravenous bolus injection of up to 2 mg synthetic GRF in monkeys (7.5–9.5 kg body weight) or up to 1 mg in rats produces no obvious behavioral effect, save perhaps for a mild tranquilization of the animals. At these extremely high doses there is in rats a transient (5 minute) minimal fall of blood pressure (5–10 mm Hg), as shown by direct recording of aortic pressure in animals with chronic

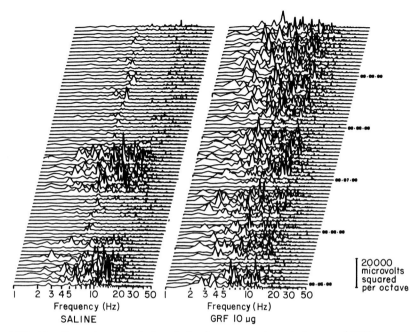

FIG. 16. Computer-generated analysis of compressed spectral array of EEG recorded for 15 minutes after icv injection of saline or GRF-44 (Ehlers *et al.*, unpublished results).

catheters. This is accompanied by a rise in pulse rate, probably reflexively induced. Acute iv injection of these large doses of GRF produces no change in blood-sugar levels. Intracerebral injection of GRF (1–10 µg) in the lateral or third ventricle again produces little obvious effect, except again a general quietening of the animals.

In early studies Ehlers *et al.* (1984) observed with continuous EEG monitoring that intraventricular injection of hpGRF-44 tends to maintain the EEG in the stage of slow-wave sleep (Fig. 16). Other computer treatment of the EEG (power spectral band time series) shows GRF to increase EEG stability.

This overall tranquilizing effect of large doses of GRF, the complete opposite of the excitatory effects of CRF, a peptide of similar size, is reminiscent of the clinical comportmental makeup of all acromegalics, described by physicians as quite, unhurried, "the smiling apathy" of the acromegalics, in the terms of Bleuler (1951). Mandell (1984) has gone so far as to propose that GRF could be the substrate of the neuroendocrine trophotropic functions of the hypothalamus, while CRF would be the ergotropic counterpart, in the terminology and concept of Walter Hess (1948).

VII. Localization of GRF-Containing Cells Using Immunohistochemistry

The first and basic question addressed was whether there would be any immunological community between hpGRF and hypothalamic GRF. Indeed we found that antibodies raised against hpGRF-40-OH and hpGRF-44-NH$_2$ specifically stained discrete neurons in primate hypothalamus, the topography and organization of which were characteristic of a neuronal system producing a hypophysiotropic releasing factor. Structures stained with hpGRF antibodies were, both in human and monkey, dense bundles of fibers in the median eminence that terminate in contact with portal capillaries and immunoreactive cell bodies that were found essentially in the mediobasal hypothalamus, mainly in the infundibular arcuate nucleus. The ventromedial nucleus contained few neurons, or none at all, according to the samples. These cells bodies were found in small amounts and inconsistently in the monkey, while they were invariably numerous and intensely immunoreactive in human (Figs. 17 and 18) (Bloch *et al.*, 1983c).

Controls of inhibition by hpGRF or fragments thereof demonstrated the specificity of the immunostaining in both species and also supplied information about antigens recognized by these antibodies. Antibodies against hpGRF-40 were inhibited by hpGRF-40, hpGRF-44-NH$_2$, and hpGRF28-44-NH$_2$, indicating that this antibody recognizes both hpGRF-40 and hpGRF-44-NH$_2$ in their C-terminal region. Antibody against hpGRF-44-NH$_2$ was inhibited by hpGRF-44-NII$_2$ but not by hpGRF-

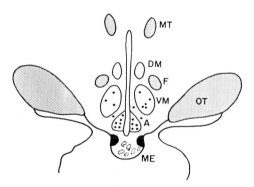

FIG. 17.   Topographical representation of neurons containing hpGRF immunoreactivity in monkey hypothalamus. Coronal section. Small black circles represent cell bodies. The two black areas in the median eminence indicate the fiber bundles and the small dots represent the endings in contact with portal vessels. OT, Optic tract; ME, median eminence; A, arcuate nucleus; VM, ventromedial nucleus; DM, dorsomedial nucleus; F, fornix; MT, mamillothalamic tract.

40 or hpGRF-44-OH, showing that it was specific of the 1–44 amidated full-length form of GRF in its C-terminal ending. Since these antibodies recognized hpGRF in two different epitopes located outside sequence common with other neuropeptides (PHI, VIP, etc., see Table VI), it appears that the staining in the brain was indeed due to genuine GRF or related metabolic compounds. Stainings of neurons with antibodies specific for hpGRF-44-NH$_2$ showed the presence of the full-length form of amidated GRF in the brain, in accordance with radioimmunological detection in human hypothalamus of a peptide indistinguishable from hpGRF-44-NH$_2$.

Neurons containing hpGRF immunoreactivity give projections in the anterior hypothalamus, especially in the paraventricular nucleus. Some fibers terminate as perisomatic endings, suggesting that, in addition to its neurohumoral role, GRF could be involved in interneuronal relationships. Comparative topographical studies showed that neurons producing GRF were different from those producing LRF, somatostatin, CRF, and pro-

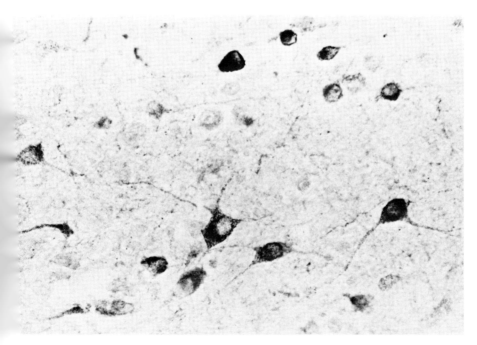

FIG. 18.   GRF-immunoreactive neurons in the adult human hypothalamus (arcuate nucleus). Indirect immunoenzymatic technique. The polyclonal antiserum was raised in rabbits against synthetic hpGRF-44-NH$_2$. (From Bloch *et al.*, unpublished.)

opiocortin, each of them having their own specific and expected location in the hypothalamus.

Study of the ontogenesis of GRF neurons in human fetal hypothalamus (Bloch *et al.*, 1983) showed that they first became detectable at the twenty-ninth week of intrauterine life, as neuroblastic cells without processes. Endings in the median eminence and fibers in the hypothalamus became detectable from the thirty-first week. Neurons producing GRF remain immature in aspect until birth, in contrast to other neuronal categories producing hypophysiotropic hormones, which differentiate months earlier. Since growth hormone-producing cells appear in the eighth week of fetal life in the pituitary and growth hormone becomes detectable in the blood in the tenth week, these results indicate that first stages of differentiation and activity in somatotropic cells are independent of fetal hypothalamic stimulation in the human.

Both antibodies against hpGRF presently used did not stain any structure in rat hypothalamus, showing that antigenic determinants recognized were species-specific, a finding later confirmed on the basis of the primary structure of rat hypothalamic GRF. Using antibodies against synthetic rat GRF, we have found staining in fibers and endings of rat median eminence with cell bodies located mainly in the arcuate nucleus and in ventral and dorsolateral hypothalamus. Ventromedial nucleus contains only very occasional neurons. The same investigations in rats treated neonatally with monosodium glutamate that destroyed the arcuate nucleus showed a selective disappearance of GRF neurons in the arcuate nucleus, together with disappearance of GRF fibers in the median eminence, while CRF, LRF, and somatostatin fibers produced normal staining (Bloch *et al.*, 1983). These results suggest that the arcuate nucleus is the source of GRF fibers projecting to the median eminence and establish monosodium glutamate-treated rats as a model for studying growth hormone secretion in rats permanently deprived of GRF stimulation. Very low abundance of GRF neurons in the human, monkey, and rat ventromedial nucleus suggests that this area plays only a minor role in GRF production, contrary to what was hypothesized on the basis of electrical stimulation and destruction experiments. Since most hypothalamic GRF neurons are located in areas contiguous to the ventromedial nucleus, effects observed upon stimulation or destruction of this area must be mainly attributed to diffusion of the effect, included in the arcuate nucleus, the region that appears to be the primary source of GRF in the hypothalamus.

The search for the presence of hpGRF immunoreactivity in normal primate pancreas and gut gave negative results, suggesting in particular that the pancreas is not physiologically involved in GRF production. Finally, hpGRF antibodies can be used for retrospective diagnosis of putative ectopic GRF-producing tumors. Not only did we find hpGRF immunoreactivity in cells of the tumor from which hpGRF was isolated, but we also found it in two other tumors, one in the lung, the other in the digestive tract, both of which had produced acromegaly in the patients.

VIII. Clinical Studies with GRF

Clinical interest in a "true" GRF, i.e., a substance that would directly stimulate secretion of GH at the pituitary level, has always been considerable, since all current methods to stimulate secretion of GH in human subjects (i.e., hypoglycemia, L-Dopa, infusion of amino acids, etc.) are indirect, i.e., mediated by some brain center. As soon as synthetic hpGRF became available and clearance had been obtained from the FDA, many clinical studies were promptly started and are currently expanding. The results have not been disappointing. Intravenous injection into normal young adults, male or female, of synthetic hGRF (Rosenthal *et al.*, 1983; Chatelain *et al.*, 1983; Wood *et al.*, 1983; Gelato *et al.*, 1983) or of the fragment hGRF(1–40) (Thorner *et al.*, 1983) is doses ranging from 0.1 to 10 μg/kg body weight regularly produces elevation of plasma immunoreactive GH, with a peak response at 15–30 minutes and lasting for 1–2 hours (Fig. 19). The response to GRF is highly specific for the secretion of GH, with no effect on plasma levels of all the other pituitary hormones or gut peptides (Thorner *et al.*, 1983). Obviously synthetic GRF should and will replace the indirect methods currently used to assess GH secretion or

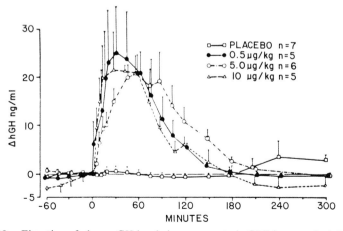

FIG. 19.   Elevation of plasma GH levels in response to hpGRF in normal adult human volunteers. The responses to 0.5, 5, and 10 μg/kg doses of hpGRF-44 were all significantly higher than the placebo. GH levels rose within 5 minutes and reached peak concentrations at 30–45 minutes (0.5 μg/kg), 45–90 minutes (5 μg/kg), and 30–120 minutes (10 μg/kg). Results are expressed in ng hGH/ml (mean ± SEM). (From Rosenthal *et al.*, 1983.)

will be used in conjunction with them to finalize a diagnosis. Since all the current GH secretion tests work indirectly, i.e., through the central nervous system, none of them being truly hypophysiotropic, they do not permit a diagnosis of GH pituitary insufficiency as truly pituitary or hypothalamic in origin. Indeed, injection of GRF into "hypopituitary dwarfs" has already led to the recognition of GH-secretory deficiencies truly pituitary in origin (no response to GRF) and of a second category which is best qualified as suprapituitary (most likely hypothalamic) in origin (positive response to GRF) (Takano et al., 1984). Chronic administration of GRF should be the treatment of choice for these cases on "hypothalamic dwarfism." Early studies indicate that the acute pituitary response to GRF in human subjects may be highly age-dependent, the response being quasi abolished after age 40 (Shibasaki et al., 1984a). This remarkable observation remains to be confirmed and explained.

Clinical interest in GRF extends over its use as a diagnostic tool and a treatment of hypothalamic dwarfism: the use of GRF can be contemplated to promote anabolism in chronic debilitating diseases, so long as the dietary intake is adequate, and to promote the healing of wounds and bone fractures. The availability of GRF with its highly specific effect in stimulating GH secretion should permit once and for all investigations of the proposed role of GH in diabetic retinopathy. Structural analogs of GRF acting as competitive antagonists, as we have already reported in an early series (Ling and Brazeau, 1983), may be of major clinical significance in the treatment of these accidents of juvenile diabetes, something that somatostatin eventually could not offer in view of its too numerous sites of action as they came to be recognized.

IX. Conclusions

In the space of 12 months following the characterization of human GRF from the islet cell tumor of these two acromegalic patients, one in France, the other in the United States, most of the pioneering studies on the mechanism of GRF *in vivo* and *in vitro* were described and, for some of them, completed; immunocytochemical mapping of GRF neurons in the human brain was carried out; structure–function studies were initiated; clinical trials were started and confirmed the potent GH-releasing activity of GRF in man. The effect of the peptide on specific GH-mRNA levels was described and molecular cloning was used to establish the structures of human preproGRF. The primary structure of hypothalamic GRF from several species (porcine, bovine, and murine) was determined.

Thus all the hypothalamic releasing factors which had been postulated in the early 1950s as humoral regulators of the secretion of each pituitary hormone have now been characterized.

ACKNOWLEDGMENTS

Research supported by program grants from the National Institutes of Health (HD-09690 and AM-18811) and from the Robert J. Kleberg, Jr. and Helen C. Kleberg Foundation. The authors are happy to acknowledge the collaboration of the technical staff of the Laboratories for Neuroendocrinology: B. Alford, D. Angeles, F. Castillo, K. Cooksey, T. Durkin, D. Fuller, R. Klepper, D. Lappi, D. Martineau, M. Mercado, B. Phillips, M. Regno, R. Schroeder, and K. von Dessonneck. The services of the secretarial staff of the laboratories in typing and handling the manuscript are also highly appreciated.

REFERENCES

Arimura, A., Matsumoto, K., Culler, M., Turkelson, C., Luciano, M., Obara, N., Thomas, R., Groot, K., Shibata, T., and Shively, J. (1983). *Endocrinology* **112**, A291.

Barinaga, M., Yamonoto, G., Rivier, C., Vale, W., Evans, R., and Rosenfeld, M. G. (1983). *Nature (London)* **306**, 84.

Beck, C., Larkins, R. G., Martin, T. J., and Burger, H. C. (1973). *J. Endocrinol.* **59**, 325.

Berelowitz, M., Szabo, M., Frohman, L. A., Firestone, S., Chu, L., and Hintz, R. L. (1981). *Science* **212**, 1279.

Bleuler, M. (1951). *J. Nerv. Ment. Dis.* **113**, 497.

Bloch, B., Brazeau, P., Ling, N., Böhlen, P., Esch, F., Wehrenberg, W. B., Benoit, R., Bloom, F., and Guillemin, R. (1983). *Nature (London)* **301**, 607.

Bloch, B., Gaillard, R. C., Brazeau, P., Lin, H. D., and Ling, N. (1984a). *Reg. Peptides* (in press).

Bloch, B., Ling, N., Benoit, R., Wehrenberg, W. B., and Guillemin, R. (1984b). *Nature (London)* **307**, 273.

Böhlen, P., and Mellet, M. (1979). *Anal. Biochem.* **94**, 313–321.

Böhlen, P., and Schroeder, R. (1982). *Anal. Biochem.* **126**, 144.

Böhlen, P., Stein, S., Stone, J., and Udenfriend, S. (1975). *Anal. Biochem.* **67**, 438–445.

Böhlen, P., Thorner, M., Cronin, J., Shively, J., and Scheithauer, B. (1982). *Endocrinology* **110**, A540.

Böhlen, P., Brazeau, P., Bloch, B., Ling, N., and Gaillard, R. (1983a). *Biochem. Biophys. Res. Commun.* **114**, 930.

Böhlen, P., Brazeau, P., Esch, F., Ling, N., Wehrenberg, W. B., and Guillemin, R. (1983b). *Reg. Peptides* **6**, 343.

Böhlen, P., Esch, F., Brazeau, P., Ling, N., and Guillemin, R. (1983c). *Biochem. Biophys. Res. Commun.* **116**, 726.

Boyd, A., Sanchez-Franco, E., Spencer, E., Patel, Y. C., Jackson, I. M. D., and Reichlin, S. (1978). *Endocrinology* **103**, 1075.

Brazeau, P., Vale, W., Burgus, R., Ling, N., Butcher, M., Rivier, J., and Guillemin, R. (1973). *Science* **179**, 77.

Brazeau, P., Ling, N., Esch, F., Böhlen, P., Benoit, R., and Guillemin, R. (1981a). *Reg. Peptides* **1**, 255.

Brazeau, P., Böhlen, P., Ling, N., Esch, F., Benoit, R., and Guillemin, R. (1981b). *Endocrinology* **108**, A837.

Brazeau, P., Ling, N., Böhlen, P., Esch, F., Ying, S.-Y., and Guillemin, R. (1982a). *Proc. Natl. Acad. Sci. U.S.A.* **79**, 7909.

Brazeau, P., Ling, N., Böhlen, P., Esch, F., Ying, S.-Y., and Guillemin, R. (1982b). *Endocrinology* **111**, 2149.

Brazeau, P., Guillemin, R., Ling, N., van Wyk, J., and Humbel, R. (1982c). *C. R. Acad. Sci. (Paris)* **295**, 651.

Brazeau, P., Ling, N., Wehrenberg, W., Jones, K., and Guillemin R. (1984). *Neuroendocrinology* (submitted).
Caplan, R. H., Koob, L., Abellera, R. M., Pagliara, A. S., Kovacs, K., and Randall, R. V. (1978). *Am. J. Med.* **64**, 874.
Chatelain, P., Cohen, H., Sassolas, G., Exclerc, J. L., Ruitton, A., Cohen, R., Claustrat, B., Laporte, S., Laferre, B., Elcharfi, A., Ferry, S., and Guillemin, R. (1983). *Ann. Endocrinol. (Paris)* **44**, A25.
Cronin, M. J., Rogol, A. D., Dabney, L. G., and Thorner, M. O. (1982). *J. Clin. Endocrinol. Metab.* **55**, 381.
De Lean, A., Munson, P. J., and Rodbard, D. (1978). *Am. J. Physiol.* **235**, E97.
Dhariwal, A. P. S., Krulich, L., Katz, S. H., and McCann, S. M. (1965). *Endocrinology* **77**, 932.
Drouin, J., DeLean, A., Rainville, D., LaChance, R., and Labrie, F. (1976). *Endocrinology* **98**, 914.
Dubois, P., Mesguich, P., and Morel, G. *Neuroendocrinology* (in press).
Ducommun, P., Vale, W., Sakiz, E., and Guillemin, R. (1967). *Endocrinology* **80**, 953.
Ehlers, C. L., Henriksen, S., Reed, T. K., and Bloom, F. E. (1984). *EEG J.,* submitted.
Esch, F. S., Böhlen, P., Ling, N. C., Brazeau, P. E., Wehrenberg, W. B., Thorner, M. O., Cronin, M. J., and Guillemin, R. (1982). *Biochem. Biophys. Res. Commun.* **109**, 152.
Esch, F., Böhlen, P., Ling, N., and Brazeau, P. (1984). *Nature (London)*, submitted.
Faden, V. B., Huston, J., Munson, P., and Rodbard, D. (1980). "Logit-log Analysis of Radio Immunoassay." NICHD RRB NIH.
Frohman, L. A., Szabo, M., Berelowitz, M., and Stachura, M. E. (1980). *J. Clin. Invest.* **65**, 43.
Gelato, M. C., Pescovitz, O., Cassola, F., Loriaux, L., and Merrian G. (1983). *J. Clin. Endocrinol. Metab.* **57**, 674.
Gick, G. G., Zeytinoglu, F. N., Esch, F. S., and Bancroft, F. C. (1983). *Endocrinology* **112**, A295.
Gubler, U., Monahan, J. J., Lomedico, P. T., Bhatt, R. S., Collier, K. J., Hoffman, B. J., Böhlen, P., Esch, F., Ling, N., Zeytin, F., Brazeau, P., Poonian, M. S., and Gage, L. P. (1983). *Proc. Natl. Acad. Sci. U.S.A.* **80**, 4311.
Guillemin, R. (1978). *Science* **202**, 390.
Guillemin, R., Ling, N., and Vargo, T. (1977). *Biochem. Biophys. Res. Commun.* **77**, 361.
Guillemin, R., Brazeau, P., Böhlen, P., Esch, F., Ling, N., and Wehrenberg, W. (1982). *Science* **218**, 585.
Hess, W. R. (1948). "Die funktionelle Organization des vegetativen Nervensystems." Schwabe, Basel.
Hewick, R. M., Hunkapiller, M. W., Hood, L. E., and Dreyer, W. J. (1981). *J. Biol. Chem.* **15**, 7990.
Hunkapiller, M. W., and Hood, L. E. (1983). *In* "Methods of Enzymology" (W. C. H. Hirs and S. N. Timasheff, eds.), Vol. 91, p. 487. Academic Press, New York.
Hunkapiller, M. W., Hewick, R. W., Dreyer, W. J., and Hood, L. E. (1983). *In* "Methods in Enzymology" (W. C. H. Hirs and S. N. Timasheff, eds.), Vol. 91, p. 399. Academic Press, New York.
Johansson, K., Currie, B., Folkers, K., and Bowers, C. Y. (1974). *Biochem. Biophys. Res. Commun.* **60**, 610.
Kadikani, H., Furutani, Y., Tarahashi, H., Noda, M., Morimoto, Y., Hirose, T., Asai, M., Inayama, S., Nakanishi, S., and Numa, S. (1982). *Nature (London)* **298**, 245.
Krulich, L., Dhariwal, A. P. S., and McCann, S. M. (1968). *Endocrinology* **83**, 783.
Leveston, A., McKeel, D. W., Buckley, P. J., Deschryver, K., Greider, M. H., Jaffe, B. M., and Daughaday, W. H. (1981). *J. Clin. Endocrinol. Metab.* **53**, 682.

Lewin, M. J. M., Reyl-Desmars, F., and N. Ling. (1983). *Proc. Natl. Acad. Sci. U.S.A.* **80**, 6538.

Ling, N., and Brazeau, P. (1983). *Endocrinology* **112**, A295.

Ling, N., Esch, F., Davis, D., Mercado, M., Regno, M., Böhlen, P., Brazeau, P., and Guillemin, R. (1980). *Biochem. Biophys. Res. Commun.* **95**, 945.

Luben, R. A., Brazeau, P., Böhlen, P., and Guillemin, R. (1982). *Science* **218**, 887.

Malacara, J. M., Valverde, R. C., Reichlin, S., and Bollinger, J. (1972). *Endocrinology* **91**, 1189.

Mandell, A. J. (1984). *Int. Rev. Neurobiol.* (in press).

Mayo, K. E., Vale, W., Rivier, J., Rosenfeld, M. G., and Evans, R. M. (1983). *Nature (London)* **306**, 86.

Minamino, N., Kangawa, K., Fukuda, A., and Matsuo, H. (1980). *Biochem. Biophys. Res. Commun.* **95**, 1475.

Nair, R. M. G., de Villier, C., Barnes, M., Antalis, J., and Wilbur, D. L. (1978). *Endocrinology* **103**, 112.

Reyl, F. J., and Lewin, M. J. M. (1981). *Proc. Natl. Acad. Sci. U.S.A.* **79**, 978.

Rivier, J. (1978). *J. Liq. Chromatogr.* **1**, 343–366.

Rivier, J., Spiess, J., Thorner, M. O., and Vale, W. (1982). *Nature (London)* **300**, 276.

Rodbard, D. (1974). *Clin. Chem.* **20**, 1255.

Rosenthal, S., Schriock, E., Kaplan, S., Guillemin, R., and Grumbach, M. (1983). *J. Clin. Endocrinol. Metab.* **57**, 677.

Rubinstein, M., Stein, S., Gerber, L., and Udenfriend, S. (1977). *Proc. Natl. Acad. Sci. U.S.A.* **74**, 3052.

Sachar, E. J. (1975). *In* "Topics in Neuroendocrinology" (E. J. Sachar, ed.), p. 135. Grune & Stratton, New York.

Sakiz, E. (1964). *Excerpta Med. Int. Congr. Ser.* **83**, 225.

Sassolas, G., Rousset, H., Cohen, R., and Chatelain, P. (1983). *C. R. Acad. Sci. (Paris)* **296**, 527.

Schally, A. V., Sawano, S., Arimura, A., Barrett, J. F., Wakabayashi, I., and Bowers, C. Y. (1969). *Endocrinology* **84**, 1493.

Schally, A. V., Baba, Y., Nair, R. M. G., and Bennett, C. D. (1971). *J. Biol. Chem.* **246**, 6647.

Selye, H. (1946). *J. Clin. Endocrinol.* **6**, 117.

Shibasaki, T., Shizume, K., Nakahara, M., Masuda, A., Jibiki, K., Demura, H., Wakabayashi, I., and Ling, N. (1984a). *J. Clin. Endocrinol.* **58**, 212.

Shibasaki, T., Shizume, K., Masuda, A., Nakahara, M., Hizuka, N., Miyakawa, M., Takano, K., Demura, W., Wakabayashi, I. and Ling, N. (1984b). **58**, 215.

Sinha, Y. N., Selby, F. W., Lewis, U. J., and Vanderlaan, W. P. (1972). *Endocrinology* **91**, 784.

Spiess, J., Rivier, J., and Vale, W. (1983). *Nature (London)* **303**, 532.

Stachura, M. E., Dhariwal, A. P. S., and Frohman, L. A. (1972). *Endocrinology* **91**, 1071.

Sykes, J. E., and Lowry, P. J. (1983). *Biochem. J.* **209**, 643.

Takano, K., and Hizuka, N., Shizume, K., Asakawa, K., Miyakawa, M., Hirose, N., Shibasaki, T., and Ling, N. (1984). **58**, 236.

Tannenbaum, G. S., and Martin, J. B. (1976). *Endocrinology* **98**, 562.

Tannenbaum, G. S., Epelbaum, J., Colle, E., Brazeau, P., and Martin, J. B. (1978). *Endocrinology* **102**, 1909.

Thorner, M. O., Perryman, R. L., Cronin, M. J., Draznin, M., Johanson, A., Rogol, A. D., Jane, J., Rudolf, L., Horvath, E., Kovacs, K., and Vale, W. (1982). *Clin. Res.* **30**, 555A.

Thorner, M., Spiess, J., Vance, M., Rogol, A., Kaiser, D., Webster, J., Rivier, J., Borges,

J., Bloom, S., Cronin, M., Evans, W., Macleod, R., and Vale, W. (1983). *Lancet* **1**, 24.
UzZafar, M. S., Mellinger, R. C., Fine, G., Szabo, M., and Frohman, L. A. (1979). *J. Clin. Endocrinol. Metab.* **48**, 66.
Vale, W., Burgus, R., and Guillemin, R. (1968). *Neuroendocrinology* **3**, 34.
Vale, W., Rivier, C., Brazeau, P., and Guillemin, R. (1974). *Endocrinology* **95**, 968.
Veber, D. F., Bennett, C. D., Milkowski, J. D., Gal, G., Denkewalter, R. G., and Hirschmann, R. (1971). *Biochem. Biophys. Res. Commun.* **45**, 235.
Wehrenberg, W. B., and Ling, N. (1983). *Neuroendocrinology* **115**, 525.
Wehrenberg, W. B., Ling, N., Brazeau, P., Esch, F., Böhlen, P., Baird, A., Ying, S., and Guillemin, R. (1982a). *Biochem. Biophys. Res. Commun.* **109**, 382.
Wehrenberg, W. B., Ling, N., Böhlen, P., Esch, F., Brazeau, P., and Guillemin, R. (1982b). *Biochem. Biophys. Res. Commun.* **109**, 562.
Wehrenberg, W. B., Brazeau, P., Luben, R., Böhlen, P., and Guillemin, R. (1982c). *Endocrinology* **111**, 2147.
Wehrenberg, W. B., Brazeau, P., Luben, R., Ling, N., and Guillemin, R. (1983a). *Neuroendocrinology* **36**, 489.
Wehrenberg, W. B., Bloch, B., Zhang, C.-L., Ling, N., and Guillemin, R. (1983b). *Reg. Peptides* (in press).
Wehrenberg, W. B., Baird, A., Ying, S.-Y., Rivier, C., Ling, N., and Guillemin, R. (1984). *Endocrinology* (in press).
White, B. A., and Bancroft, F. C. (1983). *J. Biol. Chem.* **258**, 4618.
Wilber, J. F., Nagel, T., and White, W. F. (1971). *Endocrinology* **89**, 1419.
Wilson, M. C., Steiner, A. L., Dhariwal, A. P. S., and Peake, G. T. (1974). *Neuroendocrinology* **15**, 313–327.
Wood, S. M., Ching, J. L. C., Adams, E. F., Webster, J. D., Jopling, F., Mashiter, K., and Bloom, S. R. (1983). *Br. Med. J.* **286**, 1687.
Yudaev, N. A., Utesheva, Z. F., Novikova, T. E., Shvachki, Y. P., and Smirnova, A. P. (1973). *Dan. SSSR* **210**, 731.
Zeytinoglu, F., Ling, N., Mougin, C., and Esch, F. (1983). *Endocrinology* **112**, A293.

DISCUSSION

F. Labrie: Thank you very much for this very elegant presentation which is now open for discussion and comments. What is your explanation of the effect of GRF on the secretory granules in terms of phosphorylation? Do you think that there is a receptor and a cyclase in the granules?

R. Guillemin: I cannot add anything to what I reported here. Both the biochemical results of Lewin and collaborators and those of the group of Paul Dubois with his immunocytochemistry at the electron microscope level, if they are confirmed by others or additional methods, would all lead to the consideration of some locus of action of GRF at the level of the GH secretory granules. We have not done cyclase measurements, but these are on the books.

R. N. Anderson: Is there any evidence for GRF in the placenta; and do you think that it might function in the release of HPL?

R. Guillemin: In one experiment we looked for GRF activity by bioassay in an extract of human placenta after G-75 filtration. We did not find any GRF activity. Similarly we had negative results with immunocytochemistry. We have not looked for GRF with radioimmunoassay and we don't know whether GRF might stimulate the secretion from placental cells.

R. N. Anderson: If I may extend the question? In regard to your last statement, my impression is that with LRF it is difficult to get a standardized response; that is, the hormonal milieu affects the response in the pituitary to LRF. So is it not possible that it might be necessary to get what one might call standardized conditions of blood levels of various hormones with feedback activity before one can have really completely satisfactory tests with all of these factors simultaneously?

R. Guillemin: You are quite right; the absolute values of the response to a standard dose of LRF in women, in terms of gonadotropins, in a pituitary reserve test are dependent on the day of the cycle. Regarding the response to GRF in similar clinical tests, I do not know of any data as yet to answer your question. That will have to be studied.

J. Geller: The clinical implications of what you presented are enormous. I cannot resist asking you several questions. (1) Have you or others done appropriate experiments to see whether there is a possibility of down-regulation of GH release following repetitive GRF stimulation? This would represent potential use for GRF in acromegalics. It would be very exciting if we had a way of suppressing growth hormone as well as stimulating it. (2) Is it known whether growth hormone-producing tumors even have a GRF receptor? They respond in very diverse ways to other releasing factors.

R. Guillemin: That's a good and complex question. In the case of the patients with the ectopic GRF-secreting tumors releasing GRF in high amounts continuously for several years, there certainly were enough functional GRF receptors in their pituitary since they were full-bloomed acromegalics with elevated levels of plasma GH. In animal studies we can observe both down-regulation and evidence for depletion of the pituitary GH stores. These are experiments still in progress in our laboratory. I would like to ask Bill Wehrenberg, who is conducting these, to expand on this answer and, if it is all right with the Chairman, to show a couple of slides with some recent results on this subject.

W. Wehrenberg: We cannot directly address the question of down-regulation since thus far we have been unable to develop receptor assays for GRF due to the difficulties in labeling GRF. However, I would like to show two slides on the effects of chronic GRF administration on pituitary GH secretion. We studied the pituitary GH response during a 24-hour iv infusion of GRF (15 μg/hour) and during a subsequent bolus injection of GRF (2 μg) in conscious freely moving male rats pretreated with somatostatin antibodies to eliminate interference with the GH response to GRF by endogenous somatostatin. Within 2 hours of initiation of GRF infusion, plasma GH concentrations rose from less than 200 ng/ml to 2465 $\pm$ 307 ng/ml (Fig. A). By 6 hours plasma GH concentrations began to fall. They decreased slowly and reached a nadir of 490 $\pm$ 107 ng/ml by 12 hours. Rats infused for 24 hours with GRF failed to respond to a 2 μg bolus injection of GRF iv while rats infused for 24 hours with saline responded with a normal increase in plasma GH. Pituitary GH content of rats treated with saline was significantly greater than that of rats treated with GRF (Fig. B). These results indicate that the capacity of pituitary to respond to GRF can be exhausted following chronic administration of GRF and that this lack of response appears to be due, in part, to a depletion of pituitary stores of GH.

F. Labrie: It is certainly very different from LHRH agonists where you can block secretion completely after a long-term treatment. In the response to GRF, if there is desensitization, it is much weaker than the one observed with LHRH agonists.

R. Guillemin: As Bill said, we have no good data at the moment on a cell or membrane receptor assay for GRF. We have not been able to solve the problem of marking GRF in a way that would not destroy the biological activity. Remember that the N-terminal tyrosine is necessary for biological activity. Nicholas Ling has synthesized several analogs for iodination, such as His[1]-GRF or GRF with an additional tyrosine at the C-terminal. We do not have enough results at the moment to comment upon them.

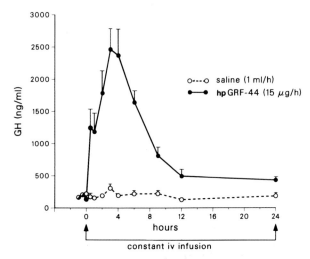

FIG. A.   Plasma GH levels during a 24-hour infusion of saline or GRF in male rats.

S. M. Russell: We have some data I would like to show on the effects of synthetic human GRF–44 on the secretion by rat pituitaries of two low-molecular-weight peptides, one of which has prolactin biological activity and the other of which has growth hormone bioactivity. This work was done in collaboration with Greg Mayer. Figure C shows the results of two separate *in vitro* incubations of rat anterior pituitary explants. The media were electrophoresed on SDS polyacrylamide gels. The two columns on the left show the patterns of proteins secreted in one experiment with control medium on the far left and medium containing 15 μmol GRF in the column next to it. The numbers on the left represent the positions of

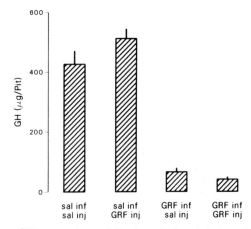

FIG. B.   Pituitary GH content in rats following a 24-hour infusion of saline or hpGRF-44 (15 μg/hour) and a bolus injection of saline or hpGRF-44 (2 μg).

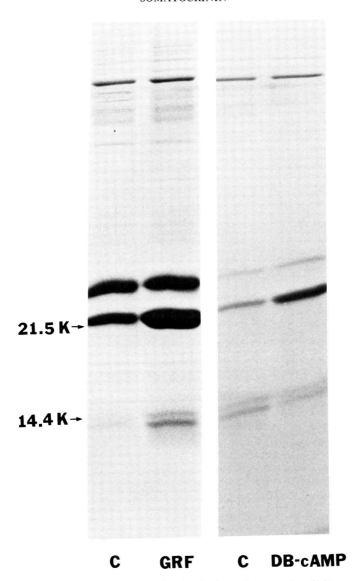

FIG. C.   Results of two separate *in vitro* incubations of rat anterior pituitary explants.

the molecular weight markers. The major bands in the medium are rat growth hormone with a molecular weight of about 22,000 (22K), and prolactin (24K). As expected, the secretion of 22K growth hormone was stimulated by the GRF. Note the two small proteins in the range of 14 to 15K. The secretion of both of these was also stimulated by the GRF. We have evidence that the smaller protein, with a molecular weight of about 14,000, has prolactin activity in the pigeon crop-sac bioassay, but it has no immunoactivity in an RIA for rat prolactin. The slightly larger, 14.5–15K protein has growth promoting activity in the rat tibia test, but little or no activity in the rat growth hormone RIA. The second two columns on the right show protein patterns from media from a similar experiment in which we studied the effects of dibutryl cyclic AMP. Again we saw stimulation of the secretion of 22K growth hormone by the cyclic nucleotide but the secretion of the two lower molecular weight proteins appeared to be inhibited. These results indicate that although GRF and cyclic AMP stimulate secretion of 22K growth hormone, they have opposite effects on the secretion of the low-molecular-weight proteins with prolactin and growth hormone bioactivities.

R. Guillemin: This is very interesting and I'm happy to hear you say that this material, whatever it is, the secretion of which was stimulated by GRF, was active in the tibia test. On that account, wouldn't you call it grown hormone?

S. M. Russell: Yes, because it has growth hormone activity.

R. Guillemin: By the way, what was the age of the animals from which you obtained the pituitaries for these studies?

S. M. Russell: These were young female rats, but we've looked at animals over a variety of ages.

R. Guillemin: So it's not a matter of the ages of the animals as compared to what we do usually, which is to use pituitaries from young male rats 100–120 g body weight. While we have never seen an effect of any dose of GRF on prolactin secretion in the *in vitro* pituitary monolayer assay, or *in vivo* in normal rats. Dr. Geneviève Sassolas, the clinician who had recognized the islet cell tumor from which we isolated GRF, tells me that in normal human subjects receiving GRF there is often a small but significant peak of plasma PRL which appears very early after the iv injection of GRF (5 minutes) and is gone at 15 minutes. This is PRL by a standard RIA.

M. Selmanoff: I wonder if you have characterized, either by immunohistochemistry or by microdissection and radioimmunoassay, any neuronal fiber pathways containing GRF outside of the medial basal hypothalamic tracts that you showed us this evening.

R. Guillemin: The results of the studies by Bertrand Bloch in our laboratory clearly indicate that with the antisera available to us there are no ir-GRF-containing neurons other than those I have mentioned here in the arcuate nucleus, the ventromedial nucleus of the hypothalamus, with occasional scattered cells outside these two nuclei but still in the ventral hypothalamus. Fibers are seen reaching to the primary plexus of the portal vessels in the median eminence. GRF-reacting fibers are also seen ending on neurons in the paraventricular nucleus. This suggest that GRF may have some role in interneuronal relationships besides being hypophysiotropic, i.e., releasing pituitary GH.

N. Samaan: In severe renal disease and liver disease the basal growth hormone level in the peripheral circulation is elevated which may show paradoxical rise or no suppression after glucose. Also in these conditions the growth hormone may rise after TRH administration similar to what is seen in patients with acromegaley. I wonder if you have had a chance to find out the status of the growth hormone releasing factor in these conditions.

R. Guillemin: This is a very interesting clinical problem for which, to my knowledge, there is no answer at the moment. We don't know the status of circulating GRF in these patients; neither do we know what the pituitary response of these patients to GRF would be. But this can now be studied with the availability of both a good radioimmunoassay for plasma GRF and the peptide to study their pituitary responses. When GRF is injected into acromegalics with a recognized pituitary tumor, early studies show that most of the patients will respond to GRF by an increase in the secretion of growth hormone, sometimes also of prolactin. That is why I referred earlier to the specificity of the peptide with normal pituitary tissues *in vitro* and in normal animals and normal subjects.

M. Saffran: In view of the chemical similarities of GRF to the secretin-glucagon family, are there any metabolic effects of GRF in hypophysectomized animals? Do you get an increase in blood sugar? Is there an effect on the gastrointestinal tract?

R. Guillemin: We have studied the question, not in hypophysectomized rats, but in normal animals, and so far we have found no effect whatsoever. At the doses of GRF injected, we have seen no increase in blood sugar. Because of the homologies in the primary structures that you mentioned and that we had recognized early on, we have, in collaboration with Jack Gerich, studied whether GRF would stimulate the secretion of glucagon and/or insulin both *in vitro* and in the perfused pancreas. Results have been negative. In the one paper you will recall that Thorner published (Thorner *et al.,* 1983) a few months ago, with Bloom in London, on the injection of GRF-40 into human subjects, they measured a large number of circulating GI peptides. They also reported no effect of GRF-40 on the plasma levels of these GI peptides. We have some results with Aaron Briskin in our laboratory showing that GRF would increase the amplitude of the spontaneous contractions of a piece of isolated rat ileum—while somatostatin does the opposite, as we have known for some time.

O. H. Pearson: Have you measured GRF in the serum of patients who presented you with the tumors that gave you this compound?

R. Guillemin: Yes, actually I have a slide with the numbers which I will spare you. We had obtained plasma of the patient in Lyons before and after surgery. The preoperative levels of ir-GRF were 200–300 ng/ml; 1 week after surgery they were 1–2 ng/ml. Normal subjects read 50 pg/ml or less. His levels never totally dropped to normal values. Three months ago, i.e., 15 months after the surgery, Paul Brazeau, who is running the RIA, was surprised to read something in the 50–100 ng range. This was mentioned to his physicians; Dr. Sassolas has now advised us that the patient is again showing an aberrant GH response to TRF (which had disappeared after surgery). They have evidence from the high-resolution scanner and ultrasound echography that the patient is now showing multiple nodules in his liver. Thus it is possible that he is getting new tumoral masses in the liver; the tumor had been diagnosed by the pathologists as an adenocarcinoma. By the way, I am puzzled as to what it is that we are measuring with the RIA for GRF in the blood of normal subjects. It is too early to say, in the early stages of the method. It may be real (that would be surprising) or, more probably, this threshold background is not due to GRF.

H. Friesen: In the very interesting blunted response to GRF in subjects after age 40 was there any sex difference in that phenomenon?

R. Guillemin: I'm not sure, but I think all the subjects in those studies of Shizume and Shibasaki were men.

H. Friesen: I'm curious to know whether men age faster than women?

R. Guillemin: Shizume and Shibasaki have studied young boys and girls in the response to GRF. In these normal children there was no difference in the response to GRF.

H. Friesen: In the light particularly of Dr. Russell's comment about enhanced release by GRF of another form of growth hormone from the rat pituitary, I was curious whether Dr. Grumbach or you had observed as Thorner *et al.* reported recently that despite a very small increase in growth hormone in a number of hypopituitary patients, a very significant elevation of somatomedin C. These data suggest other novel forms of hGH are secreted, forms not detected by current RIAs. Has that been your experience?

R. Guillemin: I suppose that you are referring to the recent data of Thorner *et al.* (1983b). Mel Grumbach and Selna Kaplan tell me that they have not seen elevations of somatomedin C in the subjects to whom they have given GRF.

H. Friesen: The effect of exogenous GRF on increasing SWS sleep was of interest. I wondered if you had an opportunity to look at whether there was the expected decrease in

SWS when rats were treated with antibodies to GRF. Such an effect might suggest that endogenous GRF might influence SWS patterns.

R. Guillemin: We have been talking about that. Except that I am not sure how the antibody will get to where you would like it to go, i.e., in the CNS.

H. Papkoff: Are the shorter GRFs derived from the larger 1–44 form? Second, what is the species specificity of GRF; is it active in all mammalian species? Finally, what is known about the stability of GRF in the blood? Is there a specific degradation system involved?

R. Guillemin: We do not know what the significance is of GRF–37 and GRF–40. I would like to propose one of two possibilities: either that they are genuinely processing products of what we call the mature peptide, or of the precursor, and that they are genuinely secreted; or that they are the products of some degree of proteolysis after the tissue was removed. In the case of the tissue from Lyons, we know that the tissue was diced into small fragments in liquid nitrogen within a couple of minutes of excision from the patient, but even that perhaps is no absolute guarantee. Indeed, even in the tumor collected in Lyons, the peptide present in largest amounts was GRF–40 (40 vs 30 nmol for GRF–44 for 7 g tissues). In the Charlottesville tumor we found only GRF–40; so did Rivier *et al.* Moreover, I am still puzzled that hpGRF–44-NH$_2$, hpGRF–40, and hpGRF–37, while of different potencies *in vitro,* are equipotent *in vivo* in the rat. On the other hand, the hypothalamic GRFs that we have characterized so far (porcine, bovine) are carboxyl terminal amidated 44-residue peptides. It is puzzling that the rat hypothalamic GRF as seen by Spiess *et al.* (1983) should be a free carboxyl terminal, 43-residue peptide. I would not be surprised if another method of extraction or cDNA sequencing should one day yield a rat hypothalamic GRF which will also be 44 residues. What is also puzzling is that such high potencies are found in analogs of hpGRF–44 when you keep deleting amino acid from the COOH-terminal end. GRF–30 has definitely measurable GRF potency. So why would nature make a "mature" peptide with 44 residues and an amidated C-terminal, while so much activity would still be available in a much smaller N-terminal fragment? It may be that GRF has roles other than that of being hypophysiotropic, in which the complete molecule of the mature form will be exclusively active. Your other question was about the stability of GRF. If you add *in vitro* either native GRF or synthetic GRF to whole human serum or whole human plasma, it is perfectly stable, as measured by bioactivity, for as long as 60 minutes; very much like β-endorphin, not like TRF—so it is not rapidly destroyed in blood *in vitro.* What I showed, of course, were curves of the disappearance after intravenous injection; you remember that the first exponential shows a half-life of ca. 5 minutes, while the slow compartment would indicate a half-life of 50–80 minutes. We have no good mathematical analysis of these results as yet. We know that murine, bovine, porcine, and human GRF have closely related but clearly different primary structures. We know that all four GRFs are active in rat pituitaries, *in vitro* and *in vivo.* Human GRF is active in bovine pituitary cells *in vitro,* and also *in vivo* when injected into cows. I have heard by the grapevine that human GRF is also active in chickens, and as you know, I have talked to you about the possibility of measuring its activity on the pituitaries of fish and other species. So it looks as if the species specificity is not going to be terribly limiting in terms of the bioactivity, and I hope that you are going to get even more of an answer now from Dr. Peter.

R. E. Peter: I have had the opportunity to test hpGRF–44 from Wylie Vale and Jean Rivier in the goldfish. The experiments were intraperitoneal injections of different dosages followed by time based blood sampling. It is clear that hpGRF–44 does stimulate growth hormone release in the goldfish. I think it is remarkable that the receptors on GH cells in goldfish recognize this peptide, if you consider the phylogenetic distance between goldfish and humans. I think that studies on the evolution of this family of peptides would be very interesting, and I hope that such studies will proceed.

R. Guillemin: Thank you, Dr. Peter. I have been looking for you all afternoon to ask you whether you would be interested in doing these experiments. Obviously you have done them and the results are quite exciting.

K. Sterling: I have a question relating to the specificity of the releasing factors. All of them seem to be limited principally to one hormone except TRF which releases TSH as well as prolactin. I wonder what your present opinion is about this and whether you think that it is probably the main regulator of prolactin secretions?

R. Guillemin: I cannot let you go without reminding you that LRF stimulates the secretion of both LH and FSH. Now in the case of TRF and prolactin, you know it's a long time since I have been really reading the literature on that subject. But a few years ago at least I was perfectly satisfied that one could explain a great deal, if not all of the physiology and control the secretion of prolactin, with TRF and dopamine. I'll be happy to add VIP to that. I don't know that I would feel inclined to search for a non-TRF PRF. I don't think I would, any more than I would look for an FSH-releasing factor other than LRF, at least until some really novel physiological data appeared to warrant it.

D. Schulster: Can you tell us anything more about the effect of GRF on the synthesis of GH or the secretion of GH?

R. Guillemin: No, Dr. Schulster; as I said earlier, I am embarrassed that these rather obvious and straightforward experiments have not been done in our laboratory. The only thing we know and that I showed is that, if you incubate rat pituitary cells as a monolayer with GRF for 3 days, you can show that you have released in the medium, at the end of the 72 hours, six times more GH than there was in the cells at time zero.

G. Moll, Jr.: I am curious about your observed release of growth hormone to GRF-40 and GRF-44. Your data strongly indicate that GRF is the final common pathway to growth hormone release, but given that there are so many stimuli to growth hormone release, is it possible that your exogenous GRF is enhancing endogenous GRF release *in vivo?*

R. Guillemin: In what circumstances and what situation?

G. Moll, Jr.: In am referring to your observation that GRF-40 and GRF-44 release growth hormone in a similar manner *in vivo.*

R. Guillemin: The two forms hpGRF-44 and hpGRF-40 have full biological activity in rats with passive neutralization of their own endogenous GRF by pretreatment with a monoclonal antibody against rat hypothalamic GRF. Now it is quite possible that any of the exogenously administered GRF-active peptides will add but not potentiate the activity of endogenous GRF, if administered at the time of a spontaneous pulse of GH release. I thought you were driving at another type of potentiation which may very well exist *in vivo* and which, we have seen *in vitro;* that is the potentiation of GRF with norepinephrine, without again going into the problem with the glucocorticoids and also of T_3. All these treatments potentiate the acute response to GRF. Similar results regarding potentiation of GRF by norepinephrine have been seen by Fusun Zeytin in our laboratory with the MTC cells (a cell line derived from a medullary thyroid carcinoma that releases neurotensin in response to GRF).

G. Moll, Jr.: This is with your GRF-44 as well as GRF-40 *in vitro?*

R. Guillemin: I don't think it would make any difference.

K. vonWerder: We have some very preliminary data in the human similar to the one which was presented in the rat which may suggest that there is some receptor down-regulation or desensitivization. We have given a bolus of 50 μg of hpGRF–44 followed by an infusion of 100 μg/hour over 2 hours to two normal male volunteers. Despite continuous infusion of hpGRF growth hormone decreased after 1 hour (Fig. D, panel a). In 4 other male subjects we gave a 50 μg bolus of hpGRF followed by the hpGRF-infusion for 2 hours followed by another bolus of 50 μg hpGRF (Fig. D, panel b). In only one subject who had a

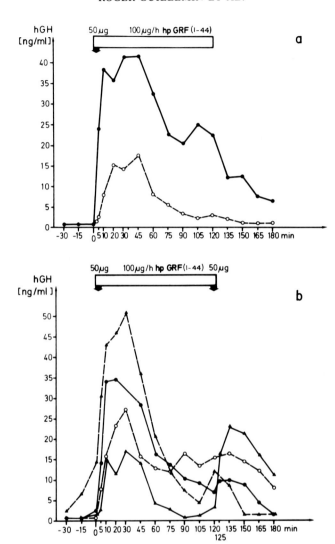

FIG. D. Growth hormone levels in 6 normal male volunteers (22–26 years of age) after the administration of 50 µg hpGRF–44 as a bolus, followed by 100 µg hpGRF–44 per hour over 2 hours (a) followed by an additional bolus of 50 µg hpGRF–44 (b). Despite continuous infusion of hpGRF–44 hGH levels decrease after 1 hour and the second GRF bolus does not lead to a second hGH surge with one exception, who had the smallest increase of hGH after the first GRF bolus.

minor initial response to the first hpGRF bolus a significant rise in response to the second hpGRF bolus was observed. In the other 3 volunteers there was no response to the second bolus. This may suggest receptor down-regulation of desensitization since it is very difficult to imagine that there is GH depletion of the pituitary considering that there are 5 mg of growth hormone in the anterior pituitary lobe, though not all of it may be readily available for secretion. Since one comment was referring to acromegaly, I would like to show a slide (Fig. E) showing two examples of acromegalic patients behaving very differently. One patient has a prompt rise of growth hormone to the appropriate releasing hormone GRF whereas all the other stimulatory agents like TRH, GnRH, CRF, and insulin hypoglycemia did not result in significant changes of GH-levels (Fig. E, panel a). The other active acromegalic patient has no response to GRF though there was prompt inappropriate rise to GnRH/TRH and to 100 g of oral glucose (Fig. E, panel b). We have been looking at 14 acromegalics so far and out of these 14, 4 had no GH response to 100 μg of hpGRF–44 whereas 10 had a very dramatic rise with the maximum within 15 to 30 minutes after GRF injection to at least the doubling of basal levels. Therefore, we feel that GRF administration may not be useful for determining the activity of acromegaly, though it may be of benefit in documenting successful therapy. Thus, in two patients who had a GH rise after GRF injection, the latter was not seen after transphenoidal surgery leading also to normalization of the basal GH levels.

R. Guillemin: Well thank you, Dr. Werder, for these very interesting observations. Let me come back to the case of the patient in Lyons as it is described by Geneviève Sassolas before and after his surgery. Even though he did not have a pituitary adenoma the man had an abnormal response to TRF in terms of elevation of growth hormone; that disappeared when the tumor of the pancreas was removed. Absence of GH response to TRF persisted until a year after surgery but has recently reappeared. There is recent evidence from the scanner and ultrasound echography studies that there are nodules appearing in the liver. These may be metastases or new tumors secreting GRF. Remember that I said earlier that we have seen his levels of plasma ir-GRF getting elevated again at about the same time. By the way, throughout the postoperational period his response to iv GRF has been normal and still is normal. I think that the next few years will see the appearance of a number of clinical studies in which this problem is investigated further with the availability of GRF to see what pattern might emerge, if any, between the specific GH response (to GRF) and the nonspecific GH response (to TRF, LRF). I would hope that similar clinical studies would also proceed regarding the same problem in uremic patients or patients with liver diseases.

S. Cohen: I am a little bit worried about the pancreatic origin of your tumor. I am no pathologist but is there any way one can tell whether the origin was actually pancreatic tissues or whether it might have originated from metastatic cells that became lodged in the pancreas.

R. Guillemin: I am no pathologist either, but I would say that, as you phrased it, it is an extremely complex question. I have discussed it at some length with the people in Lyons, including the pathologist. What we can say is that the GRF-producing tumor was macroscopically in the pancreas. No doubt about that. The pathologists call the tumor an adenocarcinoma. What we can say also is that inside the tumoral tissue there were no cells containing immunoreactive insulin or glucagon; that tumor was essentially composed of endocrine-looking cells all immunoreactive with the antibody to GRF. They were cells immunoreactive to glucagon and insulin, respectively, as thin peripheral layers, some sort of capsular layers, so to speak, while there were cells immunoreactive to somatostatin as clusters in the middle of the GRF-secreting cells. Thus the question you ask is indeed very complex: what is the true origin of that tumor? Raising the question of the neural crest origin of these tissues is too complex to discuss in a meaningful way. But along those lines we were

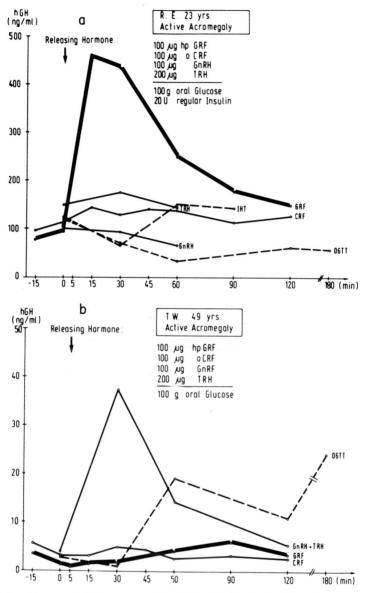

FIG. E.   Divergent hGH responses to hpGRF–44 in 2 patients with active acromegaly. One patient has a prompt response to 100 μg hpGRF–44 but no response to other releasing hormones, oral glucose or insulin-hypoglycemia (a), whereas the other patient (b) has an inappropriate hGH rise to GnRH/TRH and after 100 g of oral glucose as evidence for active acromegaly though there is no hGH rise in response to 100 μg of hpGRF–44.

very puzzled that we could not find GRF-immunoreactive cells in normal human or simian pancreas, fetal or adult, certainly not with the antisera currently available—and which we know read very well in hypothalamus and median eminence.

S. Cohen: It would seem to me that that would tend to rule out the fact that it originated from pancreatic cells.

R. Guillemin: But don't forget that part of that GRF tumor also contained somatostatin cells, so it is very complex and nobody doubts that somatostatin comes from pancreatic D cells. Sorry I do not have a better answer.

G. Merriam: I wanted to make some clinically related comments and ask a question. After we read Vale's and your reports of the structure of GRF we started clinical studies with these compounds. Like Dr. vonWerder, we observed a great heterogeneity in the response of acromegalic patients. In a multicenter collaboration, we have now tested some 20 patients with GRF–40. Some of them who have a brisk response to TRH show no response to GRF, despite active acromegaly. Others have very large and specific response to GRF. We have studied the response to both GRF–40-OH$_1$ and GRF–44-NH$_2$ in normal and GH-deficient subjects and in normal rhesus monkeys. The results suggest that there may be differences between rodents and primates in the specificity of the action of human GRF. When high doses of GRF 10 μg/kg or higher were given, we saw a rise in prolactin as well as growth hormone. At first we doubted our data because the effects of GRF in rodents were so specific; but now we have data both from Dr. Almeida's experiments in rhesus monkeys and from our human studies, both showing the rise in PRL without any elevation of cortisol to suggest a generalized stress response. My final comment is that in hypopituitary subjects injected with GRF–40-OH$_1$ in collaboration with Dr. Thorner's group, or with GRF–44-NH$_2$, we observed a rise in somatomedin C concentrations 24 hours after injection. When GRF was given repeatedly over 5 days we saw a further somatomedin rise and a potentiation of the growth hormone response to GRF. My question is this: doubtless you know the reports in from the groups of Momenee and Bowers describing a group of peptides, met-enkephalin analogs, which have a high potency for growth hormone release *in vitro*. I wondered whether you believe that these peptides have any relationship to the physiologic GRFs and conversely whether there is any interaction of the GRFs with the endorphin or enkephalin systems?

R. Guillemin: First of all, thank you, Dr. Merriam, for your comments about the clinical results, which obviously are very interesting. I hope that will be expanded upon, particularly regarding the effect on prolactin, which is peculiar and rather unique apparently to your observations. Now when you are referring to the synthetic pentapeptides related to met-enkephalin claimed to be growth hormone releasing peptides are you referring to a very recent report, namely a few hours or days old, or are you referring to the molecular structures that were reported last year or two years ago by Cy Bowers and his collaborators?

G. R. Merriam: The papers appeared about 2 or 3 years ago, one of them in *Endocrinology*.

R. Guillemin: So we are safe. Nicholas Ling has synthesized in our laboratory several of these enkephalin-related peptides as described by Bowers and collaborators. We have never been able to find any activity of these peptides, at any dose level in the *in vitro* system (the monolayer rat pituitary cells in which GRF is active in picomolar concentrations). I have discussed this extensively with Cy Bowers and we recently sent him some synthetic hGRF-44, which he finds active as described by us. In their original reports Bowers *et al.* were not using the monolayer assay system, but hemi- or quartered rat pituitaries. I don't know what to say, except that the hemipituitary assay is a system I would not trust, especially when one has the monolayer system, which is so adequate. I talked with Cy Bowers at the Endocrine Society Meeting in San Antonio and he told me that they now have another compound the structure of which they still cannot release because of the patent business but which is active, he says, both in his hemipituitaries and in the monolayer system, with very high potency; so I don't know what else to say.

D. Schulster: I was very intrigued by the declining response you got in the presence of continuous infusions of GRF and this is pertinent to another comment that was made in the discussion. You attributed it to a possible down-regulation of receptors, but I would just like to point out that it could also be due to effects on other membrane entities and their coupling or other aspects of desensitization, not just down-regulation of receptors.

R. Guillemin: If you are referring to the data shown by Bill Wehrenberg, we prefer explaining the decrease and even the quasi-total disappearance in the acute response to GRF as a depletion of the pituitary GH stores. In these animals given enormous doses of GRF over 24 hours, if you calculate the amount of growth hormone that they have secreted, based on the blood volume of the animal and GH concentrations at the end of the experiment, they have released several hundred micrograms of GH. This is corroborated by the measurement of pituitary GH content, confirming a true depletion of the pituitary GH stores. I think these results (the disappearance of the response to GRF) are best explained, as Bill proposed, by perhaps a combination of less sensitivity which one may or may not call down-regulation and/or decrease in the available pool of growth hormone.

H. Papkoff: While your data show that older males no longer respond to GRF, I presume that they would respond to other known stimuli for growth hormone release. If this is the case, does it imply that there are at least two mechanisms for growth hormone release?

R. Guillemin: Well, I can tell you that some time ago, as part of the clinical program of Mel Grumbach, I received iv 700 μg of GRF, i.e., 10 μg/kg (that was before we knew of the results of Shizume and Shibasaki) and I had no GH response to GRF, though I noticed the peculiar facial flush and tachycardia and I'm obviously over 30. I don't know what is, for instance, the GH response of a man of your age or my age to arginine infusion or to L-Dopa. That would be very interesting if the indirect system would work well on GH release and not GRF. That would be terribly puzzling.

E. L. Marut: Taking into consideration the paradoxical effect of dopaminergic stimulation on growth hormone release in acromegalics, how does the dopaminergic neurotransmitter system interact with GRF secretion?

R. Guillemin: Dr. Marut, we have no data *in vivo* or *in vitro* to answer your question. It certainly is a question well worth following.

U. Zor: In regard to the inability of GRF to release GH in elderly persons—the patient that has a tumor containing GRF is around 50 years old and he is acromegalic. So it may mean that he responds very well to GRF. Maybe in a normal person above 40 years old it may be essential to induce priming with GRF. Let us say to give GRF over several days and to examine serum GH only after this period of treatment with GRF.

R. Guillemin: It is possible. Obviously, the patient with the GRF-secreting pancreas tumor had a chronic sustained availability or presence of GRF. That is a good point, Dr. Zor.

P. K. Donahoe: I was very interested in the response of slow wave sleep to growth hormone releasing factor. Manfred Karnovsky is purifying sleep factor. Could GRF be causing the release of sleep factor?

R. Guillemin: Well, there's no muramic acid in GRF, that much we know. I can't say anything else. It's a provoking thought. If Karnofsky's group has a sensitive method to measure their sleep factor, it certainly could be investigated (by them, that is) in response to GRF.

W. Wehrenberg: I would again like to address the question of age-related changes in the pituitary response to GRF raised by Dr. Papkoff. We have studied the capability of the anterior pituitary gland to secrete GH in response to an iv injection of GRF in anesthetized male rats ranging from 22 days to 24 months of age. The increase in plasma GH concentrations following a submaximal dose of GRF (1.5 μg/kg) was similar among the different aged rats suggesting there is no age-related change in pituitary sensitivity to GRF. Likewise, the response to a maximal dose of GRF (25 μg/kg) was not different in young and old animals indicating there is no decrease in the readily releasable pool of GH. We have previously reported that the anesthetized animal model is ideal for the study of GRF since it appears that in these animals endogenous somatostatin release is interrupted. Since the effects of endogenous somatostatin, or for that matter endogenous somatomedins, were not considered in the human study discussed by Dr. Guillemin and since they have an important role in mediating GH secretion, it is possible that the absence of a GH response to GRF in old humans is due to these factors rather than pituitary insensitivity to GRF.

Phospholipid Turnover in Hormone Action

Yasutomi Nishizuka, Yoshimi Takai, Akira Kishimoto,
Ushio Kikkawa, and Kozo Kaibuchi

*Department of Biochemistry, Kobe University School of Medicine, Kobe, Japan, and
Department of Cell Biology, National Institute for Basic Biology, Okazaki, Japan*

I. Introduction

Pleiotropic actions of hormone are frequently initiated by interaction with specific cell surface receptor, and the biochemical basis of the signal transduction across the membrane has long been a subject of great interest. It is now firmly established that a group of hormones utilize cyclic AMP as an intracellular mediator for controlling physiological cellular processes. On the other hand, evidence has accumulated in recent years that a large number of other hormones, neurotransmitters, secretagogues, chemoattractants, growth factors, and many biologically active substances exemplified in Table I appear not to be related to cyclic AMP, but Ca^{2+} is essential for their actions in respective target tissues. The involvement of phospholipid in the receptor mechanism has been suggested first by Hokin and Hokin (1953), who have shown that acetylcholine induces rapid breakdown and resynthesis of phosphatidylinositol in some secretory tissues such as pancreas. Since then, a wide variety of extracellular messengers mentioned above are repeatedly shown to induce similar membrane phospholipid turnover (for reviews see Michell, 1975, 1979; Hawthorne and White, 1975). In general, inositol phospholipid is a relatively minor component, and comprises less than 10% of the total phospholipids in mammalian membranes. One of the characteristics of this phospholipid is that it contains most often arachidonic acid at position 2 (Holub *et al.*, 1970). It is also known that a small portion of this phospholipid contains an additional one or two phosphates at position 4 or positions 4 and 5 of the inositol moiety as shown in Fig. 1. These extremely minor lipid components are referred to as phosphatidylinositol monophosphate (diphosphoinositide) and phosphatidylinositol bisphosphate (triphosphoinositide), respectively. These additional phosphates attached to the inositol moiety have been known for a long time to turn over even more rapidly during the activation of cellular functions (Dawson, 1954). Re-

301

TABLE I

Two Major Groups of Extracellular Messengers

Cyclic AMP system	Non-cyclic AMP system (Ca^{2+} system)
Norepinephrine (β)	Acetylcholine (m)
Epinephrine (β)	Norepinephrine (α)
Dopamine (D1)	Epinephrine (α)
Histamine (H2)	Dopamine (D2)
	Histamine (H1)
ACTH	Cholecystokinin
Vasoactive intestinal polypeptide	Cerulein
Secretin	Gastrin
	Bombesin
	Substance-P
Prostaglandins	Thromboxane
Prostacyclin	Thrombin
	Collagen
	Platelet-activating factor
	Chemoattractants
	Secretagogues
	Growth factors
	Mitogens

cently, it was proposed that in some mammalian tissues (Kirk, 1982; Agranoff *et al.*, 1983, Imai *et al.*, 1983; for a review see Michell, 1982) and insect salivary gland (Berridge, 1982) phosphatidylinositol bisphosphate is the immediate target of the receptor-linked reaction, and a possible pathway of the signal-induced turnover of these phospholipids is schematically shown in Fig. 2. In any case, the reaction is initiated by the cleavage of phosphodiester linkage, which is catalyzed by phospholipase C (Daw-

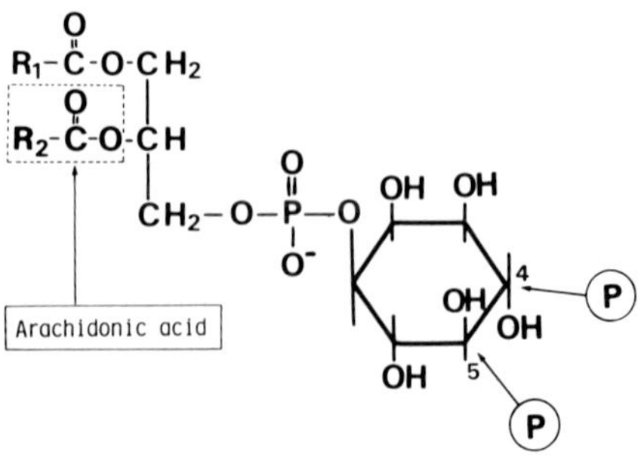

FIG. 1.   Structure of inositol phospholipid.

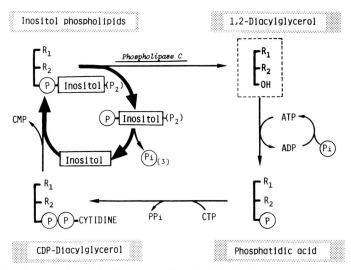

FIG. 2.   Inositol phospholipid turnover. P-inositol, inositol monophosphate; and P-inositol-P_2, inositol trisphosphate.

son *et al.*, 1971). The primary products of this reaction are diacylglycerol and inositol monophosphate or inositol trisphosphate.

Some years ago Michell (1975) postulated that the inositol phospholipid turnover may open the Ca^{2+} gate. It was also proposed that diacylglycerol acts as a membrane fusigen or perturber in some exocytotic processes (Allan and Michell, 1975). Phosphatidic acid derived from diacylglycerol has often been proposed to act as a Ca^{2+} ionophore (Tyson *et al.*, 1976; Michell *et al.*, 1977; Serhan *et al.*, 1981). However, none of these possibilities has been unequivocally established. On analogy to cyclic AMP there have been efforts to explore a possible role of inositol monophosphate, although all attempts have been unsuccessful. Very recently, inositol trisphosphate that is produced from phosphatidylinositol bisphosphate has been proposed as an intracellular mediator for signal-induced Ca^{2+} mobilization (Streb *et al.*, 1983).

Protein kinase C has been found first as a proteolytically activated protein kinase that is distributed in many tissues (Takai *et al.*, 1977; Kishimoto *et al.*, 1977), and later shown to be a Ca^{2+}-activated, phospholipid-dependent enzyme (Takai *et al.*, 1979a,b; Kishimoto *et al.*, 1980). The enzyme appears to be directly linked to the inositol phospholipid turnover. When cells are stimulated, this protein kinase is activated by diacylglycerol that is transiently produced in membranes during the signal-induced turnover of inositol phospholipids as described above. A series of analyses with several cell types suggests that the activation of this protein kinase is a prerequisite requirement, and acts synergistically with Ca^{2+} mobilization to elicit full physiological cellular responses. It is also clarified that tumor-promoting phorbol esters such as 12-O-tetradecanoyl-phorbol-13-acetate (TPA) are intercalated into the membrane, substitute for diacylglycerol, and activate this protein kinase directly. This article will outline some aspects of protein kinase C, and discuss its possible roles in hormone action. Cyclic AMP-dependent and cyclic GMP-dependent protein kinases will be tentatively referred to as protein kinase A and protein kinase G, respectively.

II. Activation and Properties of Protein Kinase C

The principal pathway of signal translation to protein phosphorylation is schematically given in Fig. 3. Under resting conditions in most tissues protein kinase C is present as an inactive form presumably in soluble cytosol or loosely bound to membranes, and is activated by tight association with membranes in a signal-dependent manner (Takai *et al.*, 1979b; Kishimoto *et al.*, 1980). The enzyme absolutely requires Ca^{2+} and phospholipid for its activation. Diacylglycerol is normally almost absent from membranes, but is transiently produced from inositol phospholipids. Kinetically, a small amount of diacylglycerol dramatically increases the affinity of this enzyme for Ca^{2+} as well as for phospholipid, and thereby renders the enzyme fully active without a net increase in the concentration of this divalent cation. For instance, in the experiment given in Fig. 4, it is shown that in the presence of phospholipid alone, protein kinase C

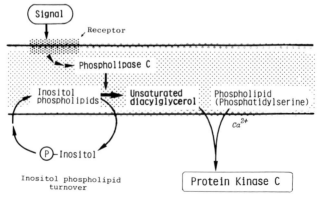

FIG. 3.   Principal pathway of signal translation to protein phosphorylation.

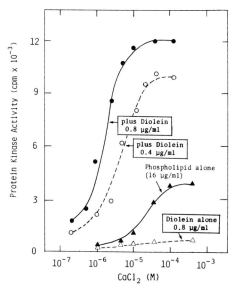

FIG. 4.   Activation of protein kinase C by diacylglycerol in the presence of Ca²⁺ and phospholipid. Protein kinase C was assayed in the presence of various concentrations of Ca²⁺ by measuring the incorporation of the radioactive phosphate of [γ-³²P]ATP into calf thymus H1 histone as a model substrate. Where indicated, diolein and a mixture of phospholipids prepared from erythrocytes were added. Detailed assay conditions were described elsewhere (Kishimoto *et al.*, 1980). (Adapted from Takai *et al.*, 1982c.)

requires extremely higher concentrations of Ca²⁺. If, however, a small quantity of diacylglycerol, diolein in this experiment, is added, the enzymatic activity is greatly enhanced with concomitant decrease in the Ca²⁺ concentration giving rise to the maximum enzyme activation. This unique effect is specific for diacylglycerol. Other neutral lipids such as triacylglycerol, monoacylglycerol, and free fatty acid are totally inactive as shown in Table II. The diacylglycerol active in this role appears to contain at least one unsaturated fatty acid irrespective of the chain length of the other fatty acyl moiety. The 1-stearoyl-2-arachidonyl-glycerol backbone which occurs most frequently in inositol phospholipids is highly active to support the enzyme activation.

  Table III shows specificity of phospholipid for the enzyme activation. At physiologically lower concentrations of Ca²⁺ only phosphatidylserine is active, and no other phospholipid is able to activate protein kinase C under comparable conditions (Takai *et al.*, 1979b). However, various other membrane phospholipids which are inert by themselves show positive or negative cooperativity for this enzyme activation, and a typical experiment is shown in Fig. 5. When phosphatidylethanolamine is supple-

TABLE II

Specificity of Neutral Lipid for Activation of Protein Kinase C[a]

Experiment	Neutral lipid added	Protein kinase activity (cpm)
1	None	980
	Triolein	970
	Diolein	6500
	Monoolein	990
	Tripalmitin	980
	Dipalmitin	970
	Monopalmitin	980
2	None	980
	Diolein	6500
	Dilinolein	5510
	Diarachidonin	6220
	1-Stearoyl-2-oleoyl-glycerol	4610
	1-Oleoyl-2-stearoyl-glycerol	4820
	Distearin	950

[a] Protein kinase C was assayed at 6 μM CaCl$_2$ with calf thymus H1 histone as a model substrate in the presence of a mixture of phospholipids isolated from erythrocyte membranes (16 μg/ml) and various neutral lipids (0.8 μg/ml each) as indicated. Detailed assay conditions were described elsewhere (Kishimoto *et al.*, 1980).

TABLE III

Specificity of Phospholipid for Activation of Protein Kinase C[a]

Phospholipid added	Protein kinase activity (cpm)
Phosphatidylserine	6940
Phosphatidylinositol	350
Phosphatidic acid	200
Phosphatidylcholine	110
Sphingomyelin	80
Phosphatidylethanolamine	30

[a] Protein kinase C was assayed at 2 μM CaCl$_2$ with calf thymus H1 histone as a model substrate in the presence of diolein (0.8 μg/ml) and various phospholipids (8 μg/ml each) as indicated. Detailed assay conditions were described elsewhere (Takai *et al.*, 1979b).

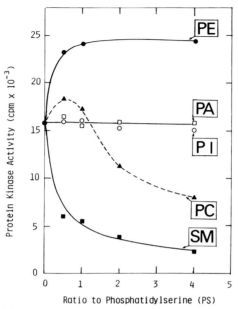

FIG. 5.   Effect of further supplement of various phospholipids to phosphatidylserine on activation of protein kinase C. Protein kinase C was assayed with calf thymus H1 histone as a model substrate in the presence of a fixed amount of phosphatidylserine (20 μg/ml), various amounts of other phospholipids as indicated, and fixed amounts of diolein (0.8 μg/ml) and $CaCl_2$ (10 μM). Detailed assay conditions were described elsewhere (Kaibuchi et al., 1981). PE, Phosphatidylethanolamine; PA, phosphatidic acid; PI, phosphatidylinositol; PC, phosphatidylcholine; SM, sphingomyelin; and PS, phosphatidylserine.

mented to phosphatidylserine, the enzyme activity is increased further, and the full activation is observed at the 10^{-7} M range of Ca^{2+}. Phosphatidylcholine and sphingomyelin show opposing effects. Thus, asymmetric distribution of various phospholipids in the membrane lipid bilayer likely favors the activation of protein kinase C. The kinetic properties of enzyme activation mentioned above are obviously highly important. In fact, as described below in detail, protein kinase C may be activated in a manner dependent solely on diacylglycerol, because its Ca^{2+} sensitivity is greatly modulated. Membrane phospholipids may not be limited in physiological processes.

Protein kinase C is found in all tissues and organs in mammals so far tested (Inoue et al., 1977; Nishizuka et al., 1979; Nishizuka, 1980; Minakuchi et al., 1981). Table IV shows relative activities of this enzyme in some of mammalian tissues, with platelets, brain, some smooth muscles, and lymphocytes having higher specific activities. Kuo and his associates (1980) have also found this enzyme in many tissues of mammals and other

TABLE IV

Relative Activities of Protein Kinases C and A in Mammalian Tissues[a]

Tissue	Protein kinase C (units/mg protein)	Protein kinase A (units/mg protein)
Platelets	6300	340
Brain	3270	250
Vas deference muscle	2210	500
Lymphocytes	1060	320
Intestinal muscle	770	560
Neutrophils	530	150
Liver	180	130
Adipocytes	170	270
Skeletal muscle	80	110

[a] Rat tissues were employed except for platelets, lymphocytes, and neutrophils which were obtained from human blood. The enzymes were assayed under comparable conditions with calf thymus H1 histone as a common model substrate, although these enzymes phosphorylate different amino acyl residues in this histone molecule (see text). Detailed assay conditions were described elsewhere (Minakuchi *et al.*, 1981). Values are units per mg of protein. One unit of protein kinase activity is defined as the amount of enzyme that incorporated 1 pmol of phosphate from ATP into H1 histone per minute.

organisms. In many tissues the activity of protein kinase C far exceeds that of protein kinase A when assayed with calf thymus H1 histone as a common model substrate. In brain, a large portion of protein kinase C is localized in the synaptosomal fraction, implying its roles in the neuronal functions (Kikkawa *et al.*, 1982). The enzyme apparently lacks tissue and species specificities at least in its kinetic and catalytic properties. The enzyme has been purified to homogeneity from the soluble fraction of rat brain (Kikkawa *et al.*, 1982), and more recently by Schatzman *et al.* (1983) from pig spleen extracts.

Protein kinase C is a single polypeptide chain with no subunit structure. The enzyme is essentially homogeneous upon electrophoresis on polyacrylamide gel in the presence of sodium dodecyl sulfate and a sulfhydryl compound. The molecular weight is estimated to be about 77,000 (Kikkawa *et al.*, 1982). Some of other physical and kinetic properties are given in Fig. 6. This polypeptide chain appears to be composed of two functionally different domains. One is a hydrophobic domain that may bind to membranes, and the other is a hydrophilic domain that carries the catalytically active center. These two domains are cleaved by Ca^{2+}-dependent neutral proteases designated as calpains (Murachi *et al.*, 1981) to produce an enzyme fragment having an approximate molecular weight of

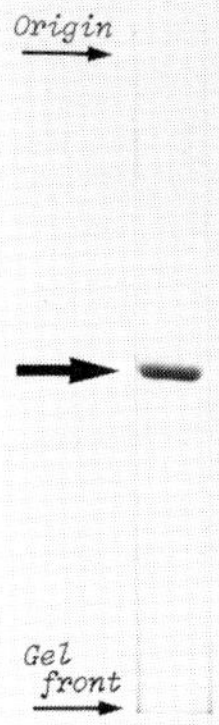

Molecular weight	77,000
Stokes radius	42 Å
S value	5.1 S
Isoelectric point	pH 5.6
Optimum pH	7.5 ∿ 8.0
Optimum Mg^{2+}	5 mM
Nucleotide specificity	ATP

Activators	K_a value
Phosphatidylserine	36 μg/ml
Diacylglycerol	0.5 μg/ml
Ca^{2+}	4×10^{-7} M

FIG. 6. Physical and kinetic properties of protein kinase C. The single protein band shown by an arrow is a homogeneous preparation of protein kinase C purified from rat brain soluble fraction by the method of Kikkawa *et al.* (1982). The physical and kinetic parameters were obtained under the conditions specified elsewhere (Inoue *et al.*, 1977; Takai *et al.*, 1977, 1979b; Kaibuchi *et al.*, 1981; Kikkawa *et al.*, 1982).

51,000 (Takai *et al.*, 1977; Inoue *et al.*, 1977; Kishimoto *et al.*, 1983). This fragment is enzymatically fully active and does not require Ca^{2+}, phospholipid, or diacylglycerol. The protein kinase fully activated proteolytically shows kinetic and catalytic properties similar to those of the enzyme that is activated nonproteolytically. It is also noted that protein kinase C which is attached to membranes is preferentially cleaved by a new class of Ca^{2+}-dependent neutral proteases active at the micromolar range of calcium (Kishimoto *et al.*, 1983). This class of proteases has been first found in dog heart by Mellgren (1980), and subsequently in virtually any tissues and organs (Murachi *et al.*, 1981; Suzuki *et al.*, 1981; Kishimoto *et al.*, 1981; Murachi, 1983). However, evidence is unavailable at present indicating that this mechanism of irreversible activation of protein kinase C does operate in physiological processes.

III. Link with Protein Phosphorylation

To obtain evidence that the signal-induced breakdown of inositol phospholipids is directly linked to the activation of protein kinase C, most of the experiments have been undertaken with platelets unless otherwise specified. Platelets are often used as a model system for understanding the mechanism of hormone action, since many extracellular messengers such as thrombin, collagen, and platelet-activating factor induce aggregation as

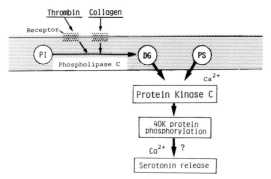

FIG. 7. A possible mechanism of receptor-linked phosphorylation of 40K protein in platelets. PI, Phosphatidylinositol; DG, diacylglycerol; and PS, phosphatidylserine. (Adapted from Nishizuka, 1983b.)

well as release reactions of various constituents of dense bodies, α-granules, and lysosomes. This activation of cellular functions is normally antagonized by prostaglandins and prostacyclin which are known to increase cyclic AMP. When platelets are stimulated, an endogenous protein having a molecular weight of about 40,000 (40K protein) is heavily phosphorylated, and this reaction appears to be associated with the release of

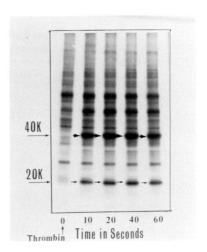

FIG. 8. Stimulation of phosphorylation of platelet endogenous proteins by thrombin. Human platelets were isolated, labeled with $^{32}P_i$, and then stimulated by thrombin (0.05 unit/ 10^8 platelets) at 37°C for various periods of time as indicated. The radioactive proteins were directly subjected to polyacrylamide gel electrophoresis in the presence of sodium dodecyl sulfate, dried on a filter paper, and exposed to an X-ray film to prepare the autoradiograph. Detailed experimental conditions were described elsewhere (Kawahara *et al.*, 1980).

serotonin (Lyons *et al.*, 1975; Haslam and Lynham, 1977). Although the function of this protein is unknown, protein kinase C is responsible for its phosphorylation as schematically shown in Fig. 7 (Kawahara *et al.*, 1980; Sano *et al.*, 1983). Figure 8 illustrates a typical autoradiograph of platelet endogenous phosphoproteins which are separated on sodium dodecyl sulfate–polyacrylamide gel electrophoresis. It is shown that, in addition to 40K protein, another protein having a molecular weight of 20,000 (20K protein) is phosphorylated upon stimulation by thrombin. The latter protein has been identified as myosin light chain, and the reaction is catalyzed by a specific enzyme, myosin light chain kinase which absolutely requires Ca^{2+} for its activity (Hathaway and Adelstein, 1979). Thus, as soon clarified below, the phosphorylation of 40K and 20K proteins may be used as the markers of protein kinase C activation and Ca^{2+} mobilization, respectively.

Under resting conditions diacylglycerol is not detected. When platelets are stimulated by thrombin or collagen, this neutral lipid is immediately produced and disappears very quickly as shown in Fig. 9. It is important

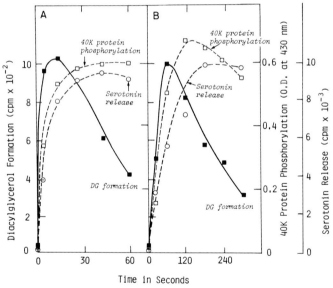

FIG. 9. Activation of platelets by thrombin (A) and collagen (B). Human platelets were isolated, labeled with either [³H]arachidonic acid, ³²P$_i$, or [¹⁴C]serotonin, and then stimulated by thrombin (0.05 unit/10⁸ platelets) or collagen (50 μg/ml) at 37°C for various periods of time as indicated. Diacylglycerol produced and serotonin released were determined by measuring the radioactivity, and radioactive 40K protein was determined by autoradiography followed by densitometric tracing at 430 nm as described elsewhere (Sano *et al.*, 1983). (Adapted from Sano *et al.*, 1983.)

to note that the diacylglycerol is probably derived mostly from phosphatidylinositol as described by Rittenhouse-Simmons (1979), Bell and Majerus (1980), and Kawahara *et al.* (1980). In addition, quantitative analysis has revealed that the amount of diacylglycerol accumulated is less than that of phosphatidylinositol expended. This poor stoichiometry as well as the rapid disappearance of diacylglycerol is due to its conversion to inositol phospholipids by way of phosphatidic acid (inositol phospholipid turnover) and also due to its further degradation to arachidonic acid for thromboxane synthesis. Thus, in platelets at least, phosphatidylinositol is the major source of diacylglycerol accumulated, even if the primary target of the signal-induced breakdown is phosphatidylinositol bisphosphate. Presumably, these inositol phospholipids are in a state of rapid equilibrium. The transient appearance of diacylglycerol in membranes is followed by immediate phosphorylation of the 40K protein and release of serotonin. Essentially similar results have been obtained with platelet-activating factor instead of thrombin and collagen (Ieyasu *et al.*, 1982).

Platelets obtained from either human or rabbit contain a large quantity of protein kinase C as mentioned above. Figure 10 shows relative activities of protein kinases C and A with calf thymus H1 histone as a common model substrate. It is found that protein kinase C phosphorylates preferentially 40K protein *in vitro* which is purified from human platelets, and this reaction is absolutely dependent on the simultaneous presence of Ca^{2+}, phospholipid, and diacylglycerol (Sano *et al.*, 1983). Fingerprint analysis of the radioactive 40K protein which is phosphorylated *in vivo* and *in vitro* suggests that protein kinase C is responsible for this protein phosphorylation which is observed in the platelets stimulated by thrombin, collagen, and platelet-activating factor (Ieyasu *et al.*, 1982; Sano *et al.*, 1983).

In another series of experiments, attempts are made to activate protein kinase C in intact cell systems by direct addition of diacylglycerol. It has been previously shown that various synthetic diacylglycerols are able to activate this enzyme *in vitro*, if diacylglycerols contain one unsaturated long-chain fatty acyl moiety, irrespective of the chain length of the other (Mori *et al.*, 1982). In intact cell systems, diacylglycerols having two long-chain fatty acyl moieties such as diolein may not be dispersed in a form suitable for presentation to intact cells. If, however, one fatty acyl moiety esterified to either position 1 or 2 is replaced by an acetyl grouping, then the resulting diacylglycerol is found to gain access to protein kinase C (Kaibuchi *et al.*, 1982a, 1983). For instance, 1-oleoyl-2-acetyl-glycerol suspended in a dilute dimethyl sulfoxide solution appears to be readily intercalated into the membrane phospholipid bilayer, and directly activates protein kinase C without interaction with cell surface receptors. In

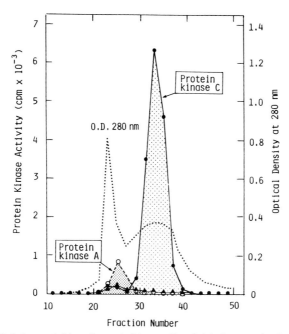

FIG. 10.   Relative activities of protein kinases C and A in human platelets. The soluble fraction of human platelets was prepared in the presence of EGTA, and then directly subjected to gel filtration on a Sephadex G-150 column (2 × 80 cm). Protein kinases C and A were assayed under the respective standard conditions with calf thymus H1 histone as a common model substrate. Detailed assay procedures were described elsewhere (Kawahara *et al.*, 1980). Triangles indicate blank values. (Taken from Takai *et al.*, 1982b.)

the experiment given in Fig. 11, it is shown that this synthetic diacylglycerol induces rapid phosphorylation of the 40K protein in platelets just as it is by natural extracellular messengers such as thrombin. Under these conditions neither the formation of endogenous diacylglycerol nor the breakdown of inositol phospholipids has been demonstrated. Dimethyl sulfoxide alone is rather inhibitory, and there is no indication that this effect of exogenous diacylglycerol is simply due to damage of the cell membrane. The fingerprint of tryptic phosphopeptides of the 40K protein isolated from the activated platelets is identical with that prepared from the 40K protein phosphorylated *in vitro* by homogeneous protein kinase C. It is also shown that, during the activation of protein kinase C, this synthetic diacylglycerol is rapidly converted *in situ* to the corresponding phosphatidic acid, 1-oleoyl-2-acetyl-3-phosphoryl-glycerol, presumably by the action of diacylglycerol kinase as shown in Fig. 12. This newly produced phosphatidic acid has been isolated from the platelets, and iden-

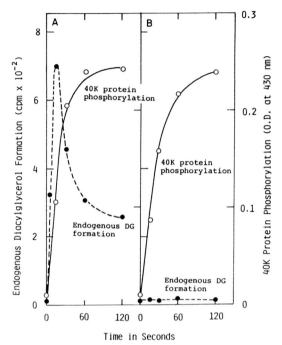

FIG. 11. Direct activation of protein kinase C in platelets by exogenous addition of synthetic diacylglycerol. Human platelets were labeled with either [³H]arachidonic acid or ³²Pᵢ, and then stimulated at 37°C by thrombin (A) (0.2 unit/ml) or 1-oleoyl-2-acetyl-glycerol (B) (50 μg/ml) for various periods of time as indicated. The final concentration of dimethyl sulfoxide was 0.1%. Endogenous diacylglycerol formation and 40K protein phosphorylation were assayed under the conditions similar to those described in Fig. 9. Detailed experimental procedures were described elsewhere (Kaibuchi et al., 1983). DG, Diacylglycerol.

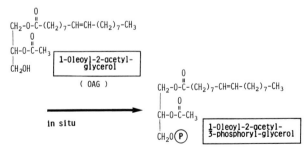

FIG. 12. A biologically active synthetic diacylglycerol and its conversion to phosphatidic acid.

tified as such by comparison with an authentic sample of the synthetic product (Kaibuchi *et al.*, 1983). Figure 13 shows an autoradiograph of this unique phosphatidic acid isolated by thin layer chromatography.

Based on the foregoing discussions it seems possible to conclude that in platelets the receptor-mediated breakdown of inositol phospholipids may be directly linked to protein phosphorylation through activation of protein kinase C. Although cell surface receptors of various extracellular messengers are presumably different, protein kinase C seems to lie on a common pathway that eventually leads to the activation of cellular functions such as release reactions. The experimental support has resulted from studies with a limited tissue, but there is no reason to expect platelets to be exceptional. In fact, the transient accumulation of diacylglycerol has been observed in several types of other tissues, such as acetylcholine-stimulated pancreas (Banschbach *et al.*, 1974), polycationic compound 48/80-stimulated mast cells (Kennerly *et al.*, 1979b), thyrotropin-stimulated thyroid follicles (Igarashi and Kondo, 1980), platelet-derived growth factor-stimulated Swiss 3T3 cells (Habenicht *et al.*, 1981), concanavalin A-stimulated lymphocytes (Hasegawa-Sasaki and Sasaki, 1982), zymosan-stimulated neutrophils (Gil *et al.*, 1982), and bradykinin-stimulated aortic endothelial cells (Hong and Deykin, 1982). It may be anticipated that this transmembrane signal pathway leading to the protein phosphorylation may operate in physiological processes in many tissues, which have receptors related to inositol phospholipid breakdown.

IV. Synergistic Role with Calcium Action

It has been repeatedly documented that stimulation of receptors related to inositol phospholipid breakdown mentioned above usually mobilizes Ca^{2+} immediately (for reviews see Michell, 1975, 1979; Hawthorne and White, 1975). Although protein kinase C absolutely requires Ca^{2+} for its activation, synthetic diacylglycerol directly added to intact platelets induces full activation of this enzyme without causing Ca^{2+} mobilization as described above (Kaibuchi *et al.*, 1982a, 1983). This is presumably due to the fact that diacylglycerol greatly increases the affinity of protein kinase C for Ca^{2+} to the 10^{-7} M range, and thereby renders this enzyme fully active without a net increase in the Ca^{2+} concentration (Kaibuchi *et al.*, 1981). Therefore, it is possible to induce protein kinase C activation and Ca^{2+} mobilization independently by the exogenous addition of synthetic diacylglycerol and Ca^{2+} ionophore such as A23187, respectively, as schematically shown in Fig. 14. An additional advantage to use platelets is that these two events may be specifically determined by measuring the phosphorylation of 40K and 20K proteins as already mentioned above. In

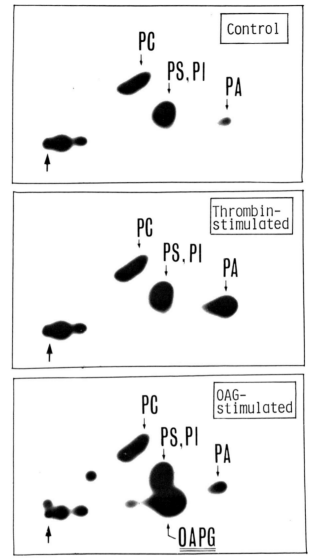

FIG. 13. Autoradiograph of various phospholipids in platelets stimulated by either thrombin or synthetic diacylglycerol. Human platelets were labeled with $^{32}P_i$, and then stimulated for 3 minutes by either thrombin or 1-oleoyl-2-acetyl-glycerol under conditions identical with those given in Fig. 11. Phospholipids were extracted directly from the platelets, separated by two-dimensional thin-layer chromatography, and autoradiographs were prepared. Detailed experimental conditions were described elsewhere (Kaibuchi *et al.*, 1983). OAG, 1-Oleoyl-2-acetyl-glycerol; OAPG, 1-oleoyl-2-acetyl-3-phosphoryl-glycerol; PC, phosphatidylcholine; PS, phosphatidylserine; PI, phosphatidylinositol; and PA, phosphatidic acid.

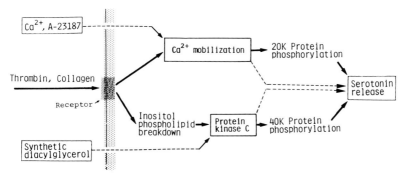

FIG. 14. Independent induction of protein kinase C activation and Ca^{2+} mobilization by synthetic diacylglycerol and Ca^{2+} ionophore and their synergistic roles for causing full physiological response. Platelets are used as a model system.

the experiment given in Fig. 15, human platelets labeled with radioactive phosphate are stimulated by either thrombin, 1-oleoyl-2-acetyl-glycerol, or A23187. Then, the radioactive 40K and 20K proteins are quantitated by sodium dodecyl sulfate–polyacrylamide gel electrophoresis, followed by autoradiography and densitometric tracing. When platelets are stimulated by thrombin, both 40K and 20K proteins are phosphorylated concomitantly. If, however, platelets are stimulated by synthetic diacylglycerol, only 40K protein is phosphorylated to an extent that is very similar to that induced by thrombin. The 20K protein is not phosphorylated to a measurable extent, suggesting that Ca^{2+} is not mobilized under these conditions. This has been recently confirmed by the direct measurement of Ca^{2+} using quin 2 by Rink *et al.* (1983). In contrast, at lower concentrations of A23187 the 20K protein is selectively phosphorylated, presumably owing to the increase in the Ca^{2+} concentration. As already noted above, the phosphorylation of the 20K protein is catalyzed by a calmodulin-dependent protein kinase specific for this protein, that is myosin light chain kinase (Hathaway and Adelstein, 1979). These results suggest that, under the limited conditions, inositol phospholipid breakdown and Ca^{2+} mobilization are not causally related to each other, although the possibility may not be ruled out that one of these events is a prerequisite requirement of the other.

The next set of experiments given in Fig. 16 is designed to show that both protein kinase C activation and Ca^{2+} mobilization are essential and act synergistically to cause full physiological cellular responses such as release of serotonin. Namely, when platelets are stimulated by synthetic diacylglycerol in the presence and absence of a low concentration of A23187, 40K protein is phosphorylated almost equally irrespective of the

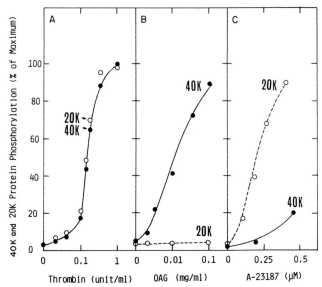

FIG. 15. Selective phosphorylation of platelet 40K and 20K proteins in platelets by exogenous addition of synthetic diacylglycerol and Ca^{2+} ionophore. Human platelets were labeled with $^{32}P_i$, and then stimulated for 1 minute by various amounts of either thrombin (A), 1-oleoyl-2-acetyl-glycerol (B), or A23187 (C) as indicated. The phosphorylation of 40K and 20K proteins was quantitated under conditions similar to those given in Fig. 9. Detailed experimental conditions were described elsewhere (Kaibuchi *et al.*, 1983). 40K, 40K protein; 20K, 20K protein; and OAG, 1-oleoyl-2-acetylglycerol.

presence and absence of the Ca^{2+} ionophore. However, serotonin is released only slightly by the addition of diacylglycerol alone, and the full response is observed when diacylglycerol and the Ca^{2+} ionophore are simultaneously added. The Ca^{2+} ionophore alone at the concentration used does not induce formation of endogenous diacylglycerol, nor does it cause release of serotonin. However, the Ca^{2+} ionophore alone at higher concentrations such as more than $5 \times 10^{-7} M$ causes a significant phosphorylation of the 40K protein in addition to the 20K protein, and also releases serotonin. This is probably due to the fact that a large increase in the Ca^{2+} concentration activates protein kinase C in the absence of diacylglycerol (see Fig. 4), and also induces nonspecific degradation of phospholipid to produce diacylglycerol. Likewise, the synthetic diacylglycerol alone at higher concentrations such as more than 50 μg/ml causes release of a significant amount of serotonin (Kaibuchi *et al.*, 1982a, 1983; Rink *et al.*, 1983). The exact reason of this enhanced release reaction is not known, but it is possible that the diacylglycerol or phosphatidic acid

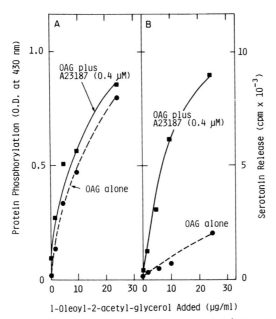

FIG. 16.   Synergistic effects of synthetic diacylglycerol and Ca^{2+} ionophore on serotonin release. Human platelets were labeled with either $^{32}P_i$ or [^{14}C]serotonin, and then stimulated by various amounts of 1-oleoyl-2-acetyl-glycerol in the presence or absence of A23187 (0.4 μM) as indicated. The phosphorylation of 40K protein (A) and release of serotonin (B) were quantitated under the conditions similar to those given in Fig. 9. Detailed experimental conditions were described elsewhere (Kaibuchi *et al.*, 1983). OAG, 1-Oleoyl-2-acetyl-glycerol.

therefrom may act as a membrane fusigen or a week Ca^{2+} ionophore as mentioned above. It is also alternatively possible that under limited conditions Ca^{2+} mobilization and protein phosphorylation are compensatory for each other to some extent. Nevertheless, the results outlined above indicate that the receptor-mediated protein phosphorylation and Ca^{2+} mobilization are equally essential and synergistically effective for causing a full physiological response (Kaibuchi *et al.*, 1982a, 1983). A similar result has been recently obtained for *N*-acetylglucosaminidase release from platelet lysosomes (Kajikawa *et al.*, 1983). At present, no direct evidence is available that 40K and 20K proteins are ultimately related to the release reactions, but it is obvious that Ca^{2+} and protein kinase C may each play diverse roles in this cellular response. It is possible, as suggested recently by Knight *et al.* (1982), that the proposed mechanism of signal transduction is probably responsible for the signal selectivity which

320 YASUTOMI NISHIZUKA ET AL.

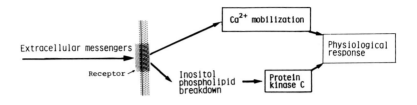

Cell system	Extracellular messenger	Physiological response
Platelets	Thrombin, Collagen, Platelet-activating factor	Serotonin release Lysosomal enzyme release
Mast cells	Concanavalin A plus PS	Histamine release
Neutrophils	Chemoattractant	Lysosomal enzyme release

FIG. 17. Synergistic effects of protein kinase C activation and Ca²⁺ mobilization in various cell types.

is observed for secretion of various constituents of different platelet granules.

The synergistic effects of protein kinase C activation and Ca²⁺ mobilization are also demonstrated for many other cell types exemplified in Fig. 17. In rat neutrophils the lysosomal enzyme release may also be observed in the presence of both synthetic diacylglycerol and A23187 (Kajikawa *et al.*, 1983). Similarly, the maximum release of histamine from rat mast cells is observed in the presence of both diacylglycerol and the Ca²⁺ ionophore, and none of these materials alone causes the full cellular response. The potential importance of protein kinase C has been recently suggested not only for various exocytotic processes but also for many other cellular functions. These include insulin release from rat pancreatic islets (Tanigawa *et al.*, 1982), catecholamine synthesis in cultured chromaffin cells (Raese *et al.*, 1979; Haycock *et al.*, 1982), various membrane processes of human neutrophils (Helfman *et al.*, 1983), contraction of smooth and heart muscles (Limas, 1980; Katoh *et al.*, 1981, 1983; Endo *et al.*, 1982), blastogenesis of lymphocytes (Ogawa *et al.*, 1981; Ku *et al.*, 1981), action of epidermal growth factor in A431 human epidermoid carcinoma cells (Sahai *et al.*, 1982), glycogenolysis in hepatocytes (Garrison, 1983), and neuronal functions (Zwier *et al.*, 1980; Takai *et al.*, 1982c; Kikkawa *et al.*, 1982), although the evidence for all of these proposals is not convincing at present. Nevertheless, it is highly possible that protein kinase C together with Ca²⁺ may play roles in the transmembrane control of various cellular functions and proliferation.

V. Inhibitors and Target Proteins for Phosphorylation

It has been described earlier (Mori *et al.*, 1980) that a large number of phospholipid-interacting drugs including local anesthetics and tranquilizers profoundly inhibit protein kinase C. For instance, trifluoperazine, chlorpromazine, dibucaine, imipramine, and many other drugs which are known as calmodulin inhibitors strongly inhibit the enzyme activation by competing with phospholipid (Mori *et al.*, 1980; Kuo *et al.*, 1980; Schatzman *et al.*, 1981). These drugs do not interact with the active site of the enzyme, since the catalytically active enzyme fragment that is obtained by limited proteolysis as described above is not susceptible to any of these drugs. Most drugs show affinity to acidic phospholipids, particularly phosphatidylserine and phosphatidylethanolamine (Seeman, 1972; Papahadjopoulos, 1977). Figure 18 shows that the thrombin-induced phosphorylation of the 40K protein in platelets is blocked almost completely by prior incubation with either dibucaine or chlorpromazine. Under these conditions the signal-induced breakdown of inositol phospholipid to produce diacylglycerol is not susceptible to these drugs (Sano *et al.*, 1983). It is also noted that the inhibition of phosphorylation of the 40K protein is more remarkable than that of phosphorylation of the 20K protein which is dependent on calmodulin. A quantitative analysis shown in Fig. 19 indicates that the *in vitro* as well as the *in vivo* phosphorylation reaction is progressively and profoundly inhibited in a parallel fashion by increasing concentrations of dibucaine and chlorpromazine (Takai *et al.*, 1981b). None of these drugs inhibits protein kinases A and G under comparable conditions. Thus, the experiments with calmodulin inhibitors do not distinguish the processes that are dependent on this particular Ca^{2+}-binding protein from those of protein kinase C-catalyzed reactions.

Recognition of phosphate acceptor proteins is one of the current problems of protein kinase C. When tested in cell-free systems, this enzyme shows a broad substrate specificity, and phosphorylates seryl and threonyl residues of many endogenous proteins, particularly those associated with membranes in most tissues. Protein kinases C and A often utilize same phosphate acceptor proteins, although the relative reaction velocities for various substrates greatly differ from one another (Nishizuka, 1980). For instance, both enzymes phosphorylate, to various extents, histone, protamine, myelin basic proteins, vinculin, microtubule-associated proteins, troponins, and many other nuclear, membrane as well as cytoskelton-associated proteins, although the physiological significance of these phosphorylation reactions is yet to be clarified. Analysis of the phosphorylation sites in some of these proteins has revealed that

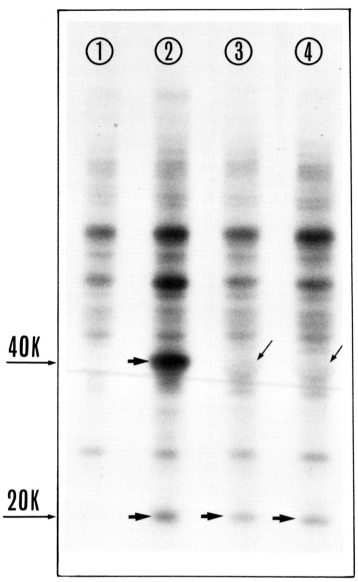

FIG. 18.   Selective inhibition of 40K protein phosphorylation by dibucaine and chlorpromazine. Human platelets were labeled with $^{32}P_i$, preincubated for 2 minutes at 37°C with
either dibucaine (2 mM) or chlorpromazine (0.5 mM), and then stimulated for another 1
minute with thrombin (0.2 unit/ml). The autoradiograph of the platelet proteins was prepared
under conditions similar to those given in Fig. 8. 1, Preincubated without drug and stimulated by saline; 2, preincubated without drug and stimulated by thrombin; 3, preincubated
with dibucaine and stimulated by thrombin; and 4, preincubated with chlorpromazine and
stimulated by thrombin. 40K, 40K protein; and 20K, 20K protein. (Adapted from Nishizuka
and Takai, 1981.)

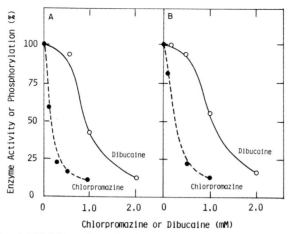

FIG. 19.   Parallel inhibition of protein phosphorylation *in vivo* and *in vitro* by dibucaine and chlorpromazine. In *in vitro* assay systems (A), protein kinase C was assayed with calf thymus H1 histone as a model phosphate acceptor in the presence of various concentrations of dibucaine or chlorpromazine. In *in vivo* assay systems (B), human platelets were labeled with $^{32}P_i$ and then stimulated by thrombin in the presence of various concentrations of dibucaine or chlorpromazine. The phosphorylation of 40K protein was quantitated under conditions similar to those given in Fig. 9. (Adapted from Takai *et al.*, 1981b.)

protein kinases C and A recognize each specific, but sometimes again same seryl and threonyl residues in common substrate proteins. For instance, for calf thymus H1 histone, protein kinase A phosphorylates the seryl residue (Ser-38) in the N-terminal portion, whereas protein kinase C preferentially phosphorylates the seryl and threonyl residues located near the C-terminal (Iwasa *et al.*, 1980). Obviously, as will be clarified soon below, protein kinases C and A may play distinctly different functions in physiological processes, but the precise nature of target proteins of protein kinase C in most tissues remains largely unexplored. It is noted that protein kinase C can phosphorylate itself, but the significance of this autophosphorylation is not known. The enzyme reacts with neither its own tyrosyl residues nor those in any phosphate acceptor proteins so far tested.

VI. Arachidonic Acid Release and Cyclic Nucleotides

Stimulation of the receptors that are related to inositol phospholipid turnover described above frequently releases arachidonic acid, and often increases cyclic GMP but not cyclic AMP (for reviews see Michell, 1975, 1979; Hawthorne and White, 1975). Thus, phospholipid degradation, Ca^{2+}

mobilization, arachidonic acid release, and cyclic GMP increase appear to be integrated together in a single receptor cascade system. Although Ca^{2+} sometimes causes direct activation of guanylate cyclase (for a review see Murad *et al.*, 1979), it is more likely that arachidonic acid peroxide and prostaglandin endoperoxide may serve as activators for this enzyme (Hidaka and Asano, 1977; Graff *et al.*, 1978).

It is generally accepted that the liberation of arachidonic acid from membrane phospholipids is rate-limiting, and that this reaction is regulated strictly by extracellular messengers. Arachidonic acid is shown to be derived from inositol phospholipids through two consecutive reactions catalyzed by phospholipase C followed by diacylglycerol lipase (Bell *et al.*, 1979; Rittenhouse-Simmons, 1980; Billah *et al.*, 1980). It is proposed that in platelets arachidonic acid may be released also from phosphatidic acid, which is derived from diacylglycerol, by its specific phospholipase A2 (Lapetina, 1982). However, inositol phospholipids appear to be relatively minor sources for arachidonic acid supply, although the pathways mentioned above specifically provide this unsaturated fatty acid. It seems clear that in many tissues a single extracellular messenger induces the activation of both phospholipase C and phospholipase A2 reactions and, as a result, causes release of arachidonic acid from various other phospholipids as well. One of the puzzles at present is that phospholipase A2 thus far found in mammalian tissues is not specific for arachidonic acyl moiety. A possibility has sometimes been discussed that the arachidonic acyl moiety of various other phospholipids is transferred selectively to lysophosphatidylinositol (Irvin and Dawson, 1979) or to lysophosphatidic acid (Lapetina, 1982) as schematically shown in Fig. 20, but the precise physiological picture remains unknown. Nevertheless, the receptor-linked breakdown of inositol phospholipids is at least one of the main pathways eventually leading to arachidonic acid release for prostaglandin synthesis.

It has been proposed for many years that cyclic GMP is a positive messenger for various hormones, neurotransmitters, growth factors, and other extracellular messengers (for a review see Goldberg and Haddox, 1977). However, it remains a problem that protein kinase G shows very similar, if not identical, catalytic properties to those of protein kinase A (Hashimoto *et al.*, 1976), and the role of cyclic GMP in cellular regulation has not yet been clarified. In human platelets this cyclic nucleotide has been suggested to be a negative rather than positive messenger to provide an immediate feedback control that prevents over-response as schematically given in Fig. 21 (Haslam *et al.*, 1980; Takai *et al.*, 1981a). This assumption is based primarily on the observation that sodium nitroprusside, a potent platelet inhibitor, markedly increases cyclic GMP. The

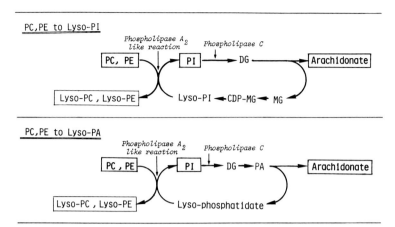

FIG. 20.   Hypothetical transarachidonyl pathways for arachidonic acid release from various membrane phospholipids. PC, Phosphatidylcholine; PE, phosphatidylethanolamine; PI, phosphatidylinositol; DG, diacylglycerol; MG, monoacylglycerol; and PA, phosphatidic acid.

experiment shown in Fig. 22 shows that both sodium nitroprusside and 8-bromo cyclic GMP block the thrombin-induced breakdown of inositol phospholipid to produce diacylglycerol as well as the phosphorylation of the 40K protein and release of serotonin in parallel ways (Takai *et al.*, 1981b, 1982c). Although sodium nitroprusside is known to increase cyclic AMP slightly, at most 2-fold, the observed inhibitory action of this compound may not be mediated by this slight increase in cyclic AMP. Sodium nitroprusside causes a marked increase in cyclic GMP, and concomitantly

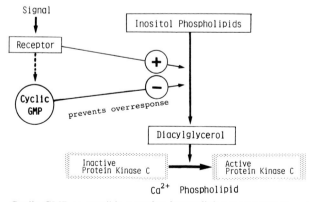

FIG. 21.   Cyclic GMP as possible negative intracellular messenger to prevent overresponse. (Adapted from Kaibuchi *et al.*, 1984.)

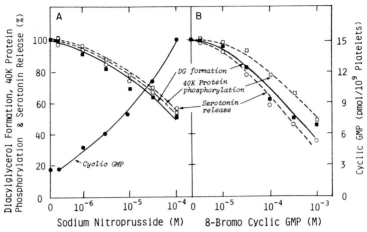

FIG. 22.   Inhibition of thrombin induced diacylglycerol formation, 40K protein phosphorylation, and serotonin release by sodium nitroprusside (A) and 8-bromo cyclic GMP (B). Human platelets were labeled with either [³H]arachidonic acid, ³²Pᵢ or [¹⁴C]serotonin, and then stimulated at 37°C by thrombin (0.2 unit/ml) in the presence of sodium nitroprusside or 8-bromo cyclic GMP as indicated under the conditions similar to those given in Fig. 9. Cyclic GMP was determined by radioimmunoassay. Detailed experimental conditions were described elsewhere (Takai et al., 1981a). DG, Diacylglycerol.

inhibits platelet activation under the conditions where cyclic AMP is not measurably increased. A similar inhibitory action of cyclic GMP on inositol phospholipid turnover is observed for rat aortic smooth muscle which is stimulated by norepinephrine (Nishizuka, 1983b). Schultz et al. (1977) have previously postulated that cyclic GMP may act as a negative messenger in smooth muscle as well, since sodium nitroprusside, nitroglycerol, and 8-bromo cyclic GMP all cause relaxation, although α-adrenergic and muscarinic cholinergic stimulators enhance cyclic GMP as well as inositol phospholipid breakdown upon contraction. Obviously, however, the proposed function of cyclic GMP described above does not necessarily exclude other possible roles of this cyclic nucleotide in biological regulation.

Although in receptor mechanisms there should be dramatic variations and heterogeneity from tissue to tissue, most tissues seem to possess at least two major classes of receptors as shown in Fig. 23. In *bidirectional control* systems in most tissues such as platelets, lymphocytes, neutrophils, and mast cells, the receptors that induce inositol phospholipid breakdown usually promote activation of cellular functions and proliferation, whereas the receptors that produce cyclic AMP normally antagonize such activation. In contrast, in *monodirectional control* systems in some

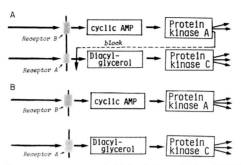

FIG. 23.   Two major receptor systems in biological regulation. (A) Bidirectional control; (B) monodirectional control.

tissues such as hepatocytes and adipocytes, the two receptors mentioned above do not appear to interact with each other but function independently. A quantitative analysis with platelets reveals that the thrombin-induced diacylglycerol formation, 40K protein phosphorylation, and serotonin release are all inhibited by prostaglandin E1, and that this inhibition appears to be proportional to the amount of cyclic AMP produced as shown in Fig. 24. Dibutyryl cyclic AMP reproduces this inhibitory action of prostaglandin E1 (Takai *et al.*, 1981b, 1982a,c). The interaction of the two receptors mentioned above is observed in many other *bidirectional control* systems. For instance, in human peripheral lymphocytes activated by a plant lectin as well as in rat neutrophils activated by a chemoattractant, the signal-induced inositol phospholipid turnover is blocked by dibutyryl cyclic AMP and prostaglandin E1 which markedly elevates cyclic AMP (Kaibuchi *et al.*, 1982b; Takai *et al.*, 1982c). In mast cells prostaglandin E1 inhibits inositol phospholipid turnover and histamine release simultaneously, which are induced by concanavalin A plus phosphatidylserine (Kennerly *et al.*, 1979a). However, the mechanism of this inhibition by cyclic nucleotides is not clear at present. It does not appear simply due to the phosphorylation of phospholipases. In platelets, the phosphorylation of the 40K protein that is induced by synthetic diacylglycerol mentioned above is not susceptible to cyclic AMP nor to cyclic GMP.

On the other hand, in hepatocytes it seems well established that glycogenolysis is enhanced by glucagon as well as by β-adrenergic stimulators through a cyclic AMP-dependent pathway. It is also well known that α-adrenergic stimulators, vasopressin and angiotensin II, equally induce glycogenolysis without any detectable increase in cyclic AMP levels and without protein kinase A activation (Scherline *et al.*, 1972; Keppens and De Wulf, 1975, 1976; Saitoh and Ui, 1976; Van de Werve *et al.*, 1977;

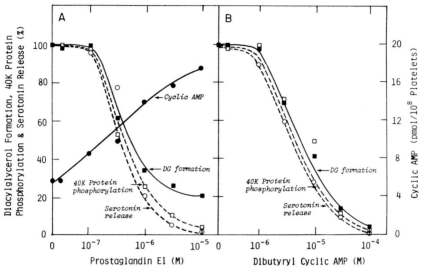

FIG. 24.   Inhibition of thrombin-induced diacylglycerol formation, 40K protein phosphorylation, and serotonin release by prostaglandin El (A) and dibutyryl cyclic AMP (B).
Human platelets were labeled with either [³H]arachidonic acid, ³²P_i or [¹⁴C]serotonin, and
then stimulated at 37°C by thrombin (0.2 unit/ml) in the presence of prostaglandin El or
dibutyryl cyclic AMP as indicated under conditions similar to those given in Fig. 9. Cyclic
AMP was determined by radioimmunoassay. Detailed experimental conditions were described elsewhere (Kawahara *et al.*, 1980). DG, Diacylglycerol. (Adapted from Takai *et al.*,
1982c.)

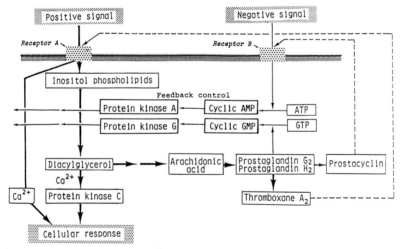

FIG. 25.   A proposed pathway of signal transduction. Platelets are used as a model
system. (Adapted from Nishizuka, 1983a.)

Birnbaum and Fain, 1977). The stimulation of the latter class of receptors is shown to provoke inositol phospholipid breakdown (Kirk *et al.,* 1979, 1981; Tolbert *et al.,* 1980), and a possible importance of protein kinase C in hepatic glycogenolysis has been very recently suggested (Garrison, 1983). However, in such a isolated hepatocyte system it is noted that the receptor-induced turnover of inositol phospholipid is not blocked by glucagon, β-adrenergic stimulators, nor by dibutyryl cyclic AMP (Kaibuchi *et al.,* 1982b).

Based on the discussions outlined above, it is attractive to suggest that cyclic AMP and cyclic GMP do not antagonize each other, but play integrated parts in the extra- and intracellular circuits, which lead eventually to feedback control of the receptor-linked phospholipid degradation, and perhaps also Ca^{2+} mobilization as well, as schematically given in Fig. 25.

VII. Hormone Action and Tumor Promotion

A potent tumor promoter, TPA first isolated from croton oil, elicits a variety of biological and biochemical responses very similar to those to hormones. In most cases Ca^{2+} is indispensable for such cellular responses, and a number of kinetic studies with various cell types suggest that the primary site of action of the tumor-promoting phorbol esters is located on cell surface membranes (for reviews see Van Duuren, 1969; Hecker, 1971; Boutwell, 1974; Weinstein *et al.,* 1979; Blumberg, 1980, 1981). Evidence recently provided from this laboratory has shown that the tumor promoter directly activates protein kinase C both *in vivo* and *in vitro,* and that this enzyme is most likely a receptive protein for tumor-promoting phorbol esters (Castagna *et al.,* 1982; Yamanishi *et al.,* 1983; Nishizuka, 1983a). This proposal has been immediately supported by Niedel *et al.* (1983), who have shown that a phorbol ester-binding protein may be purified together with protein kinase C from rat brain.

TPA has a diacylglycerol-like structure in its molecule as shown in Fig. 26. Thus, it is found that this tumor promoter can substitute for diacylglycerol and dramatically increases the affinity of protein kinase C for Ca^{2+} to the 10^{-7} M range, resulting in the full activation of this enzyme without significant mobilization of the divalent cation (Castagna *et al.,* 1982; Yamanishi *et al.,* 1983; Kikkawa *et al.,* 1983). A typical experiment given in Fig. 27 shows that TPA is active at extremely low concentrations, and that both Ca^{2+} and phospholipid are absolutely necessary for the enzyme activation. TPA alone shows practically no effect. A series of studies with a homogeneous preparation of protein kinase C indicates that [³H]phorbol-12,13-dibutyrate (PDBu), which is another potent tumor-promoting phorbol ester, may bind to the enzyme only in the presence of Ca^{2+} and

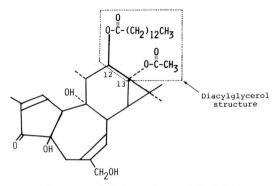

FIG. 26.   Structure of 12-O-tetradecanoylphorbol-13-acetate.

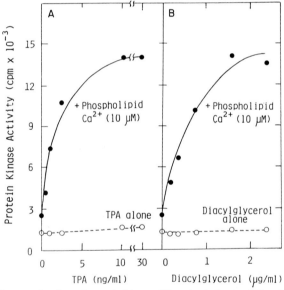

FIG. 27.   Direct activation of protein kinase C by phorbol ester (A) and diacylglycerol (B) in the presence of Ca^{2+} and phospholipid. Protein kinase C was assayed with calf thymus H1 histone as a model substrate. The reaction mixture (0.25 ml) contained 5 μmol of Tris/ HCl at pH 7.5, 2.5 nmol of $CaCl_2$, 1.25 μmol of magnesium nitrate, 2.5 nmol of [γ-^{32}P]ATP (1 $\times$ 10^5 cpm/nmol), 50 μg of histone, 5 μg of phospholipid, either TPA or diolein as indicated, and 0.5 μg of a purified preparation of rat brain protein kinase C. The incubation was carried out for 3 minutes at 30°C, and the acid-precipitable radioactivity was determined. Detailed experimental conditions were described elsewhere (Castagna *et al.*, 1982). (Adapted from Nishizuka, 1983a.)

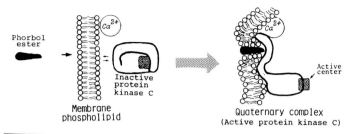

	Intact cell system	Cell-free system
Phorbol ester (PDBu)		
Binding constant (K_d)	6 - 10 nM	8 nM
Activation constant (K_a)	——	8 nM
Amount of receptor	12 pmol/mg brain	——
Amount of protein kinase C	——	16 pmol/mg brain

FIG. 28. Schematical representation of phorbol ester-binding and activation of protein kinase C. Kinetic values were obtained under the conditions described elsewhere (Kikkawa et al., 1983).

phospholipid (Kikkawa et al., 1983). This radioactive phorbol ester does not bind to protein kinase C nor to phospholipid per se irrespective of the presence and absence of Ca^{2+}, and all four components mentioned above are needed simultaneously for the binding as well as for the enzyme activation as schematically illustrated in Fig. 28. An apparent dissociation binding constant (K_d) of PDBu is estimated to be 8 nM, and this value is exactly identical with the activation constant (K_a) for the enzyme that is calculated to be 8 nM by Lineweaver–Burk double reciprocal plot. Consistent with these observations, Ashendel et al. (1983), Sando and Young (1983), Blumberg et al. (1983), and Shoyab and Boaze (1983) have recently reported that both Ca^{2+} and phospholipid are necessary for the binding of tumor promoter to its specific binding protein that is presumably protein kinase C.

It has been shown that various phorbol derivatives which show tumor-promoting activity are capable of activating protein kinase C in in vitro systems, and that the structural requirements of phorbol-related diterpenes for tumor promotion appear to be similar to those for protein kinase C activation (Castagna et al., 1982; Kikkawa et al., 1984b). It has been also reported that in intact cell systems TPA is a potent competitor for [3H]PDBu binding, whereas phorbol and 4α-phorbol-12,13-didecanoate which lack tumor-promoting activity do not inhibit the binding of [3H]PDBu (Shoyab and Todaro, 1980; Horowitz et al., 1981; Solanki and

TABLE V
Effects of Various Phorbol Derivatives on Activation of Protein Kinase C and
[³H]PDBu Binding[a]

Phorbol derivative added	Tumor-promoting activity	Activation of protein kinase C (%)	Inhibition of [³H]PDBu-binding (%)
TPA	+++	100	100
PDBu	++	88	100
Phorbol-12,13-didecanoate	++	81	100
Phorbol-12-tetradecanoate	−	0	18
Phorbol-13-acetate	−	0	0
4α-Phorbol-12,13-didecanoate	−	0	0
Phorbol	−	0	23

[a] Protein kinase C was assayed at 10 μM CaCl$_2$ in the presence of phospholipid (20 μg/ml) and various phorbol derivatives (10 ng/ml each) as indicated. Inhibition of [³H]PDBu binding to protein kinase C was assayed in the presence of a 100-fold excess of each nonradioactive phorbol derivative. Detailed experimental conditions were described elsewhere (Kikkawa *et al.*, 1983).

Slaga, 1981; Goodwin and Weinberg, 1982). Experiments in purified cell-free systems indicate, as given in Table V, that TPA, nonradioactive PDBu, and phorbol-12,13-didecanoate, which are all known as potent tumor promoters, equally compete with [³H]PDBu for the binding to the homogeneous enzyme, whereas phorbol derivatives having no tumor-promoting activity are all unable to activate protein kinase C nor to compete with [³H]PDBu for the binding. Diacylglycerols such as diolein compete with [³H]PDBu to produce the quaternary complex, whereas neither monoolein, triolein, nor free oleic acid is active in this capacity under similar conditions.

Scatchard analysis of the [³H]PDBu binding to a homogeneous preparation of protein kinase C reveals that, as shown in Fig. 29, approximately one molecule of the tumor-promoting phorbol ester binds to each molecule of protein kinase C in the presence of a physiological concentration of Ca^{2+} and apparently an excess of phospholipid (Kikkawa *et al.*, 1983). This stoichiometry does not necessarily indicate the binding of PDBu directly to the enzyme. Using a photoaffinity probe of the phorbol ester, Delclos *et al.* (1983) have suggested that the tumor-promoting diterpene interacts with phospholipid rather than with protein. Among various membrane phospholipids tested phosphatidylserine is most effective to support the binding, and relative activities of various phospholipids are nearly equal to those for this protein kinase activation described above.

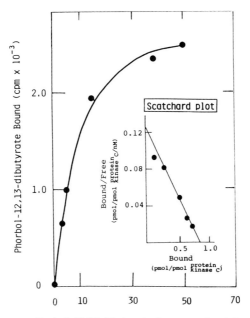

FIG. 29.   Binding of [³H]phorbol-12,13-dibutyrate to protein kinase C and its Scatchard analysis. A homogeneous preparation of protein kinase C was mixed with various concentrations of [³H]PDBu as indicated in the presence of Ca^{2+} and phospholipid. The radioactivity of [³H]PDBu bound was determined after gel filtration on a column equipped to a high-pressure liquid chromatograph. Detailed experimental conditions were described elsewhere. (Adapted from Kikkawa et al., 1984a.)

Presumably, tumor-promoting phorbol esters are intercalated into the membrane, and modify the microenvironment of phospholipid bilayer in such a way that protein kinase C recognizes this tiny change and tends to be fully activated to exhibit its apparently multifunctional catalytic activity. Kraft et al. (1982) have observed that, when TPA is added to intact cells, protein kinase C is indeed recovered in a form tightly associated with membrane fraction. These results obtained with tumor promoters may raise a possibility that, in hormone actions, one molecule of diacylglycerol which is produced from inositol phospholipids may activate one molecule of protein kinase C in a similar manner. If this is true, then it is possible to assume that, upon breakdown, phosphatidylinositol bisphosphate may provide an adequate amount of diacylglycerol to activate nearly all molecules of protein kinase C within the cell, even though this phospholipid is a very minor component in the membrane. However, it is difficult at present to prove the mechanism in which protein kinase C senses such a tiny change in the phospholipid bilayer. It may be added that mezerein, which is known as a "second stage" tumor promoter (Slaga *et al.*, 1980; Fürstenberger *et al.*, 1981), also activates protein kinase C at relatively higher concentrations (Kikkawa *et al.*, 1984b). Teleocidin, which is another type of potent tumor promoter structually unrelated to phorbol esters (Fujiki *et al.*, 1981), apparently has a potential to activate protein kinase C (Kume *et al.*, 1981). Presumably, these tumor promoters may cause analogous changes in membranes to activate protein kinase C.

The high-affinity binding site of tumor-promoting phorbol esters is distributed in many tissues and organs (Shoyab and Todaro, 1980; Shoyab *et al.*, 1981). This distribution pattern is apparently similar to that of protein kinase C, with brain tissue being richest in quantity. For instance, in rat brain homogenates 1 mg of protein binds approximately 12 pmol of [^{3}H]PDBu (Shoyab *et al.*, 1981). This value is roughly the same order of magnitude to the amount of protein kinase C in this tissue, that is estimated to be about 16 pmol/mg of protein in crude extract assuming the molecular weight as 77,000 with an overall purification of 800-fold (Kikkawa *et al.*, 1982) (see Fig. 28). It is also noted that the K_d value of PDBu mentioned above for the homogeneous preparation of protein kinase C is remarkably similar to the K_d value of 5.6 nM which has been described for the binding site in brain particulate fractions (Dunphy *et al.*, 1981), and also to the K_d values of 6–10 nM which are estimated for the specific binding sites located on intact cell membranes of rat embryo fibroblasts (Horowitz *et al.*, 1981) and mouse epidermal cells (Solanki and Slaga, 1981).

In another series of experiments tumor-promoting phorbol esters such as TPA and PDBu are shown to be intercalated into the membranes and ipso facto directly activate protein kinase C in intact cell systems in a manner similar to synthetic diacylglycerol described above (Castagna *et al.*, 1982; Yamanishi *et al.*, 1983; Kikkawa *et al.*, 1984b). For instance, when platelets are stimulated by TPA or PDBu, the 40K protein is rapidly and heavily phosphorylated as it is by natural extracellular messengers such as thrombin. Neither the breakdown of inositol phospholipids nor the formation of endogenous diacylglycerol is observed during the entire periods of stimulation. Fingerprint analysis of the radioactive 40K protein isolated from the platelets indicates that protein kinase C is indeed activated by the action of these tumor promoters. However, the activation of this protein kinase by tumor-promoting phorbol esters appears to be a prerequisite but not a sufficient requirement for causing full physiological responses in an analogous manner to that described for diacylglycerol. It is shown that TPA and A23187 act synergistically to cause full cellular responses such as release of serotonin (Yamanishi *et al.*, 1983). The tumor promoter alone at higher concentrations such as more than 30 ng/ml causes release of serotonin in a significant quantity (Castagna *et al.*, 1982). The reason of this enhanced release is not known, but it is possible that the phorbol ester at higher concentrations may act as a membrane perturber or weak Ca^{2+} ionophore by generating superoxide.

Based on several lines of evidence described above, it is reasonable to propose that protein kinase C is a receptive protein of tumor-promoting phorbol esters, and that pleiotropic actions of the tumor promoters, if not all, may be mediated through the action of protein kinase C. It seems obvious that this unique protein kinase may fulfill the requirements for a receptor eventually leading to activation of cellular functions and proliferation. In the experiment given in Fig. 30, it is clear that neither cyclic AMP nor cyclic GMP blocks the TPA-induced activation of protein kinase C in intact platelets, although both cyclic nucleotides are inhibitory for the thrombin-induced activation of this protein kinase as described above. Perhaps, the tumor-promoting phorbol esters stay in membranes

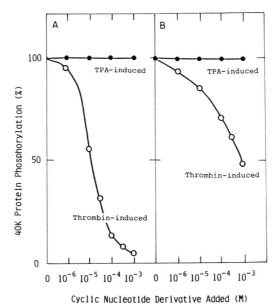

FIG. 30.   Effects of dibutyryl cyclic AMP (A) and 8-bromo cyclic GMP (B) on protein kinase C activation by natural messenger and phorbol ester. Human platelets were labeled with $^{32}P_i$, and then stimulated by either thrombin or TPA in the presence of various concentrations of dibutyryl cyclic AMP or 8-bromo cyclic GMP under conditions similar to those given in Figs. 22 and 24. Detailed experimental conditions were described elsewhere. (Adapted from Yamanishi *et al.*, 1983.)

for prolonged periods of time since the diterpenes are hardly metaboliz-able. It is possible that under these circumstances the cell tends to func-tion and proliferate when Ca^{2+} is available, because protein kinase C is always active despite the feedback control of cyclic nucleotides. In con-trast, in hormone action, diacylglycerol is produced only transiently and disappears quickly when cell surface receptors are stimulated.

VIII. Coda and Conclusion

Although the experimental support outlined in this article has resulted from studies with a limited number of specific tissues such as platelets, it is highly suggestive that the signal-induced turnover of inositol phospho-lipids is a sign of the transmembrane control of cellular functions and proliferation through activation of a novel protein kinase, that is protein kinase C. Diacylglycerol that is transiently produced from inositol phos-pholipids in membranes is crucially important for this enzyme activation. The stimulation of these receptors normally causes an immediate mobili-zation of Ca^{2+}. A series of studies with synthetic diacylglycerol and Ca^{2+} ionophore suggests that this receptor-linked protein kinase C activation and Ca^{2+} mobilization are both essential, and synergistically effective for causing full cellular responses. Obviously, protein kinase C and Ca^{2+} each play diverse roles in the biological regulation, and the precise targets of protein kinase C as well as those of Ca^{2+} in many tissues will be clarified by further investigations. It is noted that inositol trisphosphate, which is one of the products of phosphatidylinositol bisphosphate cleavage, is re-cently proposed to be a possible candidate for the intracellular mediator of Ca^{2+} mobilization, but the physiological picture remains to be clarified.

In most tissues such as platelets, cyclic AMP appears to inhibit strongly this receptor-linked whole cascade as schematically shown in Fig. 31. However, the detailed mechanism of this inhibitory action is totally un-known at present. Cyclic GMP, which is frequently increased by stimula-tion of the receptors, also serves as a negative rather than a positive intracellular messenger, providing a feedback control that prevents an overresponse. This proposed function may not necessarily exclude other functions of this cyclic nucleotide. The present article indicates that pro-tein kinase C is a possible receptor protein of tumor-promoting phorbol esters. The evidence available to date strongly suggests that pleiotropic hormone-like actions of tumor promoters, if not all, may be mediated through activation of this enzyme. It seems possible to conclude that protein kinase C may be located on the crossover point of various path-ways to exploring the roles of Ca^{2+}, inositol phospholipid turnover,

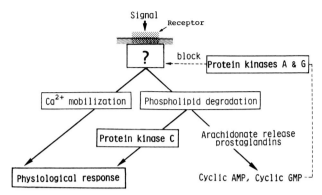

FIG. 31.   A receptor-linked cascade and feedback control by cyclic nucleotides.

arachidonic acid, prostaglandins, cyclic nucleotides, as well as phorbol esters in hormone action and tumor promotion. The underlying principles and mechanisms outlined in this article may be modified by the sum of the individual pieces of knowledge that will accumulate rapidly in the next few years.

ACKNOWLEDGMENTS

This article is a part of the lecture presented at the Laurentian Hormone Conference at Mont Tremblant on August 28–September 2, 1983. The author (N.Y.) wishes to express deep gratitude to Dr. Roy O. Greep and the program committee for the invitation to this conference. The authors also express indebtedness to their collaborators present and past who have so efficiently and actively carried out the experiments presented in this article. The authors are particularly grateful to Drs. K. Sano, K. Nishiyama, J. Yamanishi, M. Castagna, N. Kajikawa, K. Hirasawa, M. Sawamura, R. Miyake, Y. Katakami, Y. Yasue-Uratsuji, Y. Takeyama, Y. Tanaka, H. Nakanishi, and T. Tsuda. The skillful secretarial assistance of Mrs. S. Nishiyama, Mrs. K. Kikkawa, and Miss T. Kamiya is also greatly acknowledged. This investigation has been supported in part by research grants from the Scientific Research Fund of the Ministry of Education, Science and Culture; the Intractable Diseases Division, Public Health Bureau, the Ministry of Health and Welfare; a Grant-in-Aid of New Drug Development from the Ministry of Health and Welfare; the Science and Technology Agency; and the Yamanouchi Foundation for Research on Metabolic Disorders.

REFERENCES

Agranoff, B. W., Murthy, P., and Seguin, E. B. (1983). *J. Biol. Chem.* **258,** 2076.

Allan, D., and Michell, R. H. (1975). *Nature (London)* **258,** 348.

Ashendel, C. L., Staller, J. M., and Boutwell, R. K. (1983). *Biochem. Biophys. Res. Commun.* **111,** 340.

Banschbach, M. W., Geison, R. L., and Hokin-Neaverson, M. (1974). *Biochem. Biophys. Res. Commun.* **58,** 714.

Bell, R. L., and Majerus, P. W. (1980). *J. Biol. Chem.* **255**, 1790.
Bell, R. L., Kennerly, D. A., Stanford, N., and Majerus, P. W. (1979). *Proc. Natl. Acad. Sci. U.S.A.* **76**, 3238.
Berridge, M. J. (1982). *Cell Calcium* **3**, 385.
Billah, M. M., Lapetina, E. G., and Cuatrecasas, P. (1980). *J. Biol. Chem.* **255**, 10227.
Birnbaum, M. J., and Fain, J. N. (1977). *J. Biol. Chem.* **252**, 528.
Blumberg, P. M. (1980). *CRC Crit. Rev. Toxicol.* **8**, 153.
Blumberg, P. M. (1981). *CRC Crit. Rev. Toxicol.* **8**, 199.
Blumberg, P. M., Jaken, S., Jeng, A. Y., Konig, B., Leach, K. L., Sharkey, N. A., and Yeh, E. (1983). *Abstr. of Cold Spring Harbor Conf. Cell Prolif. Cancer, 11th* p. 76.
Boutwell, R. K. (1974). *CRC Crit. Rev. Toxicol.* **2**, 419.
Castagna, M., Takai, Y., Kaibuchi, K., Sano, K., Kikkawa, U., and Nishizuka, Y. (1982). *J. Biol. Chem.* **257**, 7847.
Dawson, R. M. C. (1954). *Biochim. Biophys. Acta* **14**, 374.
Dawson, R. M. C., Freinkel, N., Jungalwala, F. B., and Clarke, N. (1971). *Biochem. J.* **122**, 605.
Delclos, K. B., Yeh, E., and Blumberg, P. M. (1983). *Proc. Natl. Acad. Sci. U.S.A.* **80**, 3054.
Dunphy, W. G., Kochenburger, R. J., Castagna, M., and Blumberg, P. M. (1981). *Cancer Res.* **41**, 2640.
Endo, T., Naka, M., and Hidaka, H. (1982). *Biochem. Biophys. Res. Commun.* **105**, 942.
Fujiki, H., Mori, M., Nakayasu, M., Terada, M., Sugimura, T., and Moore, R. E. (1981). *Proc. Natl. Acad. Sci. U.S.A.* **78**, 3872.
Fürstenberger, G., Berry, D. L., Sorg, B., and Marks, F. (1981). *Proc. Natl. Acad. Sci. U.S.A.* **78**, 7722.
Garrison, J. C. (1983). *In* "Isolation, Characterization, and Use of Hepatocytes" (R. A. Harris and N. W. Cornell, eds.), p. 551–559. Elsevier, Amsterdam.
Gil, M. G., Alonso, F., Chiva, V. A., Crespo, M. S., and Mato, J. M. (1982). *Biochem. J.* **206**, 67.
Goldberg, N. D., and Haddox, M. K. (1977). *Annu. Rev. Biochem.* **46**, 823.
Goodwin, B. J., and Weinberg, J. B. (1982). *J. Clin. Invest.* **70**, 699.
Graff, G., Stephenson, J. H., Glass, D. B., Haddox, M. K., and Goldberg, M. D. (1978). *J. Biol. Chem.* **253**, 7662.
Habenicht, A. J. R., Glomset, J. A., King, W. C., Nist, C., Mitchell, C. D., and Ross, R. (1981). *J. Biol. Chem.* **256**, 12329.
Hasegawa-Sasaki, H., and Sasaki, T. (1982). *J. Biochem.* **91**, 463.
Hashimoto, E., Takeda, M., Nishizuka, Y., Hamana, K., and Iwai, K. (1976). *J. Biol. Chem.* **251**, 6287.
Haslam, R. J., and Lynham, J. A. (1977). *Biochem. Biophys. Res. Commun.* **77**, 714.
Haslam, R. J., Salam, S. E., Fox, J. E. B., Lynham, J. A., and Davidson, M. M. L. (1980). *In* "Cellular Response Mechanisms and Their Biological Significance" (A. Rottman, F. A. Meyer, C. Gilter, and A. Silberberg, eds.), pp. 213–231. Wiley, New York.
Hathaway, D. R., and Adelstein, R. S. (1979). *Proc. Natl. Acad. Sci. U.S.A.* **76**, 1653.
Hawthorne, J. N., and White, D. A. (1975). *Vitam. Horm.* **33**, 529.
Haycock, J. W., Meligeni, J. A., Bennett, W. F., and Waymire, J. C. (1982). *J. Biol. Chem.* **257**, 12641.
Hecker, E. (1971). *Methods Cancer Res.* **6**, 439.
Helfman, D. M., Appelbaum, B. D., Vogler, W. R., and Kuo, J. F. (1983). *Biochem. Biophys. Res. Commun.* **111**, 847.
Hidaka, H., and Asano, T. (1977). *Proc. Natl. Acad. Sci. U.S.A.* **74**, 3657.

Hokin, M. R., and Hokin, L. E. (1953). *J. Biol. Chem.* **203**, 967.

Holub, B. J., Kuksis, A., and Thompson, W. (1970). *J. Lipid Res.* **11**, 558.

Hong, S. L., and Deykin, D. (1982). *J. Biol. Chem.* **257**, 7151.

Horowitz, A. D., Greenebaum, E., and Weinstein, I. B. (1981). *Proc. Natl. Acad. Sci. U.S.A.* **78**, 2315.

Ieyasu, H., Takai, Y., Kaibuchi, K., Sawamura, M., and Nishizuka, Y. (1982). *Biochem. Biophys. Res. Commun.* **108**, 1701.

Igarashi, Y., and Kondo, Y. (1980). *Biochem. Biophys. Res. Commun.* **97**, 759.

Imai, A., Nakashima, S., and Nozawa, Y. (1983). *Biochem. Biophys. Res. Commun.* **110**, 108.

Inoue, M., Kishimoto, A., Takai, Y., and Nishizuka, Y. (1977). *J. Biol. Chem.* **252**, 7610.

Irvin, R. G., and Dawson, R. M. C. (1979). *Biochem. Biophys. Res. Commun.* **91**, 1399.

Iwasa, Y., Takai, Y., Kikkawa, U., and Nishizuka, Y. (1980). *Biochem. Biophys. Res. Commun.* **96**, 180.

Kaibuchi, K., Takai, Y., and Nishizuka, Y. (1981). *J. Biol. Chem.* **256**, 7146.

Kaibuchi, K., Sano, K., Hoshijima, M., Takai, Y., and Nishizuka, Y. (1982a). *Cell Calcium* **3**, 323.

Kaibuchi, K., Takai, Y., Ogawa, Y., Kimura, S., Nishizuka, Y., Nakamura, T., Tomomura, A., and Ichihara, A. (1982b). *Biochem. Biophys. Res. Commun.* **104**, 105.

Kaibuchi, K., Takai, Y., Sawamura, M., Hoshijima, M., Fujikura, T., and Nishizuka, Y. (1983). *J. Biol. Chem.* **258**, 6701.

Kaibuchi, K., Kikkawa, U., Takai, Y., and Nishizuka, Y. (1984). *In* "Enzyme Regulation by Reversible Phosphorylation Further Advances" (P. Cohen, ed.). Elsevier, Amsterdam, in press.

Kajikawa, N., Kaibuchi, K., Matsubara, T., Kikkawa, U., Takai, Y., Nishizuka, Y., Itoh, K., and Tomioka, T. (1983). *Biochem. Biophys. Res. Commun.* **116**, 743.

Katoh, N., Wrenn, R. W., Wise, B. C., Shoji, M., and Kuo, J. F. (1981). *Proc. Natl. Acad. Sci. U.S.A.* **78**, 4813.

Katoh, N., Wise, B. C., and Kuo, J. F. (1983). *Biochem. J.* **209**, 189.

Kawahara, Y., Takai, Y., Minakuchi, R., Sano, K., and Nishizuka, Y. (1980). *Biochem. Biophys. Res. Commun.* **97**, 309.

Kennerly, D. A., Secosan, C. J., Parker, C. W., and Sullivan, T. J. (1979a). *J. Immunol.* **123**, 1519.

Kennerly, D. A., Sullivan, T. J., Sylwester, P., and Parker, C. W. (1979b). *J. Exp. Med.* **150**, 1039.

Keppens, S., and De Wulf, H. (1975). *FEBS Lett.* **51**, 29.

Keppens, S., and De Wulf, H. (1976). *FEBS Lett.* **68**, 279.

Kikkawa, U., Takai, Y., Minakuchi, R., Inohara, S., and Nishizuka, Y. (1982). *J. Biol. Chem.* **257**, 13341.

Kikkawa, U., Takai, Y., Tanaka, Y., Miyake, R., and Nishizuka, Y. (1983). *J. Biol. Chem.* **258**, 11442.

Kikkawa, U., Kaibuchi, K., Castagna, M., Yamanishi, J., Sano, K., Tanaka, Y., Miyake, R., Takai, Y., and Nishizuka, Y. (1984a). *Adv. Cyclic Nucleotide Res.*, in press.

Kikkawa, U., Miyake, R., Tanaka, Y., Takai, Y., and Nishizuka, Y. (1984b). *Cold Spring Harbor Conf. Cell Prolif. Cancer*, in press.

Kirk, C. J. (1982). *Cell Calcium* **3**, 399.

Kirk, C. J., Rodrigus, L. M., and Hems, D. A. (1979). *Biochem. J.* **178**, 493.

Kirk, C. J., Michell, R. H., and Hems, D. A. (1981). *Biochem. J.* **194**, 155.

Kishimoto, A., Takai, Y., and Nishizuka, Y. (1977). *J. Biol. Chem.* **252**, 7449.

Kishimoto, A., Takai, Y., Mori, T., Kikkawa, U., and Nishizuka, Y. (1980). *J. Biol. Chem.* **255**, 2273.

Kishimoto, A., Kajikawa, N., Tabuchi, H., Shiota, M., and Nishizuka, Y. (1981). *J. Biochem.* **90**, 889.

Kishimoto, A., Kajikawa, N., Shiota, M., and Nishizuka, Y. (1983). *J. Biol. Chem.* **258**, 1156.

Knight, D. E., Hallam, T. J., and Scrutton, M. C. (1982). *Nature (London)* **296**, 256.

Kraft, A. S., Anderson, W. B., Cooper, H. L., and Sando, J. J. (1982). *J. Biol. Chem.* **257**, 13193.

Ku, Y., Kishimoto, A., Takai, Y., Ogawa, Y., Kimura, S., and Nishizuka, Y. (1981). *J. Immunol.* **127**, 1375.

Kume, S., Yamanaka, M., Kaneko, Y., Kariya, T., Hashimoto, Y., Tanabe, A., Ohashi, T., and Oda, T. (1981). *Biochem. Biophys. Res. Commun.* **102**, 659.

Kuo, J. F., Anderson, R. G. G., Wise, B. C., Mackerlova, L., Salomonsson, I., Brackett, N. L., Katoh, N., Shoji, M., and Wrenn, R. W. (1980). *Proc. Natl. Acad. Sci. U.S.A.* **77**, 7039.

Lapetina, E. G. (1982). *Trends Pharmacol. Sci.* **3**, 115.

Leach, K. L., James, M. L., and Blumberg, P. M. (1983). *Proc. Natl. Acad. Sci. U.S.A.* **80**, 4208.

Limas, C. J. (1980). *Biochem. Biophys. Res. Commun.* **96**, 1378.

Lyons, R. M., Stanford, N., and Majerus, P. W. (1975). *J. Clin. Invest.* **56**, 924.

Mellgren, R. L. (1980). *FEBS Lett.* **109**, 129.

Michell, R. H. (1975). *Biochim. Biophys. Acta* **415**, 81.

Michell, R. H. (1979). *Trends Biochem. Sci.* **4**, 128.

Michell, R. H. (1982). *Cell Calcium* **3**, 285.

Michell, R. H., Jafferji, S. S., and Jones, J. M. (1977). *In* "Function and Biosynthesis of Lipids" (N. G. Bazan, R. R. Brenner, and N. M. Giusto, eds.), pp. 447–464. Plenum, New York.

Minakuchi, R., Takai, Y., Yu, B., and Nishizuka, Y. (1981). *J. Biochem.* **89**, 1651.

Mori, T., Takai, Y., Minakuchi, R., Yu, B., and Nishizuka, Y. (1980). *J. Biol. Chem.* **255**, 8378.

Mori, T., Takai, Y., Yu, B., Takahashi, J., Nishizuka, Y., and Fujikura, T. (1982). *J. Biochem.* **91**, 427.

Murachi, T. (1983). *Trends Biochem. Sci.* **8**, 167.

Murachi, T., Tanaka, K., Hatanaka, M., and Murakami, T. (1981). *Adv. Enzyme Regul.* **19**, 407.

Murad, F., Arnold, W. P., Mittal, C. K., and Braughler, J. M. (1979). *Adv. Cyclic Nucleotide Res.* **11**, 175.

Niedel, J. E., Kuhn, L. J., and Vandenbark, G. R. (1983). *Proc. Natl. Acad. Sci. U.S.A.* **80**, 36.

Nishizuka, Y. (1980). *Mol. Biol. Biochem. Biophys.* **32**, 113.

Nishizuka, Y. (1983a). *Trends Biochem. Sci.* **8**, 13.

Nishizuka, Y. (1983b). *Philos. Trans. R. Soc. London Ser. B* **302**, 101.

Nishizuka, Y., and Takai, Y. (1981). *Cold Spring Harbor Conf. Cell Prolif.* **8**, 238.

Nishizuka, Y., Takai, Y., Hashimoto, E., Kishimoto, A., Kuroda, Y., Sakai, K., and Yamamura, H. (1979). *Mol. Cell. Biochem.* **23**, 153.

Ogawa, Y., Takai, Y., Kawahara, Y., Kimura, S., and Nishizuka, Y. (1981). *J. Immunol.* **127**, 1369.

Papahadjopoulos, D. (1977). *Biochim. Biophys. Acta* **265**, 169.

Raese, J. E., Edelman, A. M., Makk, G., Bruckwick, E. A., Lovenberg, W., and Barchas, J. D. (1979). *Commun. Psychopharmacol.* **3**, 295.

Rink, T. J., Sanchez, A., and Hallam, T. J. (1983). *Nature (London)* **305**, 317.

Rittenhouse-Simmons, S. (1979). *J. Clin. Invest.* **63**, 580.

Rittenhouse-Simmons, S. (1980). *J. Biol. Chem.* **255**, 2259.
Sahai, A., Smith, K. B., Panneersalvam, M., and Salomon, D. S. (1982). *Biochem. Biophys. Res. Commun.* **109**, 1206.
Saitoh, Y., and Ui, M. (1976). *Biochem. Pharmacol.* **25**, 841.
Sando, J. J., and Young, M. C. (1983). *Proc. Natl. Acad. Sci. U.S.A.* **80**, 2642.
Sano, K., Takai, Y., Yamanishi, J., and Nishizuka, Y. (1983). *J. Biol. Chem.* **258**, 2010.
Schatzman, R. C., Wise, B. C., and Kuo, J. F. (1981). *Biochem. Biophys. Res. Commun.* **98**, 669.
Schatzman, R. C., Raynor, R. L., Fritz, R. B., and Kuo, J. F. (1983). *Biochem. J.* **209**, 435.
Scherline, P., Lynch, A., and Glinsmann, W. H. (1972). *Endocrinology* **91**, 680.
Schultz, K.-D., Schultz, K., and Schultz, G. (1977). *Nature (London)* **265**, 750.
Seeman, P. (1972). *Pharmacol. Rev.* **24**, 583.
Serhan, C., Anderson, P., Goodman, E., Dunham, P., and Weissmann, G. (1981). *J. Biol. Chem.* **256**, 2736.
Shoyab, M., and Boaze, R., Jr. (1983). *Abstr. Cold Spring Harbor Conf. Cell Prolif. Cancer, 11th* p. 77.
Shoyab, M., and Todaro, G. J. (1980). *Nature (London)* **288**, 451.
Shoyab, M., Warren, T. C., and Todaro, G. J. (1981). *Carcinogenesis* **2**, 1273.
Slaga, T. J., Fischer, S. M., Nelson, K., and Gleason, G. L. (1980). *Proc. Natl. Acad. Sci. U.S.A.* **77**, 3659.
Solanki, V., and Slaga, T. J. (1981). *Proc. Natl. Acad. Sci. U.S.A.* **78**, 2549.
Streb, H., Irvin, R. E., Berridge, M. J., and Schultz, I. (1983). *Nature (London)* **306**, 67.
Suzuki, K., Tsuji, S., Ishiura, S., Kimura, Y., Kubota, S., and Imahori, K. (1981). *J. Biochem.* **90**, 1787.
Takai, Y., Kishimoto, A., Inoue, M., and Nishizuka, Y. (1977). *J. Biol. Chem.* **252**, 7603.
Takai, Y., Kishimoto, A., Iwasa, Y., Kawahara, Y., Mori, T., and Nishizuka, Y. (1979a). *J. Biol. Chem.* **254**, 3692.
Takai, Y., Kishimoto, A., Kikkawa, U., Mori, T., and Nishizuka, Y. (1979b). *Biochem. Biophys. Res. Commun.* **91**, 1218.
Takai, Y., Kaibuchi, K., Matsubara, T., and Nishizuka, Y. (1981a). *Biochem. Biophys. Res. Commun.* **101**, 61.
Takai, Y., Kishimoto, A., Kawahara, Y., Minakuchi, R., Sano, K., Kikkawa, U., Mori, T., Yu, B., Kaibuchi, K., and Nishizuka, Y. (1981b). *Adv. Cyclic Nucleotide Res.* **14**, 301.
Takai, Y., Kaibuchi, K., Sano, K., and Nishizuka, Y. (1982a). *J. Biochem.* **91**, 403.
Takai, Y., Kishimoto, A., and Nishizuka, Y. (1982b). *In* "Calcium and Cell Function" (W. Y. Cheung, ed.), Vol. II, pp. 386–412. Academic Press, New York.
Takai, Y., Minakuchi, R., Kikkawa, U., Sano, K., Kaibuchi, K., Yu, B., Matsubara, T., and Nishizuka, Y. (1982c). *Prog. Brain Res.* **56**, 277.
Tanigawa, K., Kuzuya, H., Imura, H., Taniguchi, H., Baba, S., Takai, Y., and Nishizuka, Y. (1982). *FEBS Lett.* **138**, 183.
Tolbert, M. E. M., White, A. C., Aspry, K., Cutts, J., and Fain, J. N. (1980). *J. Biol. Chem.* **255**, 1938.
Tyson, C. A., Van de Zande, H., and Green, D. E. (1976). *J. Biol. Chem.* **251**, 1326.
Van de Werve, G., Hue, L., and Hers, H. G. (1977). *Biochem. J.* **162**, 135.
Van Duuren, B. L. (1969). *Prog. Exp. Tumor Res.* **11**, 31.
Weinstein, I. B., Lee, L. S., Mufson, A., and Yamasaki, H. (1979). *J. Supramol. Struct.* **12**, 195.
Yamanishi, J., Takai, Y., Kaibuchi, K., Sano, K., Castagna, M., and Nishizuka, Y. (1983). *Biochem. Biophys. Res. Commun.* **112**, 778.
Zwier, H., Schotman, P., and Gispen, W. H. (1980). *J. Neurochem.* **34**, 1689.

DISCUSSION

B. Posner: This was a very lovely talk Dr. Nishizuka. Just a few questions if I may. Does diacylglycerol alone produce the same degree of phosphorylation of the 40K subprotein as seen with thrombin? You presented the data as percentage maximum and I am not sure whether the percentage maximum value is the same for each condition.

Y. Nishizuka: Yes, it does. The apparent reaction rate depends on the concentration of the diacylglycerol added.

B. Posner: Do you also see serotomin release with the calcium ionophore itself?

Y. Nishizuka: At higher concentrations, the Ca^{2+} ionophore alone mobilizes a large amount of Ca^{2+} and causes by itself phospholipid breakdown to produce diacylglycerol probably due to activation of phospholipase C. In addition, a large increase in Ca^{2+} can activate protein kinase C to some extent in the absence of diacylglycerol. Thus, both 40K and 20K proteins are phosphorylated and serotonion is released.

B. Posner: But at the lower concentration of your calcium ionophore where you did not see much 40K phosphorylation I gather you do not see serotonin release.

Y. Nishizuka: No, at lower concentrations of the Ca^{2+} ionophore serotonin is not sufficiently released, although the 20K protein is substantially phosphorylated.

M. R. Clark: I wonder if you might comment relative to your concluding statements on the variety of different observations that might be made, particularly on slightly different details of the cyclic GMP and cyclic AMP interaction with PI turnover. John Davis and I have observed with rat granulosa cells that LH as well as some other substances, can stimulate both phospholipid turnover and cyclic GMP decrease rapidly, as well as increases in cyclic AMP, and some of these features seem to be not necessarily at odds but slightly different than the general hypothesis that you proposed.

Y. Nishizuka: How rapid is the cyclic GMP decrease in your system? Perhaps the time course is very important.

M. R. Clark: In particular, could you comment further on the role of cyclic GMP, as well as the potential that something that can activate cyclic AMP extremely well might also activate phospholipid turnover.

Y. Nishizuka: It is possible that your cells belong to the class of monodirectional control systems, where the two receptors function independently. In bidirectional control systems in many tissues so far examined, cyclic AMP strongly inhibits the signal-dependent breakdown of phospholipid. But, we do not have enough data to discuss whether the proposed role of cyclic GMP may be generalized for many other tissues. It is of course possible that cyclic GMP may have other functions.

M. R. Clark: So you think that perhaps increased cyclic GMP is not so tightly coupled to activation of phospholipid turnover?

Y. Nishizuka: Yes, that is my impression. We do not know as yet the precise mechanism and signal pathway to increase GMP. Also, the mechanism of inhibitory action of cyclic AMP is totally unknown.

M. P. Czech: Have you considered the possibility that natural, heretofore unidentified, lipids might be potent activators of protein kinase C? Also, do you think that the movement of protein kinase C activity from one cellular locus to another in response to stimulant might be as important or more important in cellular signaling than the kinase activation process itself?

Y. Nishizuka: Well, this is a very good point. But I do not expect that some other hitherto unidentified natural ligand may be involved as a real activator of this enzyme, because diacylglycerol is extremely insoluble in water. Thus, the amount exogenously added does not necessarily represent the efficiency of the diacylglycerol that is generated *in* *situ* from inositol phospholipids in membranes. To your second point, we do not have any evidence indicating that the substrate is activated. A large number of endogenous substrates are apparently located in membranes. Under physiological conditions the inositol phospholipid is broken down not only in plasma membranes but in many other endoplasmic membranes. It is possible that this enzyme may be activated instantaneously within the cell. If cells are treated with phorbol esters, the enzyme is mostly attached to membranes to become active within a few minutes.

M. R. Clark: In an earlier slide that you presented, you showed the ratio of protein kinase C activity to cyclic AMP-dependent protein kinase activity. If those are the measurements that you have published, they were made under conditions which are optimum for the protein kinase C activity. I wonder, since you have some idea of how much protein kinase C mass is present per milligram of brain tissue, if in fact on that basis or perhaps under optimum conditions for the two different kinases, you can comment on the ratio of protein kinase A to C in various tissues, if you have looked at this.

Y. Nishizuka: At this time it is difficult to tell. We have not compared the net amounts of these two enzymes. One of the slides which I showed you indicated the relative activities of these enzymes with calf thymus H1 histone as a common phosphate acceptor. But, the sites phosphorylated by these enzymes in this histone molecule are different, and the values do not necessarily indicate the relative amounts of protein kinases C and A. Nevertheless, on the basis of the molecular weights and purification folds, I suspect that in some tissues such as brain the amount of protein kinase C may be at least several times much higher than that of protein kinase A. A particularly interesting point is that in brain tissues approximately one-half of the total activity of protein kinase C is tightly associated with synaptic membranes. Thus, association with membranes does not necessarily indicate the enzyme activation, but implies in brain its functions in neuronal transmission.

L. J. Grandison: In your model binding of a ligand to its plasma membrane receptor causes protein kinase C to phosphorylate a 40,000 molecular weight protein. As part of a negative feedback control, you suggest that arachidonic acid may be released and converted into a metabolite which stimulates cyclic GMP or cyclic AMP accumulation. These cyclic nucleotides then inhibit further phosphorylation. You have shown that administration of exogenous cyclic AMP or cyclic GMP will inhibit phosphorylation of the 40,000 molecular weight protein. Have you examined whether blockade of arachidonic acid release or inhibition of arachidonic acid metabolism will enhance phosphorylation of the 40,000 molecular weight protein in response to a receptor ligand?

Y. Nishizuka: No, we have not done such an experiment.

R. Chatterton: You measured the dissociation constant of the phorbol esters for the purified protein kinase C. Do you also have a value to the dissociation constant of your synthetic diglycerides?

Y. Nishizuka: Well, this is a good point. Perhaps, I have not mentioned that diacylglycerol competes with phorbol esters for binding to protein kinase C. At present I wish to reserve any description of its dissociation constant because diacylglycerol is very insoluble. It is difficult to measure its accurate dissociation constant.

R. Chatterton: Is that a possible explanation for the higher concentrations of diglyceride required?

Y. Nishizuka: Yes, I think so. Experimentally, a little more than 100-times higher than phorbol esters to compete for the binding. To answer your question correctly, we have to know the real efficiency of the endogenous diacylglycerol that is generated in membranes in a signal-dependent manner.

J. H. Oppenheimer: I was just wondering whether you would care to speculate about the relationship of your system to the problem insulin action.

Y. Nishizuka: I have no idea, but this is an important question.

A. R. Means: Does protein kinase C bind calcium in the absence of phospholipids? If so does this interaction result in a conformational change in the enzyme?

Y. Nishizuka: Does protein kinase C bind calcium in the absence of phospholipid? Well, this is a very complicated problem. In the absence of phospholipids, Ca^{2+} at higher concentrations appears to inactivate the enzyme very rapidly. The action of Ca^{2+} is apparently not simple. We do not know at present the precise picture.

A. R. Means: So the possibility exists that calcium is needed to couple the phospholipids to the hydrophobic region of the enzyme rather than bind to it directly. This raises the question of whether the active fragment of protein kinase C obtained by limited proteolysis will directly bind phorbol esters. Do you know to which portion of the enzyme the tumor promoter binds?

Y. Nishizuka: That is an interesting point, but we have not done such an experiment. Perhaps, the role of Ca^{2+} may be diverse, and one of the major roles is to modulate the fine structure of the membrane phospholipid bilayer.

U. Zor: First, is it possible that the hormones that reduce cyclic AMP formation like noradrenoline and acetylcholine are performing this effect by activation of protein kinase C which may phosphorylate adenylate cyclase and thus reduce adenylate cyclase activity. Second, is it possible that hormones such as insulin or prolactin activate membrane proteases and this activates protein kinase C without the necessity of diacylglycerol.

Y. Nishizuka: We do not have evidence to discuss any possible relationship between protein kinase C and adenylate cyclase. The second is a very difficult question. Obviously, one of our major efforts is addressed to this point, but we have not obtained any direct evidence.

M. R. Clark: Could you comment on the calmodulin sensitivity of this enzyme, in particular, is it possible that you have lost the calmodulin sensitivity early on in purification or study of this enzyme.

Y. Nishizuka: We tested various possibilities, but so far no indication is available. The enzyme activation is extremely sensitive to so-called calmodulin inhibitors such as trifluoperazine, dibucaine, and chlorpromazine. But, the enzyme is essentially free of calmodulin. The activation is not affected by calmodulin nor by calmodulin antibody at all. Do you have any evidence for calmodulin involvement in this enzyme system?

M. R. Clark: We have no direct evidence other than observations very similar to yours, in ovarian systems. These are preparations with no calmodulin sensitivity that we can demonstrate. Nevertheless, the question has been raised in the literature as to whether the calmodulin sensitivity is gone by the time you get a chance to look at it. I just wondered if you had any further information on that?

Y. Nishizuka: Calmodulin-dependent processes are inhibited nonspecifically by a variety of hydrophobic reagents, particularly by phospholipid-interacting drugs. Inversely, so-called calmodulin inhibitors are not specific for the calmodulin-dependent processes. I think we have to be extremely careful to interpret any results of inhibitor experiments.

H. Friesen: Do you have any knowledge or can you provide any speculation about the nature, the locus, and function of the 40K phosphorylated protein?

Y. Nishizuka: This is one of the problems at present. The protein has been originally described by Haslam's group in Canada and by Majerus' group in the United States some years ago. Very recently, Imaoka, Lynham, and Haslam presented a poster at the Conference on Cyclic Nucleotides and Protein Phosphorylation in Milan. They showed that the 40K protein appeared to be heterogeneous and composed of at least 7–9 phosphorylated forms with an apparently identical molecular weight of 47K, but with different isoelectric points. This heterogeneity seemed to be due not to the primary sequence of the protein but to the amount of phosphate attached. This protein may be recovered in the soluble fraction. However, nobody knows its biological function at present. Also, we do not know if this protein does occur in any other tissues.

B. Littlefield: Have you used the synthetic diglyceride to see if it might mimic either the transforming or differentiating properties of phorbol esters, and if so, do you think that protein kinase C might be the major site of action of phorbol esters?

Y. Nishizuka: We have not done that yet, but synthetic diacylglycerol appears to be active to induce Epstein–Barr virus antigens just as tumor-promoting phorbol esters do. This experiment has been done recently by Prof. Y. Ito, Kyoto University Faculty of Medicine. Another point I with to mention is that mezerein which has no diacylglycerol structure, and teleocidin which is structurally unrelated to phorbol are both capable of activating protein kinase C as well. Therefore, perhaps, this protein kinase C may lie on a common pathway eventually leading to tumor promotion by these compounds.

E. J. Peck: We now recognize a number of actions of steroids that may occur at levels and through mechanisms other than the classic cytoplasmic-nuclear receptor and the genomic level. Have you or others examined the effects of sex steroids or glucocorticoids on the protein kinase C system?

Y. Nishizuka: This is a very interesting possibility. As you stated, many steroids such as glucocorticoid suggest their acute effects perhaps on membranes. But, so far no convincing evidence is available indicating such direct actions.

New Perspectives on the Mechanism of Insulin Action

Michael P. Czech

Department of Biochemistry, University of Massachusetts Medical School, Worcester, Massachusetts

I. Introduction

The critical role that insulin plays in so many cellular processes has prompted numerous efforts to understand its mechanism or mechanisms of action. Although these efforts have provided us with many structural and functional details of isolated components of the insulin effector system, a unified, well-documented concept of cellular signaling remains unavailable. There are several reasons why the task of understanding the mechanism of insulin action has proved so difficult. The extreme low abundance of insulin receptors in target cells, the lack of well-defined cell mutants deficient in insulin receptor or insulin response, and the complexity of most target enzyme or transport systems that respond to the hormone have all been difficult obstacles that have impeded progress. Continued advances in this area will almost surely depend to a large extent on our ability to deal successfully with these specific problems. The development of methodologies to probe the most penetrating questions in the field remains an important future objective.

Experimental strategies that have proved most useful in providing insight into the question of insulin action have generally related to one of four categories. These include (1) biochemical characterization of the insulin receptor itself, (2) studies on possible "mediator" substances or pathways, (3) characterization of target membrane systems for insulin action such as the glucose transporter, and (4) studies on the complex cytoplasmic enzyme systems that respond to insulin. In this progress report, I shall review advances that have been made in the first three approaches above, and shall present some new results from our laboratory using these three strategies. Recent substantive progress using experimental strategy 4 has been reviewed recently as well (Ingebritsen and Cohen, 1983; Cohen, 1980).

347

II. The Insulin Receptor Complex

It has long been appreciated that a receptor or receptor complex located in the cell surface membrane specifically binds insulin and initiates
biological responses of the hormone. Kinetic studies established that ^{125}I-
labeled insulin–receptor interaction is characterized by a binding constant
of about 1 nM and a curvilinear Scatchard plot (Roth *et al.*, 1975). A very
fruitful experimental strategy over the past several years has been the
determination of structural and functional properties of the insulin receptor. Much of the information we have learned from these studies is schematically represented in the hypothetical insulin receptor structure in Fig.
1. Many of the experimental details leading to this model have been
reviewed previously (Czech *et al.*, 1981; Jacobs and Cuatrecasas, 1981).
The intent here is to summarize the established features of the receptor
structure.

All investigators agree that receptor subunits of 125,000 daltons and
90,000 daltons are disulfide-linked in the receptor complex. We denoted
these subunits α and β, respectively, based on affinity crosslinking studies
that lead to the visualization of these receptor subunits on SDS gels
(Massague *et al.*, 1980). As a result of the experiments of Jacobs and
colleagues (1979, 1980b) using affinity purification methodology and our
studies using affinity labeling of the receptor complex, a heterotetrameric,
disulfide-linked receptor structure as shown in Fig. 1 was proposed. The
principal data supporting this model were derived from two-dimensional
gel electrophoretic analysis of the receptor complex in the presence and

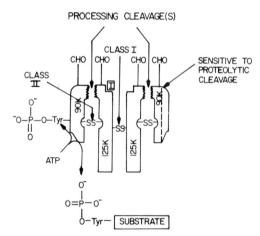

FIG. 1.   Proposed structural features of the heterotetrameric insulin receptor complex.
See text for detailed description of supporting data.

absence of reductant. These original studies indicating that the minimum covalent receptor complex consists of only α and β subunits are strongly supported by more recent data obtained with insulin receptor that is affinity purified on insulin-agarose (Fujita-Yamaguchi *et al.*, 1983) or that is immunoprecipitated with specific anti-insulin receptor antibody (Kasuga *et al.*, 1982a).

Recently, Yip and Moule (1983) have proposed that a 40,000 dalton receptor subunit may be disulfide-linked to the receptor complex in addition to the α and β subunits. This band can be visualized subsequent to photoaffinity labeling the receptor with photoactive insulin analogs. If indeed a 40,000 dalton subunit were part of the receptor structure, this component would be expected to appear in immunoprecipitates of the receptor and in purified preparations of the insulin receptor. The fact this is not the case suggests to me that the 40,000 dalton species observed in photoaffinity labeling studies may be a proteolytic fragment of one of the other receptor subunits. However, further studies will be required to clarify the nature of this 40,000 dalton species.

A well-documented property of the insulin receptor complex is the presence of two classes of intersubunit disulfides (Massague and Czech, 1982). Mild reductant treatment of the native receptor complex reduces its apparent molecular weight on dodecyl sulfate gels from the 350,000 to 400,000 dalton range to about half that size (Massague *et al.*, 1980; Massague and Czech, 1982b). As shown in Fig. 2 for a Triton X-100-solubilized affinity-labeled receptor preparation, addition of 10 or 50 mM dithiothreitol leads to the formation of a receptor species about half the apparent molecular weight of the native receptor. The partially reduced receptor fragment of about 200,000 daltons contains an α and β subunit (not illustrated). Complete reduction of the receptor complex gives rise to the highly labeled α and poorly labeled β subunits (lanes E and F, Fig. 2). The much higher degree of affinity labeling of α versus β subunit suggests that the former may contain the hormone binding site, but this is not proved. Thus, we propose that the more reductant-sensitive class of disulfide or disulfides links the two halves of the receptor complex, as shown in Fig. 1. Another class of disulfides, denoted as class 2, link α and β subunits and are highly resistant to exogenous reductants such as dithiothreitol. These disulfides are dissociated in the presence of dodecyl sulfate and high concentrations of dithiothreitol. How many disulfide linkages between the subunits in the complex are present is not yet known.

Another property of the insulin receptor relates to the extreme susceptibility of the β subunit to proteolytic nicking. In particular, a site about midway into the amino acid sequence of the β subunit is particularly sensitive to proteolytic cleavage by elastase or elastase-like proteases

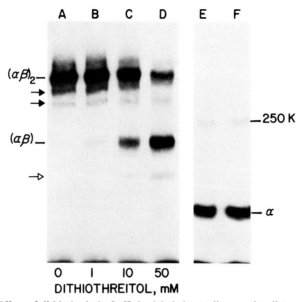

FIG. 2.   Effect of dithiothreitol of affinity-labeled rat adipocyte insulin receptor solubilized in Triton X-100. Rat adipocyte membranes were affinity labeled by successive incubation with 10 nM ^{125}I-labeled insulin and 0.2 mM disuccinimidyl suberate. The affinity-labeled membranes were resuspended (2 mg/ml of membrane protein) in a medium containing 10 mM Tris/HCl, 1 mM EDTA, pH 7.2, and 1% Triton X-100, and incubated in this medium for 45 minutes at 0°C. Nonsolubilized material was removed by centrifugation at 100,000 g for 60 minutes. Dithiothreitol was added to the solubilized membranes at the indicated concentrations (lanes A to D) and the mixtures were incubated at 23°C for 20 minutes. The action of dithiothreitol was then blocked by addition of excess N-ethylmaleimide. The samples were boiled in the presence of 1% sodium dodecyl sulfate and subjected to polyacrylamide gel electrophoresis and autoradiography (lanes A to D). Samples on lanes E and F are the counterparts of samples on lanes A and D boiled in the presence of sodium dodecyl sulfate and 10 mM dithiothreitol. Small amounts of proteolytically transformed $(\alpha\beta)(\alpha\beta_1)$, and $(\alpha\beta_1)_2$ insulin receptor forms (closed arrows), and their corresponding $(\alpha\beta_1)$ partially reduced receptor fragments (open arrow) were observed in the particular experiment shown. (From Massague and Czech, J. Biol. Chem. **257**, 6729–6738, 1982.)

(Massague et al., 1981b). Receptor forms that contain one β subunit that has been cleaved by protease or both β subunits that have been cleaved can be identified as lower molecular weight receptor complexes on nonreduced dodecyl sulfate gels (Massague et al., 1980, 1981b). Subsequent to cleavage, one fragment of the β subunit remains disulfide-linked to the receptor complex whereas the other fragment is presumably released from the complex in the presence of dodecyl sulfate. More recent studies with purified preparations of insulin receptor often show decreased amounts of recovery of the β subunit, again probably attributable to its proteolysis during preparation. Although the α subunit of the insulin receptor is much less susceptible to proteolysis than the β subunit under most conditions, the binding of insulin to the receptor complex appears to enhance the susceptibility of the α subunit to exogenous protease (Pilch and Czech, 1980). This finding indicates that a change in the conformation of the insulin receptor or in its association with a modulator component in response to insulin binding may mediate this changed sensitivity of the α subunit to proteolysis.

Both subunit types, α and β, of the insulin receptor complex contain oligosaccharide units. This property has been demonstrated by altered receptor mobility on dodecyl sulfate subsequent to neuraminidase treatment (Jacobs *et al.*, 1980a) as well as the demonstrated incorporation of labeled saccharide into the subunits (Hedo *et al.*, 1983). The latter finding has been documented in immunoprecipitates of detergent extracts from cells labeled with oligosaccharide precursors. The nature of these oligosaccharides in terms of distinct structures and their possible role in insulin function are not known. It is interesting to note that incubation of intact cells or membranes with neuraminidase does not alter insulin binding to the receptor complex (Cuatrecasas and Illiano, 1971).

Recent observations (Hedo *et al.*, 1983; Deutsch *et al.*, 1983) suggest that the α and β subunits of the mature insulin receptor may be synthesized as a single polypeptide chain. Thus, putative receptor complex components have been identified in immunoprecipitates that migrate in the 200,000 dalton region on SDS gels and are not cleaved by reductant. Results obtained in pulse-chase experiments using labeled saccharides or methionine indicate the 200,000 dalton components are rapidly labeled followed by the apparent chase of label from these components to the mature α and β subunits. Furthermore, treatment of cells with monensin has been shown to block the conversion of the noncleaved receptor precursor to the mature α and β subunits (Jacobs *et al.*, 1983a) consistent with the action of monensin to block processing of other membrane proteins. These data are consistent with the presence of a processing scheme involving proteolysis of large precursor glycopeptide structures to mature insulin receptor subunits. It is not known whether this hypothetical processing involves a single nick in the precursor polypeptide or whether a polypeptide region is exercised from the receptor precursor. Further work will be required to substantiate this processing scheme and to provide further details about it.

A final important property of the insulin receptor denoted in Fig. 1 is its association with insulin-activated tyrosine kinase activity. Experiments first performed by Kahn, Kasuga, and colleagues (Kasuga *et al.*, 1982b,e) demonstrated that incubation of ^{32}P-labeled intact cells with insulin leads to the increased incorporation of ^{32}P into the insulin receptor β subunit. The insulin-stimulated receptor phosphorylation was shown to reflect incorporation of [^{32}P]phosphate into both serine and tyrosine residues. These results are remarkably similar to experiments performed by Cohen *et al.* (1980) that showed another peptide growth factor, epidermal growth factor, stimulates phosphorylation of its receptor. The appearance of phosphotyrosine in the insulin-stimulated insulin receptor in intact cells, as well as that found in the EGF receptor, represents novel and important observations because tyrosine phosphorylations in normal cells are very rare. The effect of insulin to stimulate receptor phosphorylation in IM-9 lymphocytes (Kasuga *et al.*, 1982b), hepatoma cells (Kasuga *et al.*, 1982e), and adipocytes (Haring *et al.*, 1982) could be observed at physiological concentrations of the hormone, and appears to have other characteristics that would be expected for a physiological action of insulin. The behavior of the insulin receptor in detergent solution was also found to parallel the earlier result obtained for the EGF receptor in that an insulin-activated tyrosine phosphorylation reaction on the insulin receptor β subunit was observed (Van Obberghen and Kowalski, 1982; Petruzzelli *et al.*, 1982; Machicao *et al.*, 1982; Avruch *et al.*, Kasuga *et al.*, 1982d; Zick *et al.*, 1983). Very little or no serine phosphate could be observed in phosphorylations performed in the cell-free systems. Interestingly, Mn^{2+} appears to be required for the receptor phosphorylation reaction in detergent extracts. More recently, the ability of insulin receptor to incorporate ^{32}P in response to added insulin was demonstrated in a highly purified preparation of insulin receptor, indicating that the tyrosine kinase activity may be intrinsic to the receptor structure (Kasuga *et al.*, 1983). These studies have also shown that the receptor is capable of catalyzing phosphorylation of exogenous substrates such as histones and angiotensin upon activation by insulin. Taken together, the data are consistent with the hypothesis that the insulin receptor structure shown in Fig. 1 contains intrinsic tyrosine kinase activity that can be stimulated upon insulin–receptor interaction.

That the insulin receptor β subunit contains both the tyrosine phosphorylation sites as well as intrinsic tyrosine kinase activity is suggested by recent affinity labeling studies. Receptor preparations that are incubated with analogs of ATP that form covalent bonds with protein binding sites for ATP do label the insulin receptor β subunit (Roth and Cassell, 1983; Shia and Pilch, 1983; Van Obberghen *et al.*, 1983). Whether the ATP binding site or sites on the β subunit actually reflect catalytic sites for tyrosine kinase activity has not been unequivocally established. However, at this point, the data available strongly suggest that the insulin receptor structure itself rather than a tightly bound protein kinase carries

TABLE I

Characteristics of Insulin Receptor-Associated Kinase Activity

	References
1. Insulin stimulates receptor (β subunit) phosphorylation in serine and tyrosine residues when added to intact cells.	Kasuga *et al.* (1982b,c)
2. Insulin binding to receptors in detergent extracts leads to tyrosine phosphorylation of receptor (β subunit) and exogenous substrates.	Avruch *et al.* (1982); Kasuga *et al.* (1982d); Zick *et al.* (1983)
3. The receptor kinase appears to require Mn^{2+} or Co^{2+} activity.	Avruch *et al.* (1982); Zick *et al.* (1983)
4. Receptor phosphorylation parallels insulin occupancy and saturates when binding is saturated.	Avruch *et al.* (1983)
5. Insulin binding to purified insulin receptor stimulates autophosphorylation on tyrosine residues.	Kasuga *et al.* (1983)
6. The β subunit of the insulin receptor is affinity labeled by photoactive ATP analogs, suggesting it contains the site for kinase activity.	Roth and Cassell (1983); Shia and Pilch (1983); Van Obberghen *et al.* (1983)
7. Phosphorylation of the insulin receptor β subunit increases the activity of its associated tyrosine kinase activity.	Rosen *et al.* (1983); Czech *et al.* (1984); Yu and Czech (1984a)

the insulin-activated tyrosine kinase activity observed in cell-free systems. Table I summarizes several of the observed properties of the insulin receptor-associated kinase activity.

Another important question related to receptor phosphorylation is whether phosphorylation of the insulin receptor β subunit itself plays an important regulatory role in receptor function. The answer to this question appears to be affirmative. The receptor autophosphorylation rate was found to increase as receptor phosphorylation proceeded in in vitro incubations (Zick *et al.*, 1983). Experiments by Rosen and co-workers (1983) demonstrated that insulin receptor which had been first phosphorylated with unlabeled ATP exhibited increased tyrosine kinase activity toward histone and angiotensin compared to control receptor. These results suggest that phosphorylation of the insulin receptor β subunit leads to activation of the receptor-associated tyrosine kinase activity. Furthermore, results in the latter study suggested that tyrosine kinase activity that had been activated by prior receptor phosphorylation was no longer dependent upon insulin for stimulation.

Recent experiments in our laboratory have probed the relationship between β subunit phosphorylation and receptor-associated tyrosine kinase activation. In our studies, insulin receptor tyrosine kinase activity is assessed in a partially purified receptor preparation that is immobilized on insulin-agarose (Czech *et al.*, 1984; Yu and Czech, 1984a). The receptor preparation is readily incubated with labeled or unlabeled ATP prior to washing and a second incubation with [γ-^{32}P]ATP plus histone or other substrate. In our studies, at least seven sites on the insulin receptor were found to be phosphorylated upon addition of high concentrations of [γ-^{32}P]ATP. These phosphorylation sites are identified by tryptic hydrolysis of phosphorylated receptor and resolution of the resultant receptor peptides by high-pressure liquid chromatography. Three distinct resolved receptor peptide regions are identified by their elution profile on a propanol gradient and are referred to as receptor domains 1, 2, and 3. Interestingly, in our studies serine and tyrosine, as well as a much smaller number of threonine residues, were found to be phosphorylated by ATP during tyrosine kinase activation. When the phosphorylated insulin receptor that exhibited elevated tyrosine kinase activity was dephosphorylated by incubation with alkaline phosphatase, deactivation of the receptor-associated tyrosine kinase activity could be achieved. Under these conditions of tyrosine kinase deactivation, about 90% of the phosphate removed from the receptor could be accounted for by tyrosine phosphate in receptor domain 2. Small amounts of tyrosine phosphate were removed from the other two receptor domains with essentially no dephosphorylation of serine residues. These data are consistent with the hypothesis that tyrosine phosphorylation in domain 2 of the insulin receptor is directly regulating the receptor-associated tyrosine kinase activity *in vitro*. Whether the tyrosine phosphate groups on the receptor are strictly related to modifying the associated tyrosine kinase activity versus as yet other undetermined roles is not known.

III. Insulin Receptor Belongs to a Family of Receptor Structures

Recent evidence indicates that the general properties of the insulin receptor that are illustrated in Fig. 1 are also shared by at least one type of receptor structure with high affinity for insulin-like growth factor I. This latter receptor type also binds insulin-like growth factor II with low affinity and insulin itself with still lower affinity (Massague and Czech, 1982a; Bhaumick *et al.*, 1981; Kasuga *et al.*, 1981; Chernausek *et al.*, 1981). Interestingly, the structural homology of the receptors for insulin and IGF-I parallels the structural homologies known to be shared by insulin and the insulin-like growth peptides. Thus, the primary sequence of these peptides shows substantive similarities as do the positions of disulfide linkages within the polypeptide chains. The properties and chemistry of insulin and the insulin-like growth factors have been extensively reviewed previously (Rechler *et al.*, 1981).

Affinity labeling studies using ^{125}I-labeled peptides and crosslinking agents showed definitively that cell surface receptors with highest affinity for IGF-I contained subunit types remarkably similar to the α and β insulin receptor subunits in respect to electrophoretic mobility (Massague and Czech, 1982a). As shown in Fig. 3, a major receptor type that is affinity crosslinked to a greater extent with ^{125}I-labeled IGF-I than ^{125}I-labeled IGF-II in human placenta and fibroblast membranes exhibits a labeled subunit of about 130K under reducing conditions. In the absence of reductant, it is seen that this IGF-I receptor complex exists as disulfide-linked high-molecular-weight complexes similar to the native and pro-teolytically nicked insulin receptor complexes in respect to sizes (Fig. 3). This IGF receptor species also exhibits disulfide linkages that can be classified as class I and class II based on sensitivity to reductant. Two-dimensional SDS gel electrophoresis of the affinity labeled IGF-I receptor complex in the presence and absence of reductant leads to the identifica-tion of receptor fragments and receptor subunit species that are remark-ably similar to those for the insulin receptor complex (Massague and Czech, 1982b).

Recent studies by Jacobs and colleagues has suggested that the IGF-I receptor α and β subunits, like the insulin receptor α and β subunits, are synthesized as a single precursor polypeptide chain that is cleaved to mature subunits upon cellular processing (Jacobs *et al.*, 1983a). Addition of monensin to intact cells inhibited the apparent conversion of the high-molecular-weight precursor material to mature α and β subunits. Furthermore, in a separate series of experiments it was also found that ^{125}I-labeled IGF-I binding to its receptor complex stimulates autophosphorylation of the IGF-I receptor β subunit (Jacobs *et al.*, 1983b). *In vitro* phosphorylation of the IGF-I receptor in response to IGF-I reflects predominantly tyrosine phosphate. Although these characteris-tics of the IGF-I receptor have not been studied as extensively as have those for the insulin receptor, all the evidence available suggests that these two receptor complexes share multiple structural and functional properties.

An intriguing extension of the above concept is that multiple rather than just two heterotetrameric structures exist in cells which bind insulin and IGF-I with varying affinities. Support for the concept that more than two distinct receptor types are present for insulin and IGF-I arises from data suggesting striking heterogeneity among IGF-I receptors in different cell types in respect to affinity for IGF-II. Thus, while the IGF-I receptor has

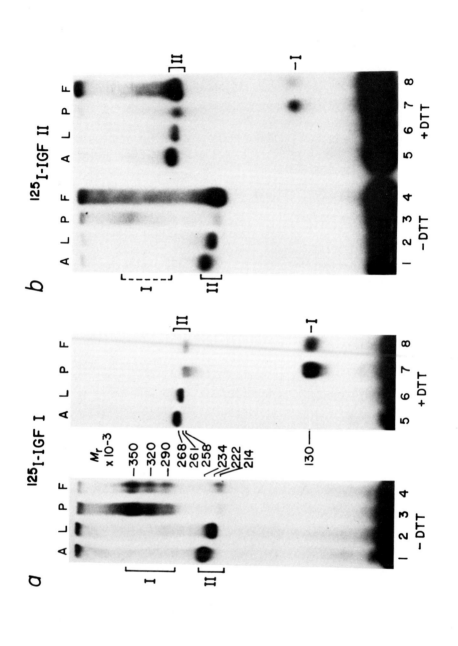

a characteristic very high affinity for ^{125}I-labeled IGF-I, its affinity for IGF-II can vary from nearly equal (Kasuga et al., 1982c) to much less than its affinity for IGF-I (Massague and Czech, 1982a). The prospect that multiple receptors for insulin and IGF-I with subtle structural and affinity differences must be considered highly speculative until more complete structural data are available on these receptor types. It is not yet known, for example, whether significant amino acid sequence similarities exists for insulin and IGF-I receptors.

Experiments in our laboratory first demonstrated (Massague et al., 1981a) yet another receptor species that could bind IGF-I and IGF-II, but had no detectable subunits that were disulfide linked. This receptor species exhibited highest affinity for IGF-II, a lower affinity for IGF-I, and no affinity for insulin. As shown in Fig. 3, it is readily affinity labeled by addition of ^{125}I-labeled IGF-II or ^{125}I-labeled IGF-I plus crosslinking agent in many cell types and migrates with an apparent molecular weight of about 250,000 on dodecyl sulfate gels. Interestingly, the apparent molecular weight varies somewhat from among cell types and is affected by the presence of reductant (Fig. 3). As illustrated in Table II, the properties of this 250,000 dalton IGF-II receptor, denoted as the type II IGF receptor, exhibits strikingly different properties compared to the insulin and IGF-I receptor types. In addition to the lack of multiple disulfide-linked subunits contained in the IGF-II receptor complex and the inability to bind insulin even at low affinity, it is not demonstrably effected by a cellular mutation or mutations that markedly decrease the expression of insulin and IGF-I receptors in parallel (Massague et al., 1983). Furthermore, experiments in our laboratory with purified receptor have indicated the lack of detectable protein kinase activity associated with this receptor under conditions where insulin and IGF-I receptors clearly exhibit associated tyrosine kinase activity (Mottola and Czech, unpublished).

FIG. 3. Dodecyl sulfate polyacrylamide gel electrophoresis of membranes from various rat and human tissues crosslinked to ^{125}I-labeled IGF-I (a) and ^{125}I-labeled IGF-II (b). Membranes from rat adipocytes (A), rat liver (L), human placenta (P), or human skin fibroblasts (F) were incubated with 5 nM ^{125}I-labeled IGF-I (a) or 5 nM ^{125}I-labeled IGF-II (b) at 10°C for 60 minutes in Krebs–Ringer phosphate buffer, pH 7.4, containing 1% bovine serum albumin. After washing out the unbound hormone, membranes were incubated with 0.2 mM disuccinimidyl suberate at 0°C for 15 minutes, and the crosslinking reaction was stopped by addition of excess Tris buffer, pH 7.4. Samples (100 μg membrane protein) of the crosslinked membranes were electrophoresed on 5% polyacrylamide slab gels in the absence (lanes 1 to 4) or presence (lanes 5 to 8) of 50 mM dithiothreitol (DTT). Autoradiograms from the fixed, dried gels are shown. Two distinct types (type I and II) of affinity labeled bands were revealed on the autoradiograms as described in the text. (From Massague and Czech, J. Biol. Chem. **257**, 5038–5045, 1982.)

TABLE II

Characteristics of the Insulin and IGF Receptor Family

Property	Insulin receptor	IGF-I receptor	IGF-II receptor	Representative reference
Apparent mass on gels	350–400K	350–400K	230–270K	Massague *et al.* (1982a)
Disulfide-linked α and β subunits	Yes	Yes	No	Massague *et al.* (1982a)
Tryptic peptide map homology	Yes	Yes		Heinrich and Czech (unpublished)
Linked to rapid bioactions	Yes	Yes	No	Yu and Czech (1984b)
Affected similarly due to mutation	Yes	Yes	No	Massague *et al.* (1983)
Tyrosine kinase activity	Yes	Yes	No	Mottola and Czech (unpublished)
Increased expression in response to insulin	No	No	Yes	Oppenheimer *et al.* (1983)

Another contrast between IGF-II receptor and the heterotetrameric receptor structures is the inability of the former receptors to catalyze acute cellular responses such as hexose transport activation in adipocytes. This contrasts with our recent demonstration that the IGF-I receptor in isolated soleus muscles is capable of mediating this acute response (Yu and Czech, 1984b). Unequivocal documentation that the type II IGF receptor actually mediates a stimulation of cell proliferation in culture is also lacking (Massague *et al.*, 1982). Furthermore, insulin action in isolated adipocytes or H-35 hepatoma cells leads to a marked stimulation of IGF-II binding to the type II receptor species (Zapf *et al.*, 1978; King *et al.*, 1982; Oppenheimer *et al.*, 1983) while no evidence is available indicating the type I IGF receptor responds to insulin in this manner. In summary then, we are left with one class of IGF receptors that is structurally and functionally very similar to the insulin receptor and another class of IGF receptors that differs markedly from the insulin receptor. The precise roles that the IGF receptors play in cellular growth and metabolism remain to be elucidated.

IV. Regulation of Insulin Receptor Function

A major thrust in our laboratory over the past year has been to examine the potential role of the insulin receptor as a target for other hormone or cellular signalling mechanisms. One of the model systems we chose to study in this regard is the known antagonism of β-catecholamine action and insulin action in isolated adipocytes (Fain, 1980). It is well documented that biological effects in these cells mediated through the β-catecholamine receptor and the resultant increased levels of cellular cyclic AMP include such responses as glycogen synthase inactivation and increased lipolytic rates. Insulin action, on the other hand, activates glycogen synthase and inhibits catecholamine-stimulated lipolysis. Such antagonism probably involves the opposing effects of the respective signaling mechanisms on the kinases and phosphatases that regulate glycogen synthase. Our experimental strategy, on the other hand, has been to evaluate the hypothesis that the signaling mechanism of the β-catecholamines (i.e., cyclic AMP) modulates the insulin receptor structure itself and thereby antagonizes insulin action at the earliest step of signal initiation.

In studying the above hypothesis, we found that adipocytes incubated with isoproterenol exhibit a markedly diminished ability to bind ^{125}I-labeled insulin (Pessin *et al.*, 1983). Using affinity crosslinking methodology, we could demonstrate that the isoproterenol effect in intact adipocytes indeed inhibits the binding of ^{125}I-labeled insulin to the α subunit of the insulin receptor complex, as shown in Fig. 4. This effect of isoproterenol is extremely rapid and measurable within a minute of addition of the hormone to the fat cells. The effect is also temperature dependent. Further, it is mimicked by addition of dibutryl cyclic AMP and potentiated by the addition of known phosphodiesterase inhibitors when added with catecholamine. These results and other recent studies (Lonnroth and Smith, 1983) strongly indicate that the effect of isoproterenol to decrease insulin receptor binding results from a cyclic AMP-dependent process, presumably mediated via the cyclic AMP-dependent protein kinase. Of further interest is the fact that ^{125}I-labeled EGF but not ^{125}I-labeled IGF-II binding to adipocytes was also strikingly inhibited by isoproterenol (Pessin *et al.*, 1983).

In analyzing the ^{125}I-labeled insulin binding to particulate fractions of adipocytes treated with and without catecholamine plus phosphodiesterase inhibitor, we find that the inhibitory effect survives homogenization of fat cells (Pessin and Czech, unpublished). Insulin receptors in the plasma membrane fraction are inhibited in their ability to bind hormone when obtained from catecholamine-treated cells, whereas low-density microsomes and other cellular fractions do not exhibit this effect. Thus, the effect of catecholamine on insulin receptors is quite different than the effect of insulin on the IGF-II receptor (see Section III) in that the cAMP effect is localized to insulin receptors in the membrane fraction that appear to be derived from the cell surface membrane. These data are consistent with the postulate that a cyclic AMP-dependent mechanism alters the insulin receptor itself, or a regulatory component of the receptor, such

ISOPROTERENOL   —   —   +   +

INSULIN   —   +   —   +

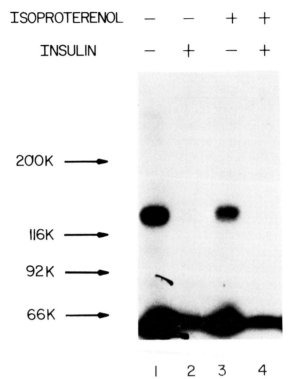

| I   2   3   4

FIG. 4.   Affinity labeling of the insulin receptor from control and isoproterenol-treated cells. Adipocytes were incubated in the absence (lanes 1 and 2) or presence (lanes 3 and 4) of 1.0 μM isoproterenol for 30 minutes at 37°C; 10 nM ^{125}I-labeled insulin (lanes 1 and 3) or 10 nM ^{125}I-labeled insulin + 5 μM unlabeled insulin (lanes 2 and 4) was added to the adipocytes for 30 minutes at room temperature. The affinity crosslinking was initiated by the addition of 50 μM disuccinimidyl suberate for 15 minutes at 10°C, and terminated by washing the cells 2 times in 5 mM Tris, 1 mM EDTA, 250 mM sucrose, pH 7.4. Cells were then homogenized and 150 μg of membrane protein was prepared for a 6% sodium dodecyl sulfate polyacrylamide gel with electrophoresis under reducing conditions. This experiment was independently performed 2 times. The arrows depict the location of standard molecular weight markers. (From Pessin *et al.*, *J. Biol. Chem.* **258**, 7386–7394, 1983.)

that binding to ^{125}I-labeled insulin is either blocked or lowered by a decrease in receptor affinity.

Attempts to evaluate the above concept by analyzing the kinetics of ^{125}I-labeled insulin binding to its receptor in control versus catecholamine-treated cells or in membranes derived from such cells has proved to be difficult. The basis for this difficulty is the curvilinearity of Scatchard plots which complicate the interpretations. Interestingly, with the EGF receptor system, isoproterenol decreased the apparent affinity of the hormone for receptor (Pessin *et al.*, 1983). In this receptor system, the Scatchard plot is linear. In any case, the kinetic data illustrate striking inhibition of binding at low ^{125}I-labeled insulin concentrations caused by isoproterenol, but a marked diminution if not elimination of this effect at high ^{125}I-labeled insulin concentrations. Thus, in simplest terms, either catecholamine action inactivates a class of high-affinity receptors without an effect on a lower affinity receptor class or catecholamine action decreases the affinity of a single class of insulin receptors which exhibits the characteristic of negative cooperativity.

Recent results in our laboratory have also demonstrated a potent inhibitory effect of the catecholamine treatment on the insulin-activated tyrosine kinase activity of the insulin receptor (Pessin and Czech, unpublished). Immunoprecipitates of the insulin receptor using insulin receptor antibody kindly provided by Dr. C. R. Kahn exhibit no change in the ability to incorporate ^{32}P when incubated with [γ-^{32}P]ATP in the absence of insulin. However, insulin receptors derived from catecholamine-treated cells showed a markedly decreased rate of autophosphorylation in such immunoprecipitates incubated with [γ-^{32}P]ATP. These experiments were conducted at very high ^{125}I-labeled insulin concentrations such that binding of the hormone to receptors was similar in the control versus isoproterenol-treated conditions. Thus the data are consistent with the hypothesis that catecholamine action leads to a decreased ability of the insulin receptor-associated tyrosine kinase activity to respond to insulin binding.

The results from our laboratory presented in this and the previous sections coupled with the data by Rosen *et al.* (1983) lead to the hypothesis illustrated in Fig. 5. Two types of positive regulatory control affect the tyrosine kinase activity associated with the insulin receptor—binding of hormone and phosphorylation of one or more tyrosine residues of the insulin receptor. The incorporation of tyrosine phosphate into the receptor appears to activate the associated tyrosine kinase activity independent of the continued presence of bound insulin (Rosen *et al.*, 1983). In contrast, one or more cAMP-dependent serine phosphorylations either on the receptor itself or on other unknown cell components have a significant inhibitory effect on both ^{125}I-labeled insulin binding to the receptor complex and the ability of insulin to activate the associated tyrosine kinase activity. Whether this latter action is the result of a direct inhibition of the effect of insulin itself or the receptor tyrosine phosphate on the tyrosine kinase is unknown. The locus of the hypothetical serine phosphate or phosphates requires further investigation. Nevertheless, the data we now

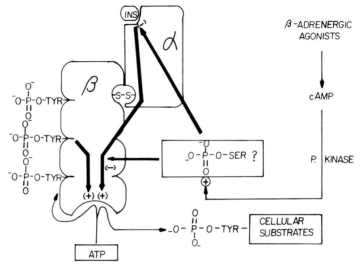

FIG. 5.   Roles of phosphotyrosines and phosphoserines in the regulation of insulin receptor functions. It is proposed that phosphorylation of the β subunit on one or more tyrosine residues leads to activation of receptor-associated tyrosine kinase activity. In contrast, cAMP-dependent protein kinase catalysis of serine phosphorylation on the insulin receptor itself or on a receptor modulator protein is proposed to lead to the inhibition of insulin binding (by lowering receptor affinity) and to a decrease in the activation of receptor tyrosine kinase activity by the hormone. In this schematic representation, only half of the proposed $\alpha_2\beta_2$ insulin receptor structure is depicted.

have available strongly suggest that a network of tyrosine and serine phosphorylations is involved in the control of the insulin receptor-associated tyrosine kinase activity and its activation by insulin.

V. Regulation of Membrane Components by Insulin

An experimental strategy that has provided novel and useful information on the mode of insulin action involves the study by which target membrane components are regulated by insulin. The insulin-sensitive membrane system that has been most carefully studied is the glucose transport system of adipocytes, although muscle has also been used. These facilitated diffusion systems transport glucose in a stereospecific manner and exhibit the expected saturation kinetics for hexoses (Czech, 1980). Insulin increases the transport of glucose or nonmetabolizable glucose analogs into these cells by up to 10-fold or more within minutes. A detailed discussion about the characteristics of the insulin-sensitive hexose transporters can be found in a previous review (Czech, 1980).

An important question related to the regulation of hexose transport by insulin has been whether activation involves an increased number of transporters in the cell surface membrane or an increased activity of the same number of transporters that occurs in control cell membranes. Important observations made independently by Kono and colleagues (Suzuki and Kono, 1980) and Cushman and Wardzala (1980; Karnieli *et al.*, 1981) have suggested the former mechanism. These workers demonstrated that plasma membranes isolated from adipocytes that had been treated with insulin exhibited higher glucose transport activity or binding sites for [³H]cytochalasin B, which appears to bind tightly to hexose transporters. Most importantly, these workers discovered that a concomitant decrease in transporter activity or [³H]cytochalasin B binding occurs in a low-density microsomal fraction prepared from insulin-treated cells compared to control cells. The insulin-stimulated increase in plasma membrane glucose transporters due to insulin action could be accounted for quantitatively by the decrease in low-density microsome transporters. These results led to the proposal that insulin action results in the mobilization or recruitment of intracellular transporters to the plasma membrane where they are exposed to the extracellular medium and where they can operate to transport hexoses. The details of these studies have been reviewed in the previous volume of this series (Kono, 1983).

The recruitment hypothesis described above relies on the assumption that transporters residing in the plasma membrane fraction and low-density membrane fraction of homogenized fat cells actually represent cell surface and intracellular loci, respectively, in the intact cell. Although this assumption is reasonable, the data available have not been conclusive in eliminating the possibility that microdomains of the plasma membrane might shear during homogenization and fractionate with low-density microsomes upon sucrose density centrifugation. Although the recruitment model is very attractive and fits with increasing evidence for similar transport activation mechanisms in other cells (Lienhard, 1983), the lack of direct evidence for increased transporters on the surface of intact cells has been problematic in our view. We therefore set out to develop methodology that would allow a direct test of this assumption of the model. This goal has been achieved with the development of a photoaffinity labeling technique which is specific for hexose transport systems.

Photolabeling of hexose transporters was first established in our laboratory (Carter-Su *et al.*, 1982) for the red cell system. Red cell membranes were incubated with [³H]cytochalasin B in the presence and absence of sorbitol or D-glucose until equilibrium was achieved and then irradiated with high-intensity UV light. Electrophoretic analysis of these membranes reveals the labeling of a broad band of apparent 55,000 daltons

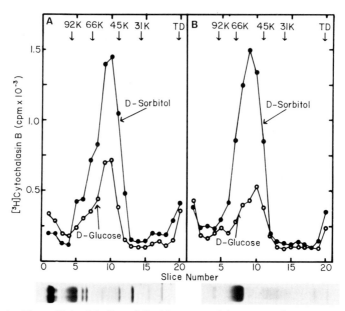

FIG. 6. Photoaffinity labeling of freshly prepared human erythrocyte proteins with [³H]cytochalasin B. Erythrocyte ghosts (A) or dimethylmaleic anhydride-extracted ghosts (B) were incubated with 1.0 μM [³H]cytochalasin B in the presence of 500 mM D-sorbitol (●) or 500 mM D-glucose (○). After equilibrium binding was reached, the samples were irradiated, washed, and electrophoresed on a 9% sodium dodecyl sulfate polyacrylamide gel. Arrows depict the location of molecular weight markers. The Coomassie blue stained gel profiles were representative of several experiments. (From Carter-Su et al., J. Biol. Chem. **257**, 5419–5425, 1982.)

(Fig. 6), as is expected for the hexose transporter in this cell system (Sogin and Hinkle, 1980). Furthermore, the labeling of this protein is inhibited by D-glucose but not by sorbitol which has no affinity for the transporter (Fig. 6). Unlabeled cytochalasin B and 3-O-methylglucose but not nontransported analogs such as L-glucose also inhibit photoaffinity labeling of this protein. This method has now been applied to membranes from chick embryo fibroblasts (Pessin et al., 1982), human placenta (Johnson and Smith, 1982), rat skeletal muscle (Klip et al., 1983), and rat fat cells (Oka and Czech, 1984a; Shanahan et al., 1982). These studies have identified transporter components of 45,000–60,000 daltons in these various cell types. The labeled fat cell transporter migrates as a relatively sharp peak at 46,000 daltons on dodecyl sulfate gels. These studies are summarized in Table III. The efficiency of covalent labeling of the red cell hexose transporter component by this method appears to be about 1%. This result agrees with previous data indicating that antiserum against the

TABLE III

Hexose Transporter Components Identified by Photoaffinity Labeling

Cell type	Apparent mass (M_r) on dodecyl sulfate gels	Reference
Red cell	44,000 to 70,000	Carter-Su *et al.* (1982)
	47,000 and 51,000	Shanahan (1982)
Chick fibroblast	46,000 and 52,000	Pessin *et al.* (1982)
Rat adipocytes	46,000	Shanahan *et al.* (1982)
	46,000	Oka and Czech (1984a)
Human placenta	52,000	Johnson and Smith (1982)
Rat skeletal muscle	45,000	Klip *et al.* (1983)

purified human red cell glucose transporter crossreacts with a 46,000 dalton protein of the adipocyte membrane (Wheeler *et al.*, 1982).

An important observation in our laboratory is that hexose transporters in intact fat cells that have been photoaffinity labeled with [³H]cytochalasin B remain sensitive to the action of insulin. Thus, addition of insulin to cells subsequent to the photoaffinity labeling procedure still leads to the redistribution of labeled hexose transporters from the low-density microsome fraction to the plasma membrane fraction upon homogenization of cells and preparation of membrane fractions. These results therefore allow transporters to be labeled prior to manipulating intact cells with various hormones or other reagents and then assessing the effects of such manipulations on transporter redistribution between the two membrane fractions.

In order to distinguish between transporters that reside on the cell surface versus in intracellular domains, we utilized a hexose analog that is known to bind to hexose transporters and inhibits [³H]cytochalasin B binding to the transporter, but cannot itself be transported by the transport system. This analog is ethylidene glucose and has been shown in red cells to specifically bind to a site on the red cell transporter that is on the extracellular side of the cell surface membrane (Baker and Widdas, 1973; Gorga and Lienhard, 1981). It is interesting to note that in red cells [³H]cytochalasin B binding appears to be on a hexose transporter site that is on the inner side of the membrane. It is thought that a transported hexose such as D-glucose has both an "outside" and "inside" binding site on the transporter. Binding of ethylidene glucose to the glucose binding site on the "outside" position appears to confer a change in the ability of a second "inside" site of the transporter to bind [³H]cytochalasin B.

When we incubated 50 mM ethylidene glucose with intact fat cells for 1 minute in the presence of [³H]cytochalasin B prior to photolysis, we found that affinity labeling of hexose transporters that fractionate into the plasma membrane upon homogenization was inhibited by the glucose analogue (Oka and Czech, 1984a,b). The affinity labeling of transporters that reside in the low-density microsome fraction was not inhibited by ethylidene glucose. Because under the conditions of our experiments the ethylidene glucose concentration was 50 mM in the extracellular medium and only about 2 mM inside the cells, these data indicate that the differential effect of the glucose analog to inhibit hexose transporter labeling in the two fractions reflects the intracellular, nonexposed position of the low-density microsome transporters. Thus these experiments demonstrate for the first time that the bulk of hexose transporters in control adipocytes resides in a position that is not exposed to the extracellular medium. Furthermore, we were able to show that insulin treatment leads to exposure of the transporters to the extracellular medium where their affinity labeling can be blocked by ethylidene glucose. These results are consistent with the original proposal presented by the laboratories of Cushman and Kono (Suzuki and Kono, 1980; Cushman and Wardzala, 1980; Karnieli *et al.*, 1981).

Recent results from our laboratory on the mechanism by which insulin modulates a second membrane component—the IGF-II receptor—have led to basically the same conclusion as described above for the glucose transporter. Previous studies had demonstrated an increased binding of ^{125}I-labeled IGF to the IGF-II receptor in adipocytes (Zapf *et al.*, 1978; King *et al.*, 1982) and H-35 hepatoma cells (Massague *et al.*, 1982). We then showed that insulin treatment of intact adipocytes increased the binding of ^{125}I-labeled IGF-II to the plasma membrane fraction and decreased binding to the low-density membrane fraction, similar to what was known for the glucose transporter (Oppenheimer *et al.*, 1983). Our approach in probing the question of whether increased numbers of IGF-II receptors versus an increased affinity of the same number of receptors on the cell surface reflects insulin action was to probe this receptor with specific antibody. Our strategy in this endeavor was predicated on the concept that a polyvalent antibody population against the IGF-II receptor would most likely bind the receptor at several sites, independent of any possible changes in the affinity of the receptor for IGF-II itself that insulin may cause. Thus, if anti-IGF-II receptor immunoglobulin binding to intact fat cells were to increase in response to insulin, in parallel with the increase in ^{125}I-labeled IGF-II binding, the results would be consistent with an increase in receptor number on the fat cell surface.

During the past year, we have been able to successfully carry out these experiments. IGF-II receptor was purified to homogeneity from rat placenta in our laboratory using an affinity purification technique (Oppenheimer and Czech, 1983). Rat IGF-II was immobilized on agarose and was found to effectively adsorb IGF-II receptor from Triton X-100 extracts. The purified receptor has also been shown to bind immobilized lectins and is therefore probably a glycoprotein (August et al., 1983). We have been able to raise potent antiserum against this receptor in rabbits and can demonstrate a positive ELISA test against purified receptor after a 5000-fold dilution of the antiserum. Interestingly, the anti-IGF-II receptor antibody that we obtained in rabbits markedly inhibits the binding of IGF-II to its receptor when added prior to the ligand (Oka and Czech, unpublished). The antiserum most potently blocks ^{125}I-labeled IGF-II binding to rat IGF-II receptor preparations and to a lesser degree to mouse preparations. It is not effective in blocking the binding of ^{125}I-labeled IGF-II to human IGF-I receptor. Importantly, immunoprecipitation lines formed in agar by the reaction of the anti-receptor antiserum preparation with purified IGF-II receptor were not affected when the receptor binding site for IGF-II was saturated by high concentrations of the growth factor. Thus the anti-receptor immunoglobulins in the polyvalent antiserum are able to bind the IGF-II receptor to the same extent whether or not the ligand binding site is occupied.

When fat cells were incubated with or without insulin prior to incubation with the immunoglobulin fraction from the anti-IGF-II receptor antiserum, increased specific binding of anti-IGF-II receptor immunoglobulins was found to adsorb to the fat cell surface (Oka and Czech, 1984c). The anti-receptor immunoglobulin binding was determined by addition of ^{125}I-labeled goat anti-rabbit immunoglobulin subsequent to reaction of cells with the anti-receptor rabbit immunoglobulin. We do not believe that the increased anti-receptor immunoglobulin binding to fat cells in response to insulin is due simply to a change in conformation of IGF-II receptors with a resultant exposure of new antigenic sites. The reason for this view is the fact that control cells were able to adsorb virtually all of the anti-IGF-II receptor immunoglobulins from the rabbit antiserum preparation. Thus the IGF-II receptor on control cells contains all the antigenic sites required to bind the various anti-receptor antibodies in the immunoglobulin population. These data strongly support the hypothesis that increased numbers of IGF-II receptors are expressed on the cell surface of adipocytes in response to insulin action.

Two possible mechanisms whereby insulin action might increase the expression of the glucose transporter and the IGF-II receptor on the cell surface of adipocytes is illustrated in Fig. 7. According to Fig. 7A, these membrane components might be cycling via endocytotic and exocytotic processes. Thus, insulin action to inhibit internalization of the glucose transporter in membrane vesicles or to stimulate the exocytosis of trans-

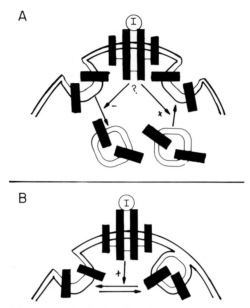

FIG. 7. Two models (A, B) whereby insulin action could lead to increased expression of glucose transports and IGF-II receptors on the intact cell surface. See text for details. I denotes insulin binding to the insulin receptor.

porter-rich intracellular vesicles fusing with the plasma membrane would achieve an increased number of cell surface transporters at steady state. Alternatively, as depicted in Fig. 7B, it is possible that a microdomain of the cell surface membrane might alter its structure such that components within the domain could either be exposed or not exposed to the bulk extracellular medium. If these two structural states of such a microdomain were in equilibrium, insulin might act to shift the equilibrium to the open or exposed state. Experiments designed to localize the glucose transporter and IGF-II receptor to specific cellular loci will be important in deciding upon these two mechanisms or other possible explanations for the data available.

VI. Mediating Actions of the Insulin Receptor

Although we have learned considerable information about the structural aspects of insulin and related receptors as well as target enzymes and transporters that respond to the hormone, we are still left with an unsatisfactory understanding of the biochemical linkages between receptor function and target proteins. A leading hypothesis to explain this linkage involves the possible action of the receptor-associated tyrosine kinase activity on cellular substrates that lead directly or indirectly to the modulation of serine protein kinases and phosphatases in the cell. The fact that certain proteins such as the ribosomal-S-6 protein expresses an increased phosphorylation state in response to insulin while others such as glycogen synthase express decreased phosphorylation suggests that both kinases and phosphatases may be activated by the hormone. As yet, there is no direct evidence that tyrosine phosphorylation directly modulates the activity of serine kinases or phosphatases, but further work on this issue is required. The fact that receptors for EGF, PDGF, insulin, and IGF-I have associated ligand-activated tyrosine kinase activity suggests an important role of this activity in receptor function.

An alternative model for the mechanism of insulin action is the possible involvement of soluble low-molecular-weight factors that may be released from the cell surface membrane in response to insulin–receptor interaction. According to this hypothesis, the intracellular concentration of such insulin-dependent factors directly acts to modify the activities of kinases or phosphatases that act on target enzymes for insulin action. This hypothesis is somewhat analogous to the mediation of hormone responses through the action of intracellular cyclic AMP. Results obtained over a decade ago by Larner's laboratory (for review, see Larner *et al.*, 1982) is consistent with this hypothesis, and more recent data from Jarett's laboratory (Seals and Jarett, 1980; Kiechle *et al.*, 1981) indicate a factor or factors is released from isolated plasma membranes by insulin action. This material was shown to be capable of activating a known insulin-dependent enzyme, pyruvate dehydrogenase *in vitro*. Substantial data from several laboratories are now available on these phenomena and several reviews (Larner, 1982; Czech, 1981; Seals and Czech, 1982) are available that summarize recent progress.

Our approach to testing this hypothesis has involved attempts at fully purifying a factor or factors that are increasing in cell extracts due to insulin action and have the capability of activating mitochondrial pyruvate dehydrogenase *in vitro*. Our basic premise has been that isolation and structural analysis of such factors are required prior to effective evaluation of the mediator hypothesis. We have made substantive progress at purifying such factors, but have not yet succeeded in obtaining complete purification and structural analysis.

In our experiments, fat cells are incubated with or without insulin, washed quickly, and disrupted by homogenization in the presence of trifluoroacetic acid (1%), EDTA (1 M), and dithiothreitol (1 mM). After centrifugation, the extracts are lyophilized and resuspended prior to testing for the ability to stimulate pyruvate dehydrogenase in isolated adipocyte mitochondria. These extracts exhibit the ability to increase the activity of this enzyme, and by serial dilution can be shown to have greater activity when derived from insulin-treated cells. A basic observation that is very reproducible in our laboratory is that two clearly resolved peaks of activity can be obtained upon high-pressure liquid chromatography of the extracts using gradient anion exchange. Extracts that are injected onto a Whatman SAX column equilibrated with water are eluted from the column with a gradient ultimately containing 2.5% trifluoroacetic acid, 50% acetonitrile, and 25% isopropanol. A first peak of insulin-dependent pyruvate dehydrogenase stimulating activity has the capacity to bind onto a second C_{18} reverse-phase high-pressure liquid chromatography system, while a second peak of activity does not bind to the C_{18} column. Using the combination of ion-exchange and reverse-phase chromatography, the first peak of activity has been purified to a single peak that adsorbs light at 210 nm. We do not yet know what specific chemical substance in this purified peak actually contains the biological activity.

Because we still lack the structural identity or identities of the factors that are involved in insulin-dependent enzyme regulation *in vitro*, we are not yet in a position to clearly evaluate the hypothesis that one or more mediators might be involved in insulin signaling. Further progress in evaluating this hypothesis will be dependent on the single issue of purifying this factor or factors in my opinion.

VII. Concluding Remarks

The recent research progress on insulin action summarized in this review reflects substantive new insights into the cellular machinery involved in signaling by the insulin receptor. Investigators in the field are now in a position to approach several critical questions with biochemical approaches. Some of the most important of these questions include Does insulin receptor-associated tyrosine kinase activity participate directly in cellular signaling? What are the mechanisms by which ligand binding and tyrosine kinase activities of insulin receptor are regulated by other signaling pathways? What are the mechanisms by which certain cell surface components (e.g., glucose transporters and IGF-II receptors) are rapidly expressed on the cell surface in response to insulin? Are there soluble cellular components that participate in mediating the actions of insulin? Recent rapid progress in the field provides hope that the answers to these questions will be forthcoming.

ACKNOWLEDGMENTS

The work from the author's laboratory described in this article is supported by Grants AM 30648, AM 30676, and AM 30898 from the National Institutes of Health.

REFERENCES

August, G. P., Nissley, S. P., Kasuga, M., Lee, L., Greenstein, L., and Rechler, M. M. (1983). *J. Biol. Chem.* **258**, 9033–9036.

Avruch, J., Nemenoff, R. A., Blackshear, P. J., Pierce, M. W., and Osathanondh, R. (1982). *J. Biol. Chem.* **257**, 15162–15166.

Baker, G. F., and Widdas, W. F. (1973). *J. Physiol. (London)* **231**, 129–142.

Bhaumick, B., Bala, R. M., and Hollenberg, M. D. (1981). *Proc. Natl. Acad. Sci. U.S.A.* **78**, 4279–4283.

Carter-Su, C., Pessin, J. E., Mora, R., Gitomer, W., and Czech, M. P. (1982). *J. Biol. Chem.* **257**, 5416–5425.

Chernausek, S. D., Jacobs, S., and Van Wyk, J. J. (1981). *Biochemistry* **20**, 7345–7350.

Cohen, P. (1980). *In* "Molecular Aspects of Cellular Regulation," Vol. 1, pp. 1 and 255. Elsevier, Amsterdam.

Cohen, S., Carpenter, G., and King, L., Jr. (1980). *J. Biol. Chem.* **255**, 4834–4842.

Cuatrecasas, P., and Illiano, G. (1971). *J. Biol. Chem.* **246**, 4938–4946.

Cushman, S. W., and Wardzala, L. J. (1980). *J. Biol. Chem.* **255**, 4758–4762.

Czech, M. P. (1980). *Diabetes* **29**, 399–409.

Czech, M. P. (1981). *Am. J. Med.* **70**, 142–149.

Czech, M. P., Massague, J., and Pilch, P. F. (1981). *Trends Biochem. Sci.* **6**, 222–225.

Czech, M. P., Massague, J., Seals, J. R., and Yu, K.-T. (1984). *In* "Biochemical Actions of Hormones" (G. Litwack, ed.), Vol. 11, pp. 93–125. Academic Press, New York.

Deutsch, P. J., Wan, C. F., Rosen, O. M., and Rubin, C. S. (1983). *Proc. Natl. Acad. Sci. U.S.A.* **80**, 133–136.

Fain, J. N. (1980). *In* "Biochemical Actions of Hormones" (G. Litwack, ed.), Vol. 7, pp. 120–204. Academic Press, New York.

Fujita-Yamaguchi, Y., Choi, S., Sakamoto, Y., and Itakura, K. (1983). *J. Biol. Chem.* **258**, 5045–5049.

Gorga, F. R., and Lienhard, G. E. (1981). *Biochemistry* **20**, 5108–5113.

Haring, H. U., Kasuga, M., and Kahn, C. R. (1982). *Biochem. Biophys. Res. Commun.* **108**, 1538–1545.

Hedo, J. A., Kahn, C. R., Hayashi, M., Yamada, K. M., and Kasuga, M. (1983). *J. Biol. Chem.* **258**, 10020–10026.

Ingebritsen, T. S., and Cohen, P. (1983). *Science* **221**, 331–338.

Jacobs, S., and Cuatrecasas, P. (1981). *Endocrinol. Rev.* **2**, 251–263.

Jacobs, S., Hazum, E., Schnechter, Y., and Cuatrecasas, P. (1979). *Proc. Natl. Acad. Sci. U.S.A.* **76**, 4918–4921.

Jacobs, S., Hazum, E., and Cuatrecasas, P. (1980a). *Biochem. Biophys. Res. Commun.* **94**, 1066–1073.

Jacobs, S., Hazum, E., and Cuatrecasas, P. (1980b). *J. Biol. Chem.* **255**, 6937–6940.

Jacobs, S., Kull, F. C., and Cuatrecasas, P. (1983a). *Proc. Natl. Acad. Sci. U.S.A.* **80**, 1228–1231.

Jacobs, S., Kull, F. C., Earp, H. S., Svoboda, M. E., Wan Wyk, J. J., and Cuatrecasas, P. (1983b). *J. Biol. Chem.* **258**, 9581–9584.

Johnson, L. W., and Smith, C. H. (1982). *Biochem. Biophys. Res. Commun.* **109,** 408–413.
Karnieli, E., Zarnowski, M. J., Hissan, P. J., Simpson, I. A., Salans, L. B., and Cushman, S. W. (1981). *J. Biol. Chem.* **256,** 4772–4777.
Kasuga, M., Van Obberghen, E., Nissley, S. P., and Rechler, M. M. (1981). *J. Biol. Chem.* **256,** 5305–5308.
Kasuga, M., Hedo, J. A., Yamada, K. M., and Kahn, C. R. (1982a). *J. Biol. Chem.* **257,** 10392–10399.
Kasuga, M., Karlsson, F. A., and Kahn, C. R. (1982b). *Science* **215,** 185–187.
Kasuga, M., Van Obberghen, E., Nissley, S. P., and Rechler, M. M. (1982c). *Proc. Natl. Acad. Sci. U.S.A.* **79,** 1864–1868.
Kasuga, M., Zich, Y., Blithe, D. L., Crettaz, M., and Kahn, C. R. (1982d). *Nature* (*London*) **298,** 667–669.
Kasuga, M., Zich, Y., Blithe, D. L., Karlsson, F. A., Haring, H. U., and Kahn, C. R. (1982e). *J. Biol. Chem.* **257,** 9891–9894.
Kasuga, M., Fujita-Yamaguchi, Y., Blithe, D. L., and Kahn, C. R. (1983). *Proc. Natl. Acad. Sci. U.S.A.* **80,** 2137–2141.
Kiechle, F. L., Jarett, L., Rotagal, N., and Popp, D. A. (1981). *J. Biol. Chem.* **256,** 2945–2951.
King, G. L., Rechler, M. M., and Kahn, C. R. (1982). *J. Biol. Chem.* **257,** 10001–10006.
Klip, A., Walker, D., Ransome, K. J., Schroer, D. W., and Lienhard, G. E. (1983). *Arch. Biochem. Biophys.* **226,** 198–205.
Kono, T. (1983). *Recent Prog. Horm. Res.* **39,** 519–557.
Larner, J. (1982). *J. Cyclic Nucleotide Res.* **8,** 289–296.
Larner, J., Cheng, K., Schwartz, C., Kikuchi, K., Tamura, S., Creacy, S., Dubler, R., Galasko, G., Pullin, C., and Katz, M. (1982). *Fed Proc. Fed. Am. Soc. Exp. Biol.* **41,** 2724–2729.
Lienhard, G. E. (1983). *Trends Biochem. Sci.* **8,** 125–127.
Lonnroth, P., and Smith, U. (1983). *Biochem. Biophys. Res. Commun.* **112,** 972–979.
Machicao, F., Urumow, T., and Wieland, O. H. (1982). *FEBS Lett.* **149,** 96–100.
Massague, J., and Czech, M. P. (1982a). *J. Biol. Chem.* **257,** 5038–5045.
Massague, J., and Czech, M. P. (1982b). *J. Biol. Chem.* **257,** 6729–6738.
Massague, J., Pilch, P. F., and Czech, M. P. (1980). *Proc. Natl. Acad. Sci. U.S.A.* **77,** 7137–7141.
Massague, J., Guillette, B. J., and Czech, M. P. (1981a). *J. Biol. Chem.* **256,** 2122–2125.
Massague, J., Pilch, P. F., and Czech, M. P. (1981b). *J. Biol. Chem.* **256,** 3182–3190.
Massague, J., Blinderman, L. A., and Czech, M. P. (1982). *J. Biol. Chem.* **257,** 13958–13963.
Massague, J., Freidenberg, G. F., Olefsky, J. M., and Czech, M. P. (1983). *Diabetes* **32,** 541–544.
Oka, Y., and Czech, M. P. (1984a). *In* "Methods in Diabetes Research" (S. L. Pohl and J. Larner, eds.), Vol. 1. Wiley, New York. In press.
Oka, Y., and Czech, M. P. (1984b). In press.
Oka, Y., and Czech, M. P. (1984c). *Proc. Natl. Acad. Sci. U.S.A.,* in press.
Oppenheimer, C. L., and Czech, M. P. (1983). *J. Biol. Chem.* **258,** 8539–8542.
Oppenheimer, C. L., Pessin, J. E., Massague, J., Gitomer, W., and Czech, M. P. (1983). *J. Biol. Chem.* **258,** 4824–4830.
Pessin, J. E., Tillotson, L. G., Yamada, K., Gitomer, W., Carter-Su, C., Mora, R., Isselbacher, K. J., and Czech, M. P. (1982). *Proc. Natl. Acad. Sci. U.S.A.* **79,** 2286–2290.
Pessin, J. E., Gitomer, W., Oka, Y., Oppenheimer, C. L., and Czech, M. P. (1983). *J. Biol. Chem.* **258,** 7386–7394.

Petruzzelli, L. M., Ganguly, S., Smith, C. J., Cobb, M. H., Rubin, C. S., and Rosen, O. M. (1982). *Proc. Natl. Acad. Sci. U.S.A.* **79**, 6792–6796.

Pilch, P. F., and Czech, M. P. (1980). *Science* **210**, 1152–1153.

Rechler, M. M., Nissley, S. P., King, G. L., Moses, A. C., Van Obberghen-Schilling, E. E., Romanus, J. A., Knight, A. B., Short, P. A., and White, R. M. (1981). *J. Supramol. Struct. Cell. Biochem.* **15**, 253–286.

Rosen, O. M., Herrera, R., Olowe, Y., Petruzzelli, L. M., and Cobb, M. H. (1983). *Proc. Natl. Acad. Sci. U.S.A.* **80**, 3237–3240.

Roth, J., Kahn, C. R., Lesniak, M. A., Gorden, P., DeMeyts, P., Megyesi, K., Neville, D. M., Jr., Gavin, J. E., III, Soll, A. H., Freychet, P., Goldfine, I. D., Bar, R. S., and Archer, J. A. (1975). *Recent Prog. Horm. Res.* **31**, 95–139.

Roth, R. A., and Cassell, D. J. (1983). *Science* **219**, 299–301.

Seals, J. R., and Czech, M. P. (1982). *Fed. Proc. Fed. Am. Soc. Exp. Biol.* **41**, 2730–2735.

Seals, J. R., and Jarett, L. (1980). *Proc. Natl. Acad. Sci. U.S.A.* **77**, 77–81.

Shanahan, M. F. (1982). *J. Biol. Chem.* **257**, 7290–7293.

Shanahan, M. F., Olson, S. A., Weber, M. J., Lienhard, G. E., and Gorga, J. C. (1982). *Biochem. Biophys. Res. Commun.* **107**, 38–43.

Shia, M. A., and Pilch, P. F. (1983). *Biochemistry* **22**, 717–721.

Sogin, D. C., and Hinkle, P. C. (1980). *Proc. Natl. Acad. Sci. U.S.A.* **77**, 5725–5729.

Suzuki, K., and Kono, T. (1980). *Proc. Natl. Acad. Sci. U.S.A.* **77**, 2542–2545.

Van Obberghen, E., and Kowalski, A. (1982). *FEBS Lett.* **143**, 179–182.

Van Obberghen, E., Rossi, B., Kowalski, A., Gazzano, H., and Ponzio, G. (1983). *Proc. Natl. Acad. Sci. U.S.A.* **80**, 945–949.

Wheeler, T. J., Simpson, I. A., Sogin, D. C., Hinkle, P. C., and Cushman, S. W. (1982). *Biochem. Biophys. Res. Commun.* **105**, 89–95.

Yip, C. C., and Moule, M. L. (1983). *Fed. Proc. Fed. Am. Soc. Exp. Biol.* **42**, 2842–2845.

Yu, K.-T., and Czech, M. P. (1984a). *J. Biol. Chem.*, submitted.

Yu, K.-T., and Czech, M. P. (1984b). *J. Biol. Chem.*, in press.

Zapf, J., Schoenle, E., and Froesch, E. R. (1978). *Eur. J. Biochem.* **87**, 285–296.

Zick, Y., Kasuga, M., Kahn, C. R., and Roth, J. (1983). *J. Biol. Chem.* **258**, 75–80.

DISCUSSION

N. Samaan: Dr. Czech, in your introductory slides you showed insulin, IGF-I, and IGF-II and mentioned that IGF-I and II formation may be related to growth hormone and formed in the liver. You also showed an overlap between the insulin receptors and IGF-I and IGF-II receptors. Later on, it was referred to IGF-I and IGF-II as the insulin peptides or the insulin family peptides.

For clarification of this complex subject, IGF-I and IGF-II were called in the past "non-suppressible insulin-like activity (ILA) or atypical ILA" which was first described by us in 1963. We have shown that nonsuppressible ILA as measured by the fat pad assay decrease significantly or disappear from the peripheral circulation after pancreatectomy depending on the degree of pancreatectomy. We also showed that the nonsuppressible ILA is increased in the hepatic vein of dogs after infusion of regular insulin in the portal circulation of pancre-atectomized animals. Furthermore, we showed that in patients with severe liver cirrhosis and porta-caval shunts, the total ILA was normal but the nonsuppressible ILA was signifi-cantly low although the growth hormone level in these patients was higher than that found in normal subjects. These experiments indicated that nonsuppressible ILA is formed in the liver and is related to pancreatic insulin. These observations have been since confirmed by other investigators.

Other workers showed that IGF-I was increased in the circulation after injection of growth hormone *in vivo* and suggested that IGF-I formation is dependent on growth hormone and formed in the liver. We should be aware of the fact that growth hormone stimulates insulin secretion by both direct action on the islet cells and indirect action through peripheral resistance to the action of insulin due to increased lipolysis. The increase of IGF-I after growth hormone injection may be a result of increased insulin secretion rather than the growth hormone itself. We should also recognize that the liver has a high content of non-suppressible ILA.

So it appears from the experimental evidence that IGF-I and IGF-II are related to pancreatic insulin and formed in the liver, but growth hormone has a synergetic effect particularly in the formation of IGF-I. We should note that both IGF-I and IGF-II structurally (amino acid sequence) are related to proinsulin but have no relation whatsoever to growth hormone molecule. This explains the overlap between the insulin receptors IGF-I and IGF-II demonstrated by your study.

M. P. Czech: I hope I made it clear that the structural homologies of the insulin family peptides are substantial, and extending that concept, the receptors themselves share at least certain structural homologies. In relation to your question, we have data that quite rigorously address the question of biological potency of the three receptor structures that I showed you. It turns out that the structurally homologous insulin receptor and IGF-I receptor, at least in muscle, are both linked to the rapid activation of hexose transport activity that we normally associate with insulin action. Thus, rather than divorcing the actions of the three peptides, I would argue that they are very related and in fact the two receptor structures for insulin and IGF-I both are capable of modulating the exact same responses, at least in muscle. Whether indeed IGF-I plays an important role in muscle physiology I think remains to be demonstrated, but I think the biochemistry would favor that may be the case.

B. Posner: I just wanted to clarify if the nonsurface available IGF-II receptor is in low-density microsomes as well?

M. P. Czech: Yes. If one looks at the quantity of the IGF-II receptor in the low-density microsomes, it's present in much higher quantities compared to the plasma membrane fraction, and the same redistribution phenomenon occurs in response to insulin.

B. Posner: And it is more concentrated in low-density microsomes than in heavier fractions?

M. P. Czech: That's correct, the heavy microsome fraction for both the transporter and the IGF-II receptor contains relatively low amounts of these components compared to the low-density microsomes.

B. Posner: I just wished to clarify whether you are convinced that the IGF-II receptor is incapable of autophosphorylation.

M. P. Czech: My point was that the IGF-II receptor, the 250K receptor structure, is a receptor structure not apparently homologous to the insulin and IGF-I receptors. In our studies with purified IGF-II receptor, we see no phosphorylation *in vitro* either on tyrosine or serine, correlated with ligand activation of that receptor. The presence of that receptor (250K type II IGF receptor) in the kind of kinase assay I showed for the insulin receptor also provides no evidence of an ability to catalyze phosphorylation. Our data I think would therefore very strongly argue against the concept that the IGF-II receptor has tyrosine kinase-associated activity. In contrast, the IGF-I receptor and the insulin receptor are homologous in that they are both associated with tyrosine kinase activity.

B. Posner: The next point is that autophosphorylation of the receptor has been demonstrated in solubilized preparations. Has anyone ever demonstrated this in membrane preparation?

M. P. Czech: That's a sticky problem and it probably relates to the presence of phosphatases in the membrane preparations we all use. It turns out that there are no published studies in isolated membranes where autophosphorylation using [γ-^{32}P]ATP is readily demonstrated for the insulin receptor. I don't think we should make too strong a conclusion based on the lack of demonstration of kinase activity in membranes.

B. Posner: Just switching to the mediator for a moment; do you see activation of mitochondrial PDH in intact freshly prepared mitochondria?

M. P. Czech: Yes, we see it in intact mitochondria or in broken freeze-thawed mitochondria.

B. Posner: Can you adsorb out this activity by pretreatment of your extracts with mitochondria?

M. P. Czech: It's a good suggestion, but we have not done that experiment.

B. Posner: If indeed the kinase is an important component of the receptor which plays a key role in mediating the biological response, how do you visualize activation of the kinase affecting a variety of intracellular enzymes often far removed from the membrane itself? Does this not imply that there is some kind of redistribution of receptor associated with biological activation?

M. P. Czech: That's one possibility. There's the possibility that the internalization of the receptor thereby brings the receptor into cellular loci required for substrate phosphorylation by the receptor. My view is that while that is of course possible, especially for the growth-related effect of insulin, the kinetics of insulin action are so rapid on many of the target enzymes that perhaps the internalization mechanism may not be necessary for the rapid, acute effects. Alternatively, is it possible that the tyrosine kinase activity initiates a cascade by phosphorylating membrane kinases or phosphatases which are then released into the cell and which then are able to catalyze phosphorylation or dephosphorylation of the ultimate target enzymes. Such a proposed mechanism, is, for example, related to the previous talk where we saw that the C kinase was redistributed in cellular location in response to its activation by phorbol esters. I think that this is another perhaps more subtle variation of the theme. Basically, at present we can't really say at all whether indeed the tyrosine kinase activity is involved in mediating cellular signals or whether it's involved in modulating other receptor functions such as internalization, deactivation of the receptor, or desensitization. I think we have to be careful about leaving open several possibilities for the function of tyrosine kinase activity. I think that's where many workers in the field are now directing their attention.

G. D. Aurbach: I would like to congratulate you on an excellent review and on the apparent real progress in identifying the mediator. In terms of the two different potential mechanisms of insulin action which is the most sensitive? In dose–response studies, how does the tyrosine kinase activity respond versus the mediator production?

M. P. Czech: Good question. The answer is that the tyrosine kinase activity, unlike all of the responsive targets for insulin action, responds in a linear fashion related to occupancy of the receptor by insulin. In other words, the dose–response curve for activation of the tyrosine kinase activity does not saturate until the receptor is saturated by ligand. All the other responses to insulin action in intact cells always appear to saturate well before saturation of the receptor. The putative mediator appears to be maximally released from membranes at 100 μU/ml of insulin or less which is well below the saturation of the insulin receptor in terms of binding. However, we must be careful that in such studies only activity is measured, not structurally characterized factors, and this could mislead us.

G. D. Aurbach: One further question. When the receptor is phosphorylated does it have a lower affinity for insulin than the nonphosphorylated receptor? In fact, does phosphorylation correlate with the negative cooperativity effects of insulin on the insulin receptor?

M. P. Czech: There are two basic responses to the question. The first is that upon addition of ATP and phosphorylation of the receptor, one can see changes in receptor binding which are not overly dramatic but in the 20 to 30% range. We can't be confident that the effect on binding is causally related to receptor phosphorylation, however. More interestingly, I think a very dramatic effect we have recently discovered and recently published in the *J. Biol. Chem.* shows that increases in cyclic AMP will rapidly modulate a decrease in insulin binding to its receptor in intact adipocytes. That is, β-catecholamines or any other agent added to fat cells which increase cyclic AMP will desensitize the insulin receptor very rapidly. The effect is substantial—up to 60% inhibition of insulin binding. It really was quite amazing to us that this phenomena was not discovered much earlier since we know that the antogonism between β-catecholamines and insulin action is very dramatic in the adipocyte. It would appear that one contributing aspect of the antoganism relates to this inhibitory effect of cyclic AMP action on the insulin receptor. The data we have generated would suggest that this effect of cyclic AMP is mediated through the cAMP-dependent protein kinase and is secondary to a phosphorylation, perhaps of the insulin receptor itself or some other modulatory of the insulin receptor.

P. A. Kelly: The very exciting data you presented on the purification of the mediator hopefully will lead to some information on whether this really is the factor which is responsible for insulin action. Could you tell us something about the second peak which you see on ion-exchange chromatography, in terms of mediator activity, and second, could you perhaps describe what might contribute to the various problems that some investigators in different laboratories have had reproducing mediator data?

M. P. Czech: The reasons for problems with reproducibility of data on putative mediator activities are unknown. Our laboratory has also experienced difficulties in reproducibly obtaining insulin-dependent enzyme regulator released from plasma membranes. There is no doubt that this is a major problem in the field. In our laboratory, we find the extractions of intact cells lead to more uniform results.

We have looked at the second peak in some detail. The amino acid composition of what appears to be substantially purified peak 2 seems to have some intriguing relationship to the amino acid composition for peak 1. Interestingly, the second peak of activity does not bind the C-18 reverse phase column in our hands and so there are clear characteristic differences between those two peaks and we have therefore utilized ion-exchange HPLC columns to obtain purity. We really can't say any more about the relationship other than that. I think the critical issue is to determine whether indeed the material that we have purified really relates to a novel peptide or protein or whether it may be a fragment or a piece of a protein of trivial nature which is present in the preparation. I think there are a tremendous number of hurdles yet to cross, and I think we should take the most conservative position possible in this area.

J. H. Oppenheimer: You have shown very nicely the cellular redistribution of the glucose transport units and IGF-II receptor. Have you had a chance to examine as controls other components of the membrane systems which do not directly relate to insulin and glucose homeostasis?

M. P. Czech: Controls that have been done by Dr. Kono's group and Dr. Cushman's group initially, and also our lab more recently, involve the measurement of marker enzymes. While these marker enzymes have been assayed by activity measurements rather than by the actual mass of the enzyme present, I think they lead quite well to the conclusion that all marker enzymes studied, other than the glucose transporter and the IGF-II receptor, do not redistribute in response to insulin.

K. Sterling: I wonder if you could provide some further idea of how the tyrosine phosphate or the mediator could produce a very rapid effect on the plasma membrane such as inward movement of glucose.

M. P. Czech: No, I cannot.

Y. Nishizuka: I have a very quick question. I wonder if insulin tyrosine kinase reaction is intramolecular or intermolecular; in other words, crosswise reactive with other tyrosine kinases such as EGF kinase.

M. P. Czech: It appears to be intramolecular, based on dilution experiments. I do not know whether the EGF receptor or other receptor kinases serve as substrates for the insulin receptor kinase.

C. Sonnenschein: I wonder whether you could briefly comment on some remarks you made in your first three of four slides in which you relate the effects of insulin to DNA synthesis or cell proliferation.

M. P. Czech: I don't know how it happens certainly but again we have looked at this issue very carefully in terms of the linkage between each receptor structure and growth control, and the conclusion from those studies is that (1) the insulin receptor is not capable in many cell types of modulating the growth response, that is, the cell proliferative response, but in some cell types such as the H35 hepatoma cell line insulin receptor is very competent in modulating that response. (2) The IGF-I receptor seems to be associated with growth control in a variety of cell types in which it resides. That is interesting because it may be the first crack in the concept that I have tried to convey that the receptors for insulin and IGF-I are homologous in virtually every way we have looked. (3) While the data I think are supportive of the notion that IGF-II receptor structure mediates a growth effect there really are no data that demonstrate this unequivocally. We are currently hopeful that antibodies we have produced which inhibit binding of IGF-II receptor to IGF-II specifically should be very useful probes addressing that particular question. Your remark seems to relate more to the molecular basis of the growth response, and since we have very little information on the actual mechanism of receptor signaling, your question unfortunately cannot be answered at this point.

The Interaction of Prolactin with Its Receptors in Target Tissues and Its Mechanism of Action

PAUL A. KELLY, JEAN DJIANE,* MASAO KATOH, LOUIS H. FERLAND,
LOUIS-MARIE HOUDEBINE,* BERTRAND TEYSSOT,* AND
ISABELLE DUSANTER-FOURT*

*Laboratory of Molecular Endocrinology, Royal Victoria Hospital, Montreal, Quebec,
Canada, and * Laboratoire de Physiologie de la Lactation, Institut National de la
Recherche Agronomique, C.N.R.Z., Jouy-en-Josas, France*

I. Introduction

Prolactin is a hormone secreted by the anterior pituitary gland, whose primary action involves the development of the mammary gland and production of milk, which is essential for the survival of newborn mammals. Prolactin was first discovered by Stricker and Grueter in 1928. These investigators demonstrated that bovine pituitary extracts could induce milk secretion in castrated rabbits treated with corpora lutea extracts (Stricker and Grueter, 1928). Independently, Corner (1930) demonstrated that milk secretion could be induced in the mammary glands of adult ovariectomized virgin rabbits by the injection of sheep pituitary extracts. Soon thereafter, Riddle *et al.* (1932) identified a fraction from bovine pituitary extracts which was capable of stimulating the growth of pigeon crop sacs, and named the factor prolactin. Studies which followed these original investigations demonstrated that the effect seen in birds was due to the same hormone that induced lactation in rats and rabbits.

Prolactin has since been identified and purified from a number of species, including human, sheep, cattle, pig, rat, rabbit, dog, chicken, and fish. In addition, it has been shown to be present in horses, whales, cats, guinea pigs, hamsters, amphibians, reptiles, and birds (Li, 1980). This ubiquitous hormone appears to exist in all vertebrates and over 85 biological functions have been attributed to prolactin (Nicoll and Bern, 1972). In mammals, prolactin is primarily involved in the regulation of reproduction and lactation and to a lesser extent in the regulation of water and ion fluxes.

The mechanisms by which prolactin induces its numerous actions are poorly understood. Most of the work in this area has utilized the mammary gland as a model, where prolactin is the essential hormone which

379

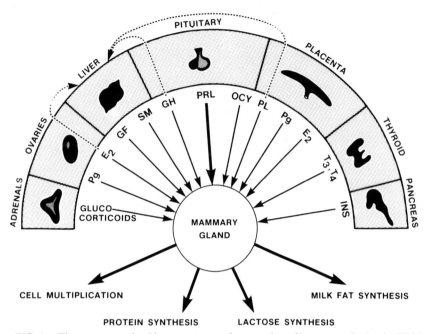

FIG. 1. The mammary gland is a target organ for a number of hormones. Prolactin (PRL) is the primary hormone controlling mammary activity. In some species, placental latogen (PL) appears to play a similar role to PRL in stimulating mammary activity directly. In addition, PL possesses properties like the pituitary growth hormone (GH) which is responsible for the stimulation of somatomedin (SM) production by the liver. These SM along with insulin (INS) are involved in cell multiplication. The ovary and placenta (in certain species) secrete the steroid hormones estrogen (E_2) and progesterone (Pg) which are responsible for the differentiation of the mammary gland. Pg also plays an important role as a syncronizing agent, blocking the secretory activity of the gland during pregnancy. Estrogens also have a direct effect on the production of growth factors (GF). Adrenal glucocorticoids amplify all the effects of prolactin. The thyroid hormones (T_3 and T_4) can be either stimulatory or inhibitory, dependent on the dose utilized. Oxytocin (OCY) is responsible for milk let-down through its action on the myoepithelial cells which surround the mammary alveoli and can also stimulate the movement of secretory vesicles within the mammary cell.

controls the activity of mammary cells. As can be seen in Fig. 1, however, the action of prolactin on cell multiplication and the synthesis of milk proteins, lactose, and milk fats, is affected by a number of other hormones either directly or indirectly. Although the model is somewhat complex, the action of prolactin is definite and easily measured.

A schematic representation of the effects of prolactin on the mammary cell is shown in Fig. 2. Following binding of prolactin to its receptor at the level of the plasma membrane, a number of effects within the cell can be

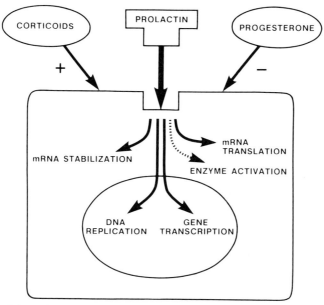

FIG. 2.   Schematic representation of the action of prolactin on a mammary cell and its modulation by glucocorticoids and progesterone.

observed: these include, at the nuclear level, a stimulation of mitotic activity and an activation of transcription of milk protein genes; within the cytoplasm, the transcriptional products (mRNA) are stabilized and the translation of messenger RNA is stimulated. Although as yet unclear, these modifications are probably mediated by a modification in various enzyme activities. The two major hormones which modulate the actions of prolactin are glucocorticoids which are synergistic to most actions of prolactin and progesterone, which is the major inhibitor of prolactin's actions (Houdebine *et al.*, 1984b).

II. General Characteristics of the Prolactin Receptor

Prolactin receptors have been localized in a number of tissues including mammary gland, liver, kidney, adrenals, ovaries, testes, prostate, seminal vesicles, hypothalamus and choroid plexus, pancreatic islets, and lymphoid tissue (Posner and Khan, 1983). Although the action of prolactin in all these tissues is not known, most of the biochemical characterization and physiological regulation have been carried out in the mammary gland and liver.

A. DISSOCIATION OF PROLACTIN FROM ITS RECEPTOR

The interaction of a hormone with its receptor is the initial event leading to the formation of a hormone receptor complex. Under equilibrium conditions, this reaction has been considered to be freely reversible (Kahn *et al.*, 1974; De Meyts *et al.*, 1976). However, for an increasing list of hormones, including PRL, hGH, TSH, insulin, LH, and β-adrenergics (Kelly *et al.*, 1980; Van der Gugten *et al.*, 1980; Donner *et al.*, 1978, 1980; Donner and Corin, 1980; Powell-Jones *et al.*, 1979; Katikineni *et al.*, 1980; Ross *et al.*, 1977), it appears that dissociation of the hormone receptor complex is difficult and that an irreversibility of the complex is established with an increase in the time of association of the hormone with its receptor.

A difference in the dissociability of prolactin from rat liver and rabbit mammary gland prolactin receptors has been observed. ^{125}I-labeled oPRL dissociates more readily from rat liver than from rabbit mammary prolactin receptors (Kelly *et al.*, 1980; Van der Gugten *et al.*, 1980; Perry and Jacobs, 1978). In addition, the longer a labeled hormone is allowed to associate with its receptor, the more tightly it appears to be bound resulting in the decreased ability to dissociate.

In rat liver, where dissociability can be more easily measured, there are marked differences in the dissociability of receptors normally found at the cell periphery (plasma membrane) and in microsomes, of which a major component in rat liver preparations is the intracellular Golgi membranes (Bergeron *et al.*, 1973, 1978). Figure 3 shows that ^{125}I-labeled oPRL dissociates from plasma membrane receptors much more readily than from microsomes following 1 hour of association. The dissociation curves, which can be resolved into fast and slow components based on logarithmic transformation (Williams and Lefkowitz, 1978) reveal a greater than two-fold increase in the faster component of the dissociation rate constant (k_2) in plasma membranes compared to microsomes with no change in the slow component (Table I).

However, with increased association times, plasma membranes preferentially develop a slowly dissociating component. Figure 4 shows a similar dissociation study carried out with membranes which have been allowed to associate with labeled prolactin for 10 hours. The difference between plasma membrane and microsome component is less apparent. It appears that with longer periods of association (10 hours), prolactin receptors in plasma membranes develop dissociation characteristics similar to those observed in microsomes following just 1 hour of association. This shift is confirmed in Table I (Kelly *et al.*, 1983b).

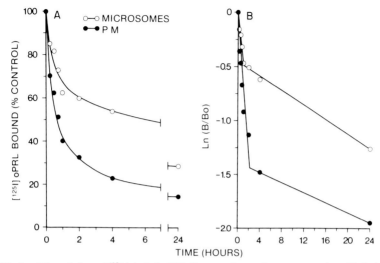

FIG. 3. Dissociation of ^{125}I-labeled oPRL from rat liver microsomes and purified plasma membranes (PM) at 23°C following 1 hour of association. A shows the dissociation as a percentage of specific binding at time 0 (after 1 hour of association) which is 11,180 and 8980 cpm for microsomes and PM, respectively. B shows the data transformed to linearize the curve. The slope of these curves is used to calculate the dissociation rate constant (k_2).

Although not shown here, Scatchard plots of purified Golgi and plasma membrane fractions revealed a more than two-fold lower dissociation constant for prolactin receptors in plasma membrane. The decreased affinity would allow prolactin to more readily dissociate from its receptors.

TABLE I

Dissociation Rate Constants (k_2) ^{125}I-Labeled oPRL from Rat Liver Microsomes and Purified Plasma Membranes as a Function of Time[a,b]

Fraction	1 hour association[c]		10 hour association[c]	
	Fast component	Slow component	Fast component	Slow component
Microsomes	0.44	0.03	0.34	0.02
Plasma membranes	0.91	0.02	0.38	0.03

[a] The labeled ligand was allowed to associate with the binding sites.

[b] Rate constants were calculated from the dissociation data shown in Figs. 3 and 4 (Williams and Lefkowitz, 1978). These data are the mean of two separate dissociation experiments.

[c] Rate constant (k_2), per hour.

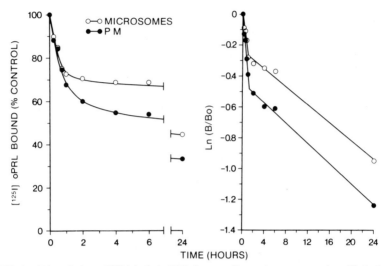

FIG. 4.   Dissociation of ^{125}I-labeled oPRL from rat liver microsomes and purified plasma membranes (PM) at 23°C following 10 hours of association. Conditions are as described in Fig. 3. Specific binding at time 0 (after 10 hours of association) is 25,800 and 18,380 cpm for microsomes and PM, respectively.

These studies could have important implications in terms of cellular function. A large percentage of prolactin receptors in rat liver is located within the cell (Josefsberg *et al.*, 1979). These results confirm the differential subcellular localization of PRL receptors and suggest that receptors in the PM and Golgi are in different forms, with the affinity of the receptor being dependent on the subcellular localization.

B. RECEPTOR REGULATION BY PROLACTIN

1. Up-Regulation

The hormonal regulation of prolactin receptors is complex (Kelly *et al.*, 1978). Estradiol injection into male or female rats leads to an increase in hepatic prolactin binding sites (Posner *et al.*, 1974a; Kelly *et al.*, 1975). The fact that prolactin binding can be stimulated by estrogens, fluctuates with the estrous cycle, and is reduced by ovariectomy implies a direct physiological involvement of estradiol.

The loss of prolactin binding in rat liver following hypophysectomy implied the importance of a pituitary factor in the maintaince of these binding sites (Kelly *et al.*, 1975). A direct effect of prolactin on its own receptor was first implied when we demonstrated that prolactin binding to rat liver in hypophysectomized rats given a pituitary implant under the kidney capsule began to increase approximately 3 days following the increase in serum prolactin levels (Posner *et al.*, 1975). A direct stimulatory effect of prolactin injected in polyvinylpyrrolidone to retard absorption has more recently been reported (Manni *et al.*, 1978; Kelly *et al.*, 1980).

The up-regulatory effect of prolactin on prolactin receptors in rabbit mammary gland has also been demonstrated (Djiane and Durand, 1977). Pseudopregnant rabbits injected with 100 IU oPRL showed a marked increase in prolactin receptor levels. This increase could be prevented by simultaneous administration of progesterone, suggesting that part of the progesterone block of lactation during pregnancy could be mediated by a reduction in prolactin receptor levels in the mammary gland.

2. Down-Regulation

As just described, in contrast to the inhibitory effect of a large number of hormones on the level of their own receptor, a stimulatory effect of prolactin on its receptor in both rabbit mammary gland and rat liver has been observed (Posner *et al.*, 1975; Djiane and Durand, 1977). Using 4 M $MgCl_2$ to dissociate bound prolactin from its receptor (Kelly *et al.*, 1979), we investigated the short-term action of prolactin on its receptor in target tissues with the goal of evaluating if prolactin, in addition to its ability to up-regulate prolactin receptors, is, like most other hormones studied so far, capable of inducing a down-regulation of its own receptor.

Lactating, New Zealand rabbits were injected every 12 hours over a 36-hour period with 2 mg of the dopamine agonist, CB-154, to lower circulating prolactin levels (Djiane *et al.*, 1977) after which the animals were anesthetized with 50 mg/kg of sodium pentobarbital. Three milligrams bovine prolactin (bPRL) was injected intravenously and 2 g biopsies of mammary gland tissue were removed at the indicated times between 0 and 30 hours after prolactin injection.

As illustrated in Fig. 5, injection of 3 mg of prolactin led to a maximal occupancy of free rabbit mammary gland prolactin receptors 15 minutes after the intravenous injection, corresponding to periods just following maximal serum concentrations. The highest serum levels were seen 1 minute after injection with values rapidly declining thereafter. Although saturating concentrations of circulating prolactin were present 15 minutes after injection, 20% of the prolactin receptors remained free to bind ^{125}I-labeled oPRL. This could be due to an inaccessibility of the receptors to the circulating prolactin or to some dissociation occurring while membranes were isolated from the tissue. Total prolactin receptor levels assayed following *in vitro* desaturation with 4 M $MgCl_2$ declined progres-

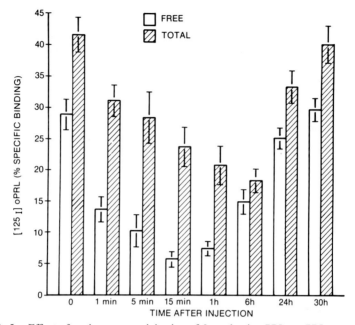

FIG. 5.   Effect of an intravenous injection of 3 mg bovine PRL on PRL receptors in rabbit mammary glands. Biopsies (2 g) were removed at the indicated times after PRL injection from lactating rabbits. Free and total (MgCl$_2$-treated) PRL receptor levels were determined. Binding is expressed as a percentage of specific binding per 400 μg protein. Values are means ± SEM of 7 animals.

sively up to 6 hours after the intravenous injection of prolactin and returned to normal at 24 to 30 hours. The difference in total prolactin binding between time 0 and 6 hours was statistically significant ($p < 0.01$). A difference was observed between the pattern of occupation (free receptors) and the down-regulation reflected by total receptors. In addition, free receptors increased between 1 and 6 hours, whereas total receptors continued to decline until 6 hours (Djiane et al., 1979a).

It has been well established that the mammary gland can be maintained in organ culture and responds well to hormones. In addition, mammary explants can be used as an experimental model to study the steps involved in the mechanisms of hormone action (Devinoy et al., 1978). The following study was undertaken to verify the maintenance of PRL receptors in mammary glands in organ culture, to assess the apparent turnover of receptors, and to describe the effect of large doses of prolactin on the levels of its own receptor.

Figure 6A illustrates the maintenance of prolactin receptors in mammary gland explants cultured in the presence of insulin. Binding increased

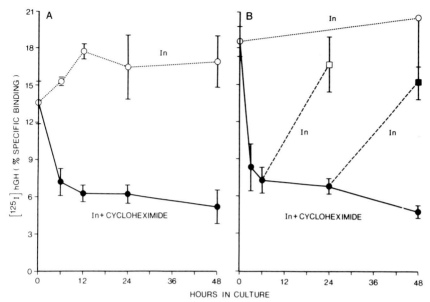

FIG. 6.   Maintenance of PRL receptors and the effect of cycloheximide on PRL receptors in rabbit mammary gland explants. (A) Mammary explants were cultured for different times in the presence of insulin (In) or In + cycloheximide. (B) Explants cultures in the presence of In + cycloheximide after which the media was changed at 6 or 24 hours and cycloheximide was removed. Values are means ± SEM of 3 cultures.

slightly up to 12 hours and remained constant up to 48 hours (Djiane *et al.*, 1979b). Addition of cycloheximide (1 μg/ml) resulted in a rapid decline of binding during the first 6 hours and remained low until 48 hours. Figure 6B shows another experiment and demonstrates the reversibility of the effect of cycloheximide (1 μg/ml). In the presence of insulin only, the level of receptors was maintained up until 48 hours as shown previously. The addition of cycloheximide resulted in a rapid decrease of receptors which was almost maximal at 3 hours. Removal of cycloheximide from the culture medium at either 6 or 24 hours by replacement with a medium deficient in cycloheximide resulted in a return of prolactin binding to near control levels 18–24 hours later.

A down-regulation of prolactin receptors in rabbit mammary gland in organ culture has also been observed. Inclusion of PRL (1 μg/ml) in the incubation medium resulted in a 80% saturation of free receptors and down-regulation of total prolactin receptors.

For a number of polypeptide hormones, binding is followed by an internalization of the hormone–receptor complex (Bergeron *et al.*, 1978; Conn *et al.*, 1978; Kolata, 1978), after which the labeled ligands become associated with lysosomal components in the cells (Conn *et al.*, 1978; Gordon *et al.*, 1978). Lysosomotropic agents such as chloroquine, methylamine, or ammonium chloride have been shown to reduce clustering for α_2-macroglobulin and epidermal growth factor (EGF) on cell surface of fibroblasts (Maxfield *et al.*, 1979). ^{125}I-labeled hCG which has been internalized and is associated with lysosomes is rapidly degraded to monoiodotyrosine. This process of degradation could be inhibited by lysosomotropic agents (Ascoli and Puett, 1978).

In order to examine if the down-regulation of prolactin receptors in rabbit mammary gland involved a lysosomal-mediated step, mammary explants were cultured in the presence of ammonium chloride (10 mM). Figure 7 shows that PRL binding after 24 hours in explant culture in the presence of In alone was similar to binding values in explants which were prepared but were immediately frozen at −20°C rather than cultured. PRL induced a 60% down-regulation of total PRL receptors. Ammonium

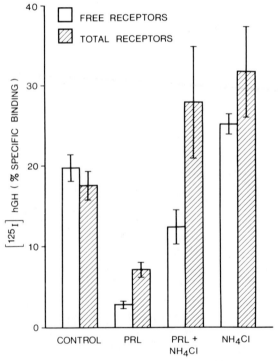

FIG. 7. Free and total prolactin receptor levels in mammary explants cultured for 24 hours in the presence of insulin (1 μg/ml) alone (control) or insulin plus prolactin (1 μg/ml) or ammonium chloride (10 mM) or a combination of both.

chloride alone markedly increased the basal level of prolactin binding and also reduced the ability of prolactin to induce a down-regulation of its receptors.

Similar experiments using mammary explants were carried out with lysosomotropic agents, and microfilament and microtubule-disrupting drugs. Houdebine and Djiane (1980) reported that although lysosomotropic agents were effective in blocking down-regulation of prolactin receptors, they were without effect on the level of casein gene expression. Cytocalasin B had no effect on down-regulation of receptors (Djiane *et al.*, 1980) nor on casein gene expression, whereas the microtubule disruption drug, colchicine, had very little effect on down-regulation, but almost completely blocked prolactin action (Houdebine and Djiane, 1980).

C. INTRACELLULAR PROLACTIN RECEPTORS

It is clear that receptors are located not only at the cell periphery, but within the cell, in Golgi elements (Josefsberg *et al.*, 1979), and also in lysosomes (Khan *et al.*, 1981).

We have identified and characterized prolactin receptors in highly purified lysosomes and light, lysosome-like structures and compared them with previously characterized Golgi and plasma membrane receptors. We also studied the internalization of labeled prolactin into liver cells by following its incorporation *in vivo* into subcellular fractions. Our results demonstrate that internalized radioactivity is observed initially in the Golgi and subsequently in the light lysosomes-like vesicles and mature lysosomes and suggest a role of lysosomes in the degradation of the hormone-receptor complex.

Lysosomes and light lysosome-like structures (the L-1 fraction from Wattiaux *et al.*, 1978) were isolated from estradiol pretreated rats (5 μg, sc twice a day for 7 days) by a modification of the method of Wattiaux *et al.* (1978) on a discontinuous Metrizamide gradient. Plasma membranes were isolated by the method of Ray (1970) and Golgi fraction by a modification of the method of Bergeron *et al.* (1978): rats were not given ethanol and the density gradient had only three stages (densities 1.20, 1.15, and 1.03 g/ml) so that all three subfractions described were mixed together.

Lysosomal fractions L-1 and L-2, although containing a very small percentage of total homogenate protein, bore somewhat larger proportions of homogenate acid phosphatase activity. L-2 had the highest relative specific activity of acid phosphatase activity. Chloroquine treatment of rats markedly reduced acid phosphatase activity in all lysosomal fractions but not in other fractions (Ferland *et al.*, 1984). Contamination of

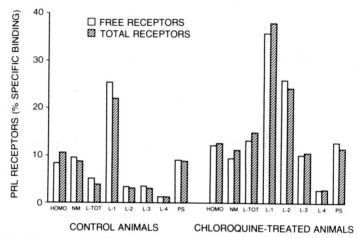

FIG. 8. Livers from female rats treated with estradiol and CB-154 (control animals) and further treated or not with chloroquine were processed for lysosome isolation. Each fraction and subfraction was assayed for prolactin receptors using 400 μg protein for the homogenate and NM, L-TOT, and PS fractions and 200 μg protein for subfractions L-1 to L-4. All values are expressed per 200 μg protein. MgCl₂ treatment was performed on separate aliquots of each fraction to desaturate the binding sites for measurement of total receptors. Homo, total liver homogenate; NM, nuclei and mitochondria (unpurified); L-TOT, "light mitochondrial fraction" of De Duve et al. (1955); L-1 to L-4, subfractions of L-TOT, including purified secondary lysosomes (L-2); PS, microsomes and soluble matrix (unpurified).

purified fractions of all four organelles studied by marker enzymes was relatively low.

Figure 8 shows prolactin binding to prolactin receptors in fractions from the isolation of lysosomes. MgCl₂ had little effect on receptor levels in any fraction, probably due to the CB-154 treatment of the animals. On the other hand, chloroquine increased hGH binding to prolactin receptors in lysosomal fractions with the maximum effect in the most purified fraction (L-2), probably the result of reducing degradation of lysosomal receptors. The L-1 fraction was high in prolactin binding activity in control animals while other lysosomal fractions were very low (Ferland et al., 1984).

Uptake of ¹²⁵I-labeled oPRL in various organelles from rat liver, after injection of 30 × 10⁶ cpm into the jugular vein was examined. Maximum incorporation in the homogenate was observed at 15 minutes as previously reported by Josefsberg et al. (1979) (Fig. 9A). It has been previously shown that intracellular receptors could account for as much as 70% of the receptors of the total liver cell (Bergeron et al., 1978). In this study, we demonstrated that most of the labeled hormone was internalized into

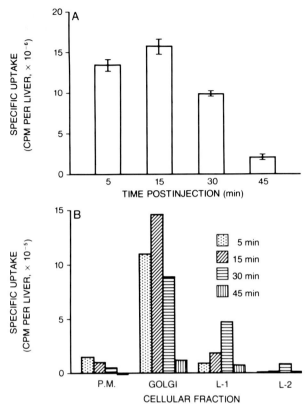

FIG. 9. Uptake of ^{125}I-labeled oPRL in liver homogenate (A) and purified fractions (B) following injection of 30×10^6 cpm ^{125}I-labeled oPRL (approx. 7.5 pmol) via the jugular vein. Female rats treated with estradiol and CB-154 were anesthetized with Surital, the jugular vein was exposed and the labeled hormone injected in a volume 0.2 to 0.4 ml. Other animals were given 500 μg unlabeled prolactin in addition to ^{125}I-labeled oPRL to determine the level of nonspecific uptake. At the times indicated, livers were rapidly removed, cut into pieces, weighed, and processed as described. Values are expressed as the counts per liver specifically bound to the homogenate or to fractions. PM, plasma membranes; Golgi, Golgi membranes; L-1, L-1 fraction; L-2, mature, secondary lysosomes.

the Golgi (Fig. 9B). About half of the injected radioactivity was taken up by the liver at 15 minutes, 10% of which was concentrated in the Golgi. The internalized material could well be in the form of hormone–receptor complexes since large amounts of hGH binding sites have been shown to be present in those vesicles (Bergeron et al., 1978). In contrast to what was observed in the homogenate and in the Golgi fraction, maximum incorporation in lysosomes and in L-1 fraction was seen at 30 minutes.

Prolactin receptors have been previously observed in rat liver lysosomes and tritosomes (Khan *et al.*, 1981). In the present study, two classes of lysosome-like vesicles were identified. L-1 fraction was rich in acid phosphatase and contained a great many intact receptors. Binding activity of L-1 fraction was only moderately augmented by chloroquine treatment of the animals, suggesting that these vesicles bear little degradative activity. Typical secondary lysosomes (L-2 fraction) were twice as rich in acid phosphatase as L-1 fraction yet very poor in receptors in control animals. The fact that chloroquine treatment considerably enhanced receptor levels in secondary lysosomes (7- to 8-fold) suggests that degradative processes may occur in these organelles.

Khan *et al.* (1981) and more recently, Baenzinger and Fiete (1982) reported insulin, lactogen, and asialoglycoprotein receptors to be internalized into uncoated vesicles of density higher than that of Golgi vesicles and comparable to that of plasma membrane. Khan *et al.* (1982) reported these vesicles to have lysosome-like features. They could correspond to the small, homogeneous lysosomes with which receptosomes appear to fuse, about 30 minutes after internalization of α_2-macroglobulin (Willingham and Pastan, 1980). The L-1 fraction in the present studies appears to closely resemble these vesicles. Nevertheless, despite the lysosome-like morphology of this fraction, it cannot be defined simply as "light lysosomes" since it is only half as enriched in acid phosphatase activity as the true lysosomal fraction yet about 7 times richer in prolactin receptors in control animals and resistant to the action of chloroquine. We suggest it may consist of immature lysosomes, or prelysosomes, in which proteolytic activity would be less than that of mature, secondary lysosomes (fraction L-2). Such an hypothesis is supported by the facts that the L-1 fraction is enriched in 5' nucleotidase, less rich in acid phosphatase activity than secondary lysosomes, that prolactin receptors remain largely intact and that receptors are only minimally affected by treatment of the animals with the lysosomotropic agent chloroquine (Fig. 8). In contrast, the mature lysosomes (L-2 fraction) are very rich in acid phosphatase activity (and presumably in general proteolytic activity), poor in intact prolactin receptors in control animals (due to degradative processes occurring within lysosomes), and rich in prolactin receptors following blockage of lysosomal degradation by chloroquine (Fig. 8). Because the L-1 fraction consists largely of lysosome-like vesicles, it seems likely that receptor activity in this fraction is related to receptor activity measured in the lysosomal compartment.

Hizuka *et al.* (1981) pointed out that lysosomotropic agents such as NH_4Cl and chloroquine increased cell associated ^{125}I-labeled hGH in cultured lymphocytes by a mechanism that involves inhibition of degradation. The present study shows that not only the hormone, but also the internalized receptors that reach the lysosomal compartment are protected by chloroquine (Fig. 8).

Iodinated prolactin was taken up *in vivo* by the liver (maximum incorporation at 15 minutes in the homogenate). It was found to be associated with both Golgi, as first reported by Josefsberg *et al.* (1979) and with lysosomes (Khan *et al.*, 1981). The kinetics of internalization differed between Golgi and lysosomes with a maximum at 15 minutes in the Golgi fraction and at 30 minutes in both prelysosomes and lysosomes. This suggests either that ^{125}I-labeled PRL is sequentially internalized into Golgi and then reaches the lysosomal compartment, as suggested by Khan *et al.* (1982) for ^{125}I-labeled insulin internalization or, alternatively, that there exist two independent paths of internalization, one toward the Golgi complex (for receptors to be recycled) and the other going directly, although less rapidly toward the lysosomes (for the receptors to be degraded). Such a model has been suggested by Geisow (1982) and is supported by the high content of plasma membrane marker enzyme found in prelysosomes.

These data, taken together, demonstrate that although following binding of the hormone to its receptor, there is an internalization of the hormone–receptor complex, and that prolactin receptors are concentrated within the Golgi and lysosomes, the lysosomal compartment does not appear to be directly involved in the mechanism of prolactin action in the mammary gland. At this point, however, the possibility cannot be ruled out that the internalized hormone–receptor complex may be somehow involved in the activation of prolactin-sensitive cells.

III. Prolactin Receptor Occupancy and Hormonal Responses

The interaction of prolactin with its receptor in mammary cells results in a cascade of events resulting finally in an increase in milk protein synthesis and cell multiplication. The effect of increasing concentrations of prolactin on explant cultures of rabbit mammary tissue is shown in Fig. 10. There is a clear occupation of free receptors and a concomitant down-regulation of total prolactin receptors as has already been described. These changes are most pronounced at high concentrations of hormone, but are easily detectable at the lower concentrations tested. Along with the occupation of free receptors and down-regulation of total receptors a progressive increase in casein and DNA synthesis was observed. The maximal effect for both casein and DNA synthesis occurred at about 100 ng/ml, whereas at higher concentrations, a desensitization of

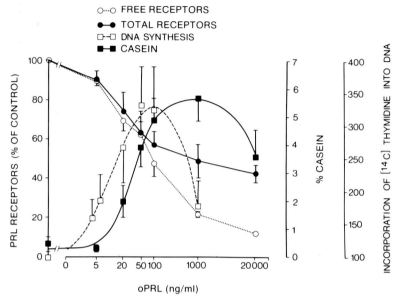

FIG. 10. Variations of total and free PRL receptors and induction of casein and DNA synthesis under the influence of increasing concentrations of PRL. The PRL was added to culture medium of rabbit mammary gland explants. Free and total receptors were estimated in crude microsomes after 24 hours cultures by estimating the ability of the membranes to specifically bind ^{125}I-labeled PRL before and after treatment by 4 M MgCl$_2$, respectively. Results are expressed for casein as the percentage of labeled proteins which are precipitable with the anticasein antibodies and for DNA as percentage of stimulation of the incorporation of [^{14}C]thymidine into DNA and are calculated as a percentage of values obtained without PRL.

the mammary cell to the hormonal stimulus was observed. It is interesting that this desensitization was not accompanied by a further decrease in prolactin receptor content (Djiane *et al.*, 1982).

IV. Molecular Characteristics of Prolactin Receptors

A. PURIFICATION OF PROLACTIN RECEPTORS

A crude microsomal membrane preparation from lactating rabbit mammary glands, suspended in 25 mM Tris–HCl, buffer, pH 7.4, 10 mM MgCl$_2$ at a final protein concentration of 5–8 mg/ml, was solubilized with the zwitterionic detergent, CHAPS. After stiring for 30 minutes, at room temperature, the suspension was centrifuged at 105,000 g for 60 minutes at 4°C. The clear supernatant was removed and used at once or stored frozen at −20°C to avoid the formation of precipitates. For purification, microsomes were pretreated with 1 mM CHAPS and the supernatants were discarded since this fraction did not contain the PRL binding activity. The resulting pellets were suspended in the original buffer and solubilized with 5 mM CHAPS.

Purification of mammary gland prolactin receptors was carried out using affinity chromatography. Briefly, oPRL was coupled to Affi-Gel 10 according to the method of Shiu and Friesen (1974). Ten milligrams of PRL was used per 25 ml Affi-Gel 10 with a coupling efficiency of 73–98%. The CHAPS extracts, containing 1 mM phenylmethyl sulfonyl fluoride, were applied to 25 ml oPRL Affi-Gel 10 packed in a 3 × 30-cm column at a flow rate of 1 bed volume per hour at room temperature. The column was washed with 10 to 20 volumes of 0.1 M borate buffer, pH 7.4, containing 1 mM CHAPS (column buffer) followed by 1 volume of 4 M urea disolved in column buffer and 4 volumes of column buffer. The receptor was eluted with one volume of 5 M MgCl$_2$ in column buffer. Ten or twenty milliliter fractions were collected from the beginning of the elution and active fractions (50–70 ml) were combined and applied to Sephadex G-100 columns (180–300 ml), previously equilibrated with column buffer, to remove the MgCl$_2$. The fractions eluted in the void volume were combined, concentrated 20 to 30 times by lyophilization after dialysis against 0.01 M borate buffer, pH 7.4 0.1 mM CHAPS, and stored at −20°C. Repeated lyophilization of partially purified receptor resulted in a loss of approximately 6% of binding activity after each lyophilization.

Generally, Triton X-100 has been used for solubilization of PRL receptor (Shiu and Friesen, 1974; Haeuptle et al., 1983). Although this detergent has the merit that it can solubilize receptors efficiently and in a nondenaturing form, aggregation of the PRL molecule is induced (Shiu and Friesen, 1974) resulting in a decrease of affinity for its receptor. Therefore, initially CHAPS, a newly developed zwitterionic detergent was tested in this study. This detergent has already been reported not to induce aggregation of the PRL molecule (Liscia et al., 1982) and to be effective in solubilizing membrane receptors (Hjelmeland, 1980) or protein (Simonds et al., 1980) in a nondenaturing state.

CHAPS, at the concentration between 0.8 and 6 mM in the incubation mixture with ^{125}I-labeled oPRL did not affect the binding activity of PRL receptor, suggesting that PRL receptors from mammary tissues do not require an optimum concentration of CHAPS as was observed for prolactin receptors from mouse liver (Liscia et al., 1982) and opiate receptors (Simonds et al., 1980) which were solubilized with the same detergent.

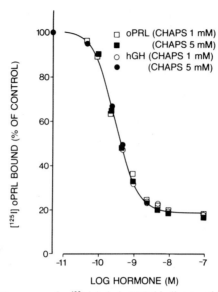

FIG. 11. Competition curves for ^{125}I-labeled oPRL binding to rabbit mammary prolactin receptors in the presence of increasing concentrations of oPRL or hGH at two concentrations of CHAPS.

The optimum concentration of polyethylene glycol to precipitate hormone receptor complexes was 16% (w/v), slightly higher than that for Triton X-100 solubilized mammary PRL receptor.

In particulate fractions, lactogenic receptors have the same affinity for hGH and oPRL (Shiu et al., 1973; Posner et al., 1974b). A similar observation was made for the CHAPS solubilized PRL receptor, in the presence of 1 or 5 mM CHAPS. Figure 11 shows that similar inhibition curves of the binding of ^{125}I-labeled oPRL to the soluble receptors were obtained for both oPRL (30.5 IU/mg) and hGH (2.2 IU/mg). Affinity constants calculated from Scatchard plots (not shown) were $11.6 \times 10^9 \, M^{-1}$ (1 mM CHAPS) and $12.2 \times 10^9 \, M^{-1}$ (5 mM) for hGH, and $16.0 \times 10^9 \, M^{-1}$ (1 mM) and $14.7 \times 10^9 \, M^{-1}$ for oPRL, respectively. Complete inhibition was achieved by as little as $10^{-8} \, M$ (approximately 200 ng/ml) of unlabeled hormone.

Since it has become clear that oPRL has a similar binding affinity with hGH to CHAPS solubilized receptors in the presence of up to 5 mM CHAPS as shown above, this hormone can be used as a ligand for affinity chromatography. PRL binding activity was not eluted in the 4 M urea fraction but rather in the 5 M MgCl$_2$ fraction from oPRL Affi-Gel 10 columns. Active MgCl$_2$ fractions were collected, separated from MgCl$_2$

TABLE II

Summary of Purification of PRL Receptor from Rabbit Mammary Gland[a]

	Protein recovery (%)	PRL binding capacity (pmol/mg)	Purification (fold)	Binding sites recovered (%)	K_a (nM^{-1})
Crude microsome	100	0.37 ± 0.15	(1)	100	3.8 ± 1.7
CHAPS extract	22.6 ± 3.4	0.72 ± 0.33	(1.87)	43.0 ± 9.5	27.6 ± 9.5
Affinity purified	0.014 ± 0.002	258 ± 126	(655)	8.9 ± 1.7	16.2 ± 7.2

[a] Crude microsomes from 3 different preparations of lactating rabbit mammary gland (680, 1600, and 3300 mg protein, respectively) were solubilized and purified. PRL binding capacity and affinity constants were determined by Scatchard analysis. The values represent the mean ± SEM.

on a Sephadex G-100 column, and concentrated by lyophilization followed by determination of protein concentration and PRL binding capacity. Table II shows the summary of purification of PRL receptor from 3 different preparations of mammary tissues. Only 0.014% protein was recovered in $MgCl_2$ fraction and an average 650-fold purification from microsomes was achieved, resulting in a recovery of total binding capacity at 8.9%. These values are comparable to those we previously obtained using Triton X-100 as a detergent and hGH as a ligand for affinity chromatography with 0.11% protein recovery, 836-fold purification, and 9% recovery of binding sites (Katoh et al., 1984).

B. ELECTROPHORETIC ANALYSIS OF PARTIALLY PURIFIED RECEPTOR

Partially purified receptors were dialyzed against 2 ml Tris–HCl, pH 7.4, 0.1% SDS, and lyophilized before electrophoresis. The powders were dissolved in electrophoresis sample buffer and boiled for 2 minutes in the absence or presence of 10 mM DTT.

Electrophoresis was performed on a 5–15 or 9–15% gradient gel slab of 1.5 mm thickness according to the method of Laemli (1970). Gels were stained by 0.2% Coomassie Brilliant Blue R-250 or by silver as described by Wray et al. (1981). Affinity labeled or radiolabeled receptors were electrophoresed similarly.

Three techniques were employed to detect the proteins separated by SDS–polyacrylamide electrophoresis, that is, Coomassie Brilliant Blue staining, Silver staining, and autoradiography of the gel containing radioiodinated purified receptor on Kodak X-Ray film XAR-5 for 2–4 days

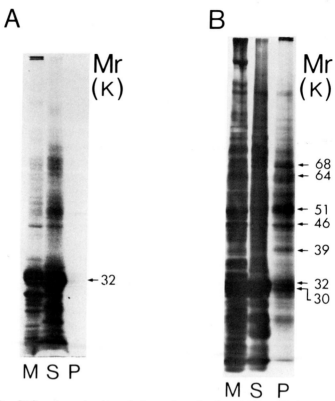

FIG. 12. SDS–polyacrylamide gel electrophoresis of partially purified PRL receptors. Ten (A) or five (B) micrograms partially purified receptor (lanes P), dialyzed against 2 m*M* Tris–HCl, pH 7.4, 0.1% SDS overnight and concentrated by lyophilization, were run on a 9–15% gradient SDS–electrophoresis gel under reducing condition. Staining was carried out in 2 manners, by Coomassie Brilliant Blue (0.2%) for 1 hour (A) and silver staining (B). Crude preparations (20 µg), microsome (lanes M), and CHAPS solubilized proteins (lanes C) were also indicated. The M_r of each band was determined using standard marker proteins.

at $-70°$C. One faint band at $M_r = 32,000$ was occasionally detected by Coomassie Brilliant Blue staining (Fig. 12). However, silver staining, which is much more sensitive, detected at least 7 major bands of $M_r =$ 30,000, 32,000, 39,000, 46,000, 51,000, 64,000, and 68,000. In some preparations, a larger $M_r = 114,000$ band was observed. This indicates that further purification is necessary to obtain a more homogeneous preparation (Kelly *et al.*, 1983a).

As shown in Fig. 13, when this affinity-purified material was iodinated and analyzed by SDS–polyacrylamide gel electrophoresis and autoradio-

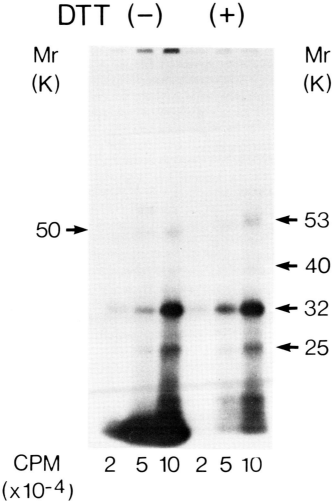

FIG. 13. SDS–polyacrylamide gel electrophoresis of ^{125}I-labeled partially purified receptor. Affinity purified receptor was iodinated with chloramine T and increasing concentrations of ^{125}I-labeled receptor was applied to the gel. Samples were pretreated with electrophoresis sample buffer in the presence or absence of 10 mM DDT at 100°C for 2 minutes. After electrophoresis, the gel was dried and an autoradiograph was taken.

graphy, an $M_r = 32,000$ band was the most intense. In addition, faint $M_r = 25,000$, 40,000, and 53,000 bands could be observed under reducing condition. The largest $M_r = 53,000$ band migrated somewhat faster under nonreducing condition.

C. AFFINITY LABELING OF MICROSOMAL PRL RECEPTOR

The effect of increasing the concentration of the photoactive cross-linker N-hydroxysuccinimidyl-4-azidobenzoate (HSAB) is shown in Fig. 14. As can be seen, a single band at $M_r = 32,000$ is seen. The only effect of increasing the HSAB concentration is to increase nonspecific background. The molecular weight of the binding component is calculated as

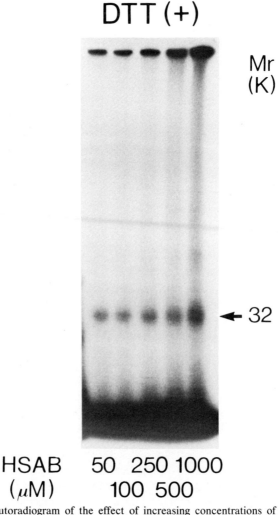

FIG. 14. Autoradiogram of the effect of increasing concentrations of HSAB on the affinity labeling of rabbit mammary gland microsomal proteins with ^{125}I-labeled oPRL. Microsomes were photoaffinity labeled and electrophoresed on a 7.5% gel.

the difference in the molecular weight of this prolactin–receptor complex and that of prolactin. The nonphotoactive agent, disuccinimidyl suberate (DSS), also resulted in good affinity labeling of the receptor although the bands were less intense than with HSAB.

To elucidate the significance of disulfide linkages among the components of PRL receptor, the effect of increasing concentration of DTT, which was used to reduce S–S bonds were added when samples were boiled with the electrophoresis sample buffer (Fig. 15). In the absence of

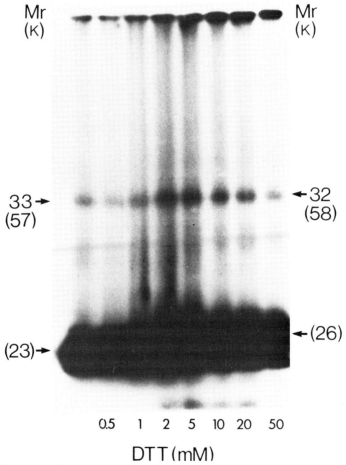

FIG. 15.   Autoradiogram of the effect of increasing DTT concentrations on the migration of affinity labeled PRL binding components with ^{125}I-labeled oPRL on a 9–15% gradient SDS–electrophoresis gel. Mammary gland microsomes were photoaffinity labeled with ^{125}I-labeled oPRL using 500 μM HSAB and treated with electrophoresis sample buffer containing various concentrations of DTT indicated.

TABLE III

Summary of Molecular Weight of the Microsomal PRL Binding Component from Rabbit Mammary Gland Determined by Affinity Labeling

	DTT (+) ($n = 9$)	DTT (−) ($n = 6$)
Binding site–PRL complex	$58,000 \pm 300^a$	$56,000 \pm 700^a$
oPRL	$27,200 \pm 200$	$23,600 \pm 200$
Binding site	$31,300 \pm 400$	$32,900 \pm 700$

[a] Mean ± SEM.

DTT, the oPRL, which was freed from complexes during solubilization and electrophoresis, appeared at $M_r = 23,000$ and hormone–receptor complexes appeared at $M_r = 57,000$. No other binding components were observed. When more than 2 mM DTT was present, oPRL molecule migrated more slowly indicating its M_r at 26,000. Hormone–receptor complex also migrated at a higher M_r of 58,000. The average M_r of oPRL and the PRL binding component, observed in several experiments, is summarized in Table III. Similar to the results described in Fig. 15, the oPRL molecule migrated somewhat more slowly after reduction by 10 mM DTT. As a result, larger M_r values were obtained for the reduced hormone-binding component complex. Accordingly, the M_r of PRL binding component was calculated at 31,300 and 32,900 under reducing and nonreducing conditions, respectively.

D. PHOTOAFFINITY LABELING OF AFFINITY-PURIFIED PRL RECEPTOR

Partially purified PRL receptors were also affinity labeled. After the incubation with ^{125}I-labeled oPRL as described above, hormone–receptor complexes were precipitated with PEG-8000 at a final concentration of 16% and the tubes centrifuged. Pellets were labeled using HSAB. After photolysis, 4 volumes of cold (−20°C) ethanol was added resulting in a final ethanol concentration of 80% and the tubes centrifuged at 2300 g for 15 minutes. Pellets were treated in a similar manner as described for particulate receptors.

One major $M_r = 33,000$ binding component can be seen in Fig. 16, whereas 2 minor components, with an M_r of 63,000 and 80,000, assuming 1 : 1 cross-linking between hormone and binding component, are also visible under reducing conditions. A single $M_r = 65,000$ was observed under nonreducing conditions.

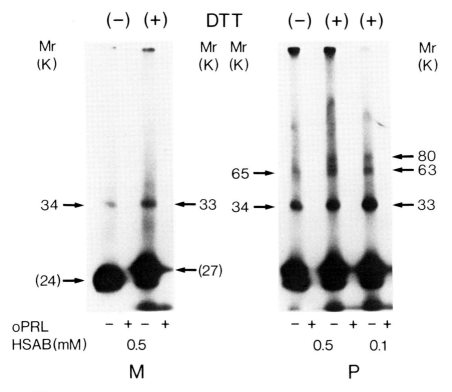

FIG. 16.   Autoradiogram comparing binding components, microsomal (M) from affinity purified (P) PRL receptors. Affinity purified receptor (1.2 μg per incubation), characterized in Table II, was photoaffinity labeled with ^{125}I-labeled oPRL using 100 or 500 μM HSAB and analyzed on a 5–15% gradient gel under reducing and nonreducing conditions. Microsomal receptors affinity labeled and electrophoresed on the same gel are indicated in the left portion of the figure (M).

The present data indicate that the major binding component in the membrane of rabbit mammary tissue has a relative molecular mass of 31,000–32,000 when affinity labeling techniques combined with SDS–polyacrylamide gel electrophoresis were employed. We have mainly used HSAB, a photoreactive reagent as a crosslinker. This reagent was more effective than DSS, an amino specific homobifunctional crosslinker, for affinity labeling of rabbit microsomal PRL receptors with ^{125}I-labeled oPRL and has been employed for direct crosslinking of hormone–receptor complexes without producing photoreactive derivatives (Johnson *et al.*, 1981; Massagué *et al.*, 1981b).

As shown in Table III, using electrophoretic analysis under reducing conditions, we obtained from rabbit mammary gland microsomes a single M_r = 58,500 binding component–[125]I-labeled oPRL complex, a similar value to that reported previously for rabbit mammary gland solubilized microsomes bound to ^{125}I-labeled hGH (M_r = 57,000) and for rat liver microsomes bound to ^{125}I-labeled oPRL (M_r = 60,000). A similar binding component–[125]I-labeled oPRL complex was observed for affinity-purified receptor as a major band (Fig. 16). This band did not disappear nor change its migration rate even when excess amount of HSAB was used or when HSAB was replaced by other crosslinkers. The band disappeared only when excess unlabeled oPRL was incubated with receptors. However, under the conditions employed, ^{125}I-labeled oPRL which was freed from complexes during solubilization or electrophoresis, migrated at the position of M_r = 27,200 under reducing conditions, resulting in the M_r of binding components at 31,300. Intact unlabeled oPRL also showed a slightly faster migration rate under the same conditions. The molecular weight of PRL can be calculated from its amino acid sequence (Li et al., 1970) and sedimentation experiments (Squire et al., 1963) as 22,500 and 23,300, respectively, and a similar value was obtained by our nonreducing electrophoresis (Table III, Fig. 15). This discrepancy between the actual M_r which appeared on SDS gels under reducing conditions and the theoretical value is considered to result from an effect of DTT on all or some of the 3 S–S bonds within the oPRL molecule. Nonreduced oPRL migrates faster as was shown for BSA (Fairbanks et al., 1971), or some of the binding components for insulin (Kasuga et al., 1982), insulin-like growth factor II (Massagué and Czech, 1982), or for multiplication stimulating activity (Massagué et al., 1981a). We therefore employed the apparent M_r of oPRL that was observed on the same gel.

This M_r = 31,000 binding component does not seem to bind to itself or to other binding components or membrane proteins through disulfide linkages, since no other binding components were observed and M_r = 31,000 band did not disappear, nor was altered in the absence of DTT. Although the amount of proteins bound with ^{125}I-labeled oPRL (not shown) or of radioactivity of labeled purified receptor (Fig. 15) which did not penetrate the gel was increased by reducing the concentration of DTT, this phenomenon was also mentioned by Haeuptle et al. (1983), the high M_r region of each gel lane was completely clear. Consequently, we do not believe that PRL receptor exists as high-molecular-weight entities that are constituted from small M_r = 31,000 binding components through S–S bonds, as have been observed for insulin receptors (Pilch and Czech, 1979; Jacobs et al., 1979; Massagué et al., 1980) suggesting a similar structure to that of insulin-like growth factor II and of multiplication stimulating activity

(Massagué *et al.*, 1981a) as well as PRL receptor, in rat liver (Borst and Sayare, 1982) which have been considered to exist as a single binding component.

Contrary to the results obtained from the electrophoretic analysis of denatured and dissociated solubilized PRL receptor, larger molecular weights (100,000 to 300,000) have been reported using gel filtration chromatography in the presence of Triton X-100 (M_r of hormone–receptor complex). More recently, we have obtained M_r = 133,000 peak of rabbit mammary receptors from high-performance liquid chromatography (HPLC) equipped with gel exclusion columns in the presence of Triton X-100 (Katoh *et al.*, 1984). Only one group has observed the small M_r binding site under nondissociating condition with an M_r = 37,000 in mouse liver which was solubilized with CHAPS (Liscia *et al.*, 1982; Liscia and Vonderhaar, 1982). It could be possible that the higher molecular weight forms of the receptor contain aggregated forms of PRL receptors or two or more M_r = 31,000 binding components, although it is not clear whether other components, which do not contribute to the hormone binding subunit, exist in the overall molecule.

V. Prolactin Receptor Antibodies

Partially purified receptor preparations were injected at monthly intervals into male sheep, goats, and guinea pigs, at a concentration of 50 μg of antigen per injection in Freund's complete adjuvant. Animals were bled at 7 to 10 days after the booster immunization. Antibodies began to become measurable after the second immunization and reached a maximum titer after 3 to 6 immunizations (Djiane *et al.*, 1981; Kelly *et al.*, 1983a).

A. INHIBITION OF BINDING OF PROLACTIN BY ANTIRECEPTOR SERUM

Sera of animals injected with partially purified receptor preparations (less than 10% pure) were assayed for their capacity to inhibit the binding of ^{125}I-labeled ovine prolactin to receptors in rabbit mammary gland membranes. As shown in Fig. 17, sera from sheep, goats, and guinea pigs were capable of inhibiting the binding of prolactin to its receptors. Significant inhibition of binding was observed at a dilution of 1 : 10,000, with the sheep antibody being the most potent. The half-maximal inhibition (IM_{50}) values for the sheep, guinea pig, and goat antisera represented a delution of 1 : 5700, 1 : 2400, and 1 : 1100, respectively. Sera of nonimmunized animals did not significantly alter the formation of the prolactin–receptor complex. That increased concentration of PRL receptor required more

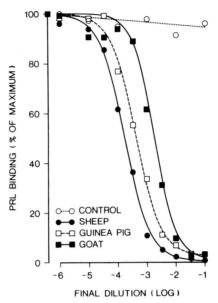

FIG. 17.   Action of anti-prolactin receptor sera on the binding of ^{125}I-labeled ovine prolactin to mammary membranes. About 100,000 cpm of the hormone was incubated for 16
hours at 20°C with rabbit mammary membranes (300 μg protein per incubate), in the presence of various concentrations of control sera or antiprolactin receptor serum from a sheep,
guinea pig, and goat. Binding values are expressed as a percentage of values in tubes
containing no antiserum.

antiserum is demonstrated by the linearity of the regression curve obtained between IM_{50} values and PRL receptor concentrations (data not
shown).

The specificity of the sheep antiserum was further examined in rabbit
ovary and adrenal and mammary tissue from a lactating pig. Figure 18
shows a similar inhibition curve for rabbit mammary tissue as has been
observed previously ($IM_{50} = 1 : 5200$). Although rabbit ovary and adrenal
and pig mammary tissues showed lower IM_{50} values ($1 : 49,000$, $1 : 23,000$,
and $1 : 16,500$, respectively), these tissues usually contain lower PRL receptor concentration (30–100 fmol/mg microsomal protein) than rabbit
mammary gland (200–500 fmol/mg microsomal protein).

B. INHIBITORY AND STIMULATORY ACTIONS OF
ANTIRECEPTOR SERA

The antireceptor antibodies which prevented the binding of prolactin to
its receptor were expected to also prevent the biological activity of the

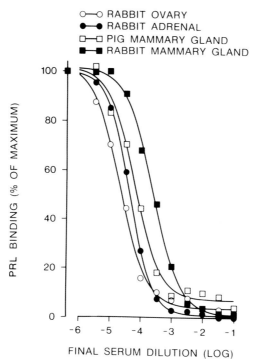

○—○ RABBIT OVARY
●—● RABBIT ADRENAL
□—□ PIG MAMMARY GLAND
■—■ RABBIT MAMMARY GLAND

FIG. 18. Specificity of sheep prolactin receptor antiserum on the inhibition of binding of ^{125}I-labeled ovine prolactin to receptors in rabbit ovary, adrenal, and pig mammary gland compared with rabbit mammary gland. Conditions were as described in Fig. 17. Three hundred micrograms microsomal protein per incubation was employed. Control (100%) values were 7750, 19,690, 8110, and 29,250 cpm for rabbit ovary and adrenal, pig and rabbit mammary gland, respectively.

hormone. This was indeed the case: guinea pig antiserum inhibited the initiation of casein synthesis as a function of the antiserum concentrations in the medium (Fig. 19A). More surprising was the fact that in the absence of prolactin, the anti-prolactin receptor containing antiserum stimulated casein synthesis, thus mimicking prolactin action. This effect was also dose-dependent: at the lowest concentrations, the antiserum was inactive, whereas at the highest concentrations, it inhibited its own action. At none of the concentrations tested did the antiserum exhibit any significant toxic effect as judged by the incorporation of ^{14}C-labeled amino acids into proteins in the explant cultures; therefore, the inhibitory effect of the antiserum at high concentrations may be considered as specific.

An examination of the activity of the sheep antiserum containing prolactin receptor antibodies revealed that it also was able to mimic prolactin

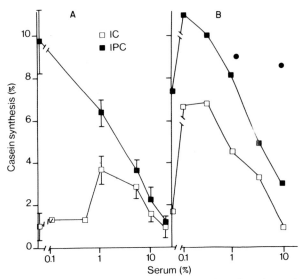

FIG. 19.   Action of anti-prolactin receptor on the induction of casein synthesis. Cultures of rabbit mammary explants were carried out in all cases in the presence of insulin and cortisol with or without ovine prolactin and serum. Results are expressed as the percentage of the labeled mammary proteins precipitated by the anticasein antibody as a function of the antiserum concentration in the medium. □, Without prolactin; ■, with prolactin; ●, with prolactin and control serum. (A) Results with guinea pig antiserum are the mean of four independent cultures. (B) Results with sheep antiserum are the mean of two experiments.

action on casein synthesis in a dose–dependent manner (Fig. 19B). This antiserum was more active in stimulating casein synthesis at low concentrations but less potent in inhibiting prolactin action at high concentrations than was the guinea pig antiserum. Control serum incubated even at high concentrations failed to inhibit the action of prolactin. Interestingly, the sheep receptor antiserum at low concentrations was even slightly but significantly capable of stimulating casein synthesis when added to prolactin at 100 ng/ml (a prolactin concentration that gives the near-maximum response in this system). This fact was observed repeatedly in other experiments not shown here. It is conceivable that the stimulation, or at least part of it, by the receptor antiserum is due to prolactin present in the antiserum. This hypothesis is not tenable in the case of sheep antiserum because all of the cultures were performed in the presence of antibodies to ovine prolactin present in the culture medium in sufficient amounts to suppress the effect of 1 μg of prolactin per ml (Djiane *et al.*, 1981).

The initiation of casein synthesis in organ culture by prolactin has been shown to be accompanied in all cases by a parallel accumulation of the corresponding mRNA (Devinoy *et al.*, 1978). This effect of prolactin was

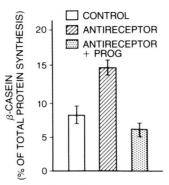

FIG. 20. The effect of *in vivo* administration of a γ-globulin fraction of prolactin antire-ceptor on casein synthesis in mammary tissue compared with tissue from uninjected animals or those which received antireceptor plus progesterone.

also blocked by a high concentration of guinea pig receptor antiserum. Similarly, this antiserum was able to mimic prolactin action at moderate concentrations and to suppress its own effect at high concentrations. Under all conditions examined, there was an excellent agreement be-tween the rate of casein synthesis and the content in β-casein mRNA (Djiane *et al.*, 1981).

In addition to stimulating casein mRNA and casein synthesis, receptor antibodies are also able to mimic the action of prolactin on DNA synthesis in mammary explant culture. Increasing concentrations of an immunoglo-bin fraction of antireceptor serum stimulated [^{14}C]thymidine incorpora-tion into DNA whereas a similar fraction prepared from a nonimmunized animal was essentially devoid of activity (Djiane *et al.*, 1981).

The *in vivo* lactogenic effects of prolactin receptor antibodies were examined in pseudopregnant rabbits. Animals twice received 200 mg of antiprolactin receptor γ-globulin fractions at 2-day intervals and were killed 4 days after the beginning of the treatment. Mammary glands were removed and frozen until measurement of β-casein was made by RIA. A marked accumulation of β-casein was observed following 4 days of treat-ment with the Ig fraction. In addition, as is shown in Fig. 20, there was a net stimulation of β-casein synthesis in mammary tissue and the appear-ance of milk in the gland. The stimulatory effect was completely abolished by simultaneous treatment of animals with progesterone (5 mg twice a day, Dusanter-Fourt *et al.*, 1983), a well-known inhibitor of prolactin stimulation of casein synthesis (Matusik and Rosen, 1978; Teyssot and Houdebine, 1981).

The effects of a serum containing PRL receptor antibodies on PRL binding sites were investigated in suspension culture of rat liver cells. In

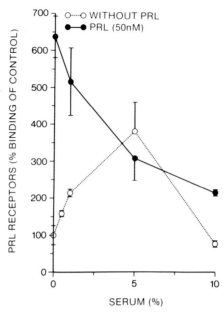

FIG. 21.   Effect of antireceptor serum on PRL binding sites of rat liver cells in continuous suspension culture. Cells were cultured in L-15 medium in the absence or presence of PRL (50 n*M*) and increasing concentrations of antireceptor serum for 48 hours. Values are expressed as a percentage of control (cells cultured without PRL) and are the means ± SEM of 3 independent cultures.

this model, PRL binding sites decline rapidly with time, with 50% of the sites lost in 10 hours and 90% at 24 to 48 hours of culture. This loss can be prevented by the inclusion of 50 n*M* oPRL in the incubation medium, resulting in a sixfold increase in PRL receptor number compared to control cultures after 48 hours of culture. Figure 21 illustrates that anti-PRL receptor serum, which inhibits the binding of PRL to its receptor, is capable of preventing this PRL induced increase in PRL receptors. However, when incubated alone, these PRL receptor antibodies at lower concentrations (0.5 to 5%) mimic the up-regulatory effect of PRL on its own binding sites (Rosa *et al.*, 1982).

In another model system, namely nitrosomethylurea (NMU)-induced rat mammary tumor in explant culture, the effects of antireceptor serum were investigated on lactose synthetase. As is shown in Fig. 22, prolactin stimulated lactose synthetase activity, and the antireceptor serum was able to completely inhibit the stimulatory activity of prolactin. When incubated in the absence of prolactin, the antireceptor serum was able to significantly increase the enzyme activity, although not to the level seen with prolactin (Edery *et al.*, 1983).

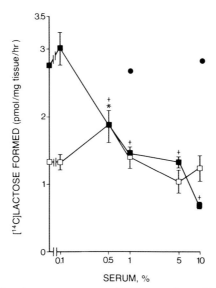

FIG. 22.   Effect of antireceptor serum on [^{14}C]lactose formed in NMU-induced mammary tumors in explant cultures. Explants were cultured in the absence or presence of 300 ng/ml oPRL and increasing concentrations of antireceptor serum for 24 hours. Values are the means ± SEM of 5 independent cultures. □, Without PRL; ■, with PRL; ●, with PRL and control serum.

Therefore, in a number of different systems, prolactin antireceptor sera are able to mimic or inhibit the various actions of prolactin.

C. EFFECT OF AND MONO- AND BIVALENT FRAGMENTS OF ANTIRECEPTOR SERUM

Bivalent fragments, F(ab')$_2$, of antiprolactin receptor antibodies were prepared by pepsin cleavage, whereas the monovalent fragment Fab', was obtained after a reduction with dithiothretol of the F(ab')$_2$ fragment. When assayed for their ability to inhibit ^{125}I-labeled oPRL binding to its receptor in rabbit mammary gland, whole antireceptor serum, immunoglobulin bivalent F(ab')$_2$, and monovalent Fab' fragments had similar potencies (Fig. 23). Half maximal inhibition was reached with 5 to 10 μg/ml for sheep antireceptor antibodies, with similar but slightly higher concentrations being effective for goat antireceptor antibodies (Dusanter-Fourt *et al.*, 1984).

Because anti-prolactin receptor immunoglobulins as well as their F(ab')$_2$ and Fab' fragments were all able to bind to prolactin receptors, we tested whether the three types of antireceptor molecules were able to induce a down-regulation of prolactin receptors. As shown in Fig. 24, prolactin, antireceptor immunoglobulins, as well as their bivalent F(ab')$_2$

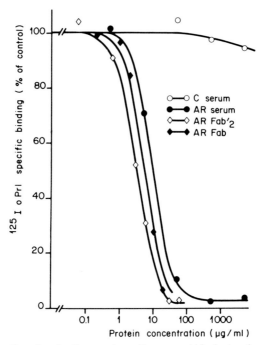

FIG. 23.   The action of prolactin receptor antiserum and bivalent and monovalent receptor antibodies on the binding of ^{125}I-labeled prolactin to rabbit mammary membranes. About
100,000 cpm of the hormone was incubated for 18 hours at 20°C with rabbit mammary
membranes (200 μg of protein per incubate) in the presence of various concentrations of
anti-prolactin receptor antibodies. ○, Control serum from nonimmunized sheep; ●, sheep
prolactin receptor antiserum; ◇, sheep bivalent anti-prolactin receptor F(ab')₂ fragments;
♦, sheep monovalent anti-prolactin receptor Fab' fragments.

fragments and monovalent Fab' fragments, were equipotent in provoking
a 50% decrease of the level of total prolactin receptors, after 24 hours
culture of mammary tissue.

Mammary gland explants were cultured for 24 hours in supplemented
Medium 199, in all cases in the presence of insulin and cortisol. When
prolactin was added at the beginning of the culture, it induced an increase
in the β-casein content of the mammary cells. Maximal β-casein accumulation was obtained at a prolactin concentration of 100 ng/ml. A desensitization was observed further with a prolactin concentration of 10 μg/ml,
in agreement with previous studies (Djiane et al., 1983). Cultures were
also performed in the presence of anti-prolactin receptor antibodies and
with the antibody fragments. Total antiserum as well as the bivalent
F(ab')₂ fragments of the antibodies were able to increase β-casein content
of the mammary cell to respectively 50 and 30% of the maximal value

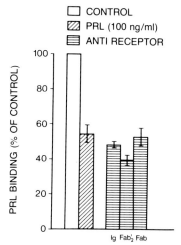

FIG. 24. Total prolactin receptor levels titrated after *in vitro* desaturation of the receptors by a treatment with 4 M $MgCl_2$ in mammary explants cultured for 24 hours in the presence of insulin and the indicated agents: prolactin, 100 ng/ml; anti-prolactin receptor antibodies or their fragments, 100 μg/ml. Results are expressed as the percentage of total prolactin receptor level in mammary explants incubated with insulin alone. Means ± SEM of three separate experiments are shown.

obtained with prolactin ($p < 0.01$), whereas monovalent Fab' fragments and control serum from a nonimmunized animal were totally devoid of activity (Fig. 25). The results depicted in Fig. 25 were obtained with sheep prolactin receptor antibodies. Similar conclusions were drawn when cultures were performed with goat anti-prolactin receptor immunoglobulins and their bivalent and monovalent fragments (results not shown). Maximal prolactin-like effects were reached at the concentration of 100–200 μg/ml bivalent antibodies, a concentration which totally inhibits prolactin binding (Fig. 23). Higher doses induce a desensitization of the mammary cell. Immunoglobulin fractions obtained from a nonimmunized animal as well as their monovalent F(ab') fragments were all devoid of activity (not shown).

In vitro, prolactin enhances thymidine incorporation into DNA in mammary explants (Houdebine, 1980). Prolactin receptor antibodies were tested to determine if they can mimic this effect. Figure 26 shows that only bivalent F(ab')$_2$ fragments were able to stimulate thymidine incorporation into DNA, with a maximal effect at the concentration of 100 μg/ml ($p < 0.01$) with a desensitization beyond 200 μg/ml ($p < 0.05$). The maximal effect induced by F(ab')$_2$ fragments represents approximately 50% of the prolactin maximal action. Neither the monovalent Fab' fragments nor

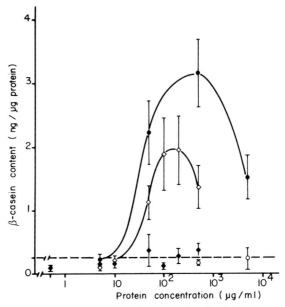

FIG. 25. Action of prolactin receptor antiserum and antibody fragments on the β-casein content of mammary cells. Cultures of mammary explants were performed for 24 hours in the presence of insulin and cortisol and increasing concentrations of the indicated agents. Agents added were ○, control serum from nonimmunized sheep; ●, sheep prolactin receptor antiserum; ◇, sheep prolactin receptor bivalent F(ab')$_2$ fragments; ◆, sheep prolactin receptor monovalent Fab' fragments. Results are the mean ± SEM of four independent experiments.

control immunoglobulins or control bivalent F(ab')$_2$ fragments, both prepared from nonimmunized serum, were able to increase DNA synthesis above basal levels.

Partially purified receptor preparations are of sufficient purity to make antibody production feasable. Whole antisera as well as bivalent F(ab')$_2$ and monovalent Fab' fragments produced in sheep, goats, and guinea pigs were capable of inhibiting the binding of prolactin to rabbit mammary gland membranes. The inhibition of binding by the antireceptor was specific for PRL or lactogenic hormones. In addition, these antisera were shown to inhibit the binding of prolactin to a number of tissues containing prolactin receptors in rabbits, rats, and even in human breast cancer biopsies (data not shown). These observations suggest some homology of the receptor molecule between species.

The prolactin receptor antibodies are potent inhibitors of at least one prolactin action on the mammary cell: the initiation of casein synthesis. This fact is in good agreement with earlier observations which reported inhibitory actions of prolactin antireceptors on the mammary gland (Shiu

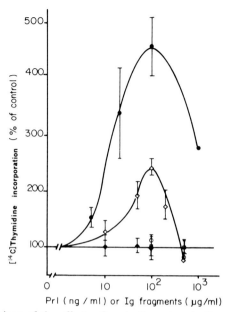

FIG. 26. Comparison of the effects of prolactin and prolactin receptor bivalent and monovalent antibodies on [³H]thymidine incorporation into DNA. Mammary explants were cultured in the presence of insulin, cortisol, and the indicated agents prior to the addition of [¹⁴C]thymidine (during the last 3 hours of culture). Results are expressed as percentage of [¹⁴C]thymidine incorporated into DNA in the presence of insulin and cortisol. ●, Prolactin; ■, control immunoglobulins; ○, F(ab')₂ fragments from control immunoglobulins; ◇, sheep prolactin receptor bivalent F(ab')₂ fragments; ◆, sheep anti-prolactin receptor monovalent Fab' fragments.

and Friesen, 1976) and on ovary (Bohnet *et al.*, 1978). They can also mimic prolactin actions on the mammary gland, namely the production of casein mRNA and casein synthesis (Djiane *et al.*, 1981). Similar dose-dependent inhibitory as well as stimulatory effects of the antisera could be seen on prolactin receptor levels in rat liver cells in suspension culture (Rosa *et al.*, 1982) and on lactose synthetase in experimentally induced mammary carcinoma (Edery *et al.*, 1983).

Stimulatory actions have been observed using anti-insulin receptors found in serum of some patients or obtained from purified receptors which can mimic insulin action on the uptake and oxidation of glucose (Flier *et al.*, 1975; Jacobs *et al.*, 1978; Baldwin *et al.*, 1980). The effects of the anti-prolactin receptor sera on the action of other tissues, such as the testis, ovary, adrenal, etc., is yet to be elucidated.

The studies with mono- and bivalent fragments demonstrate that the whole serum as well as the F(ab')₂ fragments possess prolactin-like activity, which is active in a dose-dependent fashion, with desensitization being observed at high concentrations. It is interesting to note that prolactin receptor antibodies mimic prolactin action on both casein and DNA synthesis, suggesting these two effects may involve a common mechanism, at least in their early steps.

None of the prolactin-like actions could be mediated by the monovalent Fab' fragment, although these monovalent fragments are as efficient as bivalent fragments to inhibit prolactin binding to its receptor. Clearly, these studies indicate that the anti-receptor antibodies require their bivalency to activate casein and DNA synthesis. This suggests that the prolactin receptor antibodies contribute to crosslink or to microaggregate prolactin receptors when they mimic prolactin's actions. These models are in agreement with that proposed for insulin receptor antibodies (Kahn *et al.,* 1978). The importance of receptor crosslinking or microaggregation is emphasized by other studies involving EGF (Schechter *et al.,* 1979), acetylcholine (Drachman *et al.,* 1978), and LHRH (Conn *et al.,* 1982).

In conclusion, antisera produced from partially purified prolactin receptors are able to inhibit binding of labeled hormone to all tissues thus far tested which contain prolactin receptors. It appears that microaggregation is a key step for the prolactin-like activity of prolactin receptor antibodies to be observed. It remains to ascertain if prolactin itself is a bivalent ligand, or if receptor microaggregation is induced by increased mobility of receptors in the plasma membrane, triggering the formation of chemical links between receptors or by enhancing the affinity of receptors for each other.

VI. An Intracellular Mediator for Prolactin

Figure 27 presents a schematic representation of the various mechanisms which might be involved in the recognition of prolactin at the cell surface and the transfer of the information within the cell to the nuclear compartment.

There is no question but that following binding of prolactin, there is an internalization toward the Golgi and lysosomal compartments. Blocking degradation of receptors does not affect the activity of the mammary cell. In addition, the fact that receptor antibodies can mimic the action strongly suggests that the prolactin molecule is not required inside the cell for the transmission of the hormonal message. Therefore, it became necessary to develop an alternative approach to explain the mechanism of prolactin action.

The studies described in the previous section suggest that an intracellular mediator exists which is distinct from the hormone and the receptor. It is generally admitted that neither cAMP, nor cGMP, polyamines, calcium

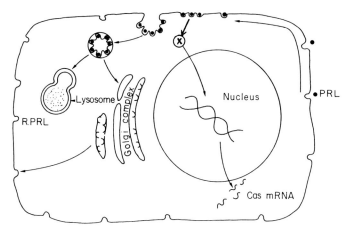

FIG. 27. Schematic representation of the various events following the binding of prolactin to the mammary cell and the transfer of information to the nuclear compartment.

ions, or prostaglandins are prolactin intracellular mediators for the activation of gene transcription (Houdebine *et al.*, 1984b). It seems, therefore that, as for insulin or growth hormone, nonclassical mechanisms should be considered to account for the transmission of the prolactin message to the nucleus.

A. IDENTIFICATION

The hypothesis that a soluble mediator is released after prolactin binding at the membrane level, and that this relay molecule can directly activate casein gene transcription after having been transferred to the nucleus, was studied as summarized in Fig. 28. Mammary microsomes prepared from lactating rabbits were incubated with or without prolactin for 1 hour at room temperature and the supernatants were saved after pelleting the membranes. This soluble fraction was incubated with mammary nuclei, isolated from rabbits treated for 4 days with the hypoprolactinemic drug, bromocriptine, a treatment which has been demonstrated to provoke a partial deinduction of the transcriptional activity in mammary cell nuclei (Houdebine *et al.*, 1984a). These isolated nuclei were incubated in the presence of the various nucleotide triphosphates, one of which was mercurated (HgCTP or HgUTP). The neosynthesized mRNA were selected by an affinity column using SH-Sepharose and their quantification was performed after an hybridization with specific cDNA probes. In the initial studies, these were ^{3}H-labeled probes produced by reverse transcriptase (Teyssot *et al.*, 1981, 1982). In some experiments, the nuclei

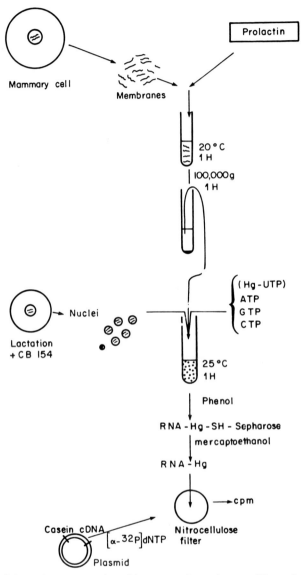

FIG. 28. Schematic representation of the preparation and assay of the prolactin intracellular mediator.

were incubated with a ^{32}P-labeled nucleotide (CTP) and the affinity column was omitted. In the later studies, the hybridization was performed with cloned cDNAs corresponding to different casein genes (α-S$_1$, β- or α-lactalbumin) inserted into plasmids which were fixed to nitrocellulose

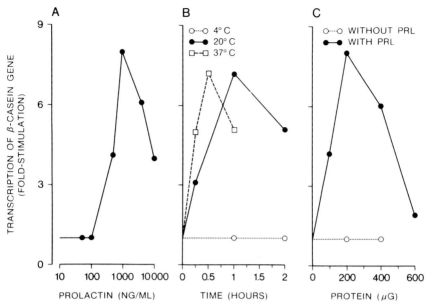

FIG. 29.   Effect of prolactin concentration (A), time and temperature (B), and protein concentration (C) on the transcription rate of β-casein genes. Mammary nuclei ($300A_{260}$ DNA) were incubated at 25°C for 1 hour (A and C) or the indicated times (B) in a final volume of 2 ml with 2 mM ATP, 1 mM UTP, 1 mM GTP, 0.37 mM Hg-CTP, 150 mM KCl, 50 mM Tris–HCl, pH 8.0, 5 mM MgCl$_2$, 1 mM MnCl$_2$, 12.5% glycerol, and 10 mM thioglycerol. At the end of the incubation, the nucleic acids were extracted at pH 9 by phenol and chloroform successively and precipitated with 2 volumes ethanol. The pellet was chromato-graphed on SH-Sepharose in 40% formamide. Mecurated RNAs were eluted with 2-mercap-toethanol. The transcription rate of the β-casein gene was estimated by hybridization with a ^{3}H-labeled β-casein cDNA probe. Results were deduced from hybridization curves not shown here and they refer to the control value obtained in the presence of a supernatant from membranes not exposed to prolactin.

filters. In experiments in which ^{32}P-labeled nucleotides were not used, the cloned probes were labeled with ^{32}P by nick translation (Houdebine *et al.*, 1984a). Results are expressed either as a fold stimulation over control incubations performed with mammary membranes incubated in the absence of prolactin, or as a percentage of actual counts hybridized to nitrocellulose filters.

B. SPECIFICITY OF ASSAY FOR MEDIATOR

The techniques utilized to assay the putative prolactin mediator have just been reviewed. Figure 29 summarizes the effects of prolactin concentration (A), time and temperature (B), and supernatant protein concentration (C) on transcription of β-casein genes. It is apparent that the optimum concentration of prolactin incubated with mammary membranes was 1000 ng/ml with concentrations greater than this resulting in a reduced effect (Fig. 29A). The mediator was released at either 20 or 37°C, with the optimum effect being observed at 1 hour and at 30 minutes, respectively. There was no release of mediator when incubations were performed at 4°C (Fig. 29B). The optimum concentration of supernatant protein was 200 μg (Fig. 29C), with greater concentrations resulting in reduced transcriptional activity (Teyssot *et al.*, 1981).

The results of Fig. 30 indicate that membrane supernatants from incubations with PRL markedly stimulated the transcription of the β-casein gene, whereas the supernatant obtained without PRL was totally devoid of stimulating activity. Various hormones with established lactogenic activity in the rabbit, such as hGH, oPRL, and oPL (a gift of Dr. H. Friesen) share the same capacity to induce the release of a mediator from membranes capable of stimulating β-casein gene transcription, whereas nonlactogenic hormones such as bGH or luteinizing hormone (LH) were totally devoid of this activity. In addition, oPRL or hGH are both ineffective when added alone to nuclei in the absence of membranes.

Prolactin receptors have been measured in many tissues. It was therefore of interest to ascertain whether nonmammary prolactin receptors

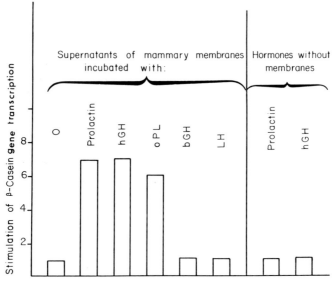

FIG. 30.   Effect of supernatants prepared after an incubation of mammary gland microsomes with various hormones on the transcription rate of the β-casein gene. Crude mammary microsomes were incubated 1 hour at 20°C with the indicated hormones. The supernatants (200 μg protein) were added to transcription media and the β-casein gene transcription carried out as described in Fig. 29.

from other tissues were able to release a mediator capable of stimulating β-casein gene transcription by isolated mammary nuclei. For that purpose, crude microsomes from various tissues were incubated with oPRL and the resulting supernatants were incubated with mammary nuclei prepared from CB-154-treated lactating rabbits. In parallel, the capacity of the various microsomal preparations to specifically bind ^{125}I-labeled prolactin was evaluated. Results of Fig. 31 indicate that membranes from the liver, ovary, and adrenal were capable of generating a factor stimulating β-casein gene transcription under the influence of PRL, whereas muscle, heart, and lung do not share this property. In all cases, there was a good correlation between the stimulatory activity of the membrane superna-

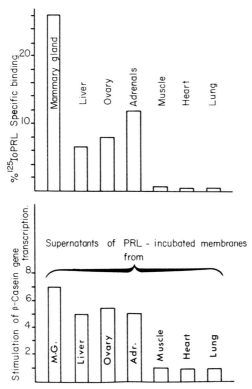

FIG. 31. Effect of microsomal supernatants obtained from membranes of various tissues incubated with PRL on the transcription rate of β-casein gene. Crude microsomes from various rabbit tissues were incubated with 4 μg/ml PRL. The supernatants were added to the transcription medium of mammary nuclei prepared from CB-154-treated lactating rabbits. Results are deduced from hybridization curves with ^{3}H-labeled β-casein cDNA. The data refer to the control values obtained from nuclei incubated without membrane supernatants. The amount of PRL receptors in the various microsomes was expressed as a percentage of ^{125}I-labeled PRL specifically bound to 200 μg microsomal proteins.

tants and the binding of PRL to the microsomal fractions (Teyssot *et al.*, 1981; Djiane *et al.*, 1983).

The specificity of the nuclei used in the *in vitro* transcription assay is shown in Fig. 32. It has been previously shown that rabbit liver cells do not synthesize casein mRNA sequences (Teyssot and Houdebine, 1980). When mammary supernatants containing the prolactin mediator were incubated with nuclei from various origins, only nuclei from mammary tissue were able to induce β-casein gene transcription, whereas nuclei from rabbit liver or red blood cells were unable to synthesize casein mRNA. In addition, this figure shows that nuclei from lactating mammary gland produced the highest level of casein mRNA, and that addition of the mediator was without additional effect. The value of the deinduction fol-

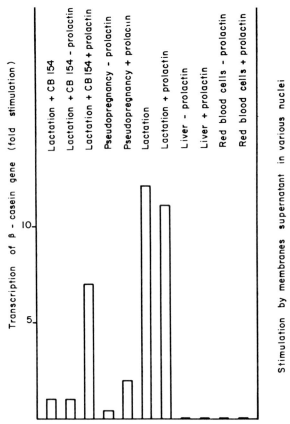

FIG. 32. Specificity of β-casein gene transcription from mammary supernatants incubated in the absence and presence of prolactin with nuclei prepared from various rabbit tissues.

lowing treatment of lactating animals for 4 days with bromocryptine (CB-154) can be seen, as it makes the system more sensitive and able to respond to the mediator. Nuclei from pseudopregnant rabbits produced less casein mRNA and were less sensitive to the mediator. Nuclei from lactating rabbits treated for 4 days with CB-154 therefore represent the most sensitive assay for the prolactin mediator (Teyssot *et al.*, 1981; Houdebine *et al.*, 1984a).

A study was carried out to compare the previous assay techniques involving SH-Sepharose column chromatography of the neosynthesized mRNA with a direct assay utilizing $[\alpha\text{-}^{32}\text{P}]\text{CTP}$ and cloned probes to $\alpha\text{-S}_1$, and β-casein and α-lactalbumin. Figure 33 shows that when nuclei are incubated with no membranes (control) or with mammary membranes in the absence of prolactin (−relay), there is no stimulation of mRNA, whereas addition of mediator (+relay) resulted in a marked stimulation of mRNA levels for all probes. The mediator was without effect on stimulation of total DNA or rRNA levels (Houdebine *et al.*, 1984a). Essentially, identical results were obtained when the neosynthesized mRNA levels were purified on a SH-Sepharose column and hybridization was measured either using ^{32}P-labeled nucleotides incorporated into the mRNA or with cloned probes labeled with ^{32}P by nick translation (Houdebine *et al.*, 1984a).

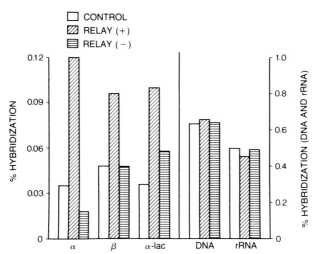

FIG. 33.   Effect of the prolactin mediator (relay) on the transcription of milk protein genes. Transcription was carried out by the incubation of nuclei with $[^{32}\text{P}]\text{CTP}$ and following extraction of the nuclei, the labeled RNA were hybridized to nitrocellulose filters containing plasmids with the specific probes for the milk protein genes, total DNA, or rRNA. Results are expressed as a percentage of the total labeled RNA which was hybridized to the filters.

C. RELEASE OF MEDIATOR FROM THE MEMBRANE

Purified plasma membrane (Ray, 1970) and Golgi-rich components (Bergeron *et al.*, 1978; Ferland *et al.*, 1984) were prepared from female rat liver, a tissue which contains high concentrations of PRL receptors, since the purification techniques of these subcellular fractions are well established for rat liver, in contrast to rabbit mammary gland. As is shown in Fig. 34, liver microsomal membranes were also capable of generating a mediator which was significantly active when added to rabbit mammary nuclei. Interestingly, purified plasma membranes from liver were more efficient in generating the mediator than microsomes or than purified

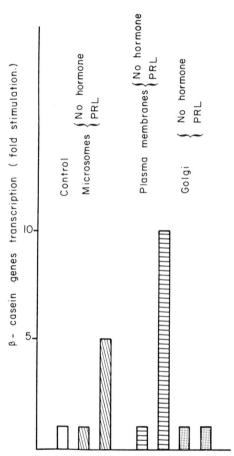

FIG. 34.   The effect of the subcellular source of prolactin receptors (microsomes, plasma membranes, or Golgi membranes) on the transcription of the β-casein gene.

Golgi membranes, although the latter contain 12- to 15-fold more PRL receptors than plasma membranes. This fact points to different roles of the various cellular membranes, and it suggests that the PRL intracellular relay is generated directly by the binding of the hormone to its peripheral receptors prior to endocytosis of the PRL receptor complex and its fusion with lysosomes (Djiane *et al.*, 1983).

Colchicine and various related drugs have been shown to inhibit the action of prolactin at the nuclear level for the induction of casein and DNA synthesis (Houdebine, 1980; Houdebine and Djiane, 1980). This effect of colchicine in explant cultures can be explained by a direct effect at the membrane level. As can be seen in Fig. 35, colchicine is able to block the generation of the intracellular mediator. Colchicine alone had no effect on the transcription rate of the β-casein gene when included in the incubation mixture with mammary microsomes; however, it completely blocked the stimulation of β-casein gene transcription induced by prolactin. Interestingly, colchicine was also able to block the generation of the

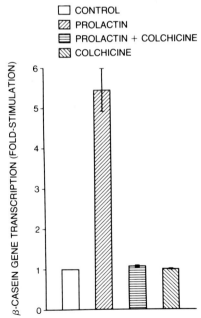

FIG. 35.   Effect of colchicine on the generation of the mediator stimulating β-casein gene transcription by prolactin. Mammary membranes were incubated with or without prolactin (4 μg/ml) in the presence or absence of colchicine (5 μM). Supernatants (200 μg) were incubated with isolated nuclei and β-casein mRNA synthesis was measured. The values are means ± SEM of four independent experiments.

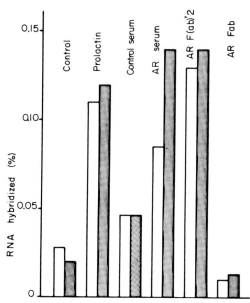

FIG. 36. Comparison of the effect of prolactin, prolactin receptor antibodies, and their fragments on the generation of the factor stimulating α-S$_1$- and β-casein gene transcription in mammary cell nuclei. Mammary microsomes were incubated either with buffer alone, or in the presence of prolactin (2 μg/ml), serum from nonimmunized sheep (1%), sheep prolactin receptor antiserum (1%), sheep prolactin receptor bivalent F(ab')$_2$ fragments (100 μg/ml), or the corresponding monovalent Fab' fragments (100 μg/ml). The supernatants were then added to transcriptional media of isolated mammary nuclei. The transcription rates of α-S$_1$- and β-casein were estimated by using an α-S$_1$- or β-casein cDNA probe. Results are expressed as a percentage of hybridization with α-S$_1$- (open bars) or β-casein (cross-hatched bars) cDNA probe.

mediator from rat liver membranes, suggesting a similar mechanism is occurring in these two different species and tissues. Colchicine added directly to isolated nuclei had no effect on casein gene transcription (Teyssot *et al.*, 1982). Colchicine clearly appears to be acting at an early step in the mechanism of action of prolactin.

It has been recently demonstrated that the prolactin mediator, when added directly to rabbit mammary cells in primary culture, stimulates transcription of the β-casein genes (Servely *et al.*, 1982). It was somewhat surprising, but the most feasible explanation is that the small mediator was able to penetrate the mammary cells and activate nuclear transcription.

Prolactin receptor antibodies have been shown to mimic prolactin action when added to the culture medium of explants (Djiane *et al.*, 1981). The bivalent fragments, as discussed previously, have maintained their capacity to stimulate casein and DNA synthesis whereas the monovalent fragments are devoid of these activities. In order to determine if the action of these mono- and bivalent fragments is mediated via the prolactin intracellular mediator, crude rabbit mammary gland microsomes were incubated with anti-prolactin receptor antibodies. The supernatants of the incubation mixtures were added to isolated mammary nuclei and transcription was allowed to proceed. As depicted in Fig. 36, the membrane supernatants obtained with anti-receptor antiserum or with bivalent anti-prolactin receptor F(ab')$_2$ fragments were able to markedly stimulate the transcription of both α- and β-casein genes. In contrast, monovalent anti-receptor Fab' fragments were never able to induce a stimulation of gene transcription.

D. PHYSICOCHEMICAL CHARACTERISTICS OF THE MEDIATOR

The fractionation on Sephadex G-15 of membrane supernatants obtained from incubations of mammary membranes with prolactin revealed an apparent molecular weight of less than 1000 (Teyssot *et al.*, 1982). However, it is well known that some molecules, particularly glycopeptides, may have a retarded elution on Sephadex. Other gel filtration systems were tried, such as the acrylamide-agarose gel Trisacryl GF-05. The mediator activity eluted in the void volume of the column, suggesting that a molecular weight is in excess of 3000.

The thermostability of the mediator was tested first by heating mammary membranes at 70°C for 5 minutes. Surprisingly, heat itself was able to release the mediator from membranes. In addition, the supernatant fraction containing the mediator was heated to 100°C for 10 minutes. This treatment did not affect the transcriptional activity of the mediator; therefore it appears to be thermostable (Teyssot *et al.*, 1982).

Another important characteristic of the mediator is its sensitivity to proteases. Treatment of supernatant fractions with trypsin (1 μg/ml) destroyed activity. However, trypsin at a lower concentration (0.1 μg/ml) was able to release mediator from membranes (Teyssot *et al.*, 1982) as has been shown to be the case for the insulin mediator (Seals and Czech, 1980). This suggests that the mediator is peptidic in nature and may be a part of the receptor molecule or associated with it, in such a way that proteases might be involved in its release from the membrane.

E. MECHANISM OF ACTION OF MEDIATOR ON NUCLEI

It was important to determine if the prolactin mediator is an activator of transcription at the initiation step, and not simply a factor which may

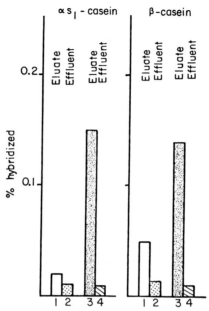

FIG. 37. Distribution of α-S_1- and β-casein sequences in effluent and eluate of the Hg-cellulose column. Conditions of transcription were those depicted in Fig. 3. Hybridization to the plasmids was carried out independently with both fractions. (1,2) Membrane supernatant without prolactin; (3,4) membrane supernatant with prolactin.

facilitate the elongation of previously (*in vivo*) initiated RNA chains. For that purpose, we analyzed the effect of the mediator on neosynthetized RNA labeled with γ-S ATP, γ-S GTP and [^{32}P]CTP. The resulting RNA were isolated using a Hg-cellulose column. Only RNA chains initiated *in vitro* were retained through their thio-phosphate 5′ end to the affinity column. Hybridization of the ^{32}P-labeled RNA retained and those not retained by the Hg-cellulose column were performed with plasmids containing cloned cDNA of casein genes bound to nitrocellulose filters. The results of Fig. 37 indicate that the transcription of casein genes was stimulated by the mediator essentially at the initiation step, since the effect of the mediator was observed only with the RNA fraction labeled by the γ-thionucleotides and retained by the column, whereas the column effluant did not respond to the mediator. Another demonstration relies on the utilization of specific inhibitors of initiation. Compounds such as AF-13, heparin, sarkosyl, and *S*-adenosyl homocysteine were added to nuclei with the mediator. In the presence of these inhibitors, the effect of the mediator on the initiation of casein mRNA synthesis was completely abolished (Fig. 38).

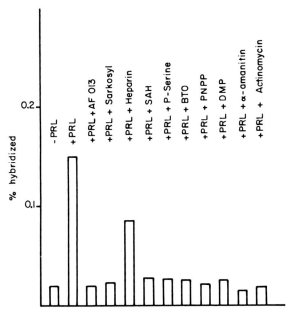

FIG. 38. Effects of various inhibitors on the initiation of the transcription by the prolactin mediator. Initiation inhibitors were AF013 (50 μg/ml); sarkosyl (0.5%); heparin (50 μg/ml); S-adenosylhomocysteine (20 mM). Phosphatase inhibitors were P-serine (10 mM); L-bromotetramizole oxalate (10 mM); p-nitrophenyl phosphate (5 mM); 2,3-dimercaptopropan-1-ol (10 mM). Inhibitors of transcription were antinomycin D (50 μg/ml) and α-amanitin (10 μg/ml).

The mechanism through which the initiation of the transcription of genes could be stimulated is an important question, for which few data are available in other biological systems. It is generally admitted that a high transcriptional activity is associated with an hyperphosphorylation of nuclear proteins. We have postulated that the prolactin mediator is acting through a modification of the phosphorylation state of nuclear proteins. For that purpose we have tested in our system the effects of inhibitors of protein phosphatase. As shown in Fig. 38, several of these compounds prevented the action of the mediator without interfering significantly with the initiation process of the transcription of whole genes. Interestingly, inhibitors of protein phosphatase acting on phosphotyrosine (Zn^{2+}, sodium vanadate) were totally inactive (not shown). These results suggest that the mediator acts on the nucleus probably via an activation of protein phosphatase and that the proteins which are dephosphorylated probably contain phosphoserine or phosphothreonine rather than phosphotyrosine.

The properties of the mediator released by insulin as described by several groups (Larner *et al.,* 1979; Seals and Jarett, 1980) share many similarities with the prolactin mediator. It has been clearly demonstrated that this mediator acts via a dephosphorylation of regulatory enzymes such as pyruvate dehydrogenase or glycogen synthetase (Larner *et al.,* 1979). The experiments on dephosphorylation of nuclear proteins induced by the prolactin mediator suggest the possibility that a common mechanism could be involved in the transfer of the stimulation of insulin or prolactin in their target cells.

F. SIMILARITY OF PROLACTIN AND INSULIN MEDIATORS

Recently, it has been reported in mouse mammary explants that prolactin does not induce casein synthesis unless insulin is present in the culture medium (Bolander *et al.,* 1981). Studies in the rabbit indicate that significant β-casein synthesis occurs in the presence of prolactin alone. However, insulin, which is quite inactive alone, markedly potentiates the lactogenic action of prolactin (Houdebine *et al.,* 1984b).

There are a number of striking similarities between the prolactin and insulin mediator. They are both small molecules which are heat stable, inactivated by trypsin, and which appear to stimulate a phosphatase. Insulin, when added to mammary membranes, produces the formation of a factor which slightly stimulates casein gene transcription when added to isolated nuclei (unpublished observations).

In order to compare the relative activities in the two systems, our laboratories have exchanged samples with those of Dr. J. Larner. We have recently observed that a Sephadex fraction of rat skeletal muscle extracts from animals treated with insulin specifically stimulated mitochondrial pyruvate dehydrogenase activity. The same fraction that stimulated pyruvate dehydrogenase activity was able, in a dose-dependent fashion, to stimulate the transcription of the α-S_1 casein gene from isolated rabbit mammary nuclei. Until the two factors are purified to homogeneity, it will be impossible to determine if the actions of insulin and prolactin are mediated by the same or different molecules. At this point, however, it appears clear that there is some homology between the two mediators.

VII. Summary and Conclusions

Prolactin receptors have been localized in a number of different tissues, although they have been most extensively studied in the mammary gland and liver. Receptor numbers differ dependent upon the physiological state of the animal. A large percentage of prolactin receptors are located within the cell in the Golgi and lysosomal compartments.

Prolactin is able to regulate its receptor number both in a positive and negative fashion. A slow up-regulation observed most generally *in vivo* following extended periods of injection, corresponding to a large extent, to the accumulation of Golgi membranes which occurs during differentiation of the mammary gland. In rat liver cells in suspension culture, this up-regulation probably represents a reduced level of degradation as well as an increased synthesis of receptors. The down-regulation of prolactin receptors is a more rapid and reversible process. It can be observed both *in vivo* and *in vitro* in rabbit mammary glands and rat liver.

Prolactin receptors have been partially purified and the binding subunit appears to be approximately 32,000 daltons, as determined by photoaffinity labeling studies.

Polyclonal antibodies to the receptor molecule have been prepared. These antibodies are able to inhibit binding of prolactin to prolactin receptors in all tissues that have been shown to contain prolactin receptors, including human breast cancer biopsies. In addition, the action of prolactin can be either mimicked or inhibited, dependent upon the dose of receptor antibody utilized. Bivalency of the receptor antibody is essential for its action, although monovalent fragments inhibit binding and induce down-regulation of receptors.

Figure 39 summarizes the current status concerning the mechanism of prolactin action. It is clear that internalization and down-regulation of the receptor are not necessary for action to be observed. However, this pathway via the Golgi and lysosomes is probably important in receptor replenishment to the plasma membrane and receptor degradation.

Both prolactin and antireceptors are able to induce the release of an intracellular relay which is capable of stimulating the transcription of milk protein genes from isolated mammary nuclei. The release of this mediator can be blocked by colchicine by a direct interaction with the membrane.

The second messenger or mediator of prolactin action appears to be a small peptide, heat stable which may be released by the action of proteases at the membrane. This raises the interesting possibility that the mediator is a portion of the receptor molecule itself. Preliminary studies have revealed that polyclonal antibodies against the receptor molecule are able, at concentrations much greater than those which provoke the liberation of mediator, to bind and prevent the action of preformed mediator. These results suggest that the prolactin mediator has been copurified with the receptor and that antibodies against the mediator are present in the antisera obtained against partially purified receptors.

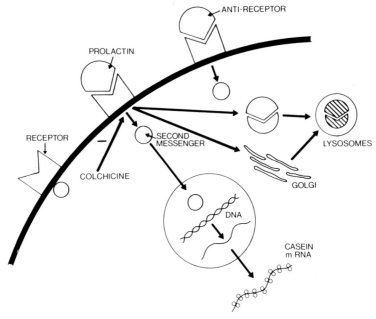

FIG. 39.   Schematic representation of the mechanism of action of prolactin in the mammary cell.

The interaction of the mediator with the nucleus involves a dephosphorylation of some nuclear proteins, as phosphatase inhibitors block the action of the mediator in isolated nuclei. In addition, the stimulation of milk protein gene transcription appears to involve initiation of mRNA sequences.

There are some interesting similarities between the prolactin and insulin mediators and these molecules must be purified to homogeneity before it will be possible to determine if the mediators are identical or related peptides.

ACKNOWLEDGMENTS

The authors wish to express their gratitude to the National Hormone and Pituitary Program, National Institute of Arthritis, Metabolism and Digestive Diseases for providing human growth hormone, ovine prolactin, and other hormones used in the experiments described in this manuscript. These studies were supported in part by grants from the Medical Research Council of Canada, the National Cancer Institute (Canada), United States Public Health Service, the Centre National de la Recherche Scientifique, the Institut National pour la Santé et la Recherche Médicale, and the Délégation à la Recherche Scientifique et Technique.

REFERENCES

Ascoli, M., and Puett, D. (1978). *J. Biol. Chem.* **253,** 4892–4899.

Baenzinger, J. U., and Fiete, D. (1982). *J. Biol. Chem.* **257,** 6007–6009.

Baldwin, D., Terris, S., and Steiner, D. F. (1980). *J. Biol. Chem.* **255,** 4028–4034.

Bergeron, J. J. M., Ehrenreich, J. H., Siekevitz, P., and Palade, G. E. (1973). *J. Cell Biol.* **59,** 73–88.

Bergeron, J. J. M., Posner, B. I., Josefsberg, Z., and Sikstrom, R. (1978). *J. Biol. Chem.* **253,** 4058–4066.

Bohnet, H. G., Shiu, R. P. C., Grinwich, D., and Friesen, H. G. (1978). *Endocrinology* **102,** 1657–1661.

Bolander, F. F., Nicholas, K. R., Wanwyck, J. J., and Topper, Y. J. (1981). *Proc. Natl. Acad. Sci. U.S.A.* **78,** 5682–5684.

Borst, D. W., and Sayare, M. (1982). *Biochem. Biophys. Res. Commun.* **105,** 194–201.

Conn, P. M., Conti, M., Harwood, J. P., Dufau, M. L., and Catt, K. J. (1978). *Nature (London)* **274,** 598–600.

Conn, P. M., Rogers, D. C., Stewart, J. M., Niedel, J., and Sheffield, T. (1982). *Nature (London)* **296,** 653–655.

Corner, G. W. (1930). *Am. J. Physiol.* **95,** 43–55.

De Duve, C., Pressman, B. C., Gianetto, R., Wattiaux, R., and Appelmans, F. (1955). *Biochem. J.* **60,** 604–617.

De Meyts, P., Bianco, A. R., and Roth, J. (1976). *J. Biol. Chem.* **251,** 1877–1888.

Devinoy, E., Houdebine, L. M., and Delouis, C. (1978). *Biochem. Biophys. Acta* **517,** 360–366.

Djiane, J., and Durand, P. (1977). *Nature (London)* **266,** 641–643.

Djiane, J., Durand, P., and Kelly, P. A. (1977). *Endocrinology* **100,** 1348–1356.

Djiane, J., Clauser, H., and Kelly, P. A. (1979a). *Biochem. Biophys. Res. Commun.* **90,** 1371–1378.

Djiane, J., Delouis, C., and Kelly, P. A. (1979b). *Proc. Soc. Exp. Biol. Med.* **162,** 342–345.

Djiane, J., Kelly, P. A., and Houdebine, L. M. (1980). *Mol. Cell. Endocrinol.* **18,** 87–98.

Djiane, J., Houdebine, L. M., and Kelly, P. A. (1981). *Proc. Natl. Acad. Sci. U.S.A.* **78,** 7445–7448.

Djiane, J., Houdebine, L. M., and Kelly, P. A. (1982). *Endocrinology* **110,** 791–795.

Djiane, J., Houdebine, L. M., Kelly, P. A., Teyssot, B., and Dusanter-Fourt, I. (1983). "Prolactin and Prolactinomas," pp. 29–42. Raven, New York.

Donner, D. B., and Corin, R. E. (1980). *J. Biol. Chem.* **255,** 9005–9008.

Donner, D. B., and Martin, D. W., and Sonenberg, M. (1978). *Proc. Natl. Acad. Sci. U.S.A.* **75,** 672–676.

Donner, D. B., Cadadei, J., Hartstein, L., Martin, D., and Sonenberg, M. M. (1980). *Biochemistry* **19,** 3293–3300.

Drachman, D. B., Angus, C. W., Adams, R. N., Michelson, J. D., and Hoffman, G. J. (1978). *N. Engl. J. Med.* **298,** 1116–1122.

Dusanter-Fourt, I., Djiane, J., Houdebine, L. M., and Kelly, P. A. (1983). *Life Sci.* **32,** 407–412.

Dusanter-Fourt, I., Djiane, J., Kelly, P. A., Houdebine, L. M., and Teyssot, B. (1984). *Endocrinology* **114,** 1021–1027.

Edery, M., Djiane, J., Houdebine, L. M., and Kelly, P. A. (1983). *Cancer Res.* **43,** 3170–3174.

Fairbanks, G., Steck, T. L., and Wallach, D. F. H. (1971). *Biochemistry* **10,** 2606.

Ferland, L. H., Djiane, J., Houdebine, L.-M., and Kelly, P. A. (1984). *Endocrinology,* in Press.

Flier, J. C., Kahn, C. R., Roth, J., and Bar, R. S. (1975). *Science* **190,** 63–65.

Geisow, J. M. (1982). *Nature (London)* **295,** 649–650.

Gordon, P., Carpentier, J. L., Cohen, S., and Orci, L. (1978). *Proc. Natl. Acad. Sci. U.S.A.* **75,** 5025–5029.

Haeuptle, M. T., Aubert, M. L., Djiane, J., and Kraehenbuhl, J. P. (1983). *J. Biol. Chem.* **258,** 305–314.

Hizuka, N., Gorden, P., Lesniak, M. A., Van Obberghen, E., Carpentier, J.-L., and Orci, L. (1981). *J. Biol. Chem.* **256,** 4591–4597.

Hjelmeland, L. M. (1980). *Proc. Natl. Acad. Sci. U.S.A.* **77,** 6368–6370.

Houdebine, L. M. (1980). *Eur. J. Cell Biol.* **22,** 755–760.

Houdebine, L. M., and Djiane, J. (1980). *Mol. Cell. Endocrinol.* **17,** 1–15.

Houdebine, L. M., Djiane, J., Teyssot, B., Devinoy, E., Kelly, P. A., Dusanter-Fourt, I., Servely, J. L., and Martel, P. (1984a). *Methods Enzymol.,* in Press.

Houdebine, L. M., Djiane, J., Teyssot, B., Dusanter-Fourt, I., Martel, P., Kelly, P. A., Devinoy, E., and Servely, J. L. (1984b). *J. Dairy Sci.,* in Press.

Jacobs, S., Chang, K. J., and Cuatrecasas, P. (1978). *Science* **200,** 1283–1284.

Jacobs, S., Hazum, E., Schechter, Y., and Cuatrecasas, P. (1979). *Proc. Natl. Acad. Sci. U.S.A.* **76,** 4918–4921.

Johnson, G. L., MacAndrew, V. I., and Pilch, P. F. (1981). *Proc. Natl. Acad. Sci. U.S.A.* **78,** 875–878.

Josefsberg, Z., Posner, B. I., Patel, B., and Bergeron, J. J. M. (1979). *J. Biol. Chem.* **254,** 209–214.

Kahn, C. R., Freychet, P., and Roth, J. (1974). *J. Biol. Chem.* **249,** 2249–2257.

Kahn, C. R., Baird, K. L., Jarrett, D. B., and Flier, J. S. (1978). *Proc. Natl. Acad. Sci. U.S.A.* **75,** 4209–4213.

Kasuga, M., Hedo, J. A., Yemada, K. M., and Kahn, C. R. (1982). *J. Biol. Chem.* **257,** 10392–10399.

Katikineni, M., Davies, T. F., Huhtaniemi, I. T., and Catt, K. J. (1980). *Endocrinology* **107,** 1980–1988.

Katoh, M., Djiane, J., Leblanc, G., and Kelly, P. A. (1984). *Mol. Cell. Endocrinol.* **34,** 191–200.

Kelly, P. A., Posner, B. I., and Friesen, H. G. (1975). *Endocrinology* **97,** 1408–1415.

Kelly, P. A., Ferland, L., and Labrie, F. (1978). "Progress in Prolactin Physiology and Pathology," pp. 59–68. Elsevier, Amsterdam.

Kelly, P. A., Leblanc, G., and Djiane, J. (1979). *Endocrinology* **104,** 1631–1638.

Kelly, P. A., Djiane, J., and DeLéan, A. (1980). *Prog. Reprod. Biol.* **6,** 124–136.

Kelly, P. A., Djiane, J., Houdebine, L. M., Katoh, M., and Rosa, A. A. M. (1983a). "Prolactin and Prolactinomas," pp. 19–28. Raven, New York.

Kelly, P. A., Djiane, J., and Leblanc, G. (1983b). *Proc. Soc. Exp. Biol. Med.* **172,** 219–224.

Khan, M. N., Posner, B. I., Verma, A. K., Khan, R. J., and Bergeron, J. J. M. (1981). *Proc. Natl. Acad. Sci. U.S.A.* **78,** 4980–4984.

Khan, M. N., Posner, B. I., Khan, R. J., and Bergeron, J. J. M. (1982). *J. Biol. Chem.* **257,** 5969–5976.

Kolata, G. B. (1978). *Science* **201,** 895–897.

Laemli, U. K. (1970). *Nature (London)* **227,** 680–685.

Larner, J., Galasko, G., Chang, K., Depaoliroach, A., Huang, L., Daygy, P., and Kellogg, J. (1979). *Science* **206,** 1408–1411.

Li, C. H. (1980). "Hormonal Proteins and Peptides, Vol. VIII, Prolactin," pp. 1–36. Academic Press, New York.

Li, C. H., Dixon, J. S., Los, T. B., Schmidt, K. D., and Pankov, Y. A. (1970). *Arch. Biochem. Biophys.* **141**, 705–737.

Liscia, D. S., and Vonderhaar, B. K. (1982). *Proc. Natl. Acad. Sci. U.S.A.* **79**, 5930–5934.

Liscia, D. S., Alhadi, T., and Vonderhaar, B. K. (1982). *J. Biol. Chem.* **257**, 9401–9405.

Manni, A., Chambers, M. J., and Pearson, O. H. (1978). *Endocrinology* **103**, 2168–2171.

Massagué, J., and Czech, M. P. (1982). *J. Biol. Chem.* **257**, 5038–5045.

Massagué, J., Pilch, P. F., and Czech, M. P. (1980). *Proc. Natl. Acad. Sci. U.S.A.* **77**, 7137–7141.

Massagué, J., Guillette, B. J., and Czech, M. P. (1981a). *J. Biol. Chem.* **256**, 2122–2125.

Massagué, J., Guillette, B. J., Czech, M. P., Morgan, C. J., and Bradshaw, R. A. (1981b). *J. Biol. Chem.* **256**, 9419–9424.

Matusik, R., and Rosen, J. M. (1978). *J. Biol. Chem.* **253**, 2343–2347.

Maxfield, F. R., Willingham, M. C., Davies, D. J. A., and Pastan, I. (1979). *Nature (London)* **277**, 661–663.

Nicoll, C. S., and Bern, H. A. (1972). "Lactogenic Hormones," pp. 299–317. Churchill, London.

Perry, H. M., and Jacobs, L. S. (1978). *J. Biol. Chem.* **253**, 1560–1564.

Pilch, P. F., and Czech, M. P. (1979). *J. Biol. Chem.* **255**, 1722–1731.

Posner, B. I., and Khan, M. N. (1983). "Prolactin and Prolactinomas," pp. 9–18. Raven, New York.

Posner, B. I., Kelly, P. A., Shiu, R. P. C., and Friesen, H. G. (1974b). *Endocrinology* **96**, 521–531.

Posner, B. I., Kelly, P. A., and Friesen, H. G. (1975). *Science* **187**, 57–59.

Powell-Jones, C. H. J., Thomas, C. G., and Nayfeh, S. N. (1979). *Endocrinology* **104**, 136A.

Ray, T. F. (1970). *Biochim. Biophys. Acta* **196**, 1–9.

Riddle, O., Bates, R. W., and Dykshorn, S. W. (1932). *Proc. Soc. Exp. Biol. Med.* **29**, 1211–1212.

Rosa, A. A. M., Djiane, J., Houdebine, L. M., and Kelly, P. A. (1982). *Biochem. Biophys. Res. Commun.* **106**, 243–249.

Ross, E. M., Maguire, M. E., Sturgill, T. W., Biltonen, R. L., and Gilman, A. G. (1977). *J. Biol. Chem.* **252**, 5761–5775.

Schechter, Y., Hernaez, L., Schlessinger, J., and Cuatrecasas, P. (1979). *Nature (London)* **278**, 835–838.

Seals, J. R., and Czech, M. E. (1980). *J. Biol. Chem.* **255**, 6529–6533.

Seals, J. R., and Jarett, L. (1980). *Proc. Natl. Acad. Sci. U.S.A.* **77**, 77–81.

Servely, J. L., Teyssot, B., Houdebine, L. M., Delouis, C., Djiane, J., and Kelly, P. A. (1982). *FEBS Lett.* **148**, 242–246.

Shiu, R. P. C., and Friesen, H. G. (1974). *J. Biol. Chem.* **249**, 7902–7911.

Shiu, R. P. C., and Friesen, H. G. (1976). *Science* **192**, 259–261.

Shiu, R. P. C., Kelly, P. A., and Friesen, H. G. (1973). *Science* **180**, 968–971.

Simonds, W. F., Koski, G., Streaty, R. A., Hjelmeland, L. M., and Klee, W. A. (1980). *Proc. Natl. Acad. Sci. U.S.A.* **77**, 4623–4627.

Squire, P. G., Starman, B., and Li, C. H. (1963). *J. Biol. Chem.* **238**, 1389–1395.

Stricker, P., and Grueter, F. (1928). *C. R. Soc. Biol.* **99**, 1978–1980.

Teyssot, B., and Houdebine, L. M. (1980). *Eur. J. Biochem.* **110**, 263–272.

Teyssot, B., and Houdebine, L. M. (1981). *Eur. J. Biochem.* **114**, 597–608.

Teyssot, B., Houdebine, L. M., and Djiane, J. (1981). *Proc. Natl. Acad. Sci. U.S.A.* **78**, 6729–6733.

Teyssot, B., Djiane, J., Kelly, P. A., and Houdebine, L. M. (1982). *Biol. Cell.* **43**, 81–88.
Van der Gugten, A. A., Waters, M. J., Murthy, G. S., and Friesen, H. G. (1980). *Endocrinology* **106**, 402–411.
Wattiaux, R., Wattiaux-De Coninck, S., Ronveaux-Dupal, M.-F., and Dubois, F. (1978). *J. Cell Biol.* **78**, 349–368.
Williams, L. T., and Lefkowitz, R. J. (1978). "Receptor Binding Studies in Adrenergic Pharmacology," pp. 27–41. Raven, New York.
Willingham, M. C., and Pastan, I. (1980). *Cell* **21**, 67–77.
Wray, W., Boulikas, T., Wray, V. P., and Hancock, R. (1981). *Anal. Biochem.* **118**, 197–203.

DISCUSSION

F. C. Bancroft: Paul, I'm very impressed with the data you have shown for the specificity of your factor. However, as you know, I think there are some aspects of your transcription assay which need to be further clarified. I have two related questions. First, do you currently think that your factor is regulating casein gene transcription in your isolated nuclei at the initiation step? If so, how does this possibility fit in with the general observation that nuclei incubated *in vitro* exhibit little reinitiation of transcription?

P. A. Kelly: Our isolated nuclei have a very low capacity to initiate new RNA chains, as has been shown in many other systems. In the presence of the mediator, general initiation is not affected at all. It is only prolactin-sensitive genes which are stimulated. Experiments using inhibitors of initiation and γ thio or β ATP and GTP strongly suggest that the action of the prolactin mediator is exerted essentially at the initiation step. Further experiments, currently in progress, using 5'-P and 3'-OH probes will demonstrate this unequivocally. Therefore, isolated nuclei are probably more capable of initiating new RNA chains than generally believed, with the condition of adding specific cytoplasmic factors which are eliminated during the preparation of the nuclei.

S. L. Cohen: I am interested in knowing whether estrogen and progesterone play any role in the formation of casein in the human mammary gland and second does prolactin have any function in egg-laying animals?

P. A. Kelly: Estrogen and progesterone, of course, are intimately involved in the development of the mammary gland. As I mentioned, progesterone is able to block the production of casein so it has an inhibitory effect during pregnancy; estrogen is involved in the development of the early glandular tissue but is not specifically involved in the production of casein.

S. L. Cohen: Both estrogen and progesterone are involved in the formation of ovalbumin in the egg-laying chicken so that they can play a role in protein formation, I wondered whether they have a role in the human?

P. A. Kelly: The development of the breast is under the control of sex steroids. We have no specific data, however, for human breast tissue.

S. L. Cohen: Do you know of any function for prolactin in egg-laying animals?

P. A. Kelly: There have been several reported functions in birds, one of which in nesting behavior. Perhaps Dr. Nicoll could respond to the question since he has worked in that area.

C. S. Nicoll: It so happens that the comments I wish to make will address the question of Dr. Cohen, and they are related to the articles of Dr. Czech and Dr. Kelly. We have been using a different prolactin-responsive system, namely the pigeon crop-sac, which is an avian target organ for the hormone. The primary response of this organ is cellular proliferation, rather than the more complex responses found in the mammary gland. We have investigated the interaction between prolactin as a mitogenic hormone and the insulin-like growth factors [Anderson *et al.,* "Insulin-like Growth Factors/Somatomedins" (E. M. Spencer, ed.). de

Gruyter, Berlin, in press]. The mucosal dry weight of the crop-sac is used as an index of the number of cells, since a high correlation exists between that index and the DNA content. A low dose of human somatomedin C (8 μg total) has a small stimulatory effect on the mucosal epithelium. Injection of a total dose of 0.5 μg of prolactin had about the same effect as the somatomedin. When we combine these two factors at the same doses we get a striking augmentation of the prolactin effect. It would require at least 10 times more prolactin to get that degree of response if it were injected alone. In a similar type of experiment we used 2.0 μg proinsulin rather than somatomedin C. Both bovine and human proinsulin have been tested and they give a similar augmentation of prolactin's response. Other insulin-like growth factors have been tested in this system. Their relative potencies as prolactin synergists, using bovine proinsulin as a reference preparation with a potency of 100%, are as follows: human somatomedin C is about 4.5 times more potent than proinsulin, and porcine relaxin is about half as potent, but insulin has very little activity. In addition, rat multiplication simulating activity (MSA), which is similar to human somatomedin-A, is totally inactive as a prolactin synergist. Accordingly, this is an unusual system because both proinsulin and relaxin are much more potent than insulin, and MSA is inactive. I think that analysis of the receptor in this system should be very interesting.

R. Chatterton: I was interested in a little further clarification of the site of action of prolactin. Have you attempted to purify membranes using enzyme markers to show that when you eliminate intracellular membranes the response to prolactin increases and is related strictly to the plasma membrane. And also the other hormone I was thinking might be included would be insulin to see whether this stimulates the mediator. The last question relates to whether you can see an effect of glucocorticoids on the membrane preparation that you have.

P. A. Kelly: In response to the first question, we have simply prepared from rat liver purified plasma membrane fractions and purified Golgi fractions, following the technique of Dr. Posner's group, and followed the purity by 5' nucleotidase and galactosyltransferase activity. It is these which we have shown to be either active or inactive in terms of the generation of the intracellular mediator. For preparation of the mediator from rabbit mammary gland, we use a mixed microsomal pellet which contains plasma membranes as well as intracellular membranes. We have shown, however, that generation of the mediator is greater in membrane fractions enriched in 5' nucleotidase, an enzyme marker for plasma membranes. Glucocorticoids certainly potentiate the effect of prolactin in terms of the release of casein messenger RNA and casein production, but they do not appear to have, at least in the rabbit, any direct effect. In response to your question about the role of insulin, we have measured the potentiation of the effect of prolactin by insulin in explant cultures of rabbit mammary glands. There is an increased sensitivity to prolactin in explants cultured in the presence of insulin, the effect being dose dependent. We have carried out a collaborative study with Dr. Larner's group in Charlottesville. They have partially purified an insulin mediator and followed its activity by measuring mitochondrial PDH stimulation. Muscle from control or insulin-treated rats was extracted and chromatographed on a Sephadex G-25 followed by a G-15 column. The column was divided into four fractions. The major PDH activity appears in fraction 2, with mediator from insulin-treated animals having the greatest activity. The same fraction is able to stimulate the generation of the casein-specific genes in isolated mammary nuclei. So it appears that there is some cross-reactivity of this insulin mediator and the prolactin mediator, however, we cannot determine at the present time whether the mediators released in response to insulin and prolactin are identical. In the mammary gland there is some release of the "prolactin mediator" or low levels of release of a mediator similar to the prolactin mediator in response to incubation with insulin. However, the release in response to insulin of a "prolactin mediator" is not always observed, and when it is, it is present at low levels. So until we reach the stage which Dr. Czech is with his material, we will be unable to say whether the insulin mediator and prolactin mediator are the same or similar molecules.

H. G. Friesen: I thoroughly enjoyed your presentation very much. It clearly represents an enormous amount of work over an extended period of time. I have a number of questions. The first relates to the rabbit mammary gland preparation used for the isolation of the nuclei in your experiments. After treatment of the rabbits with bromocriptine for a period of 4 days, what is the functional status of the mammary glands? For example, would these rabbits continue to nurse their young?

P. A. Kelly: Yes it is known—perhaps Jean you could respond.

J. Djiane: When bromocryptine is given to rabbits for 4 days at mid-lactation, milk production is reduced by only 50%, and the mother continues to nurse her young. When we remove the mammary gland at this period, it has a lower content of milk, but the ultrastructure of the mammary cells as judged by electron microscopy appears to be maintained. It is important in our nuclear transcription assay to use these CB-154-treated rabbits, however, so that these nuclei can respond to a new stimulus.

H. G. Friesen: Thank you very much. Clearly their endogenous casein gene expression is still very active at the time of the isolation of the nuclei. Is that correct?

P. A. Kelly: As you saw in that slide showing the casein mRNA production from nuclei from mammary glands during pregnancy or lactation, CB-154 treatment induces a marked reduction in casein message production. However, this level appears to be sufficient to allow some milk production.

H. G. Friesen: The induction of the putative mediator of PRL action from membranes occurred at about an hour. I wonder if you have ever attempted to centrifuge down the membrane preparation, resuspend the pellet, and reexpose the residual membranes to additional prolactin to see whether there was any evidence of down-regulation as demonstrated by decreased release of the mediator. In other words is there really a limit to the production of the mediator upon initial exposure to PRL.

P. A. Kelly: Yes, upon a second exposure to prolactin, more mediator can be produced. However, there is almost no release following a third exposure.

H. G. Friesen: I was very interested in your observation that membranes incubated with PRL and colchicine fail to generate the peptide mediator. I wonder if you have any thoughts on how colchicine acts? Does colchicine bind to a specific plasma membrane component? Have you done any studies of that kind?

P. A. Kelly: Louis-Marie Houdebine has done some studies and perhaps he could respond specifically to that question.

L. M. Houdebine: From the data that Paul has shown we might deduce that colchicine is acting by destabilizing the microtubules; in fact, we have obtained the inhibitory effect with isolated membranes, therefore microtubules are probably not involved, Another argument that we have is that various drugs which destroy microtubules such as griseofulini and tubulazole are totally unable to prevent the action of prolactin on explants and on membranes, so clearly there is no link between the integrity of cytoskeleton and the inhibitory effect of colchicine and related drugs. We have indeed found molecules which are capable of binding colchicine in the membranes in mammary glands. This binding is resistant solubilization of the membrane by Triton X-100. We have not identified this molecule but it might be tubulin, but this remains to be demonstrated.

P. K. Donahoe: Is the dephosphorylation event that occurs with the mediator a cytosol dephosphorylation or a nuclear event?

P. A. Kelly: The studies were performed with isolated nuclei, therefore the dephosphorylation is a nuclear event.

B. I. Posner: In view of the bimodal effect of prolactin in generating the mediator it would seem to be important to do a prolactin dose–response curve in Golgi preparations.

P. A. Kelly: We've only looked at two doses, and your point is well taken. We do need to do a broad range dose–response curve to be sure that we are not simply measuring the inhibitory activity of a more sensitive Golgi preparation.

P. Wynn: I have a question regarding regulation of the prolactin receptor. You have mentioned both down-regulation and up-regulation of receptors in response to prolactin administration. Could you give us some idea of the time course of down-regulation and up-regulation in this system, and how this relates to the time course of stimulation of transcription of the casein gene.

P. A. Kelly: Under *in vivo* conditions the down-regulation of prolactin receptors occurs very rapidly and within 5–15 minutes with the effect being maximal at about 1 hour, and after that period there's a slow return to control levels which is attained at about 24 hours. The up-regulation of prolactin receptors is an event which takes a longer period of time *in vivo*, a maximal effect being seen in 3 to 4 days in the rabbit and approximately 7 to 8 days in the rat. Temporally, down-regulation of receptors could be involved in prolactin stimulation of casein mRNA production, but we have shown that this is not the case. Certainly, up-regulation of receptors requires much longer periods than is required for the production of either casein messenger RNA or casein.

P. Wynn: Just one further point—may down-regulation possibly be explained by persistent occupancy of receptors by ligand in view of the increased residual binding following dissociation when the time of association of receptor and ligand is increased.

P. A. Kelly: I didn't have time during the presentation to describe the method, but we have utilized in all the studies where we were looking at receptor occupancy or down-regulation, a technique to dissociate prolactin from the membrane preparations which involves high molar concentrations of magnesium chloride, which does not destroy the receptor. Therefore, in effect, we measured total receptor levels.

C. Sonnenschein: I wonder whether you could elaborate a little further on whether prolactin has a direct proliferative effect on cell multiplication? I noticed that you did not include a possible mechanism mediated by your mediator on this particular parameter.

P. A. Kelly: Certainly in the mammary gland and mammary tumors, prolactin has an effect on the stimulation of DNA synthesis as measured by [^{3}H]thymidine incorporation. We are unable at the present time to say whether the mediator responsible for the stimulation of transcription of casein genes is the same factor which is involved in this increase in DNA synthesis. We haven't yet done those experiments but certainly it's something we want to look at.

C. Sonnenschein: I haven't seen the evidence for direct stimulatory effect on DNA synthesis by prolactin in your slides.

P. A. Kelly: I think I had two or three slides which showed that in explant cultures increasing concentrations of prolactin were able to induce the 3- to 4-fold increase in DNA synthesis.

C. Sonnenschein: But you will agree that the explants do not have a homogeneous population of target cells that could be considered all target for prolactin but in fact you have a mixture of cells, is that correct?

P. A. Kelly: That's certainly true, but the majority of cells are mammary epithelial cells.

The Hypothalamic Control of the Menstrual Cycle and the Role of Endogenous Opioid Peptides[1]

MICHEL FERIN, DEAN VAN VUGT, AND SHARON WARDLAW

International Institute for the Study of Human Reproduction and Departments of Obstetrics and Gynecology, and Medicine, Columbia University, College of Physicians and Surgeons, New York, New York

I. Introduction

The primate menstrual cycle is the result of complex interacting processes between the hypothalamus, the hypophysis, and the ovaries. At the 1970 Laurentian Hormone Conference, R. L. Vande Wiele *et al.* (1970) presented a model of the human menstrual cycle which emphasized ovarian hypophyseal feedback interactions. At that time little was known of hypothalamo-hypophyseal relationships, and of the neuroendocrine events which govern the menstrual cycle. Simulation performance of a mathematical model of the human menstrual cycle derived from that experimental report indicated however that signal frequencies, which at that time were undetected by experimental procedures, constituted an essential source of feedback information (Bogumil *et al.*, 1972a,b). Because of the inherent difficulties of conducting extensive neuroendocrine investigations in the human, several primate centers, including ours, have focused their attention on the rhesus monkey, a subhuman primate with menstrual cycles similar to the human. Significant progress toward our understanding of the neuroendocrine control of gonadotropin secretion was made during these past 10 years, including the demonstration that gonadotropin-releasing hormone (GnRH) is released from the hypothalamus in a pulsatile fashion (Carmel *et al.*, 1976) and that GnRH pulse characteristics are important determinants of gonadotropin secretion (Belchetz *et al.*, 1978).

At the 1979 Laurentian Hormone Conference, Knobil (1980) presented a model of the neuroendocrine system that governs the menstrual cycle of the rhesus monkey. In summary, the model postulated that the arcuate area of the medial basal hypothalamus (MBH) generates a signal at approximately hourly (circhoral) intervals ("arcuate oscillator") to induce the release of GnRH into the hypophyseal portal circulation. The hourly

[1] This article is dedicated to the memory of Raymond L. Vande Wiele.

441

GnRH pulses, then, stimulate the gonadotrope to release pulses of LH and FSH, which, in turn, induce morphological and secretory changes in the ovaries. Estradiol was postulated to modulate the gonadotropin response to this *unchanging* GnRH regimen through a feedback directed exclusively at the anterior pituitary. The two basic features of the model, the unchanging hourly pulsatile GnRH release and the estradiol feedback on the pituitary, were judged to be sufficient for normal cyclicity to occur.

The apparent validity of this model has been demonstrated under several experimental circumstances. These include (1) generation of normal menstrual cycles in monkeys bearing a lesion of the MBH (Nakai *et al.*, 1978) or following pituitary stalk section (Richardson *et al.*, 1984), by hourly pulses of GnRH, and (2) induction of normal menstrual cycles, including follicular maturation, a gonadotropin surge, ovulation, and a luteal phase by an unchanging GnRH therapeutical regimen in amenorrheic patients (Leyendecker *et al.*, 1981; Hoffman and Crowley, 1982). However convincing the experimental support for this menstrual cycle model is, we would like to present two lines of experimental evidence which will illustrate the need for further modifications of the model, if it is to accurately represent the phenomenon of cyclicity. This evidence includes the observations that (1) pulsatile characteristics of the arcuate oscillator vary during the menstrual cycle, and (2) ovarian steroids affect hypothalamic GnRH secretion. A significant body of experimental evidence from our laboratory as well as others indicates that endogenous opioid peptides play a significant role in these phenomena and therefore in the control of gonadotropin secretion.

This presentation will be divided into two parts. The first will review the current evidence in the rhesus monkey which demonstrates changes in the arcuate oscillator caused by ovarian steroids during the menstrual cycle. The second part will study the role of endogenous opioid peptides in the central modulation of gonadotropin secretion by ovarian steroids.

II. Modulation of Pulsatile Gonadotropin Release by Ovarian Steroids at CNS Sites

This section will examine changes in the characteristics of pulsatile gonadotropin and GnRH release during the menstrual cycle and explore the role of ovarian steroids in these phenomena.

A. CHARACTERISTICS OF PULSATILE GONADOTROPIN RELEASE DURING THE MENSTRUAL CYCLE

In 1972, it was reported that frequency and amplitude of pulsatile gonadotropin release in the human were important determinants of the observed differences in "basal" gonadotropin secretion between eugonadal and agonadal subjects. Frequency and amplitude of the LH pulse were shown to vary according to the phase of the menstrual cycle (Yen *et al.,* 1972). In our laboratory, we have compared LH pulse characteristics exhibited by rhesus monkeys in the luteal phase and early follicular phase of the menstrual cycle. Because documentation of rapid changes in hormone concentrations requires frequent blood sampling, an adequate method for restraining the animal without interfering with the phenomenon under study is required. Long-term tranquilization or anesthesia is not practical and may modify the characteristics of pulsatile release (Wehrenberg and Ferin, 1981), while restraint of animals in primate chairs is not desirable and may interfere with normal menstrual cyclicity. A more satisfactory approach appeared to be that of Nakai *et al.* (1978), in which serial blood collection from monkeys involves an indwelling cardiac catheter exteriorized to a swivel joint at the top of the cage. This system allows for frequent sampling without unduly disturbing the animal. Unfortunately, we have found that this procedure interferes with gonadotropin and ovarian hormone secretion and results in a cessation of ovarian cycles. Presumably, as suggested by Pohl *et al.* (1982), the stress caused by this manipulation may derange the hypothalamic mechanisms which control pulsatile GnRH release. To avoid this problem, we have characterized changes in pulsatile LH activity in monkeys wearing a primate vest and a mobile tether assembly, a procedure which has allowed maintenance of normal cyclicity (Sopelak *et al.,* 1983). In order to further minimize disruptions to the menstrual cycle, the monkeys were tethered only on sampling days.

The results indicate that, in the monkey as well, there are profound changes in the characteristics of the LH pulse at different phases of the menstrual cycle. Figure 1 illustrates the changing patterns of pulsatile LH secretion in the same animal sampled twice during a luteal phase and once during the subsequent early follicular phase. The changes in LH pulse frequency and amplitude in 8 monkeys from luteal phase to early follicular phase are summarized in Fig. 2. During the early follicular phase, pulse frequency was high, with an average of 0.52 LH pulse/hour. The LH pulse frequency decreased sharply following ovulation and formation of a corpus luteum, with a mean of 0.18 pulses/hour in the luteal phase. LH pulse intervals were 1.9 and 5.6 hours for the follicular and luteal phases, respectively. A comparison of LH pulse pattern between the luteal and early follicular phase shows not only striking differences in the frequency but also in the amplitude of the LH pulse. Mean pulse amplitude during the luteal phase was nearly double that in the early follicular phase (Fig. 2). Similar differences between the luteal and early follicular phase were observed by Norman *et al.* (1983). In addition, these authors re-

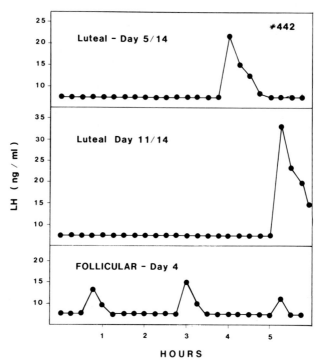

FIG. 1.   In order to document changes in LH pulse characteristics which occur during the menstrual cycle, serial blood samples were collected on the fifth and eleventh day of a 14-day luteal phase and on the fourth day of the subsequent follicular phase. The pattern of pulsatile LH secretion during the luteal phase was characterized by large, infrequent pulses. In contrast, LH pulse frequency in the same animal was markedly increased whereas pulse amplitude was significantly decreased in the follicular phase of the menstrual cycle.

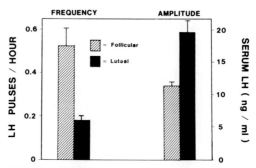

FIG. 2.   Mean LH pulse frequency and amplitude between the follicular and luteal phases are compared and represented by the vertical bars. The frequency with which LH pulses were observed during the follicular phase was approximately 1 pulse per 2 hours (26 pulses in 53 hours of sampling) as compared to approximately 1 pulse per 6 hours during the luteal phase (33 pulses in 191 hours of blood collection). Significant differences in pulse amplitude also were observed between the 2 phases of the menstrual cycle as mean pulse amplitude was significantly greater in the luteal phase (19.7 ± 1.7 ng/ml) compared to the follicular phase (11.7 ± 0.3 ng/ml).

ported that no changes in LH pulse frequency occurred across the entire follicular phase. However, the preovulatory LH surge was characterized by high-frequency, high-amplitude LH pulses (Marut *et al.*, 1981; Norman *et al.*, 1983).

There is little doubt that these changes in pulsatile LH secretory patterns during the menstrual cycle are influenced by ovarian steroids. In women, progesterone administration in the follicular phase can effect a slowing of LH pulse frequency and an augmentation in LH pulse amplitude (Soules *et al.*, 1984). In the ovariectomized monkey, the frequency of gonadotropin discharges was reduced by progesterone administration (Knobil, 1981), while their amplitude was decreased by estradiol (Knobil, 1974). An example of the estradiol effect on pulsatile LH release is illustrated in Fig. 3, which compares LH secretion in the ovariectomized monkey to that in the early follicular phase. In this typical example, there was a 10-fold reduction in the amplitude of the LH pulse, while its frequency appeared unchanged.

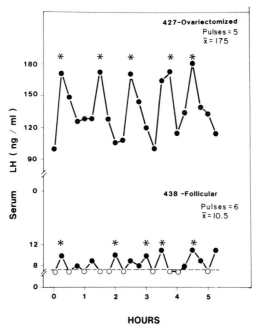

HOURS

FIG. 3.   The patterns of LH secretion in an ovariectomized and follicular phase monkey are compared. Pulses are designated by asterisks and the open circles represent samples of undetectable LH concentrations (<8 ng/ml). While LH pulse frequency is essentially the same in the 2 examples, both exhibiting circhoral release, pulse amplitude is clearly reduced in the follicular phase. These results suggest that estrogens affect LH pulse amplitude, but not LH pulse frequency.

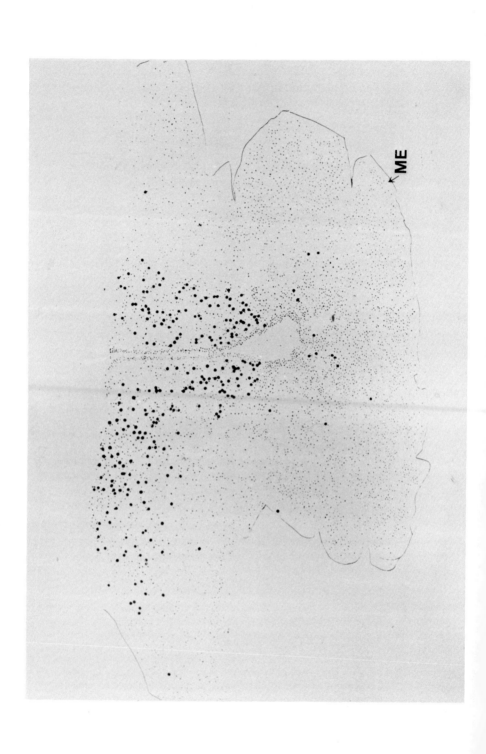

Although the physiological sequelae of these changes in LH pulse characteristics remain to be clearly defined, it is valid to assume that they do play a role in the control of cyclic events. The question that concerns us next is whether such changes in pulsatile patterns result from an action of ovarian hormones at a central site.

B. SITE OF FEEDBACK ACTION OF OVARIAN STEROIDS

Recent reviews (Knobil, 1980; Goodman and Knobil, 1981) on the subject of the site at which estradiol exerts its feedback on gonadotropin secretion (this discussion will confine itself to the *inhibitory* feedback action of estradiol) in the monkey have emphasized evidence favoring a hypophyseal site of action. The evidence is derived from experiments in monkeys bearing MBH lesions or in which the pituitary stalk has been sectioned and to which hourly GnRH pulses have been administered to elevate LH to prelesion control concentrations. Administration of estradiol to such animals in which the potential hypothalamic feedback site has been destroyed or in which the pituitary has been isolated from direct brain influences, produced a fall in LH and a decrease in pulsatile LH secretion (Plant *et al.*, 1978a; Richardson *et al.*, 1984), presumably by an action on the anterior pituitary. Similar estradiol effects on the pituitary gland were seen in intact monkeys in which systemic estradiol administration dampened the increase in serum LH observed after infusion of GnRH (Spies and Norman, 1975). The fact that this phenomenon has also been observed *in vitro* (Chappel *et al.*, 1981) indicates that this action represents a direct hypophyseal estradiol effect.

The evidence to be presented below in our view clearly indicates that ovarian steroids, in addition to their hypophyseal effects, influence menstrual cyclicity by acting at a hypothalamic site as well. The demonstration of estradiol receptors (Pfaff *et al.*, 1976; Garris *et al.*, 1981) in the MBH (with heavy labeling in the arcuate nucleus) provides the background for this conclusion (Fig. 4). A CNS site is also supported by the results of intracranial estradiol administration. In an experiment per-

---

FIG. 4.   Chart of estradiol-concentrating cells in the arcuate (infundibular) nucleus and median eminence of the female rhesus monkey. On both sides of this figure locations of all cell bodies visible with cresyl violet staining (including neurons, glia, and ependymal cells) in representative autoradiogram are shown by small dots. Cell bodies labeled with [³H]estradiol are shown by large dots. Heavily labeled cells are found in the arcuate nucleus, and their distribution spread dorsally and laterally toward the ventromedial nucleus of the hypothalamus. The median eminence (ME) itself had only a small number of labeled cells. Reprinted with permission from Pfaff *et al.* (1976). *J. Comp. Neurol.* **170,** 279.

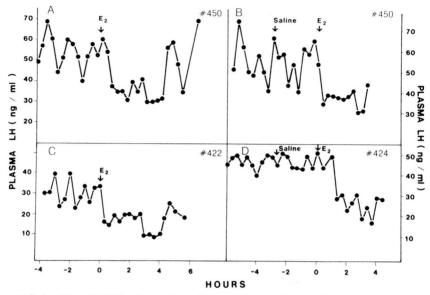

FIG. 5.   Estradiol (800 pg) was injected into several specific hypothalamic sites in ovariectomized monkeys and the LH response was monitored. Microinjection of estradiol into
the hypothalamus inhibited LH secretion similarly to systemic administration of 1000-fold
higher doses of estradiol. Injection of saline had no effect. The sites at which estradiol
produced marked inhibition of LH secretion included the premammillary nucleus (A), the
arcuate nucleus (B and D), and the ventromedial nucleus (C). These results are evidence that
the hypothalamus is a site where estradiol exerts an inhibitory effect on LH secretion.

formed in our laboratory, it was shown that single injections of small
amounts of estradiol at specific intrahypothalamic sites in monkeys bearing multiple intracranial cannulae depressed LH levels and mimicked the
effects of intravenous estrogen administration (Fig. 5). Most of the responsive sites were situated in the MBH, but extended to include the
mammillary complex and perifornical nucleus (Ferin *et al.,* 1974). Such
results provide evidence that estradiol can act at a hypothalamic site to
inhibit LH secretion. These results are most probably not due to diffusion
of the lipophilic steroid through the CNS and to an action at a pituitary
site for the following reasons. No radioactivity in the pituitary gland was
noted 40 minutes after the simultaneous injection of [³H]estradiol into 4
cannulae situated in the MBH. Also no LH response was seen when
multiple injections were made at sites closely adjacent to responsive ones
in the same animal indicating that responsive sites are located in very
circumscribed zones of the brain and that diffusion does not occur.
    Additional indirect evidence for CNS effects of estradiol includes the
observation that GnRH receptor concentrations are increased during the

negative feedback phase of estradiol (Adams *et al.*, 1981). Since there appears to be an inverse correlation between GnRH secretion and GnRH receptors, this experiment would also suggest that estradiol inhibits the release of GnRH.

Fewer experiments in the monkey have investigated the site of action of progesterone. However, as for estradiol, progesterone uptake occurs in the hypothalamus (Garris *et al.*, 1982). Progesterone was found to inhibit estrogen-induced gonadotropin surges in the monkey by acting at the level of the CNS (Wildt *et al.*, 1981a). In sheep, progesterone decreases the frequency of the LH pulse without reducing amplitude or the response to exogenous GnRH, suggesting that progesterone suppresses LH secretion by acting in the brain to decrease the frequency of GnRH pulses (Goodman, and Karsch, 1980). In Section III, evidence will be presented that, in the monkey, this effect of progesterone is exerted at a hypothalamic site and involves the endogenous opioid peptides.

In our view, the above experimental observations provide evidence that both steroids, estradiol and progesterone, act on CNS sites to modify the secretion of gonadotropins. More convincing evidence, however, would be provided by showing that these steroids influence hypothalamic output of GnRH. This evidence will be reviewed below.

C. HYPOTHALAMIC GnRH DISTRIBUTION

Pertinent to our discussion of GnRH secretory patterns and their modification by ovarian steroids is a presentation of the distribution of GnRH perikarya and neuronal networks in the monkey. Results in our laboratory (Silverman *et al.*, 1977, 1982) have indicated that GnRH neurons are present in a continuum along the midline beginning in the preoptic area and extending caudally to the premammillary region. Several distinct neuronal groups can be identified (Fig. 6). (1) Within the preoptic area, a large number of perikarya are observed in the medial and lateral preoptic nuclei, in the bed nucleus of the stria terminalis, in the organum vasculosum laminae terminalis (OVLT), and in the pericommisural region. A small but distinct group of GnRH neurons is seen within or near the supraoptic nucleus. (2) Several clusters of GnRH neurons are observed in the periventricular-arcuate region, their numbers decreasing from the anterior to the more posterior sections. (3) GnRH neurons are also seen in the premammillary nuclei.

Most of these cell groups appear to contribute to GnRH innervation of the median eminence. Axons can be traced from cell bodies to the median eminence, where they form swirls around the capillaries which collect into the long portal vessels. The portion of GnRH axons in the median

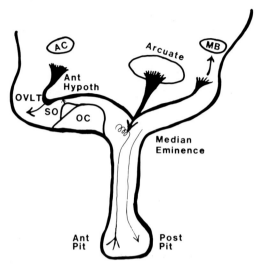

FIG. 6.   GnRH in the brain of monkeys is distributed in a continuum along the midline
from preoptic area to the premammillary region. Three major groups within this continuum
originate within the preoptic area, periventricular–arcuate region, and premammillary nuclei. Axons from all three regions can be traced to the median eminence. Anterior commis-
sure (AC); supraoptic nucleus (SO); optic chiasm (OC); mammillary body (MB).

eminence deriving from cell bodies in the anterior regions is unknown.
Several axons of these anterior cells also extend to several extrahypothalamic areas, including the OVLT and the amygdala. Although the number
of cells varies considerably, their general distribution in the hypothalamic
regions appears to be similar across primate groups (Barry and Carrette,
1975; Barry, 1976; Marshall and Goldsmith, 1980). In the rodent, however, GnRH cell bodies are usually not reported in the arcuate region
(Witkin *et al.*, 1982; Shivers *et al.*, 1983).

Present evidence in the female rhesus monkey indicates that the main
specific GnRH cell group involved in the control of gonadotropin secretion is that originating from the arcuate region since complete neural
disconnection of the MBH does not interfere with basal gonadotropin
secretion. Indeed, hourly pulsatile LH release continues to be observed in
deafferented ovariectomized monkeys (Krey *et al.*, 1975). Furthermore,
placement of discrete lesions within the arcuate region results in a precipitous fall in serum gonadotropins to undetectable levels (Plant *et al.*,
1978b), a fall similar to that observed in animals passively immunized to
GnRH (McCormack *et al.*, 1977) or following pituitary stalk section
(Vaughan *et al.*, 1980). In contrast, circhoral LH release is not affected by
large MBH lesions which spare the arcuate region.

The intermittant stimulation of LH release must be the consequence of a synchronous discharge of GnRH neurons, effected by a neural signal generator or oscillator. The circhoral oscillator may be presumed to reside in the GnRH network located within the arcuate area. In fact, recordings of multiunit electrical activity in the MBH of ovariectomized monkeys suggest the existence of electrophysiological correlates for this circhoral oscillator (Knobil, 1981). [The role of the anterior hypothalamic GnRH network in the control of the gonadotropin surge remains controversial (Knobil, 1980; Norman *et al.*, 1976; Cogen *et al.*, 1980) and is not the subject of the present discussion.]

An intriguing observation in our studies was that GnRH fibers were seen to descend along the pituitary stalk to enter the neurohypophysis, an observation which confirms the finding by RIA of large concentrations of the hormone in the posterior pituitary gland of the monkey (Neill *et al.*, 1977). It is possible, therefore, that under normal conditions, GnRH could reach the anterior pituitary, not only via the long portal vessels, but also via the short portal vessels which connect the posterior to the anterior part of the gland. This observation suggests the existence of additional control pathways for gonadotropin secretion.

D. MODULATION OF GnRH SECRETION

For several years, we have known that the decapeptide GnRH is the hypothalamic hormone responsible for LH and FSH secretion. Yet, measurement of the secretory patterns of this hormone has presented rather taxing technical problems, as GnRH is present in only minute amounts in the peripheral circulation. Direct measurements of GnRH in hypophyseal portal blood, the common secretory outlet for hypothalamic neuropeptides, are necessary. Several years ago, we developed a technique to monitor for prolonged periods of time GnRH concentrations in pituitary stalk portal blood in monkeys. Using this procedure, we were able to provide direct evidence that a hypothalamic input is the cause of the circhoral LH rhythm as we demonstrated that GnRH is released in a pulsatile fashion into hypophyseal portal blood (Carmel *et al.*, 1976). However, since this procedure necessitated complete pituitary stalk section, it was not possible to correlate GnRH and LH pulses. Recently, this technique was modified in the sheep by lesioning the hypophysial portal vessels only partially across the pituitary stalk and thereby maintaining partial pituitary function (Clarke and Cummins, 1982). This approach enabled these authors to demonstrate synchrony between GnRH and LH secretion in the ovariectomized sheep.

The technique of collecting hypophysial portal blood carries with it major problems, such as its surgical complexity, and more importantly, the fact that repeated sample collections from the same animal at various time intervals are difficult because of scar tissues surrounding the lesioned pituitary stalk. In search of an alternative method which would allow repeated comparisons of GnRH secretory patterns in the same animal, we have investigated other possible routes of GnRH secretion. In this process, we have been able to detect GnRH in cerebrospinal fluid (CSF) obtained from the third ventricle. This material was found to yield a dilution curve parallel to the RIA standard curve using the synthetic decapeptide. The detection of GnRH in the third ventricle of the rhesus monkey is in contrast to previous reports in rat and sheep (Cramer and Barraclough, 1976; Coppings et al., 1977) in which no GnRH was found. While this contrast may reflect in part improved sensitivity of the GnRH RIA used in our studies, we believe it also reflects upon the anatomical distribution of GnRH in the monkey, which, as reported above, differs in this species. Not only is there GnRH in the arcuate region, but also a substantial periventricular GnRH axonal plexus that courses very close to the ependymal wall of the third ventricle.

In the last 2 months, we have fitted monkeys with intraventricular cannulae and collected CSF from the third ventricle repeatedly. When coupled to peripheral blood sampling, this approach allows simultaneous measurements of GnRH and LH responses. Results obtained in ovariectomized monkeys indicated that GnRH secretory patterns are pulsatile, with synchrony between the LH and GnRH pulses (Van Vugt et al., 1983b). A comparison of pulsatile GnRH patterns in hypophyseal portal blood and CSF of the third ventricle in ovariectomized monkeys is shown on Fig. 7. A similar pulsatile pattern of GnRH release was seen in both CSF and portal blood. Several pulses were observed during a 5- to 6-hour sampling period. Pulses detected in portal blood were typically larger than in CSF.

A comparison of GnRH secretory patterns in ovariectomized monkeys before and after chronic estrogen treatment and in monkeys during the early follicular phase is shown in Fig. 8. As in the examples of Fig. 7, untreated ovariectomized monkeys had high levels of GnRH in CSF and portal blood, the result of several large amplitude GnRH pulses. In contrast, there was a decrease in the amplitude of the GnRH pulse in follicular phase monkeys and ovariectomized monkeys chronically treated with estradiol. The effect of estradiol on GnRH pulse amplitude is pronounced, although an effect on pulse frequency as well cannot be ruled out presently. These results indicate that estradiol inhibition of gonadotropin secretion is accomplished, at least in part, by an inhibitory effect of the steroid on GnRH secretion from the hypothalamus.

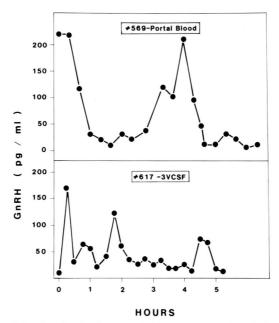

HOURS

FIG. 7.   Gonadotropin-releasing hormone (GnRH) concentrations in hypophysial portal blood and third ventricular cerebrospinal fluid (CSF) of 2 ovariectomized monkeys are compared. Large amplitude GnRH pulses occur in both portal blood and CSF with a frequency similar to LH under these conditions. The GnRH pulses are typically larger in portal blood than CSF (see Fig. 8).

The degree to which the site of estrogen action is hypothalamic or hypophyseal and whether it varies depending on endocrine conditions is not known. Recent indirect evidence has suggested that estradiol exerts its inhibitory feedback on pituitary *and* CNS, with initial effects on the pituitary and later effects on the hypothalamus (Weick *et al.*, 1982). Experiments on the acute effects of estradiol on GnRH release into stalk portal blood appear to support this observation (Carmel *et al.*, 1976).

In the monkey, distribution of ovarian steroid-concentrating neurons (Garris *et al.*, 1982; Pfaff *et al.*, 1976) and of GnRH neurons generally overlap, especially in the preoptic-anterior hypothalamic and MBH regions. In view of the role that these steroids exert on GnRH secretion, it would be logical to assume a direct cellular correlation. However, in recent studies in the rodent during which the immunocytochemical method for localizing GnRH was coupled with an autoradiographic method for detecting estrogen-concentrating neurons, doubly labeled cells were not seen (Shivers *et al.*, 1983). The results suggest that genomic regulating effects of estrogens which depend on nuclear retention, are not

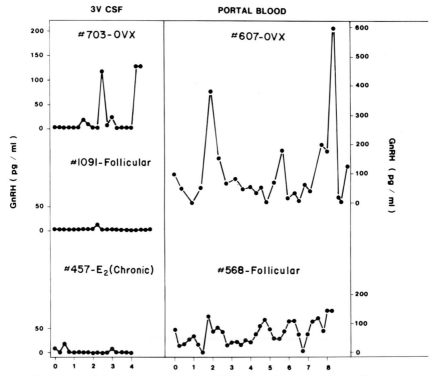

FIG. 8.   Potential effects of estrogen on GnRH secretion were examined by measuring the concentration of GnRH in CSF and portal blood of ovariectomized monkeys, with and without estrogen replacement, and follicular phase monkeys. Large amplitude GnRH pulses were present in CSF and portal blood of ovariectomized monkeys not exposed to estrogen. In comparison, the GnRH pulses were of a smaller amplitude in follicular phase and estrogen-treated monkeys. These data directly support the hypothesis that a hypothalamic site is an important component in the estrogen negative feedback.

exerted directly on most GnRH neurons, but must be mediated by other classes of neurons. Alternatively, ovarian steroids may exert their effects through nongenomic mechanisms, perhaps at the membrane level. Although this type of correlative study remains to be done in the monkey, the results suggest that the effects of ovarian steroids on GnRH and gonadotropin secretion may be relayed by neurons other than GnRH-containing ones.

III. Endocrine Role of Endogenous Opioid Peptides

Opiates are known to influence a variety of physiological processes. Among these are their effects on pain, respiration, blood pressure, behavior, temperature, and food intake (Koob and Bloom, 1983; Clement-Jones and Besser, 1983). Of importance to us are their endocrine effects. Opiates have been shown to modify the secretion of several hypophyseal hormones (Meites *et al.*, 1979; Morley, 1981; Grossman and Rees, 1983) among which are prolactin, ACTH, growth hormone, gonadotropins, vasopressin, and oxytocin.

In this section, we will consider the physiological role that endogenous opioid peptides play in the control of gonadotropin secretion in the female rhesus monkey and how these peptides affect the menstrual cycle. Several classes of endogenous opioid peptides (naturally occurring peptides with opiate-like biological properties) have been identified (Morley, 1983). Among these are the enkephalins (Hughes *et al.*, 1975), dynorphin (Goldstein *et al.*, 1981), and β-endorphin (Li and Chung, 1976), a 31 amino acid peptide. Since our work deals mainly with β-endorphin, most of our observations will be confined to this peptide.

There are presently several lines of evidence that support the conclusion that endogenous opioid peptides, and β-endorphin in particular, participate in the control of gonadotropin secretion in the monkey:

1. β-Endorphin neuronal cell bodies are preferentially concentrated in areas of the brain known to be involved in the control of gonadotropin secretion.

2. Opiate administration inhibits gonadotropin release.

3. Naloxone, a competitive inhibitor of opiates, increases the release of gonadotropins, suggesting tonic inhibition of gonadotropin release by endogenous opioids.

4. β-Endorphin secretion by the hypothalamus is modulated by ovarian steroid hormones, which also modulate gonadotropin secretion.

This evidence will now be reviewed.

A. ORIGIN AND LOCALIZATION OF β-ENDORPHIN

β-Endorphin derives from a multifunctional prohormone, known as proopiomelanocortin (POMC), which has been shown to be synthesized in the brain, pituitary, and placenta (Mains *et al.*, 1977; Roberts and Herbert, 1977; Krieger *et al.*, 1980). Upon cleavage, this 31K glycoprotein yields a 16,000 molecular weight fragment of unknown function, ACTH (39 amino acid sequence) and β-lipotropin (β-LPH) (91 amino acids sequence). β-LPH, which itself has no opiate-like activity, contains in its 61–91 carboxy terminal end, the sequence of β-endorphin. β-Endorphin 1–31 is the active compound, but several other forms devoid of opioid activity have also been identified, such as β-endorphin 1–27 and acetylated β-endorphin 1–31 (Smyth *et al.*, 1979; Zakarian and Smyth, 1982). It should be pointed out that the processing of the 31K precursor differs in various tissues to produce peptides with various biological activities. For example, in the anterior pituitary, the precursor yields predominantly ACTH and β-LPH, whereas in the intermediate pituitary, further processing yields mainly β-MSH and corticotropin-like intermediate lobe peptide (CLIP) (from ACTH), and acetylated β-endorphin (Krieger *et al.*, 1980) (Fig. 9). In the hypothalamus, the major peptides appear to be nonacetylated β-endorphin rather than β-LPH, and deacetyl α-MSH and CLIP rather than ACTH (Parker *et al.*, 1981; Donohue and Dorsa, 1982; Liotta and Krieger, 1983).

In the monkey, immunocytochemical studies have shown that CNS fibers containing POMC-derived peptides originate from neurons clustered in the arcuate region of the medial-basal hypothalamus (MBH) (Abrams *et al.*, 1980) (Fig. 9). Cell bodies are not observed at other CNS sites suggesting that, as in other species, this may be the principal site of synthesis within the brain (Bloom *et al.*, 1978; Krieger *et al.*, 1980; Hisano *et al.*, 1982). This differs from the enkephalin network, where cell bodies are scattered over several brain regions (Watson *et al.*, 1977). Direct

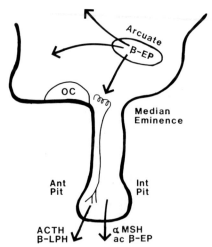

FIG. 9. Proopiomelanocortin (POMC) distribution and processing. POMC cell bodies are located in the arcuate nucleus. Axons project to different hypothalamic nuclei, as well as to extrahypothalamic areas. Large concentrations of POMC-derived peptides are found in the anterior and intermediate lobes of the pituitary. However, the processing of POMC is very different in the pituitary compared to CNS. Nonacetylated β-endorphin is the major derivative of POMC processing in the brain, whereas ACTH and β-LPH predominate in the anterior pituitary and α-MSH and acetylated endorphin in the intermediate lobe.

evidence in the rat for POMC biosynthesis in the MBH is provided by the report that arcuate neurons contain both POMC mRNA and POMC peptides (Gee *et al.*, 1983). The fiber system derived from these cell bodies is then distributed to multiple areas of the hypothalamus, as well as the preoptic area, thalamus, stria terminalis, septum, amygdala, and brainstem (Krieger *et al.*, 1980).

The location of β-endorphin within areas of the hypothalamus which in the monkey are rich in GnRH provides anatomical evidence for interactions between the two peptides. These interactions may include neuron to neuron communications within the arcuate region, an area in which cell bodies for both peptides are located, or axo-axonal influences within the median eminence which contains terminals for both GnRH and β-endorphin axons.

Our studies have also demonstrated that POMC neurons are neurosecretory. Immunocytochemical observations have shown that some of the fibers originating from the arcuate region are seen to terminate in the median eminence in contact with the portal capillaries from which the long portal vessels originate. Secretion into the hypophyseal portal circulation was demonstrated by our report of β-endorphin concentrations in samples of portal blood that are 10–100 times higher than simultaneous peripheral venous concentrations (Fig. 10) (Wardlaw *et al.*, 1980a). A hypothalamic rather than a hypophyseal origin for β-endorphin in portal blood is indicated by the fact that the hypothalamus was completely sepa-

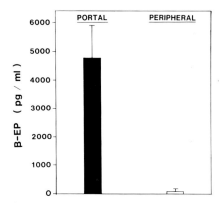

FIG. 10. β-Endorphin (β-EP) concentrations in hypophysial portal blood are compared to levels in peripheral blood. Samples were collected from 9 intact pigtailed monkeys (*Macaca nemestrina*) at random stages of the menstrual cycle. The large differences in concentrations of portal versus peripheral blood, in view of the fact that the stalk is completely severed, indicate that the source of β-EP in portal blood is hypothalamic rather than hypophysial.

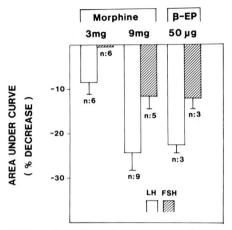

FIG. 11. Opioid inhibition of gonadotropin secretion was determined in ovariectomized monkeys injected intravenously with 3 or 9 mg morphine or intraventricularly with 50 μg β-endorphin (β-EP). Degree of inhibition was assessed by calculating the area under the LH curve 3 hours prior to and 4 hours after opioid injection. Both LH and FSH were significantly reduced by the higher dose of morphine and β-EP. Individual examples are shown in Fig. 12.

rated from the pituitary by sectioning the pituitary stalk prior to collecting the portal blood samples and that similar results were obtained in animals in which the pituitary gland had been removed immediately before portal blood collection.

B. EFFECTS OF OPIATES ON GONADOTROPIN SECRETION

In the monkey, we have shown that a single intravenous injection of morphine or an intraventricular injection of β-endorphin resulted in a decrease in circulating LH and FSH concentrations (Ferin *et al.*, 1982, 1983). The results are summarized in Fig. 11. There was a significant decrease in the surface area under the gonadotropin curve during the 4-hour period following morphine (9 mg) or β-endorphin (50 μg) injection as compared to the baseline control. Individual examples are illustrated in Fig. 12. These suggest that the reduction in LH secretion may be the result of a decreased frequency of the LH pulse. In most monkeys, the inhibitory effect of the opioid terminated abruptly with a resumption of a large LH pulse. An inhibitory effect of opiates on FSH was observed as well, although it was less pronounced. Similar results have been observed in the human (Reid *et al.*, 1981).

The above results, which are in accord with several reports in nonprimate species (Van Vugt *et al.*, 1978; Cicero *et al.*, 1979), are quite suggestive of a modulatory role for β-endorphin on basal gonadotropin secre-

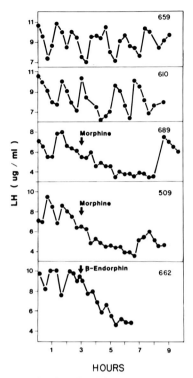

FIG. 12.   Pulsatile LH secretion in saline injected ovariectomized controls is illustrated in the top two panels. Inhibition of pulsatile LH secretion by opiates, either 9 mg morphine iv or 50 μg β-endorphin intraventricularly is shown in the lower three panels. (Differences in absolute LH levels in this figure versus previous figures are the result of a different radioimmunoassay.)

tion. Further experiments were needed however to determine whether endogenous opioids are themselves involved in controlling gonadotropin secretion.

C. EFFECTS OF ENDOGENOUS OPIOID PEPTIDE ANTAGONISM ON GONADOTROPIN SECRETION

In order to test the hypothesis that endogenous opioids are involved in the control of gonadotropin secretion, we have injected an opiate antagonist, naloxone, to block endogenous opioid activity. In the first experiment, we have examined the effects of single injections of naloxone daily throughout an entire menstrual cycle on LH secretion. The results clearly demonstrate that endogenous opioid peptides modify gonadotropin secretion, but that they do so only under specific endocrine conditions (Van

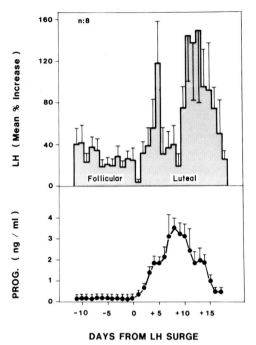

DAYS FROM LH SURGE

FIG. 13.   Monkeys with normal menstrual cycles ($n = 8$) were challenged with a single daily injection of naloxone for one complete menstrual cycle. Blood samples were collected at -1, $+20$, $+40$, and $+60$ minutes relative to the naloxone injection (2 mg). Menstrual cycles have been normalized around the midcycle gonadotropin surge so that a mean daily LH response could be calculated (mean percentage increase over preinjection concentration). Acute stimulation of LH release by naloxone was limited to the luteal phase. The small responses observed during the follicular phase were not different from responses observed in a control group, and probably reflect small frequency LH pulses associated with the follicular phase.

Vugt *et al.*, 1983a). Figure 13 illustrates the mean percentage LH increase on each day of the cycle (as normalized around the midcycle gonadotropin surge) in all 8 monkeys. LH responses to naloxone were significant only during the luteal phase. During this phase, LH was increased in approximately 60% of the naloxone trials. In contrast, naloxone was unable to stimulate LH secretion during the follicular phase. Individual LH responses to naloxone in one monkey throughout a menstrual cycle are shown in Fig. 14.

Our data in the monkey agree with observations made in the human, showing a stimulation of gonadotropin secretion by naloxone during the luteal phase, but not the early follicular phase of the menstrual cycle (Quigley and Yen, 1980). However, in this and in another study (Blankstein *et al.*, 1981), naloxone also increased LH secretion during the late

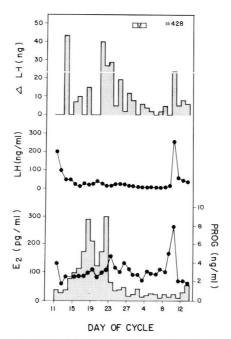

FIG. 14.   Acute effects of daily injections of naloxone (2 mg) on LH release throughout a menstrual cycle. Top bars indicate LH increments observed within 20–40 minutes following naloxone injection, while the middle and lower panels illustrate daily LH, estradiol (E_2), and progesterone (Prog) concentrations. Large LH increments resulted from naloxone injections during the luteal phase, although significant responses were not observed each day. In contrast, no significant LH responses to naloxone administration during the follicular phase were observed.

follicular phase, at a time of maximal estrogen secretion. This increase however was quite delayed when compared to the immediate one seen during the luteal phase and because of shorter sampling times could not have been detected in our own experiments.

These results provide clear evidence that, in the primate, there is an interaction between endogenous opioid peptides and LH release. This regulatory mechanism, however, is a complex one which involves gonadal hormones as well. In the monkey, LH secretion appears to be most suppressed by endogenous opioids during the luteal phase, at a time of elevated progesterone secretion.

D. MODULATION OF β-ENDORPHIN BY OVARIAN STEROIDS

Differential LH responses to naloxone administration at various times of the menstrual cycle suggested to us that endogenous opioid secretion may fluctuate with the endocrine gonadal steroid milieu. Therefore, experiments were designed to determine whether gonadal steroids modulate β-endorphin secretion. In an initial step, we were unable to demonstrate changes in peripheral venous β-endorphin concentrations following several ovarian hormone modifications. It is important, at this point, to mention that peripheral levels of β-endorphin mainly reflect the secretion of β-endorphin from the pituitary gland but not from the hypothalamus where β-endorphin synthesis and regulation are different from the pituitary. Importantly, changes in the hypothalamic β-endorphin system, perhaps sufficient to influence gonadotropin secretion *in situ*, may not be reflected by significant changes in the peripheral levels of β-endorphin.

We next attempted to monitor changes in hypothalamic β-endorphin activity by measuring concentrations of β-endorphin in hypophyseal portal blood. We believe that portal blood levels of β-endorphin reflect hypothalamic activity for several reasons : (1) axons derived from β-endorphin cell bodies in the arcuate region terminate near portal vessels; (2) high concentrations of portal blood β-endorphin are not influenced by hypophysectomy; and (3) when β-endorphin immunoactivity in monkey portal blood is characterized by gel filtration and ion-exchange chromatography, it resembles the pattern seen in monkey hypothalamic extracts, i.e., primarily β-endorphin 1–31 rather than β-LPH or the biologically less active β-endorphin derivatives (Fig. 15) (Wardlaw *et al.*, 1982a).

Changes in hypophyseal portal blood concentrations of β-endorphin following ovarian sex steroid modification were striking. First, following ovariectomy, portal blood concentrations of β-endorphin became undetectable by our RIA (Wehrenberg *et al.*, 1982) (Fig. 16). Ovarian steroid replacement in ovariectomized monkeys restored portal blood β-endorphin immunoactivity indicating that ovarian sex steroids are necessary for the release of hypothalamic β-endorphin (Wardlaw *et al.*, 1982a). Although estradiol therapy moderately increased β-endorphin concentrations in 2 of 4 animals, a combination of both estradiol and progesterone produced a large increase in β-endorphin in all 4 animals (Fig. 16). When changes in β-endorphin concentrations in portal blood throughout the menstrual cycle were studied, β-endorphin release was undetectable at menstruation, i.e., at a time when ovarian steroid concentrations are lowest. In contrast, as ovarian steroid secretion increased during the late follicular phase and luteal phase, increased amounts of β-endorphin were released into the portal circulation (Fig. 17) (Wehrenberg *et al.*, 1982). In both experiments, largest amounts of β-endorphin appear to be secreted in the presence of progesterone. However, when progesterone alone was given to ovariectomized monkeys, there was no increase in β-endorphin secretion indicating that, as in several other systems, progesterone action

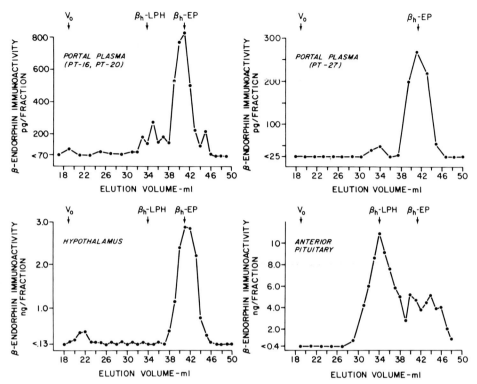

FIG. 15.   Sephadex G-50 chromatography of β-EP immunoactivity in portal plasma extracts of ovariectomized monkeys receiving estradiol and progesterone replacement. The elution patterns on Sephadex G-50 of the β-EP immunoactivity in monkey hypothalamic and anterior pituitary extracts are shown for comparison. β-LPH, human β-lipotropin; β-EP, human β-EP; V, void volume. Reprinted with permission from Wardlaw *et al.* (1982a). *J. Clin. Endocrinol. Metab.* **55,** 877.

usually is the consequence of a synergistic effect with estrogen (Maclusky *et al.*, 1980). These results clearly demonstrate that hypothalamic β-endorphin activity is modulated by ovarian sex steroids. Sex steroids have also been shown to affect hypothalamic β-endorphin immunoactivity in the rodent (Barden *et al.*, 1981; Wardlaw *et al.*, 1982b).

E. A SPECIFIC ROLE FOR β-ENDORPHIN DURING THE MENSTRUAL CYCLE

In our view, the results outlined in the previous paragraphs provide supportive evidence that endogenous opioid peptides control gonadotropin release at specific times of the menstrual cycle. Indeed, administration

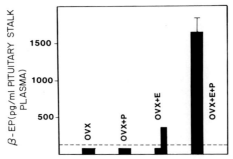

FIG. 16. Ovarian steroid modulation of β-endorphin (β-EP) secretion. Ovariectomized monkeys were replaced with physiological levels of either progesterone (P), estradiol (E), or both. Hypophyseal portal blood was collected in order to characterize steroid modulation of hypothalamic β-EP activity. Replacement of both estradiol and progesterone resulted in the greatest increase in portal blood β-EP concentration. Estrogen alone moderately increased levels in 2 of 4 animals, whereas progesterone alone had no effect. Similar effects of estrogen and progesterone were observed in cycling monkeys (see Fig. 17).

of opiates decreases LH release and antagonism of endogenous opioid peptides results in an increase in gonadotropin secretion. Furthermore, naloxone's effectiveness in modifying LH release parallels portal blood β-endorphin immunoactivity, which is maximally increased during the progesterone phase of the cycle. Naloxone is ineffective in stimulating LH

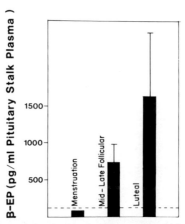

FIG. 17. Changes in hypothalamic β-endorphin activity during the menstrual cycle. β-Endorphin concentrations in portal blood were determined at 3 different stages of the menstrual cycle. This study confirms the modulatory effects of ovarian steroids on β-endorphin (Fig. 16) and reveals a cyclic pattern of β-endorphin activity that is associated with the menstrual cycle.

when administered at times when portal blood β-endorphin immunoactivity is undetectable, such as during the early follicular phase.

Our present hypothesis is that endogenous opioid peptides participate in the decrease in LH pulse frequency which has been observed during the luteal phase. To test this hypothesis, we have examined the effects of naloxone infusions on LH pulse frequency during the luteal phase. In a first experiment, LH release during a 5-hour naloxone infusion (2 mg/hour) in 11 monkeys was compared to that seen during the preceeding 5-hour control period using the vest and tethering system described in the first section to collect frequent blood samples. LH pulse frequency was clearly increased during the naloxone infusion period as compared to the preceding control period. Eight LH pulses were observed during a control period totalling 49 hours or 1 pulse per 6.1 hours. In contrast 24 pulses were observed during the naloxone infusion which consisted of 46 hours or 1 pulse/1.9 hours. LH pulse amplitude was unchanged by naloxone administration (23.5 and 25.3 ng/ml for controls and naloxone-treated, respectively). The results of 3 animals, representative of the 11 tested, are shown in Fig. 18.

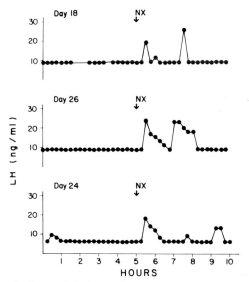

FIG. 18.   Effect of naloxone infusion on LH secretion during the luteal phase. An infusion of naloxone (2 mg/hour) was begun following a 4- to 5-hour control period in rhesus monkeys that were in the luteal phase. The frequency with which LH pulses occurred during the 5-hour infusion period was greater than during the control period. These results suggest that endogenous opiates inhibit pulsatile LH secretion during the luteal phase.

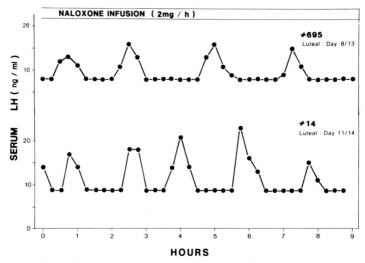

FIG. 19. Effect of a continuous naloxone infusion on LH pulse frequency during the
luteal phase. The naloxone infusion period was lengthened from previous studies in order to
determine if an increase in LH pulse frequency could be sustained by antagonism of endogenous opioid activity. Since LH pulses of fairly constant magnitude occurred at regular
intervals throughout the infusion period, we conclude that antagonism of endogenous
opioids does stimulate LH pulse frequency.

The effect of a more prolonged naloxone infusion on pulsatile LH secretion was examined in subsequent experiments in an attempt to differentiate between simply an acute LH response to naloxone and a true
increase in LH pulse frequency resulting from removal of tonic opioid
inhibition. Shown in Fig. 19 are two examples of the LH secretory pattern
during a 9-hour naloxone infusion performed in the luteal phase. Regular
pulses of LH of fairly constant amplitude were evident in both animals.
These experiments lead us to conclude that naloxone does not simply
increase LH secretion acutely, but rather has a stimulatory effect on LH
pulse frequency. Similar results were reported in women during the luteal
phase (Ropert *et al.*, 1981) as well as in normal men (Ellingboe *et al.*,
1982).

The results of these experiments in which endogenous opioid activity
was antagonized provide evidence that an increase in opioid inhibition of
the GnRH-LH system participates in the decrease in LH pulse frequency
observed during the luteal phase. A corollary to our demonstration, then,
is that the rapid increase in LH pulse frequency (from 1 pulse/6 hours to 1
pulse/1–2 hours) which is seen at menstruation is related to the abrupt
decrease in hypothalamic opioid activity at the end of the luteal phase.
This hypothesis is summarized in Fig. 20, as experimental results in an

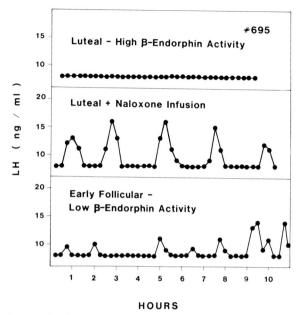

FIG. 20. The postulated role of β-endorphin in cyclic changes in pulsatile LH secretion is summarized. The changes in LH pulse frequency which occur during the menstrual cycle, along with the level of hypothalamic β-endorphin activity, are contrasted in the top and bottom panels. That high β-endorphin activity is responsible for the low LH pulse frequency during the luteal phase is indicated by the dramatic increase in LH pulse frequency by naloxone.

individual animal are illustrated. Precise day to day relationships between hypothalamic β-endorphin activity and gonadotropin pulse frequency remain to be defined.

F. SITE AND MECHANISM OF ACTION OF β-ENDORPHIN IN THE MONKEY

There are two levels at which endogenous opioids may potentially influence gonadotropin secretion. In the first, β-endorphin may compete with GnRH action at the anterior pituitary gland. In the second, β-endorphin may modulate GnRH release from the hypothalamus.

The presence of high concentrations of biologically active β-endorphin in the hypophyseal portal circulation suggests that it may exert direct effects at the anterior pituitary level. However, we were unable to demonstrate such direct hypophyseal effects in the monkey. For instance, in pituitary stalk-sectioned monkeys in which the hypophysis has been iso-

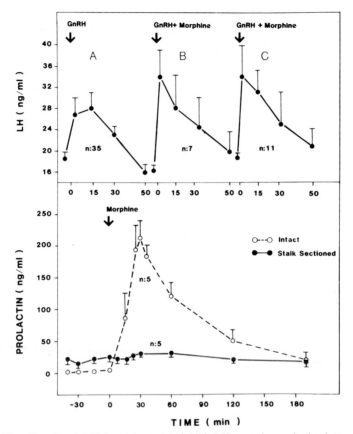

FIG. 21.   The site at which opiates act to inhibit LH secretion and stimulate prolactin secretion was tested in stalk-sectioned female monkeys. Morphine failed to alter the GnRH-induced LH pulse when administered at a dose of 9 (B) or 12 mg (C) iv. Administration of 9 mg morphine to stalk-sectioned monkeys failed to elicit the prolactin response seen in intact animals. These experiments indicate that the action of opiates on LH and prolactin is not at the anterior pituitary.

lated from direct hypothalamic influences, morphine pretreatment did not affect the LH response to GnRH stimuli (Fig. 21) (Ferin *et al.*, 1982). In these animals as well, β-endorphin failed to increase prolactin, although in intact animals it induced a rapid rise in prolactin to peak concentrations of 200–300% of baseline within 20 minutes of injection (Fig. 21) (Wardlaw *et al.*, 1980b). β-Endorphin was also unable to antagonize the inhibitory effect on prolactin secretion which L-dopa exerts at the hypophyseal level. These results support a suprahypophyseal rather than a hypophyseal site of action of β-endorphin. This conclusion is consistent with several *in vitro* studies in the rodent, which failed to show a direct opiate effect either on gonadotropes (Cicero *et al.*, 1979) or lactotropes (Grandison *et al.*, 1980; Rivier *et al.*, 1977). The unlikeliness of a hypophyseal site of action is further underlined by the absence of anterior pituitary opioid receptors (Simantov and Snyder, 1977; Wamsley *et al.*, 1982).

A hypothalamic site of action for β-endorphin must then be considered. There is good evidence in the rodent that β-endorphin modifies prolactin release by modulating the secretion of dopamine into hypophyseal portal blood. Iontophoresis into the arcuate nucleus or ventricular administration of morphine significantly reduced dopamine secretion (Haskins *et al.*, 1981; Reymond *et al.*, 1983). *In vitro*, β-endorphin reduced the efflux of dopamine from superfused MBH (Wilkes and Yen, 1980). In the monkey, it was shown that prior administration of L-dopa (the immediate precursor of dopamine) suppressed the prolactin response to morphine (Wehrenberg *et al.*, 1981), suggesting that the prolactin increase in response to β-endorphin involves a reduction in dopaminergic output.

There is presently no direct *in vivo* evidence in the monkey that the secretion of GnRH, the neuropeptide responsible for gonadotropin release, is modified by β-endorphin in such a way as to explain its effect on LH and FSH secretion. However, there is sufficient indirect evidence for such a conclusion. The *in vitro* GnRH efflux from superfused human (Rasmussen *et al.*, 1983) or rat (Wilkes and Yen, 1980) medial basal hypothalami was increased following naloxone perfusion. Conversely *in vivo* chronic morphine treatment prevents the decline of GnRH from hypothalami of castrated male and female rats (Cicero *et al.*, 1980; Van Vugt *et al.*, 1982), and the naloxone-induced release of LH in the rat was blocked by the administration of a GnRH antagonist (Blank and Roberts, 1982). On the basis of these observations, it can be concluded that endogenous opioid peptides act to suppress the secretion of GnRH from arcuate neurons into the hypophyseal portal circulation, thereby inhibiting hypophyseal secretion of gonadotropins.

The precise CNS site in the monkey at which β-endorphin might affect GnRH secretion remains to be examined. Two obvious possibilities come to mind (Fig. 22). In the first, the modification in GnRH release is the result of interactions within the confines of the arcuate nucleus between GnRH and β-endorphin cell bodies. The arcuate nucleus contains not only cell bodies for GnRH and β-endorphin but also a dense arborization of fibers. Some of the opioid peptide-containing fibers have been shown, by immunocytochemistry, to form axosomatic contact with other cells of the arcuate nucleus, presumably containing other peptides or neurotransmitters (Kiss and Williams, 1983). This observation supports the concept of local neuronal circuits, which may not only integrate the function of

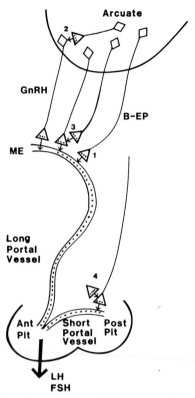

FIG. 22. Site of β-endorphin regulation of LH secretion. Four possible mechanisms by which β-endorphin could inhibit gonadotropin secretion are depicted. (1) β-Endorphin, which is released into the hypophyseal portal vessels and is transported to the pituitary, could act directly on the gonadotrope. Current experimental evidence does not support this mechanism. The three other possibilities depicted all involve an interaction with GnRH. This interaction may occur at the cell bodies in the arcuate nucleus (2), at the nerve terminal in the median eminence (3), or at the posterior pituitary gland (4).

neurons of the same type but also influence the activity of different types of neurons within the same nucleus (Rakic, 1975). In the second possibility, opioid regulation of GnRH is executed at the level of the median eminence. Intense innervation by β-endorphin and GnRH fibers, most of which originate from cell bodies in the arcuate area, can be seen in this region. This mechanism would allow for β-endorphin control at the nerve terminal at the point of GnRH release into the hypophyseal portal circulation and would also offer an explanation for our observation of high concentrations of β-endorphin in hypophyseal portal blood. This "gating" mechanism in the median eminence is similar to one that has been proposed in the posterior pituitary where there is now good evidence that opiates can control the release of magnocellular peptides from their nerve terminals (Bicknell and Leng, 1982; Clarke *et al.*, 1979). Similar presynaptic inhibition by opioids has been found in other parts of the central nervous system (Carstens *et al.*, 1978), indicating that endogenous opioid peptides may tonically inhibit the release of several neuropeptides or transmitters.

Another potential site of action of opioids on GnRH which remains to be investigated in the monkey is the posterior pituitary gland. Indeed, this pituitary lobe is rich in opioid receptors (Wamsley *et al.*, 1982), and the presence of GnRH-containing fibers in the area makes an interaction at that level possible.

Whether inhibition of GnRH release by β-endorphin is the result of a direct synapse or whether neurotransmitters (or other neuroactive substances) are intermediary remains to be examined in the monkey. The most obvious neurotransmitter candidates are norepinephrine, serotonin, and dopamine which, at least in the rodent, have been implicated in gonadotropin secretion. In the rat, normal noradrenergic activity is required in order for naloxone to stimulate LH release, since this action can be prevented by prior administration of norepinephrine synthesis inhibitors or antagonists (Kalra, 1981; Van Vugt *et al.*, 1981). β-Endorphin has been shown to decrease dopamine turnover in the median eminence (Deyo *et al.*, 1979; Van Vugt *et al.*, 1979), and to increase reuptake of dopamine into dopamine nerve endings (George and Van Loon, 1982). However, little is known about the effects of neurotransmitters on LH secretion in the monkey and further speculation on this subject is outside the scope of this article.

G. β-ENDORPHIN AND MENSTRUAL CYCLICITY

Our demonstration in the primate that endogenous opioid peptides are important determinants of gonadotropin secretion during the menstrual cycle, and that they exert their effect by modulating the neurosecretory activity of the arcuate GnRH oscillator leads us to believe that these peptides are involved in the physiological process of cyclicity. Abnormal opioid activity may in turn evoke pathological processes.

Specifically, we postulate that the alternation of high and low β-endorphin hypothalamic activity, which we have shown to occur during the menstrual cycle, is an important causal phenomenon in cyclicity. In this view, the onset of a new follicular phase may in part be the result of a sequence of events involving, first tonic opioid inhibition of GnRH and LH pulse frequency during the luteal phase, followed by disinhibition at

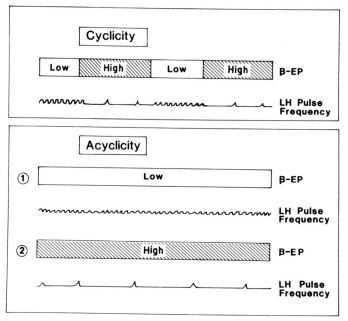

FIG. 23. Hypothetical model of how normal ovulatory cyclicity depends on β-endorphin input. The cyclic variations in hypothalamic β-endorphin activity and the resultant cyclic changes in LH pulse frequency are depicted in the top panel. We propose that alternating β-endorphin activity is an essential feature of cyclicity and that amenorrhea may arise when this feature of β-endorphin is disturbed. Two possibilities are depicted in the lower panel.

the end of the luteal phase with resultant increases in GnRH and LH frequency (Fig. 23).

In order to test this hypothesis, we have, in an on-going experiment, replaced the low-frequency GnRH oscillator of the luteal phase with a rapid (circhoral) GnRH oscillator, and are studying the effects of this pulse frequency on menstrual cyclicity. Circhoral administration of 1.5 or 3.0 μg GnRH pulses (6 minutes in duration) was begun in normally cycling monkeys during the early part of the luteal phase and continued until the onset of menstruation (approximately 10 days). Increasing the GnRH pulse frequency had profound effects on the menstrual cycle (Fig. 24). Significant delays in the next ovulation occurred in 3 of the 4 animals tested. One of these monkeys resumed normal ovulation on day 135 following the end of the treatment. The other 2 resumed ovulatory cycles on day 175 and 190, respectively. The fourth animal continued to have normal ovulatory cycles but had received only 5 days of the GnRH treatment. This striking but tentative result allows us to conclude that opioid-

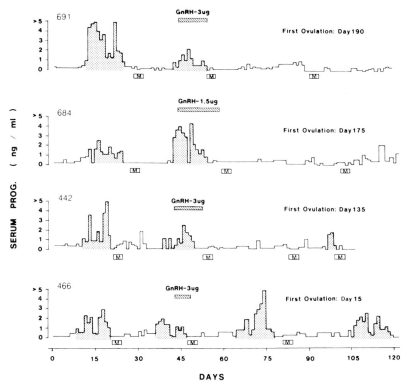

FIG. 24. The importance of a period of reduced GnRH pulse frequency on ovulatory cyclicity was tested in 4 normal cycling rhesus monkeys. After 1 control cycle, hourly GnRH pulses (1.5 or 3.0 μg in 6 minutes) were begun at the start and continued to the end of the luteal phase. Daily blood samples for progesterone measurement were collected to monitor potential effects on subsequent cycles. Circhoral GnRH pulses interrupted ovulatory cyclicity. The top 3 monkeys did not ovulate until 135–190 days posttreatment. A fourth animal did continue to exhibit normal ovulatory cycles following GnRH administration. However, in this animal, GnRH was not begun until the latter half of the luteal phase. These results support the hypothesis that a slowing down of the GnRH oscillator during the luteal phase is a prerequisite for cyclicity.

induced modifications in the frequency of the arcuate oscillator may represent an essential feature of the normal menstrual cycle. In view of a recent experiment by Wildt *et al.* (1981b), it is possible that a reduction in the frequency of the GnRH oscillator during the luteal phase is necessary for normal gonadotropin secretion at the end of the cycle and for cyclicity. These authors have shown that LH and FSH concentrations are profoundly influenced by changes in the frequency of pulsatile GnRH administration in lesioned ovariectomized monkeys lacking endogenous GnRH. For instance, a decrease in the frequency of the administered GnRH pulse from 1/hour to 1/3 hours led to a decline in plasma LH levels, but to an increase in FSH. This surprising divergent effect in the two hormones results within a few days in a reversal of their secretory ratios that now favors FSH. The increase in the FSH : LH ratio which occurs at the beginning of the follicular phase and which initiates the recruitment of the new crop of follicles may represent a similar phenomenon, and may have been prevented in our experiment, hence the ensuing months of acyclicity.

Our present hypothesis on the role of endogenous opioids in menstrual cyclicity raises the possibility that, in certain cases, amenorrhea may reflect abnormal hypothalamic β-endorphin activity. In such cases, sequential periods of high and low opioid activity may be lacking and if replaced by a continuously low or a sustained high opioid activity, and, hence, high or low GnRH oscillator frequency, proper gonadotropin ratios for normal ovarian morphology may not be achieved. That a sustained decrease in GnRH pulse frequency may be deleterious to cyclicity is suggested by an experiment in which nonovariectomized lesioned monkeys were subjected to a continuous low-frequency GnRH pulse regimen (Pohl *et al.*, 1983). In these animals, the reduction in GnRH pulse frequency was associated with a progressive decline in follicular development and anovulation. Therefore, alterations in the frequency of endogenous GnRH release may play a major role in the control of ovarian function.

Our hypothesis for a role of opioids in the etiology of amenorrhea finds support in clinical studies in which naloxone was administered to amenorrheic patients. For example, a clear increment in LH levels, in the form of an amplified pulsatile pattern of release, was observed by various authors (Grossman *et al.*, 1982; Blankstein *et al.*, 1981; Quigley *et al.*, 1980; Lightman *et al.*, 1981) in several (but not all) hyperprolactinemic patients, suggesting that acyclicity can be due, at least in part, to an increased inhibitory effect of endogenous opioids on GnRH and gonadotropin secretion. Similar effects of naloxone on LH release were seen in normoprolactinemic amenorrheic patients as well (Blankstein *et al.*, 1981) suggesting that the increase in tonic inhibition by opiates may play a role in more than one type of amenorrhea. Amenorrhea may therefore in certain cases reflect a tonic inhibitory condition, in which LH and FSH secretion is decreased because of active β-endorphin inhibition, rather than represent a deficiency syndrome in which gonadotropin secretion is low due to a lack of factors necessary for normal secretion.

The possible existence of increased opioid inhibitory tonus in amenorrheic patients suggests that opioid antagonists may be useful as a new therapeutic approach. Such treatment is under investigation in several laboratories. A potential problem with this long-term therapy relates to the anorectic properties that opiate antagonists have (Sanger *et al.*, 1983; Atkinson, 1982) and the well-known inhibitory influence that weight loss exerts on menstrual cyclicity (Warren *et al.*, 1975). The findings of increased food intake following opioid administration and decreased food intake following naloxone injection are consistent with a role of endogenous opioids in the regulation of appetite (McKay *et al.*, 1982; Morley and Levine, 1982). An interesting correlation between food intake and hypothalamic opioid activity was also found in cycling monkeys, in which we observed that the amount of food consumed was significantly greater during the luteal phase, at the time of greatest hypothalamic β-endorphin activity, than at other stages of the menstrual cycle (Rosenblatt *et al.*, 1980).

In view of these observations on the stimulatory effects of endogenous opioids on food intake, it is unlikely that, as had been postulated by some authors, excess endogenous opioid activity is the primary causative factor in the decline in gonadotropin secretion observed in anorectic patients. Indeed, attempts at increasing gonadotropin secretion in these patients with naloxone were unsuccessful (Grossman *et al.*, 1982). In apparent contradiction to this observation, elevated concentrations of opioids in CSF were found in patients suffering from anorexia nervosa at their minimum weight (Kaye *et al.*, 1982). However, rather than being the primary cause of the disease, this increase in CSF opioid activity may be the consequence of compensatory mechanisms in response to stress to decrease metabolic requirements while at the same time increasing appetite, (Margules, 1979).

Our hypothesis on the role of endogenous opioids on menstrual cyclicity may shed further light on our understanding of stress and psychological amenorrhea. In various forms of stress, there is an increased release of corticotropin-releasing factor (CRF). Data in human pituitaries have clearly demonstrated that CRF not only increases the release of ACTH, but is also a potent secretagogue for other POMC-related peptides including β-endorphin (Gibbs *et al.*, 1982; Chan *et al.*, 1982). If a similar effect of CRF on hypothalamic β-endorphin can be demonstrated, or if, as suggested by recent immunocytochemical studies, CRF and opioid-like peptides are released simultaneously from the same terminals (Hokfelt *et al.*, 1983; Roth *et al.*, 1983), it is then possible that under stress circumstances, CRF-induced increased opioid tonus may act to dampen the GnRH arcuate oscillator and alter the characteristics of GnRH pulsatile release, thereby producing anovulation and amenorrhea.

IV. Summary and Conclusions

In a previous model of the primate menstrual cycle (Knobil, 1980), it was postulated that menstrual cyclicity is the result of unvarying circhoral GnRH signals coupled with an estrogen feedback exerted exclusively on the anterior pituitary. However, in this presentation we have demonstrated that the ovarian hormones, estradiol and progesterone, both also act at a hypothalamic site to modulate GnRH signals; estradiol primarily affects the amplitude while progesterone decreases the frequency of the GnRH pulse. The modulation of GnRH and consequently LH pulsatile secretion by ovarian steroids involves to a certain degree an interaction with the hypothalamic opioid peptide network. β-Endorphin secretion into the hypophyseal portal circulation, a reflection of hypothalamic β-endorphin secretory activity, fluctuates cyclically and in accordance with the endocrine milieu. The stimulatory action of naloxone on GnRH and LH release parallels that of endogenous opioid secretion. We postulate that the sequential acceleration and deceleration of the GnRH oscillator during the menstrual cycle, brought about by these cyclic β-endorphin variations, are important determinants of menstrual cyclicity, as experimental disturbance of this sequence results in acyclicity for a prolonged period of time.

ACKNOWLEDGMENTS

The authors would like to acknowledge the collaborative efforts of: Drs. G. Abrams, J. A. Antunes, S. Araki, P. W. Carmel, I. Dyrenfurth, A. G. Frantz, J. L. Gerlach, M. S. McEwen, D. W. Pfaff, A. J. Silverman, W. B. Wehrenberg, and E. A. Zimmerman in various aspects of this research work. They also thank Mrs. Kate Hildreth for her special efforts in typing the manuscript.

This research was supported by NIH Grants HD05077 and 10873.

REFERENCES

Abrams, G. M., Nilaver, G., Hoffman, D., Zimmerman, E. A., Ferin, M., Krieger, D. T., and Liotta, A. S. (1980). *Neurology* **8**, 1106.
Adams, T. E., Norman, R. L., and Spies, H. G. (1981). *Science* **213**, 1388.
Atkinson, R. L. (1982). *J. Clin. Endocrinol. Metab.* **55**, 196.
Barden, N., Merand, Y., Rouleau, D., Garon, M., and Dupont, A. (1981). *Brain Res.* **204**, 441.
Barry, J. (1976). *Neurosci. Lett.* **3**, 287.
Barry, J., and Carrette, B. (1975). *Cell Tissue Res.* **164**, 163.
Belchetz, P. E., Plant, T. M., Nakai, Y., Keogh, E. G., and Knobil, E. (1978). *Science* **202**, 631.
Bicknell, R. J., and Leng, G. (1982). *Nature (London)* **298**, 161.
Blank, M. S., and Roberts, D. L. (1982). *Neuroendocrinology* **35**, 309.
Blankstein, J., Reyes, F. I., Winter, J. S. D., and Faiman, C. (1981). *Clin. Endocrinol.* **14**, 287.

Bloom, F. E., Rossier, J., Battenberg, E. L., Bayon, A., French, E., Henriksen, S. I., Siggins, G. R., Desal, D., Browne, R., Ling, N., and Guillemin, R. (1978). *Adv. Biochem. Psychopharmacol.* **18**, 89.

Bogumil, R. J., Ferin, M., Rootenberg, J., Speroff, L., and Vande Wiele, R. L. (1972a). *J. Clin. Endocrinol. Metab.* **35**, 126.

Bogumil, R. J., Ferin, M., and Vande Wiele, R. L. (1972b). *J. Clin. Endocrinol. Metab.* **35**, 144.

Carmel, P. W., Araki, S., and Ferin, M. (1976). *Endocrinology* **99**, 243.

Carstens, E., Tulloc, H. I., Zieglgansberger, W., and Zimmerman, M. (1978). *J. Physiol. (London)* **284**, 137P.

Chan, J. S. D., Lu, C. L., Seidah, N. G., and Chretien, M. (1982). *Endocrinology* **111**, 1388.

Chappel, S. C., Resko, J. A., Norman, R. L., and Spies, H. G. (1981). *J. Clin. Endocrinol. Metab.* **52**, 1.

Cicero, T. J., Schainker, B. A., and Meyer, E. R. (1979). *Endocrinology* **104**, 1286.

Cicero, T. J., Meyer, E. R., Gabriel, S. M., Bell, R. D., and Wilcox, C. E. (1980). *Brain Res.* **202**, 151.

Clarke, G., Wood, P., Merrick, L., and Lincoln, D. W. (1979). *Nature (London)* **282**, 746.

Clarke, I. J., and Cummins, J. T. (1982). *Endocrinology* **111**, 1737.

Clement-Jones, V., and Besser, G. M. (1983). *Br. Med. Bull.* **39**, 95.

Cogen, P. H., Antunes, J. L., Louis, K. M., Dyrenfurth, I., and Ferin, M. (1980). *Endocrinology* **107**, 677.

Coppins, R. J., Malven, P. V., and Ramirez, V. D. (1971). *Proc. Soc. Exp. Biol. Med.* **154**, 219.

Cramer, O. M., and Barraclough, C. A. (1975). *Endocrinology* **96**, 913.

Deyo, S. N., Swift, R. M., and Miller, R. J. (1979). *Proc. Natl. Acad. Sci. U.S.A.* **76**, 3006.

Donohue, T. L., and Dorsa, D. M. (1982). *Peptides* **3**, 353.

Ellingboe, J., Veldhuis, J. D., Mendelson, J. H., Kuehnle, J. C., and Mello, N. K. (1982). *J. Clin. Endocrinol. Metab.* **54**, 854.

Ferin, M., Carmel, P. W., Zimmerman, E. A., Warren, M., and Vande Wiele, R. L. (1974). *Endocrinology* **95**, 1059.

Ferin, M., Wehrenberg, W. B., Lam, N. Y., Alston, E. F., and Vande Wiele, R. L. (1982). *Endocrinology* **111**, 1652.

Ferin, M., Van Vugt, D., and Chernick, A. (1983). *ORPPC Symp. Primate Reprod. Biol.* **II**.

Garris, D. R., Billiar, R. B., Takaoka, Y., White, R. J., and Little, B. (1981). *Neuroendocrinology* **32**, 202.

Garris, D. R., Billiar, R. B., Takaoka, Y., White, R., and Little, B. (1982). *Neuroendocrinology* **35**, 388.

Gee, C. E., Chen, C. L., Roberts, J. L., Thompson, R., and Watson, S. J. (1983). *Nature (London)* **306**, 374.

George, S. R., and Van Loon, G. R. (1982). *Brain Res.* **248**, 293.

Gibbs, D. M., Stewart, R. D., Liu, J. H., Vale, W., Rivier, J., and Yen, S. S. C. (1982). *J. Clin. Endocrinol. Metab.* **55**, 1149.

Goldstein, A., Fischli, W., Lowney, L. I., Hunkapiller, R. M., and Hood, L. (1981). *Proc. Natl. Acad. Sci. U.S.A.* **78**, 7219.

Goodman, R. L., and Karsch, F. J. (1980). *Endocrinology* **197**, 1286.

Goodman, R. L., and Knobil, E. (1981). *Neuroendocrinology* **32**, 57.

Grandison, L., Fratta, W., and Guidotti, A. (1980). *Life Sci.* **26**, 1633.

Grossman, A., and Rees, L. H. (1983). *Br. Med. Bull.* **39**, 83.

Grossman, A., Moult, P. J., McIntyre, H., Evans, J., Silverstone, T., Rees, L. H., and Besser, G. M. (1982). *Clin. Endocrinol.* **17**, 379.

Haskins, J. T., Gudelsky, G. A., Moss, R. L., and Porter, J. C. (1981). *Endocrinology* **108**, 767.

Hisano, S., Kawano, H., Nishiyama, T., and Daikoku, S. (1982). *Cell Tissue Res.* **224,** 303.

Hoffman, A. R., and Crowley, W. F. (1982). *N. Engl. J. Med.* **307,** 1237.

Hokfelt, T., Fahrenkrug, J., Tatemoto, K., Mutt, V., Werner, S., Hulting, A. L., Terenius, L., and Chang, K. J. (1983). *Proc. Natl. Acad. Sci. U.S.A.* **80,** 895.

Hughes, J., Smith, T. W., Kosterlitz, H. W., Fothergill, L. A., Morgan, B. A., and Morris, H. R. (1975). *Nature (London)* **258,** 577.

Kalra, S. P. (1981). *Endocrinology* **109,** 1805.

Kaye, W. H., Pickar, D., Naber, D., and Ebert, M. (1982). *Am. J. Psychiat.* **139,** 643.

Kiss, J. Z., and Williams, T. H. (1983). *Brain Res.* **263,** 142.

Knobil, E. (1974). *Recent Prog. Horm. Res.* **30,** 1.

Knobil, E. (1980). *Recent Prog. Horm. Res.* **36,** 53.

Knobil, E. (1981). *Biol. Reprod.* **24,** 44.

Koob, G. F., and Bloom, F. E. (1983). *Br. Med. Bull.* **39,** 89.

Krey, L. C., Butler, W. R., and Knobil, E. (1975). *Endocrinology* **96,** 1073.

Krieger, D. T., Liotta, A. S., Brownstein, M. J., and Zimmerman, E. A. (1980). *Recent. Prog. Horm. Res.* **277,** 344.

Leyendecker, G., Wildt, L., and Hansmann, M. (1981). *J. Clin. Endocrinol. Metab.* **51,** 1214.

Li, C. H., and Chung, D. (1976). *Proc. Natl. Acad. Sci. U.S.A.* **73,** 1145.

Lightman, S. L., Jacobs, H. S., Maguire, A. K., McGarrick, G., and Jeffcoate, S. L. (1981). *J. Clin. Endocrinol. Metab.* **52,** 1260.

Liotta, A. S., and Krieger, D. T. (1983). *Endocrine Soc. Annu. Meet., 65th* Abstr. No. 45.

Maclusky, N. J., Lieberburg, I., Krey, L. C., and McEwen, B. S. (1980). *Endocrinology* **106,** 185.

Mains, R. E., Eipper, B. A., and Ling, N. (1977). *Proc. Natl. Acad. Sci. U.S.A.* **74,** 3014.

Margules, D. L. (1979). *Neurosci. Biobehav. Rev.* **3,** 155.

Marshall, P. E., and Goldsmith, P. C. (1980). *Brain Res.* **193,** 353.

Marut, E. L., Williams, R. F., Cowan, B. D., Lynch, A., Lerner, S. P., and Hodgen, G. D. (1981). *Endocrinology* **109,** 2270.

McCormack, J. T., Plant, T. M., Hess, D. L., and Knobil, E. (1977). *Endocrinology* **100,** 663.

McKay, L. D., Kenney, N. J., Edens, N. K., Williams, R. H., and Woods, S. C. (1981). *Life Sci.* **29,** 1429.

Meites, J., Bruni, J. F., Van Vugt, D. A., and Smith, A. F. (1979). *Life Sci.* **24,** 1325.

Morley, J. E. (1981). *Metabolism* **30,** 195.

Morley, J. E. (1983). *Br. Med. Bull.* **39,** 5.

Morley, J. E., and Levine, A. S. (1982). *Am. J. Clin. Nutr.* **35,** 757.

Nakai, Y., Plant, T. M., Hess, D. L., Keogh, E. J., and Knobil, E. (1978). *Endocrinology* **102,** 1008.

Neill, J. D., Dailey, R. A., Tsou, R. C., and Tindall, G. T. (1977). *Adv. Exp. Med. Biol.* **87,** 20.

Norman, R. L., Resko, J. A., and Spies, H. G. (1976). *Endocrinology* **99,** 59.

Norman, R. L., Lindstrom, S. A., Bangsberg, D., Ellinwood, W. E., Gliessman, P., and Spies, H. G. (1984). *Endocrinology,* in press.

Parker, C. R., Barnea, A., Tilders, F. J. H., and Porter, J. C. (1981). *Brain Res. Bull.* **6,** 275.

Pfaff, D. W., Gerlach, J. L., McEwen, B. S., Ferin, M., Carmel, P. W., and Zimmerman, E. A. (1976). *J. Comp. Neurol.* **170,** 279.

Plant, T. M., Nakai, Y., Belchetz, P., Keogh, E. J., and Knobil, E. (1978a). *Endocrinology* **102,** 1015.

Plant, T. M., Krey, L. C., Moossy, J., McCormack, J. T., Hess, D. L., and Knobil, E. (1978b). *Endocrinology* **102,** 52.

Pohl, C. R., Richardson, D. W., Marshall, G., and Knobil, E. (1982). *Endocrinology* **110**, 1454.

Pohl, C. R., Richardson, D. W., Hutchinson, J. S., Germak, J. A., and Knobil, E. (1983). *Endocrinology* **112**, 2076.

Quigley, M. E., and Yen, S. S. C. (1980). *J. Clin. Endocrinol. Metab.* **51**, 179.

Quigley, M. E., Sheehan, K. L., Casper, R. F., and Yen, S. S. C. (1980). *J. Clin. Endocrinol. Metab.* **50**, 427.

Rakic, P. (1975). *Neurosci. Res. Prog. Bull.* **13**, 291.

Rasmussen, D. D., Liu, J. H., and Yen, S. S. C. (1983). *Annu. Meet. Soc. Gynecol. Invest.*, *30th* Abstr. No. 115.

Reid, R. L., Hoff, J. D., Yen, S. S. C., and Li, C. H. (1981). *J. Clin. Endocrinol. Metab.* **52**, 1179.

Reymond, M. J., Kaur, C., and Porter, J. C. (1983). *Brain Res.* **262**, 253.

Richardson, D. W., Wildt, L., Hutchinson, J. S., Pohl, C. R., Knobil, E., Antunes, J. L., Chernick, A., Murasko, K., Wehrenberg, W., and Ferin, M. (1984). Submitted.

Rivier, C., Vale, W., Ling, N., Brown, M., and Guillemin, R. (1977). *Endocrinology* **100**, 238.

Roberts, J. L., and Herbert, E. (1977). *Proc. Natl. Acad. Sci. U.S.A.* **74**, 5300.

Ropert, J. F., Quigley, M. E., and Yen, S. S. C. (1981). *J. Clin. Endocrinol. Metab.* **52**, 583.

Rosenblatt, H., Dyrenfurth, I., Ferin, M., and Vande Wiele, R. L. (1980). *Physiol. Behav.* **24**, 447.

Rossier, J., Vargo, T. M., Minick, S., Ling, N., Bloom, F. E., and Guillemin, R. (1977). *Proc. Natl. Acad. Sci. U.S.A.* **74**, 5162.

Roth, K. A., Weber, E., Barchas, J. D., Chang, D., and Chang, J. K. (1983). *Science* **219**, 189.

Sanger, D. J., McCarthy, P. S., Lord, J. A. H., and Smith, C. F. C. (1983). *Drug Dev. Res.* **3**, 137.

Shivers, B. D., Harlan, R. E., Morrell, J. I., and Pfaff, D. W. (1983). *Nature (London)* **304**, 345.

Silverman, A. J., Antunes, J. L., Ferin, M., and Zimmerman, E. A. (1977). *Endocrinology* **101**, 134.

Silverman, A. J., Antunes, J. L., Abrams, G., Nilaver, G., Thau, R., Robinson, J. A., Ferin, M., and Krey, L. C. (1982). *J. Comp. Neurol.* **221**, 309.

Simantov, R., and Snyder, S. H. (1977). *Brain Res.* **124**, 178.

Smyth, D. G., Massey, D. E., Zakarian, S., and Finnie, M. D. A. (1979). *Nature (London)* **279**, 252.

Sopelek, V. M., Lynch, A., Williams, R. F., and Hodgen, G. D. (1983). *Biol. Reprod.* **28**, 703.

Soules, M. R., Steiner, R. A., Clifton, D. K., Cohen, N. L., Aksel, S., and Bremner, W. J. (1984). *J. Clin. Endocrinol. Metab.* **58**, 378.

Spies, H. G., and Norman, R. L. (1975). *Endocrinology* **97**, 685.

Van Vugt, D. A., Bruni, J. F., and Meites, J. (1978). *J. Med. Sci.* **7**, 56.

Van Vugt, D. A., Bruni, J. F., Sylvester, P. W., Chen, H. T., Ieiri, T., and Meites, J. (1979). *Life Sci.* **24**, 2361.

Van Vugt, D. A., Aylsworth, C. F., Sylvester, P. W., Leung, F. C., and Meites, J. (1981). *Neuroendocrinology* **33**, 261.

Van Vugt, D. A., Sylvester, P. W., Aylsworth, C. F., and Meites, J. (1982). *Neuroendocrinology* **34**, 274.

Van Vugt, D. A., Bakst, G., Dyrenfurth, I., and Ferin, M. (1983a). *Endocrinology* **113**, 1858.

Van Vugt, D. A., Diefenbach, W. P., and Ferin, M. (1983b). *Endocrine Soc. Annu. Meet.*, *65th* Abstr. No. 193.

Vande Wiele, R. L., Bogumil, R. J., Dyrenfurth, I., Ferin, M., Jewelewicz, R., Warren, M., Mikhail, G., and Rizkallah, T. (1970). *Recent Prog. Horm. Res.* **26**, 63.

Vaughan, L., Carmel, P. W., Dyrenfurth, I., Frantz, A. G., Antunes, J. L., and Ferin, M. (1980). *Neuroendocrinology* **30**, 70.

Wamsley, J. K., Zarbin, M. A., Young, W. S., and Kuhar, M. J. (1982). *Neuroscience* **7**, 595.

Wardlaw, S. L., Wehrenberg, W. B., Ferin, M., Carmel, P. W., and Frantz, A. G. (1980a). *Endocrinology* **106**, 1323.

Wardlaw, S. L., Wehrenberg, W. B., Ferin, M., and Frantz, A. G. (1980b). *Endocrinology* **107**, 1663.

Wardlaw, S. L., Wehrenberg, W. B., Ferin, M., Antunes, J. L., and Frantz, A. G. (1982a). *J. Clin. Endocrinol. Metab.* **55**, 877.

Wardlaw, S. L., Thoron, L., and Frantz, A. G. (1982b). *Brain Res.* **245**, 327.

Warren, M. P., Jewelewicz, R., Dyrenfurth, I., Ans, R., Khalaf, S., and Vande Wiele, R. L. (1975). *J. Clin. Endocrinol. Metab.* **40**, 601.

Watson, S. J., Akil, H., Sullivan, S. O., and Barchas, J. D. (1977). *Life Sci.* **21**, 733.

Wehrenberg, W. B., and Ferin, M. (1981). *Proc. Soc. Exp. Biol. Med.* **168**, 286.

Wehrenberg, W. B., McNicol, D., Frantz, A. G., and Ferin, M. (1980). *Endocrinology* **107**, 1747.

Wehrenberg, W. B., McNicol, D., Wardlaw, S. L., Frantz, A. G., and Ferin, M. (1981). *Endocrinology* **109**, 544.

Wehrenberg, W. B., Wardlaw, S. L., Frantz, A. G., and Ferin, M. (1982). *Endocrinology* **111**, 879.

Weick, R. F., Pitelka, V., and Thompson, D. L. (1982). Endocrinology **112**, 1862.

Wildt, L., Hutchinson, J. S., Marshall, G., Pohl, C. R., and Knobil, E. (1981a). *Endocrinology* **109**, 1293.

Wildt, L., Hausler, A., Marshall, G., Hutchinson, J. S., Plant, T. M., Belchetz, P. E., and Knobil, E. (1981b). *Endocrinology* **109**, 376.

Wilkes, M. M., and Yen, S. S. C. (1980). *Life Sci.* **27**, 1387.

Witkin, J. W., Paden, C. M., and Silverman, A. J. (1982). *Neuroendocrinology* **35**, 429.

Yen, S. S. C., Tsai, C. C., Naftolin, F., Vandenberg, G., and Ajabor, L. (1972). *J. Clin. Endocrinol. Metab.* **34**, 671.

Zakarian, S., and Smyth, D. G. (1982). *Nature (London)* **296**, 250.

DISCUSSION

G. B. Cutler, Jr.: One of the common causes of menstrual irregularity is high androgen levels. Do you have any evidence for what androgens do to the hypothalamic β-endorphin?

M. Ferin: We have not studied the effects of androgens on hypothalamic β-endorphin secretion. In the human, there is a syndrome, the polycystic ovarian disease, in which androgen levels are elevated. What is of interest in these patients is the high frequency of the GnRH-LH oscillator, with LH pulses usually occurring at hourly or even less than hourly intervals. This may represent an example of continuously low β-endorphin activity, although there is no evidence for it. The high LH frequency then drives the ovaries to increase androgen secretion, which may then interfere with normal feedback regulation, and result in anovulatory cycles.

I. Callard: How can you be sure that the β-endorphin that you are measuring in such large quantities in the portal plasma is of hypothalamic origin especially since there is anatomical and physiological evidence for refluxing of blood backup in the pituitary stalk, and you do not find an effect of β-endorphin on the anterior pituitary?

M. Ferin: This is a question which has concerned us a lot. There is indeed evidence of back and forth circulation between the hypothalamus and the pituitary gland. However, there are several reasons why we believe that stalk portal plasma concentrations of β-endorphin represent β-endorphin of hypothalamic origin. Some of these were mentioned in the presentation, such as the chromotagraphic pattern of β-endorphin immunoactivity in portal blood resembling that seen in hypothalamic extracts, and the fact that, in our monkeys, hypophysectomy did not reduce significantly the levels of β-endorphin in portal blood. In addition, the method of collecting stalk portal blood was such that only blood derived directly from the brain could have been collected. Indeed, the pituitary stalk was sectioned entirely and only the upper portion (hypothalamic) of the sectioned stalk was connected to the collector. Our method differs from that where portal blood is collected from individual portal vessels along the unsevered pituitary stalk, in which case blood from the pituitary gland would be aspirated as well. This was not the case in our experiments.

The absence of direct effects of β-endorphin on the anterior pituitary gland is puzzling, even more so that these large concentrations of β-endorphin in stalk portal blood are of the nonacetylated, i.e., the biological active kind. In the rodent as well, the overwhelming evidence supports a hypothalamic site of action. There are, however, a couple of articles which support a pituitary site of action. The first [Enjalbert, A., Ruberg, M., Arancibia, S., Priam, M., and Kordon, C. (1979). *Nature (London)* **280**, 595] reported that β-endorphin blocked dopamine inhibition of prolactin release by rat hemipituitaries. The second [Judd, A. M., and Hedge, G. S. (1983). *Endocrinology* **113**, 706] implies that β-endorphin can release TSH *in vitro*. The physiological significance of these observations in general and to the primate in particular is unknown. It is possible that direct action of the opioids will be demonstrated some day if tested under the right conditions. Until then, we believe that β-endorphin acts at a hypothalamic site to modulate GnRH secretion, and that β-endorphin concentrations in portal blood are a reflection of this action.

N. B. Schwartz: How do you explain Knobil's data on the GnRH pump where he has a constant frequency and amplitude and obtains a cycle from it.

M. Ferin: It is indeed well known, that ovulatory cycles can be induced with GnRH regimens of unchanging frequency and amplitude. We ourselves have been involved in such studies in the human and monkey. At first view, of course, this is difficult to reconcile with the hypothesis which we have postulated in this talk. However, there are three remarks that can be made about these unchanging GnRH regimens which have been used: (1) Most of the experiments have been performed in subjects with hypothalamic deficiencies, either in patients with so-called hypothalamic amenorrhea, or in monkeys bearing lesions of the hypothalamus or having undergone pituitary stalk section. Under such conditions, it is possible that normal servo feedback mechanisms may not be functional. (2) The long-term effects of the unchanging GnRH regimens are difficult to evaluate, since most patients were not treated continuously for months, but rather were placed on and off on the GnRH regimen. (3) Most importantly, the dose used in these treatments, i.e., the amplitude of the GnRH pulse, (6 μg over 6 minutes in the monkey), may not be representative of physiological amounts. GnRH levels following injection of a 6 μg pulse in the monkeys are indeed higher than those we observed in portal blood of ovariectomized rhesus monkeys. The LH response to such GnRH pulse, for instance during the luteal phase, is 2- to 3-fold that of spontaneous LH pulses during the phase of the cycle. The results of such experiments may therefore not be completely relevant to the physiological situation. I think that further experimental testing is in order.

N. B. Schwartz: I did not find the naloxone data particularly impressive from the few examples that you gave. I was not convinced that you showed an increase in frequency. How many monkeys have you tried the naloxone treatment on?

M. Ferin: At this point, there is no doubt in my mind that naloxone infusions during the luteal phase have a profound effect on LH pulsatile frequency. The experimental design however has been difficult, since it is usually not possible to have prolonged control and experimental periods side by side to compare frequencies.

F. J. Karsch: I would like you to expand your comments on the distribution of GnRH in the hypothalamus, as you have observed in collaboration with Ann Judith Silverman. You described three clusters of cell bodies for GnRH, one in the preoptic area, one in the arcuate nucleus, and one in the posterior hypothalamus. Your talk addressed only the cluster of cell bodies in the arcuate nucleus. Would you comment on the possible functions of the cluster of cell bodies in the preoptic area as well as the one in the posterior hypothalamus?

M. Ferin: First, I should point out that, when we measure GnRH in hypophyseal portal blood, and most probably in CSF as well, it is obviously not possible to dissect the contribution of each of the hypothalamic regions, since all pathways which you refer to terminate, at least in part, in the median eminence. As you know, there has been a long controversial history on the role of the anterior hypothalamic-preoptic area GnRH pathway on gonadotropin secretion in the rhesus monkey. Knobil and collegues believe that this area does not play a role, since complete hypothalamic deafferentation does not interfere with normal gonadotropin secretion. On the contrary, Spies and collegues believe that it is an important area for the control of cyclic gonadotropin release. Our group has shown that anterior hypothalamic disconnection results in anovulation, supporting a role for the anterior hypothalamus in cyclicity. However, these animals resume spontaneous ovulatory cycles within 2–6 months following deafferentation, casting a doubt about the degree of involvement of the anterior hypothalamus. The role of the posterior hypothalamic GnRH nerve fibers is even less known. In our hands, estradiol injection directly into these caudal hypothalamic areas has been followed by inhibition of LH secretion to a degree even greater than following injections in other brain areas. That posterior pathways may exert an inhibitory role is also indicated by reports by Terasawa and collegues of inhibitory effects by the posterior hypothalamus on puberty.

F. Karsch: One more question relative to the distribution of GnRH in nerve terminals in the posterior pituitary gland. Do these terminals originate from one of those clusters of cell bodies, in particular, or are they a mixture of neurons from more than one source?

M. Ferin: The location of the cell bodies of the fibers which descend along the pituitary stalk to terminate in the posterior pituitary in the monkey is still unknown. With Dr. A. Silverman, we are presently attempting to answer this question, using first HRP tracing techniques.

S. Cohen: In the first place, is it possible to have opiates secretion without having ACTH secretion?

M. Ferin: In stress situations, β-LPH or opioid secretion accompanies the release of ACTH from the anterior pituitary. In the intermediary lobe, ACTH is further cleaved to yield MSH, and therefore is not actively secreted. In this situation, β-endorphin release by the tissue is not accompanied by ACTH release.

S. Cohen: How do you know that your effects are not due to ACTH rather than endorphins?

M. Ferin: Our effects at which level?

S. Cohen: At any level.

M. Ferin: Well, we have shown that injection of β-endorphin itself does decrease gonadotropin secretion.

S. Cohen: The second question concerns the fact that when I was being introduced to the physiology of reproduction, this goes back nearly 50 years ago, we were taught that the feedback mechanisms took place through the pituitary itself and that estradiol inhibits the secretion of FSH and stimulates the secretion of LH. Well, this was of course before the days of purified extracts. I wondered is that still true for the relationship between estradiol and LH secretion by the anterior pituitary glands?

M. Ferin: While the emphasis in this talk was on the effects of estradiol on LH secretion by acting at a hypothalamic site, I believe that estradiol also acts at a pituitary site. Thus, there may well be 2 sites for the negative feedback effect of estradiol. In fact, in a recent paper [Weick, R. F., Pitelka, V., and Thompson, D. L. (1982). *Endocrinology* **112**, 1862] it was suggested that estradiol first may acutely suppress LH secretion by acting at a pituitary site, but that hours later, it will suppress LH by acting at a hypothalamic site. This result is borne out by some of our stalk portal blood collection in which we have shown that estradiol does not acutely (within 3 hours) affect GnRH secretion and yet LH secretion decreases. This is in contrast to the chronic effects of estradiol, demonstrated in this talk. Obviously, we deal with complex ovarian–hypothalamic–hypophyseal interactions, and I would not want to leave you with the impression that estradiol acts uniquely at the hypothalamus. Further studies are obviously needed. In regard to the separate control of FSH, there is now, as mentioned, good evidence that the ratio between LH and FSH may well be related to GnRH pulse frequency.

S. Cohen: I was thinking that if LH is stimulated by estradiol in the pituitary and inhibited through the hypothalamus, that would be like driving a car with your foot on the brake and the accelerator simultaneously.

B. Murphy: What behavioral changes did you observe in your monkeys and do you have any thoughts on the possible relationship between changes in endorphins and the premenstrual tension syndrome?

M. Ferin: We have not really made studies of changes in behavior in our animals, except for a report of changes in food intake with the menstrual cycle, most probably related to changes in endogenous opioid peptide activity. In relation to the premenstrual syndrome, some of the observations which we have reported here may be of special interest. I am thinking especially of the increase in hypothalamic β-endorphin throughout the luteal phase, associated with the abrupt decrease at menstruation. Since it is well known that opioids exert panoramic effects on the entire central nervous system, several of the symptoms associated with the syndrome may well be explained on this basis. Acute endorphin withdrawal at menstruation, associated with rebound dopamine activity, may well account for further sudden changes in mood and irritability at that time. An animal model such as the monkey, in which central changes in β-endorphin could be measured, may be a useful one in this regard.

A. Segaloff: I would like to point out that estradiol is metabolized in the body and in the brain. It has been reported [LaBella (1983). *Can. J. Physiol. Pharm.* **61**, 191] that estradiol-17α competes with naloxone for the opiate receptor and has analgesic activity equivalent to morphine in the mouse hot plate test. I wonder if some of the phenomena you are seeing would not be seen with an opiate or with an estradiol metabolite from the estradiol-17β that you are administering.

M. Ferin: This is entirely possible. We haven't studied this aspect.

M. V. Nekola: Have you or anybody else attempted to measure the β-endorphins in the pituitary stalk blood in males?

M. Ferin: No.

M. V. Nekola: You postulate a role for opiates in the control of LHRH secretion. Do you have evidence that LHRH affects the secretion of opiates?

M. Ferin: It may well be, but we have not studied this aspect.

F. Turek: My question is related to the synthesis of β-endorphin in the arcuate neurons. Do you find ACTH in these neurons also, and if not, do you think that the synthesis of β-endorphin may be different in neurons than it is in the pituitary gland?

M. Ferin: Little work has been done in the primate. In the rodent, however, it is known that POMC mRNA in the arcuate region is similar to that in the pituitary gland. The precursor is cleaved into several products, as outlined in the talk. The proportion of end products, however, differs from tissue to tissue, with nonacetylated β-endorphin the main component in the arcuate region.

F. Turek: With regard to your slide showing LHRH in the posterior pituitary gland, were you suggesting a blood or a neural route for the movement of LHRH from the hypothalamus to the posterior pituitary gland?

M. Ferin: GnRH in the posterior pituitary gland of the monkey derives from GnRH containing axons descending along the pituitary stalk. The location of the cell bodies for these axons is unknown. These axons appear to terminate within the posterior pituitary gland, near the short portal vessels.

J. Martin: You have not commented on the presence of progesterone receptors in the hypothalamus. It would be important if they are there to complete your feedback effects of progesterone on β-endorphin secretion. Do you have any evidence that progesterone receptors reside in the arcuate nucleus?

M. Ferin: We ourselves have no information on progesterone receptors, but I believe that Dr. Billiar has such evidence in the monkey, so maybe he would like to comment on that.

R. B. Billiar: We have localized by light autoradiography progesterone, both progesterone and the synthetic progestin R5020, in the arcuate and also in the ventral medial nuclei of the monkey hypothalamus. In fact, I am a little more impressed with the localization in the ventral medial nuclei than the arcuate in terms of the rhesus monkey.

D. Foster: My question concerns the temporal relationship between pulses of GnRH and pulses of LH. Although you presented data for GnRH pulses in the cerebral spinal fluid, you did not show the pattern of LH in the peripheral circulation of the same monkeys during the period of GnRH measurement. Did you measure LH, and if so, was each LH pulse preceded by a GnRH pulse? Did each GnRH pulse induce an LH pulse?

M. Ferin: The advantage of measuring GnRH in CSF is, of course, in theory that simultaneous measurements of LH in peripheral blood can be made. This is not true for portal blood, since GnRH measurements require prior pituitary stalk section and derivation of all portal blood to the collection tube.

As far as CSF, we have in most cases carried out simultaneous measurements of LH and GnRH. Our present experience is quite limited and therefore general conclusions cannot be arrived at yet. However, in most cases, we have seen a good correlation between GnRH and LH pulses. There were a few instances of a single GnRH pulse not accompanied by a corresponding LH pulse, an observation also made in sheep, where GnRH portal blood measurements were compared to LH [Clarke, I. J., and Cummings, J. T. (1982). *Endocrinology* **III**, 1737].

M. Selmanoff: I have a brief neuroanatomical question related to Fred Karsch's. You showed us autoradiograms of perikarya in the arcuate nucleus which were concentrating radioactive estradiol in the rhesus monkey. Have you been able to demonstrate in adjacent sections by immunohistochemistry that those neurons are indeed LHRH-containing neurons?

M. Ferin: This is a very interesting question. The presence of estradiol concentrating neurons in the same general area as GnRH cell bodies in the monkey has of course led us to believe that there could be a direct interaction between GnRH and estradiol. In the rodent, however, immunocytochemical studies combined with autoradiography have shown that doubly labeled cells were very rarely seen [Shivers, B. D., Harlan, R. E., Morrell, J. I., and Pfaff, D. W. (1983). *Nature* (*London*) **304,** 345], suggesting that genomic regulatory effects of estradiol do not appear to be exerted on most GnRH cells. There is no information available in the monkey.

A Role For Hypothalamic Catecholamines in the Regulation of Gonadotropin Secretion

CHARLES A. BARRACLOUGH, PHYLLIS M. WISE, AND
MICHAEL K. SELMANOFF

*Department of Physiology, School of Medicine, University of Maryland,
Baltimore, Maryland*

Introduction

The functional activity of the LHRH neuron can be affected by numerous putative neurotransmitters which stimulate or inhibit LHRH release (McCann, 1982). Further, some neurotransmitters also may activate or inhibit other primary inputs to affect, secondarily, the activity of the LHRH neuron. Coupled with these complex controls are those modulatory influences exerted within the brain by changing serum levels of sex steroids on input circuitry, genomic function, and, perhaps, even on ionic transport properties of the LHRH neuronal membrane (Fig. 1).

Since this article will emphasize our recent studies on the role of the hypothalamic catecholaminergic system in regulating LHRH secretion, our conclusions necessarily are derived from the data we obtained. However, we also recognize that other modulatory systems also may specifically affect the surge release of LHRH.

HISTORICAL

It has been over 36 years since Sawyer *et al.* (1947) suggested that norepinephrine was involved in LH release. Subsequent studies by Everett *et al.* (1949) and Sawyer *et al.* (1950) demonstrated that dibenamine and SKF-501 [N-(9-fluorenyl)-n-ethyl-β-chlorethylamine hydrochloride], a drug with 3–10 times the adrenergic blocking properties as dibenamine, blocked ovulation in cyclic rats. In 1957, Barraclough and Sawyer (1957) examined the effects of two drugs which affect different functional components of the catecholamine (CA) synapse and terminal. Chlorpromazine, an α-adrenergic receptor antagonist, when administered before the presumptive time of the gonadotropin surge on proestrus, effectively blocked LH release. Reserpine, a depletor of CAs from presynaptic ter-

487

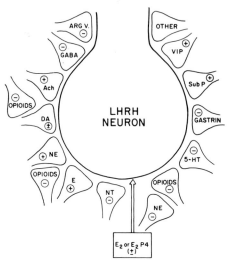

FIG. 1.   Diagrammatic representation of an LHRH neuron and some of the various neuropeptides and neurotransmitters reported to influence LHRH secretion. Stimulatory agents: norepinephrine (NE), epinephrine (E), acetylcholine (Ach), vasointestinal peptide (VIP), substance P (Sub P). Inhibitory agents: opioids, 5-hydroxytryptamine (5-HT), γ-aminobutyric acid (GABA), neurotensin (NT), gastrin. Some neurohormones may indirectly affect LHRH secretion by their action on a primary regulatory system. For example, opioids suppress DA and perhaps NE secretion. In contrast, NE may exert part of its stimulatory effects on LHRH by suppressing release of opioids and many other possible permutations also may exist which affect the function of the LHRH neurons. Estradiol (E_2) alone or in combination with progestrone (P_4) may directly affect responsiveness of the LHRH neuron or indirectly modulate its responsiveness to other putative neurotransmitters.

minals, also effectively suppressed ovulation in cyclic rats (Barraclough and Sawyer, 1957; Meyerson and Sawyer, 1968). Further, both drugs, when administered to cyclic rats, induced pseudopregnancy probably by blocking lactotroph dopamine (DA) receptors and/or by depleting median eminence (ME) terminals of DA (Barraclough and Sawyer, 1959). These early observations contributed to the concept that monoamines somehow are intimately involved in the preovulatory discharge of LHRH from ME axon terminals. Since these pioneering studies, many different investigators have evaluated a variety of drugs which seemingly affect different functional systems in the brain and which also block gonadotropin secretion. A partial list of these drugs and their effects on LH, FSH, and PRL secretion have been published in a recent review article by Barraclough and Wise (1982). Some general conclusions can be drawn from the data obtained using the pharmacological approach to study CA regulation of LH and FSH secretion. Clearly, drugs which interrupt CA synthesis or block α-adrenergic receptors also block spontaneous LH surges in proestrous rats, in estradiol (E_2) and progesterone (P_4)-treated ovariectomized (OVX) animals, and they also suppress pulsatile LH release in gonadectomized rats. What is not clear is whether it is NE, DA, or both CAs which ultimately are involved in inducing LH surges. Also, with the recent development of more specific ligands for detecting specific NE, DA, β-adrenergic, and opioid receptors it is becoming evident that many of the drugs thought to be specific to adrenergic receptors in fact lack such specificity. For example, phenoxybenzamine not only blocks pre- and postsynaptic α-adrenergic receptors but also responses to 5-hydroxytryptamine, histamine, and acetylcholine (Brittain et al., 1970). Recently, Blank et al. (1983) reported that α_1 and α_2 specific receptor blockers (prazosin and yohimbine) not only were equally effective in attenuating naloxone-induced LH release but also were effective competitors for naloxone binding sites contained on hypothalamic membranes.

Since most investigators recognize the shortcomings of the use of drugs to study CA–LHRH interactions, a variety of other in vivo and in vitro approaches have been used to determine the role of NE and/or DA in the surge release of gonadotropins. Because many of these approaches have been discussed in detail in a recent review article (Barraclough and Wise, 1982) they will not be considered in this article. Rather, we will focus this discussion on recent studies from our laboratories which correlate changes in hypothalamic catecholaminergic activity with the surge secretion of LH, FSH, and PRL.

II. Measurement of Catecholaminergic Activity in Brain

Presently, we cannot directly quantitate the rate of release of any neurotransmitter at the synaptic cleft and measuring neurotransmitter concentrations is not a sensitive index of functional activity. Resting NE and DA concentrations have been found to be remarkably constant despite very different rates of neuronal depolarization and transmitter release (Carlsson, 1964). Thus, evidence suggests that changes in the turnover rate (T/R) of the neurotransmitter pool is a mechanism by which the stable transmitter concentrations are maintained even during increased CA neuronal activity (Brodie et al., 1966; Weiner, 1974; Costa and Neff, 1970). Increased turnover rates or rates of synthesis have been equated with increased transmitter release while decreased turnover rates are associated with decreased neuronal activity. Both steady and nonsteady state methods are available to estimate T/R of NE and DA and they have been employed to correlate changes in neuronal activity with changes in gonadotropin secretion. In our studies we have employed a non-steady-state method which measures the rate of decline in CA concentrations after blockade of new CA synthesis with α-methyl-p-tyrosine, a competitive inhibitor of tyrosine hydroxylase (the rate-limiting enzyme for NE and DA synthesis). We recognize that the major theoretical disadvantage of all non-steady-state methods is that inhibition of synthesis or metabolism constitutes a gross perturbation of the system. On the other hand, these methods are advantageous, particularly when they are combined with micromodifications of the radioenzymatic assay since CA concentration changes can be measured in microdissected brain areas of individual rats. This is contrasted to less sensitive steady-state methods which do not permit selective analysis of CA dynamics in specific anatomical loci, and as such, severely limit the interpretation of data when large pieces of hypothalamus are used. Thus, if changes occur in one brain nucleus but not in another, or if T/R change in opposite directions in two different loci, such events could remain undetected if whole brain or hypothalamus is analyzed.

III. Changes in Catecholamine Turnover Rates Associated with Gonadotropin Surges

A. CYCLIC PROESTROUS AND DIESTROUS RATS

To obtain information on the dynamics of change which occur in hypothalamic catecholamine activity prior to and during the proestrous pre-ovulatory gonadotropin surge we examined NE and DA T/R in specific nuclei microdissected from the hypothalamus (Rance et al., 1981a). In these initial studies we used 4-day cyclic proestrous or diestrous day 1 rats. The methods for the brain dissections, for the radioenzymatic measurements of catecholamines, the calculations of turnover rates, and the radioimmunoassay of serum steroids, LHRH and gonadotropins previously have been published (Rance et al., 1981b).

During proestrus, LH, FSH, PRL, and progesterone (P_4) increased significantly in serum between 0900 and 1500 hours. In contrast, estradiol (E_2) was significantly elevated at 0900 hours on proestrus above diestrous day 1 (D-1) (0900 and 1500 hours) values (Table I). Median eminence (ME)–LHRH concentrations rose significantly between 0900 and 1200 hours on proestrus (before preovulatory serum gonadotropins increased) and declined during the time of the gonadotropin surge (1500 hours; $p <$ 0.05). In contrast, serum LH, FSH, PRL, and E_2 at 1500 hours D-1 were not statistically different from 0900 hour values on D-1. Only P_4 was elevated at 1500 compared to 0900 hours on D-1. Earlier studies by us

TABLE I
Hormone Concentrations[a]

Hormone	Proestrus				Diestrous day 1	
	0900 hours	1200 hours	1500 hours		0900 hours	1500 hours
ME-LHRH (pg/μg) protein	105.9 ± 8.3	161.5 ± 14.6[b]	115.7 ± 12.1		93.7 ± 10.0	70.7 ± 9.8
Serum						
LH (ng/ml)	48.4 ± 5.1	80.1 ± 21.0	2153.5 ± 91.7[c]		74.8 ± 9.9	54.3 ± 10.8
FSH (ng/ml)	122.5 ± 3.5	131.6 ± 5.5	207.9 ± 42.0[b]		127.5 ± 5.6	136.2 ± 6.5
PRL (ng/ml)[d]	58.5 ± 14.3	108.5 ± 28.7	380.1 ± 31.5[b]		31.6 ± 4.0	19.1 ± 2.1
E$_2$ (pg/ml)	43.1 ± 5.2	43.3 ± 3.4	39.7 ± 7.3		9.8 ± 1.5	8.1 ± 0.64
P (ng/ml)	3.6 ± 1.8	1.4 ± 0.2	18.7 ± 3.1[b]		8.6 ± 1.1	14.3 ± 1.5[e]

[a] Values given are the mean ± SEM (n = 6–8 rats/group).
[b] $p < 0.05$ compared to 0900 hours on proestrus.
[c] $p < 0.01$ compared to 0900 hours on proestrus.
[d] PRL, RP-1 standard.
[e] $p < 0.05$ compared to 0900 hours on diestrous day 1.

revealed that ME–LHRH concentrations at 0900, 1200, 1500, and 1800 hours did not change in D-1 rats (Wise *et al.*, 1981c).

Shown in Fig. 2 are the changes which occurred on proestrus in NE T/R in the medial preoptic (MPN), suprachiasmatic (SCN), and arcuate nuclei (AN), and in the median eminence (ME).

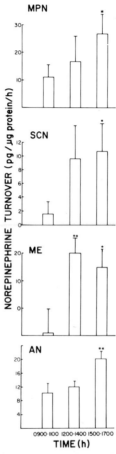

FIG. 2.　NE turnover rates (T/R) in the medial preoptic nucleus (MPN), suprachiasmatic nucleus (SCN), median eminence (ME), and arcuate nucleus (AN) during proestrus. NE T/R are low in all areas between 0900 and 1100 hours on proestrus. Between 1200 and 1400 hours, NE T/R increase significantly in the ME over 0900–1100 hour rates and remain significantly elevated through 1500–1700 hours. Also, between 1500 and 1700 hours, NE T/R are significantly increased in SCN, AN, and MPN. (**, $p < 0.01$; *, $p < 0.05$.) Verticle lines above bars in this and other figures represent SEM. (From Rance *et al.*, 1981b.)

During the interval (0900–1200 hours) that LHRH increased in ME, MPN, and SCN (Wise *et al.,* 1981c), NE T/R were low in all brain regions between 0900 and 1100 hours. However, between 1200 and 1400 hours, ME T/R increased significantly ($p < 0.01$) and remained elevated for the next 2 hours (1500–1700 hours). NE turnover rates in the MPN, SCN, and AN also were significantly increased ($p < 0.05$) at 1500–1700 hours compared to 0900–1100 hour values (Fig. 2).

In contrast to the changes observed in MPN–NE, DA T/R in the MPN remained unchanged throughout the time periods examined. However, AN and ME DA T/R increased between 1200 and 1400 hours proestrus but thereafter between 1500 and 1700 hours on proestrous T/R and rate constants were significantly depressed. In other words, ME and AN DA T/R paralleled ME–NE T/R between 1200 and 1400 hours but as NE T/R increased in the MPN, SCN, and AN there was an abrupt decline in tuberoinfundibular DA T/R (Fig. 3).

NE T/R in MPN and ME and DA T/R in ME remained unchanged at 1500 hours compared to values at 0900 hours on diestrous day 1 (Rance *et al.,* 1981b).

From these studies several interesting correlations can be made: (1) during the interval that LHRH is accumulating in ME (0900–1200 hours) both NE and DA T/R in MPN, SCN, AN, and ME are low and peripheral serum gonadotropin concentrations remain basal; (2) just before and during the beginning of the gonadotropin surge, ME–LHRH declines and ME, NE, and DA T/R are greatly increased (1200–1400 hours); (3) during the interval (1500–1700 hours) that LH, FSH, and PRL are still rising to peak serum concentrations, ME NE T/R remain elevated and increased NE T/R also are evident in the MPN, SCN, and AN. Within this same time period, DA T/R dramatically decline in the ME and AN.

Some of these data confirm previous observations in which semiquantitative microflurometric studies showed a decline in DA T/R in the ME (Löfström, 1977; Ahren *et al.,* 1971). This DA decline may represent the removal of an inhibitory influence of DA on LHRH terminals in the ventral lateral ME or the removal of PIF activity antecedent to the proestrous PRL surge.

More important to the initiation of preovulatory LH and FSH surges is the increased T/R of CAs which occur in ME. Clear temporal relationships exist among increased ME CA T/R, a decline in ME–LHRH and a rise in serum gonadotropins. Since these events do not occur on diestrous day 1, the changes in hormone patterns observed during proestrus are not part of an intrinsic diurnal rhythm. Rather, we suggest that they represent dynamic CNS events which ultimately are required for ovulation in the

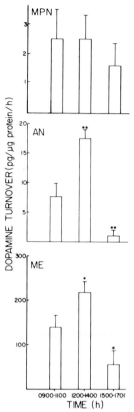

FIG. 3.   DA T/R in discrete MPN and hypothalamic regions (SCN, AN, and ME) during proestrus. Significant increases in DA T/R occur during the 1200- to 1400-hour period compared to 0900–1100 hour rates in the AN and ME but not in the MPN. Thereafter, as NE T/R increase in AN, there is a significant decline in DA T/R in AN and ME but not in MPN between 1500 and 1700 hours. (**, $p < 0.01$; *, $p < 0.05$.) (From Rance *et al.*, 1981b.)

rat. Honma and Wuttke (1980) concluded that the stimulatory action of NE on LHRH release is via its action within the MPN. We disagree, to some extent, with this conclusion and suggest instead that NE may act within the entire preoptico–suprachiasmatic–tuberoinfundibular system including the ME. Since previous studies of serum LH and FSH profiles in our rat colony showed that LH and FSH continued to rise to reach peak concentrations at about 1700 hours, it may be essential that NE release be maintained during this interval (1500–1700 hours) to affect the entire preoptico–suprachiasmatic–tuberoinfundibular system for full expression of gonadotropin surges to occur.

B. EFFECTS OF PHENOBARBITAL ON GONADOTROPIN SURGES AND HYPOTHALAMIC CATECHOLAMINE TURNOVER RATES

In the previous study we provided evidence that an increase in NE T/R could be responsible for the preovulatory release of LHRH during proestrous afternoon. In the present study we attempted to block part of the sequence of events we described on the dynamics of change in ME–LHRH concentrations and NE and DA T/R to determine which of these hypothalamic components is essential for the proestrous gonadotropin surge to occur.

One class of drugs which effectively blocks LH release is the barbiturates. These drugs, when administered prior to the proestrous "critical period," prevent gonadotropin release for 24 hours (Everett and Sawyer, 1950). Barbiturates depress excitability of the midbrain reticular activating system (RAS) (Sawyer et al., 1955; Killam, 1962) but have no effect on pituitary responsiveness to LHRH (Rance and Barraclough, 1981). Since cell bodies of the hypothalamic noradrenergic system reside, in part, within the RAS (Lindvall and Björklund, 1978) it is possible that barbiturates could affect the physiological activation of this CA system.

In the present study we examined the effects of an ovulation blocking dose of phenobarbital (PB) on three component parts of the proestrous LH surge system: (1) the ability of LHRH to induce LH release from the adenohypophysis, (2) the accumulation of LHRH in the ME on proestrous morning, and (3) CA T/R in the MPN, SCN, and ME during proestrus.

Studies in which two pulses of LHRH (50 ng/100 g body weight) were injected iv 60 minutes apart into saline or PB-treated rats revealed no effect of PB on LH release in either group after the first LHRH pulse. Following the second injection of LHRH, LH responses in PB rats were significantly greater than controls (Rance and Barraclough, 1981). Hence, PB does not diminish or abolish the responsiveness of the pituitary gland to LHRH. Further studies revealed that PB does not alter the increased accumulation of ME–LHRH which occurs between 0900 and 1200 hours proestrus. In control rats, LHRH concentrations in the ME rose significantly ($p < 0.01$) from 105.9 ± 8.3 to 181.9 ± 16.5 and in PB from 105.9 ± 8.3 to 177.9 ± 17.2 pg/μg protein between 0900 and 1200 hours confirming earlier observations (Wise et al., 1981c; Rance et al., 1981b).

PB (100 mg/kg body weight ip), when injected at 1200 hours proestrus, effectively prevented the afternoon surge of LH, FSH, PRL, and P_4 and it also significantly reduced plasma E_2 concentrations when compared to saline injection controls.

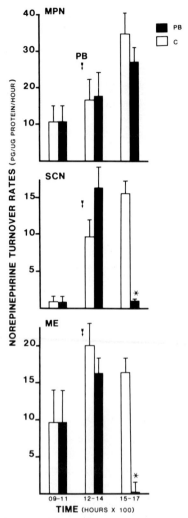

FIG. 4. NE T/R in saline and phenobarbital-treated proestrous rats. Phenobarbital (100 mg/kg body weight), when given at 1200 hours blocks preovulatory gonadotropin surges and markedly suppresses NE T/R between 1500 and 1700 hours in SCN and ME but not in MPN. (*, $p < 0.05$.) (From Rance and Barraclough, 1981.)

In Fig. 4 are shown the effects of PB on NE T/R in MPN, SCN, and ME. In control rats, NE T/R were low between 0900 and 1100 hours, increased significantly between 1200 and 1400 hours, and remained elevated between 1500 and 1700 hours proestrus. The administration of PB at 1200 hours proestrus did not affect the increase in ME–NE T/R which occurred between 1200 and 1400 hours. Further, the increase in NE T/R in MPN recorded between 1500 and 1700 hours also was not affected by PB. In contrast, PB had a dramatic suppressive effect on NE T/R, rate constants, and initial concentrations in the SCN and ME between 1500 and 1700 hours (Fig. 4).

DA T/R in ME of control animals increased significantly between 1200 and 1400 hours and then were significantly reduced between 1500 and 1700 hours confirming our previous observations (Rance et al., 1981b). PB treatment did not prevent the significant decline in ME-DA T/R from occurring between 1500 and 1700 hours.

It is obvious from these studies that the most striking effects of PB treatment are on the hypothalamic noradrenergic system. Since PB did not affect the increased NE T/R which occurred in MPN, these data support the concept that the effective site of NE in evoking LHRH release is not solely MPN as originally proposed by Honma and Wuttke (1980) but also involves other components of the preoptico–suprachiasmatic–tuberoinfundibular LHRH system. In PB-treated proestrous rats, preovulatory gonadotropin surges did not occur and in such animals a decline in both SCN and ME–NE T/R was observed. Since PB does not affect the normal 1200–1400 hour rise nor the 1500–1700 hour decline in ME–DA T/R it seems apparent that the tuberoinfundibular system remains functionally normal. These data add further support to the concept that NE and not DA is the most important CA involved in preovulatory gonadotropin surges.

C. DEVELOPMENT OF AN OVARIECTOMIZED RAT MODEL TO STUDY THE EFFECTS OF STEROIDS ON HYPOTHALAMIC CATECHOLAMINE ACTIVITY

Since rats ovulate once every 4–5 days and this event is closely linked to ovarian follicular development and the rise in serum E_2 which occurs prior to the proestrous gonadotropin surge, we reasoned that perhaps this ovarian steroid was responsible for activating both the preoptico–hypothalamic LHRH system to increase the releasable pool of LHRH in ME axon terminals and to activate the noradrenergic system to trigger the release of this peptide. We recognize that E_2 induces gonadotropin and PRL surges in ovariectomized rats when administered under a variety of experimental paradigms (Caligaris et al., 1971a; DePaolo and Barraclough, 1979a; Legan et al., 1975; Legan and Karsch, 1975). When E_2-primed OVX rats are treated with progesterone (P_4), LH surges are temporally advanced and peak concentrations are greatly amplified (Caligaris et al., 1971b; DePaolo and Barraclough, 1979a,b; Aiyer and Fink, 1974).

The present studies were designed to answer three questions: (1) What are the lowest serum E_2 concentrations which we can produce in 7 day OVX rats which will result in spontaneous LH surges. Also will further increases in serum E_2 concentrations result in the release of greater LH peak concentrations? (2) What are the minimal serum E_2 concentrations which, following P_4 treatment, will result in markedly amplified and temporally advanced LH surges? (3) What effects do various serum E_2 and P_4 levels have on ME–LHRH concentrations (Wise *et al.*, 1981a)?

Shown in Fig. 5 are the results of some of these studies. When Silastic E_2 capsules were implanted sc and changes in plasma LH concentrations were examined 2 days later (day 2), LH surges of equal magnitude (peak values ~1000 ng/ml) occurred in all rats even though plasma E_2 concentrations were increased from OVX levels of 5.4 ± 0.6 to 7.1 ± 0.6 to 9.6 ± 0.5 or even to 15.3 ± 0.9 pg/ml. Since these initial studies we have observed that even at plasma E_2 concentrations of 32.5 ± 1.2 ng/ml, peak LH concentrations on day 2 did not exceed 1000 ng/ml. When we examined the responsiveness of E_2-treated rats to P_4 48 hours later (plasma P_4 = 13.9–15.2 pg/ml) we observed that in rats with plasma E_2 levels of 7–10 pg/ml, P_4 stimulated slightly larger (by 60–80%) gonadotropin surges (Fig. 5). However, when plasma E_2 levels were raised between 15 and 19 pg/ml, the P_4-induced LH surge was 5-fold greater than in animals exposed only to E_2. Interestingly, if plasma E_2 was further increased to 35 pg/ml, P_4 did not further amplify the LH surge. Only at E_2 concentrations of 15 pg/ml or higher and only after supplementary P_4 treatment did LH surges occur which were comparable in magnitude and duration to those observed on proestrus.

ME–LHRH concentrations were significantly higher in rats with plasma E_2 levels of about 15 pg/ml than rats with lower E_2 levels. Statistical analysis of ME–LHRH concentrations revealed a significant interaction between the presence or absence of P_4 and time. When P_4 capsules were implanted at 0900 hours, ME–LHRH concentrations were higher at 1200 hours ($p < 0.05$) than in animals treated only with E_2. Seemingly, one explanation why P_4 amplifies the LH surge is that more LHRH becomes available for release from ME axon terminals and the increase in ME–LHRH in E_2P_4-treated rats represents an increase in the releasable pool size of LHRH. Pituitary responsiveness to LHRH is not different in E_2 versus E_2P_4-treated OVX rats (Blake, 1977).

Having defined a steroid-treated OVX rat model in which we could obtain spontaneous LH surges with low physiological plasma levels of E_2 and in which P_4 markedly amplifies and advances (by 1 hour) the time of onset of LH release, we next examined the effects of such steroid treatment on CA turnover rates in the hypothalamus.

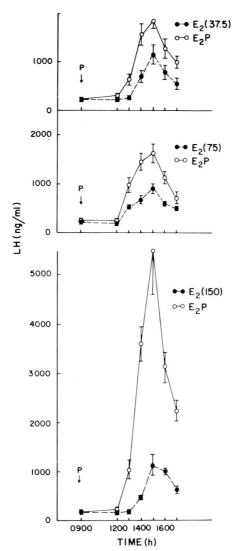

FIG. 5.   Effects of elevating plasma estradiol (E_2) on spontaneous LH surges in ovariectomized (OVX) rats. When Silastic capsules containing 37.5, 75.0, or 150 μg E_2 in oil were
implanted 7 days after OVX and plasma was collected 48 hours later (day 2), spontaneous
LH surges of equal magnitude were obtained even though plasma E_2 levels increased from
5.4 (OVX) to 7.1 (37.5) to 9.6 (75.0) to 15.3 (150) pg/ml. When two Silastic progesterone (P)
capsules (50 mg/ml oil) were placed at 0900 hours day 2, this steroid slightly amplified the
LH surge in rats with E_2 levels of 7.1–9.6 pg/ml. In rats with E_2 levels of 15.3 pg/ml, P
markedly amplified the LH surge. Further, P advanced the time of onset of the LH surge by
1 hour in all groups. (From Wise *et al.*, 1981a.)

D. EFFECTS OF E_2 AND P_4 ON CATECHOLAMINE TURNOVER RATES IN THE HYPOTHALAMUS OF OVARIECTOMIZED RATS

Animals were ovariectomized and 7 days (day 0) later Silastic E_2 capsules were implanted sc (150 μg/ml oil). These capsules produced serum E_2 levels of 13.2 ± 1.8 pg/ml. A second group of OVX rats received an E_2 capsule on day 0 and two P_4 Silastic capsules (50 mg/ml) (serum P_4 = 18.4 ± 2.2 ng/ml) at 0900 hours on day 2. Such steroid treatment resulted in LH surges on day 2 and P_4 advanced and amplified the LH surge in these rats.

Shown in Fig. 6 are the effects of the steroids on NE T/R in ME. E_2-induced LH surges on day 2 were accompanied by an increase in afternoon NE T/R in MPN, AN, SCN, and ME ($p < 0.01$). NE average rate constants in AN, MPN, SCN, and ME also were significantly higher during the afternoon LH surge compared to morning values in E_2-treated rats.

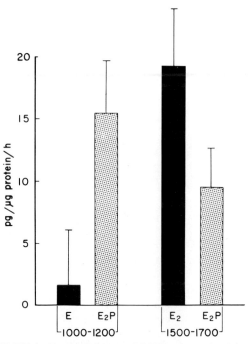

FIG. 6.   ME–NE T/R in E_2 and E_2P-treated OVX rats on day 2. LH surges could be correlated with an increase in NE T/R during the afternoon (1500–1700 hours). P treatment advanced the time of onset of the LH surge and the increase in NE T/R between 1000 and 1200 hours. (From Wise *et al.*, 1981b.)

E_2P_4-induced gonadotropin surges were correlated with increased NE turnover rates in AN and MPN during the afternoon compared to morning values and their patterns were similar to those observed in animals treated with E_2 alone. In contrast, enhanced NE T/R were observed during the morning in SCN and ME of E_2P_4-treated compared to E_2-treated rats (Fig. 6). NE T/R were significantly greater in the ME and SCN in E_2P_4-treated vs E_2-treated rats between 1000 and 1200 hours and they remained high during the afternoon hours.

In contrast to the changes observed in NE T/R, there were no significant changes in initial concentrations, average rate constants or T/R of DA from morning to afternoon in E_2- or E_2P_4-treated rats in ME, AN, or MPN (Wise *et al.*, 1981b).

E. CONCLUSIONS

From this series of studies it is apparent that a close correlation exists between the increased NE T/R observed in the preoptico–hypothalamic LHRH system, and preovulatory and steroid-induced gonadotropin surges. This increase in NE secretion occurs in proestrous and in E_2 or E_2P_4-treated OVX rats. Further, if NE T/R are blocked with phenobarbital (Rance and Barraclough, 1981) or Nembutal (Kalra *et al.*, 1981) gonadotropin surges do not occur.

We believe that several distinct neuroendocrine processes occur on proestrus. The first event is an increase in the releasable pool size of LHRH perhaps due to an increase in the synthesis of new LHRH. This event may occur as the result of rising serum E_2 concentrations and this estrogen, upon entering the LHRH neuronal nucleus, activates genomic processes responsible for the synthesis of LHRH. To date there is little convincing experimental evidence that E_2 increases LHRH synthesis or that P_4 amplifies this E_2 effect. However, the increase in ME–LHRH concentrations in E_2P_4-treated OVX rats, the lack of effect of P_4 on pituitary responsiveness to LHRH in this model, and the dramatic amplification of the LH concentrations spontaneously released by the pituitary gland in E_2P_4-treated rats all suggest that greater concentrations of LHRH are released in E_2P_4-treated versus E_2-treated OVX rats. Secondary to the increase in ME–LHRH there is a dramatic increase in noradrenergic activity (increased NE T/R) within the vicinity of preoptico–suprachiasmatic–tuberoinfundibular LHRH neurons and we suggest that NE could be the neural trigger responsible for the surge release of the gonadotropin hormones. Presumably, estrogen also could be the "zeitgeber" for activation of the hypothalamic noradrenergic system. Whether E_2 acts within NE cell bodies in mid (A_5, A_7) and hindbrain (A_1, A_2) ultimately to increase their frequency of depolarization or on terminal fields within the POA-hypothalamus to increase NE release remains to be resolved. Heritage *et al.* (1980) have identified NE cell bodies in mid and hindbrain and "estrodopaminergic" neurons in the arcuate and periventricular nuclei which concentrate E_2. As well, estrogen cytoplasmic and nuclear and progestin cytosolic receptors exist within the midbrain of rats (MacLusky and McEwen, 1980) and guinea pigs (Blaustein and Feder, 1979a,b, 1980).

We have observed that afternoon increases in NE T/R occur only if the negative feedback effects of E_2 on LH secretion first are manifested. During proestrous morning, LH levels are low and E_2 treatment of OVX rats reduces the high serum levels of LH. In such animals with low morning LH values, NE T/R increase during the afternoon and LH surges occur. In contrast, in long-term castrated rats (day 1 of life) E_2 is ineffective in suppressing the high OVX LH levels after 2 days of treatment and no change in NE T/R occurs from morning to afternoon and LH surges are not observed (Weiland and Barraclough, 1983). Recent evidence suggests that the interaction of estrogen with the central nervous opioid system may account for some of the negative feedback actions of E_2 on LH secretion. Perhaps the opioid–noradrenergic neurons interact in such a manner that suppression of the opioid system permits expression of increased hypothalamic noradrenergic activity (Meites *et al.*, 1979; Kalra and Simpkins, 1981; Korf *et al.*, 1974; Van Vugt *et al.*, 1981).

We believe that NE rather than DA is the CA primarily responsible for triggering the release of LHRH to induce pituitary gonadotropin surges. These conclusions are based upon several observations made in these studies: (1) DA T/R in AN and ME increase in proestrous rats just prior to and during the beginning of the gonadotropin surge but, as LH continues to rise to reach peak plasma LH concentrations, there is an abrupt cessation of tuberoinfundibular dopaminergic activity. DA T/R do not change in the incertohypothalamic terminal field within the preoptic area on proestrus. (2) In E_2- or E_2P_4-treated OVX rats, there are no changes in DA T/R between morning and afternoon even though LH, FSH, and PRL surges occur. (3) Phenobarbital effectively blocks proestrous gonadotropin surges on proestrus but does not affect tuberoinfundibular dopaminergic activity in control proestrous rats. These observations, coupled with those reported from several other laboratories (for review see Barraclough and Wise, 1982), support the concept that NE and not DA is the CA responsible for triggering the preovulatory release of LHRH.

IV. Negative Feedback Effects of Progesterone on Gonadotropin Secretion and Hypothalamic Catecholamine Turnover Rates

While E_2 treatment of OVX rats results in daily afternoon LH surges (Legan et al., 1975; Legan and Karsch, 1975), P_4 has biphasic effects on pituitary LH and FSH release when given to E_2-primed rats (DePaolo and Barraclough, 1979a,b; Caligaris et al., 1971b). P_4 temporally advances and amplifies LH surges on the day that it is given but once P_4-induced gonadotropin surges occur, further 24-hour rhythmic releases of LH and FSH are abolished (DePaolo and Barraclough, 1979a,b; Freeman et al., 1976; Banks and Freeman, 1978). These inhibitory effects of P_4 may serve an important physiological function in limiting the proestrous gonadotropin surge to a single day of the cycle (Freeman et al., 1976). Since hypothalamic CAs and LHRH are important modulators of gonadotropin release, conceivably a mechanism exists by which P_4's inhibitory action is expressed by inducing functional alterations in these systems.

In these studies, 7 day (day 0) OVX rats received E_2 Silastic capsules and 48 hours (day 2) or 72 hours (day 3) later the effects of P_4 on afternoon LH surges on day 2 or day 3 were examined. As is shown in Fig. 7, LH surges were amplified in rats receiving both E_2 and P_4 on day 2. Twenty-

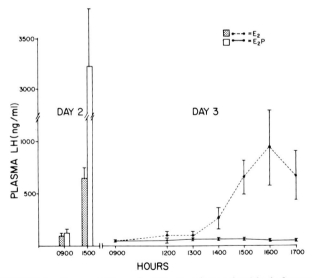

FIG. 7. OVX (7 days) rats which received E_2 capsules on day 0 had afternoon spontaneous LH surges 2 (day 2) and 3 (day 3) days later. When P was administered at 0900 hours day 2 it amplified the LH surge that day but extinguished the diurnal LH surge which normally would have occurred 24 hours later. (From Rance et al., 1981a.)

TABLE II

NE Activity on Day 3[a]

	1000–1200 hours		1500–1700 hours	
	E_2	E_2P	E_2	E_2P
MPN				
Turnover rate (pg/μg protein/hour)	5.7 ± 4.0	7.3 ± 3.6	23.9 ± 4.0[b]	12.5 ± 3.4[c]
Slope (h^{-1})	0.09 ± 0.08	0.11 ± 0.07	0.24 ± 0.05	0.16 ± 0.04
Initial conc. (pg/μg protein)	63.1 ± 4.6	66.4 ± 4.1	99.6 ± 7.8[b]	78.0 ± 3.4[c]
SCN				
Turnover rate	9.2 ± 3.8	0.71 ± 3.7[d]	40.6 ± 5.7[b]	2.2 ± 4.3
Slope	0.23 ± 0.11	0.03 ± 0.19	0.77 ± 0.12[b]	0.04 ± 0.10
Initial conc.	40.1 ± 5.1	23.8 ± 4.5[d]	52.8 ± 4.4	55.8 ± 6.5
ME				
Turnover rate	1.1 ± 3.8	5.3 ± 4.6	20.9 ± 5.8[b]	13.9 ± 6.7
Slope	0.02 ± 0.09	0.08 ± 0.09	0.22 ± 0.08	0.15 ± 0.09
Initial conc.	50.9 ± 7.6	66.4 ± 4.9	94.9 ± 6.9[b]	93.0 ± 10.4
AN				
Turnover rate	6.56 ± 3.8	14.9 ± 3.4	14.4 ± 3.1	7.86 ± 3.3
Slope	0.14 ± 0.10	0.25 ± 0.07	0.22 ± 0.06	0.11 ± 0.06
Initial conc.	46.9 ± 6.9	59.8 ± 4.1	65.3 ± 6.8	71.5 ± 6.5

[a] n = 22–24 determinations for turnover rate; n = 15–16 rats for slope; n = 7–8 rats for initial concentration.

[b] $p < 0.01$ compared values at 1000–1200 hours with same hormone treatment.

[c] $p < 0.05$ compared to E_2-oil-treated rats at the same time.

[d] $p < 0.01$ compared to E_2-oil-treated rats at the same time.

four hours later, rats with only E_2 capsules again had LH surges but the LH surge was extinguished in those animals which were exposed to P_4 on day 2. The effects of P_4 on NE T/R on day 3 are presented in Table II. Rats that received only E_2 capsules had increased NE T/R during the afternoon (1500–1700 hours) of day 3 in ME, SCN, and MPN. DA T/R declined in AN but not in the ME or MPN from morning to afternoon of day 3 in E_2-treated rats. All of these animals had LH surges on day 3. In contrast, when P_4 was administered on day 2 it extinguished the increase in NE T/R observed in E_2-treated rats on day 3 and NE T/R remained unchanged between morning and afternoon in ME (Fig. 8), SCN, and AN of E_2P_4-treated rats. A striking difference also was observed in DA T/R in E_2P_4-treated versus E_2-treated rats on day 3. MPN, AN, and ME DA T/R were markedly increased between the AM and PM hours. This result was most pronounced in the ME which exhibited a 3-fold increase in DA T/R

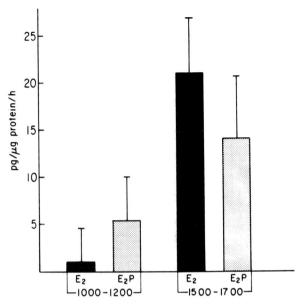

FIG. 8. NE T/R were examined on day 3 in rats which received only E_2 on day 0 or in estrogen-primed rats which also were treated with P on day 2. ME–NE T/R increased from morning to afternoon in E_2-treated rats and similar T/R increases were observed in MPN and SCN but not in AN. In contrast, in E_2P-treated rats, NE T/R did not increase in MPN, ME, SCN, or AN during the afternoon of day 3 and LH surges did not occur in these rats. (From Rance *et al.*, 1981a.)

and a 2-fold increase in rate constants and initial concentrations (Fig. 9) (Rance *et al.*, 1981a).

CONCLUSIONS

It is apparent from these studies that the diurnal release of LH in E_2-treated OVX rats is accompanied by an increased NE T/R within neuro-anatomical areas which also contain the preoptico–hypothalamic LHRH system. Presumably, if we had performed additional temporal studies on noradrenergic function in E_2-treated rats which exhibit daily afternoon LH surges for at least 5 consecutive days, we also would have detected similar temporal diurnal increases in hypothalamic NE T/R. As well, the failure of DA T/R to change in rats subjected to 2 or 3 days of E_2 treatment further argues against a stimulatory role of DA in the surge release of LHRH. Adding further support to the concept that the surge release of LHRH is triggered by an increase in the secretion of NE are the observations that 24 hours after P_4 exposure, when LH surges are extinguished,

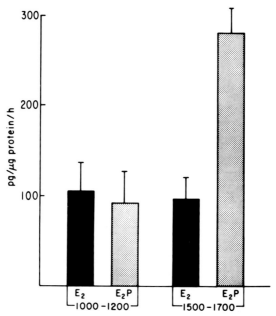

FIG. 9. ME–DA T/R in E_2-treated rats on day 3 did not change between morning and afternoon. In contrast, DA T/R were markedly increased in the afternoon in the ME, AN, and MPN of E_2P-treated OVX rats. (From Rance *et al.*, 1981a.)

afternoon increases in NE T/R also are abolished. This lack of increased NE secretion (T/R) may account for the complete failure of LHRH to be released in these E_2P_4-treated rats. Also, hypothalamic DA activity in E_2-treated rats which exhibit gonadotropin surges is considerably different from that observed in E_2P_4-treated animals on day 3. DA T/R are markedly increased in the afternoon in ME, AN, MPN of E_2P_4- versus E_2-treated rats. These observations correlate well with studies by others who reported an increase in DA concentrations in portal plasma 24 hours after the administration of P_4 to acutely OVX, adrenalectomized proestrous rats (Cramer *et al.*, 1979). Perhaps, the P_4 effect of increasing DA T/R in discrete hypothalamic areas provides another mechanism by which LH release is inhibited. Although pharmacological studies on the role of DA in releasing LHRH have been inconsistent (Sawyer *et al.*, 1978; Ojeda and McCann, 1978), increased ME DA T/R has been reported in rats made acyclic by constant light or by androgen sterilization (Fuxe *et al.*, 1972) and in OVX rats receiving pharmacological doses of E_2 to inhibit LH release (Fuxe *et al.*, 1977). However, these increases in ME DA turnovers could be due to the increased secretion of PRL which occurs secondary to the elevated plasma E_2 levels observed in the studies of

Fuxe *et al.* (1977) or in androgen-sterilized or light-induced constant estrous rats. In summary, on the day that P_4 exerts its negative feedback actions on LH release (day 3), NE T/R decrease and DA T/R increase in discrete hypothalamic nuclei. These effects may be one mechanism by which P_4 suppresses LH and FSH secretion in E_2-primed and proestrous rats.

V. Function of the Hypothalamic Catecholaminergic System in Neonatally Androgen-Sterilized Rats

A. ADULT STERILE RATS

Neonatal androgen treatment of female rats renders these animals permanently infertile as adults. Such animals exhibit persistent vaginal estrus and lack cyclic preovulatory LH and FSH surges (Barraclough, 1961; Gorski, 1971; Chappel and Barraclough, 1976). Recent studies established several facts regarding the function of the preoptico–suprachiasmatic–tuberoinfundibular system (PSTS) in adult androgen-sterilized rats (ASR): (1) the numbers of LHRH perikarya and the distribution of their processes throughout the hypothalamus do not differ in ASR and normal female rats (King *et al.*, 1980); (2) sufficient LHRH is synthesized, transported, and stored in axon terminals in the PSTS of ASR to evoke preovulatory-like LH and FSH surges when depolarizing stimuli are delivered to the MPN (Kubo *et al.*, 1975; Chappel and Barraclough, 1976); (3) pituitary responsiveness to LHRH is the same in ASR and cyclic proestrous rats (Mennin *et al.*, 1974; Boverdig *et al.*, 1972); and (4) estrogen receptor numbers and binding affinities are normal in the preoptico–hypothalamic region and E_2-induced progestin cytosol receptor concentrations also are normal in ASR (Barley *et al.*, 1977; Etgen, 1981).

In spite of apparent normal physiological processes occurring in the PSTS, the positive feedback induction of LH and FSH surges by steroids (Mennin and Gorski, 1975; Harlan and Gorski, 1977) and the spontaneous preovulatory release of these gonadotropins do not occur in ASR. Apparently, what is lacking is the neural signal responsible for the discharge of LHRH from ME axon terminals.

In the present study we evaluated the responses of hypothalamic CA neurons to estrogen in adult ASR and normal cyclic rats to establish if this system retains its steroid responsive physiological properties following prepubertal androgen exposure (Lookingland *et al.*, 1982).

All Sprague–Dawley rats were born in our colony and received either testosterone propionate (50 μg sc) or were not injected at 5 days of age. Between 100 and 120 days of age ASR or cyclic control rats were OVX and 7 days later Silastic capsules containing 150 μg E_2 in oil were implanted sc. Either 2 or 3 days later (days 2 or 3) some of these animals received P_4 Silastic capsules and their plasma hormone profiles were evaluated.

Illustrated in Fig. 10 are the plasma LH responses obtained after E_2 or E_2P_4 treatment of control and ASR. While LH surges occurred on days 3 and 4 in E_2-treated rats and P_4 amplified the LH surge on the day that it was administered (day 3), no positive feedback effects of E_2 or P_4 occurred in ASR. In OVX controls and ASR, E_2 was equally effective in suppressing high castration LH levels (Lookingland et $al.$, 1982).

The response of the hypothalamic noradrenergic system in E_2-treated

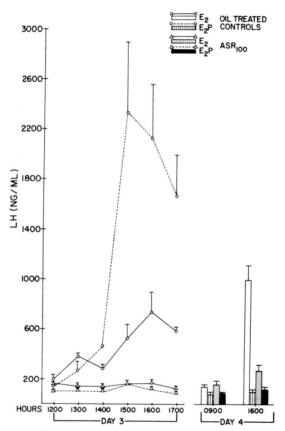

FIG. 10. Patterns of LH release in 100-day-old OVX E_2- or E_2P-treated control or androgen-sterilized rats (ASR). Spontaneous LH surges occurred in controls but not in ASR 3 and 4 days after placing Silastic E_2 capsules. P amplified and advanced the time of onset of the LH surge in E_2-treated controls and extinguished the LH surge 24 hours later in control rats but it had no effect in E_2-primed ASR. (From Lookingland et $al.$, 1982.)

OVX controls and ASR are shown in Fig. 11. In E_2-treated castrates, NE T/R increased significantly between morning and afternoon in ME, MPN, and SCN, but not in AN. In contrast, no increases in NE T/R were detected in ME or MPN of ASR. However, SCN and AN NE T/R were increased significantly between morning and afternoon in ASR. The increased T/R observed in AN of ASR should be interpreted with caution since neither initial concentrations nor rate constants changed between 1000 and 1700 hours in this region.

A second interesting observation involved differences in initial NE concentrations in ASR versus control animals. When initial NE concentrations obtained at 1000 hours were compared between groups it was observed that all microdissected brain regions in ASR contained significantly less NE than controls. Thus ME, AN, MPN, and SCN concentrations in ASR were only 40, 41, 24, and 65%, respectively, of the NE concentration measured in control rats.

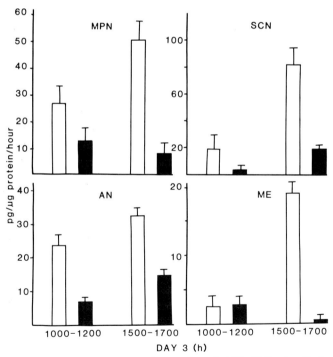

FIG. 11. NE T/R in OVX E_2-treated controls and ASR. Following E_2 treatment of controls (open bars) NE T/R increased significantly between 1000 and 1200 and 1500 and 1700 hours in MPN, SCN, AN, and ME. In contrast, only SCN and AN showed slight increases but ME and MPN had no increase in NE T/R (solid bars). (From Lookingland *et al.*, 1982.)

DA T/R in control rats showed a significant decline between morning and afternoon in ME. In AN and MPN, DA T/R were significantly increased in the afternoon versus morning. In ASR, DA T/R were less in the afternoon than the morning in ME but in AN and MPN these changes in T/R were not evident.

The data obtained on LH secretion profiles in control and adult ASR confirm previous observations (DePaolo and Barraclough, 1979a; Mennin and Gorski, 1975; Harlan and Gorski, 1977). Thus, when ASR reach adulthood (100–120 days of age) they are incapable of responding after ovariectomy to E_2 or E_2P_4 by having spontaneous LH surges which are exhibited in control rats.

Many attempts have been made to identify the pathophysiological cause for infertility produced by neonatal androgen treatment. While most investigations focused on changes which occur in the neuroanatomy or in the functional properties of the preoptico–hypothalamic LHRH system in ASR, more recent studies suggest that LHRH synthesis and release can occur in ASR but the neural trigger responsible for the discharge of this peptide is absent. In the earlier studies presented in this article we have presented evidence which suggests that the increased release of hypothalamic NE may serve as the physiological trigger for LHRH release. Consequently, we were not surprised to learn that NE T/R do not change in ME and MPN between morning and afternoon in E_2-treated ASR. Further, because of the low initial concentrations of NE in SCN, the amount of NE available for release in this nucleus is markedly less than that obtained in control animals. In the absence of any increase in NE release into the MPN and ME, the release of low NE concentrations into SCN may be inadequate to initiate the release of LHRH. Exactly how much of the preoptico–suprachiasmatic–tuberoinfundibular LHRH system must be activated by NE to induce LH surges remains to be resolved.

The cause for the reduced NE concentrations in the hypothalamus also is not known. Whether the differences in initial NE concentrations between steroid-treated OVX controls and ASR represent differential responsiveness to E_2, or are due to a defect in the NE synthesis pathway or to a loss of numbers of neurons (or all of these) requires further study. What is evident is that very little NE is available for release, particularly from axon terminals within ME and SCN.

B. DELAYED ANOVULATORY SYNDROME

The administration of low doses of androgen to neonatal female rats results in the delayed anovulatory syndrome (DAS) (Swanson and van der

Werff ten Bosch, 1964; Harlan and Gorski, 1977). In such animals, ovulatory cyclicity continues for some weeks to months after puberty before preovulatory gonadotropin surges cease prematurely and the rats become anovulatory. During the interval that lightly androgenized rats are cyclic they exhibit spontaneous LH surges in response to E_2, whereas upon becoming anovulatory, this positive feedback effect of E_2 disappears.

In this final series of studies we examined further the responsiveness of the noradrenergic system to E_2 in rats displaying the DAS. We questioned whether NE T/R increase in discrete hypothalamic areas in OVX-androgenized rats (AR) which exhibit LH surges in response to E_2 at 50–55 days of age and if this response is lost in similarly aged ASR which already have entered anovulation.

The neonatal female rats used in these studies were injected either with 50 μg of testosterone propionate at 5 days of age or with sesame oil (control) and were placed into various experimental groups between 50 and 55 days of age. A considerable number of studies were performed on these rats to define serum hormone profiles, cyclic behavior, and response to E_2 and these results previously have been published (Lookingland and Barraclough, 1982). From these studies we were able to separate AR which had normal estrous cyclicity (androgenized normal rats = ANR) from AR which displayed persistent vaginal cornification (androgen sterilized rats = ASR) not only on the basis of vaginal cytology but also by differences in ovarian weight. ANR and control rats had ovaries weighing 82–89.7 mg whereas ASR ovaries weighed only 34 ± 2.1 mg. Shown in Table III are the responses of 7 day OVX control, ASR, and ANR to 3 days of E_2 or of P_4 treatment of E_2-primed rats on day 3. All AR and control rats responded to 7 days of ovarian removal by a significant increase in serum LH and a significant reduction in prolactin (PRL). E_2 treatment for 3 days significantly lowered serum LH, and elevated serum PRL and E_2 concentrations in all groups. LH concentrations in E_2-treated controls and ANR were increased significantly by 1700 versus 1000 hours but a further elevation in serum LH in E_2P_4-treated rats was not observed in either group. However, in other groups of sequentially bled control animals (data not shown), P_4 amplified and temporally advanced the LH surge. LH surges did not occur in E_2 or E_2P_4-treated 50- to 55-day-old ASR.

NE T/R in controls, ANR and ASR are shown in Fig. 12. Significant increases in NE T/R occurred between morning and afternoon in controls and ANR in ME, MPN, and SCN, but not in AN. A similar increase in T/R was obtained in the SCN of ASR but these values were significantly less than ANR or control values. In contrast, no increases in NE T/R occurred during the afternoon in ME, AN, or MPN of ASR in response to

TABLE III

Positive and Negative Effects of E_2 or E_2P Determined in Day 3 Decapitated Ovariectomized Control Rats, ANR, and ASR

Hormones	LH (ng/ml)	PRL (ng/ml)[j]	E_2 (pg/ml)	P_4 (ng/ml)
OVX—1000 hours				
Control (7)	765.0 ± 123.3	ND (<3.0)	3.5 ± 0.3	1.1 ± 0.3
AR (5)	582.0 ± 154.7	8.8 ± 3.6	6.0 ± 0.4[e]	2.1 ± 0.4
OVX + E_2—1000 hours				
Control (7)	153.6 ± 10.3[a]	6.1 ± 2.3[a]	9.8 ± 0.8	2.2 ± 0.4[i]
ANR (9)	146.3 ± 7.2[b]	29.4 ± 5.8[c,e]	11.9 ± 0.8[b]	2.2 ± 0.4
ASR (8)	119.3 ± 9.6[b]	59.4 ± 18.4[e,f]	9.5 ± 0.4[a]	2.2 ± 0.5
OVX + E_2P—1700 hours				
Control (13)	1513.8 ± 196.9[c]	211.8 ± 45.2[c]	10.4 ± 0.5[a]	1.5 ± 0.3
ANR (7)	818.1 ± 170.3[d]	71.9 ± 24.8	8.2 ± 0.9[e]	1.5 ± 0.4
ASR (12)	134.8 ± 17.8	99.5 ± 28.4	9.1 ± 0.7	1.5 ± 0.3
OVX + E_2—1700 hours				
Control (9)	2239.2 ± 313.4[c]	190.7 ± 31.0[c]	12.8 ± 0.8[a]	8.7 ± 0.9[h]
ANR (3)	1314.3 ± 390.2[d]	227.0 ± 84.0[g]	17.0 ± 1.0[e,f]	8.7 ± 0.8[h]
ASR (5)	88.8 ± 30.9	147.5 ± 42.4	11.6 ± 0.9	10.9 ± 1.0[h]

[a] $p < 0.001$ vs OVX control 1000 hours.
[b] $p < 0.01$ vs OVX AR 1000 hours.
[c] $p < 0.001$ vs OVX E_2-treated control 1000 hours.
[d] $p < 0.01$ vs OVX E_2-treated ANR 1000 hours.
[e] $p < 0.01$ vs OVX control 1000 hours.
[f] $p < 0.05$ vs OVX E_2-treated ASR vs ANR 1000 hours.
[g] $p < 0.001$ vs E_2-treated ANR 1700 hours.
[h] $p < 0.001$ vs E_2-treated control, ASR or ANR 1700 hours.
[i] $p < 0.05$ vs OVX control 1000 hours.
[j] PRL RP-2 standard.

E_2 treatment and plasma LH surges did not occur in these rats. Thus, there is a clear, direct correlation between those AR which respond to estrogen treatment with an LH surge and those animals which have increases in rate constants and NE T/R during the afternoon of day 3.

When NE initial concentrations at 1000 hours were compared between controls versus ANR versus ASR there were no significant differences between controls and ANR. However, in ASR all microdissected areas examined contained significantly less NE concentrations than control rats at 1000 hours and similarly reduced NE concentrations also were observed in ASR versus ANR at 1000 hours.

DA T/R more or less paralleled those obtained in control and ASR at 100 days of age and could not be correlated with whether or not LH surges occurred in response to E_2. It is doubtful if the minor DA T/R changes we observed in these studies play a major role in regulating the surge of LH.

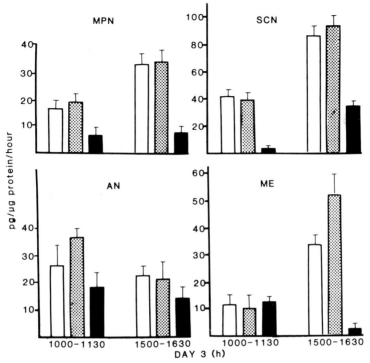

FIG. 12. NE T/R changes in OVX E_2-treated 50–55 day controls (open bars), andro-genized normal rats (ANR) (hatched bars), or ASR (black bars) which occurred between 1000 and 1130 and 1500 and 1630 hours on day 3. LH surges occurred in controls and ANR but not in ASR in response to E_2. Significant increases in NE T/R occurred between morning and afternoon in controls and ANR in MPN, SCN, and ME but not in AN. Increased NE T/R also were observed in the SCN of ASR between morning and afternoon of day 3. In contrast, no increase in NE T/R occurred in the afternoon in ME, AN, or MPN of ASR in response to E_2 treatment and plasma LH surges did not occur in these rats. (From Lookingland and Barraclough, 1982.)

C. CONCLUSIONS

These studies confirm and extend earlier reports that treatment of neo-natal female rats with a low dose of androgen results in a high percentage of rats having ovulatory cycles for a brief interval after puberty before they develop the anovulatory syndrome. It should be emphasized that *all* androgenized rats which have LH surges in response to E_2 at 50–55 days of age will become permanently unresponsive to E_2 by 100 days of age.

When initial concentrations, rate constants, and T/R of NE were com-pared between E_2-treated 50- to 55-day-old controls and ANR, no signifi-cant differences were detected in NE dynamics in most all of the micro-

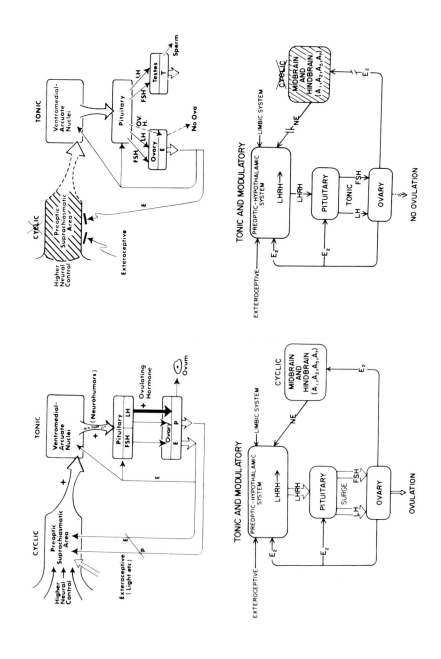

dissected brain areas examined. In contrast, in ASR which failed to respond to E_2 with LH surges, there were no changes in NE T/R or in rate constants in ME, AN, or MPN between morning and afternoon. However, an increase in rate constants and T/R occurred in SCN between morning and afternoon and these observations in ASR at 50–55 days of age are identical to those obtained by us in adult ASR.

Barraclough and Gorski (1961) previously proposed that exposure of neonatal female rats to androgen permanently disrupted normal function of the preoptic brain. As a result of these early pioneering studies, they hypothesized that the center for the cyclic control of gonadotropin secretion resides within the preoptic area whereas the tonic control of basal gonadotropin secretion was located within the arcuate-median eminence region (Fig. 13). We now recognize that lesions or retrochiasmatic transections which produce a syndrome of anovulation and persistent estrus similar to that observed in ASR may be due to a mechanical disruption of the PSTS–LHRH system rather than to an effect on the neural mechanisms involved in the surge release of the gonadotropic hormones. More recent evidence suggests that LHRH neurons in ASR and in rats exhibiting the delayed anovulatory syndrome retain most of their normal physiological properties. They synthesize, transport, and store LHRH in ME terminals; LHRH perikaryal estrogen and progestin cytosol receptors are similar in concentration to cyclic rats, and after depolarization of LHRH neurons, this peptide is released to produce LH surges equal in magnitude to those obtained in normal rats. Consequently, we believe that this original hypothesis should be revised to include the current information obtained in our studies on the function of the hypothalamic catecholaminergic system in androgen-sterilized rats.

FIG. 13. In 1961 (top), Barraclough and Gorski (1961) hypothesized that the POA-SCN area was the center for the cyclic control of gonadotropin secretion. On activation of the POA-SCN, preovulatory LH and FSH surges and ovulation occurred and this activation process involved an increase in plasma E_2 during diestrous day 2 and proestrus. At this time we proposed that neonatal androgenization deleteriously affected the POA-SCN in such a manner that normal function of this brain region was abolished and only the arcuate-median eminence control of tonic gonadotropin secretion remained functional. This basal secretion of LH and FSH was adequate to induce ovarian follicular growth and steroid production in ASR and, in male rats, it was sufficient to maintain normal testicular function. Recent evidence (1982, bottom) suggests that the preoptico–suprachiasmatic–tuberoinfundibular LHRH system in androgen-sterilized rats retains most of its normal physiological properties but the noradrenergic system fails to respond to the positive feedback effects of estrogen. We have presented considerable evidence that an increase in NE secretion may be the trigger responsible for the LHRH surge. Consequently, in the absence of an increase in hypothalamic NE T/R, the anovulatory persistent estrous syndrome ensues.

The data obtained on hypothalamic catecholamine dynamics in DAS or adult sterile rats, considered together with the changes which occur in NE T/R in other rat models we described, lead us to suggest that perhaps the noradrenergic system contains the "surge-inducing" neurons whose cell bodies and dendritic fields reside in the mid and hindbrain and whose axons project via the median forebrain bundle to terminate in the vicinity of components of the PSTS (Fig. 13). Further, we believe that these data add a new dimension to our understanding of the neural processes involved in the discharge of LH and one explanation for the cause of the DAS. If we accept the hypothesis that it is the rise in plasma estradiol on proestrus which activates both the LHRH and noradrenergic systems, and the resultant increase in hypothalamic NE T/R triggers preovulatory gonadotropin surges, then it is logical to conclude that any loss of NE neuronal responsiveness to estrogen would result in a loss of the LH surge mechanism and anovulation would occur. This is exactly what happens as neonatally androgenized rats pass through the transition phase from ovulatory cyclicity to the anovulatory persistent estrous syndrome.

VI. Summary and General Conclusions

Recently, Palkovits (1982) summarized published information on the radioimmunoassay and immunocytochemical identification of neuropeptides in the rat median eminence. Fourteen neuropeptides have been identified and of these, at least 5 have been reported to affect the function of the LHRH neuron. Coupled with these observations are other reports on the inhibitory or stimulatory effects of classical neurotransmitters as NE, DA, acetylcholine, etc. on LHRH release. Whether such reported effects of neuropeptides and of many of the neurotransmitters on LHRH secretion are physiological processes normally involved in the regulation of gonadotropin secretion or are nonspecified pharmacological effects observed when high concentrations of these substances are injected into the vicinity of the LHRH terminals (i.e., third ventricle) remains to be resolved.

In the sequence of studies presented in this article we have avoided, as much as possible, the pharmacological approach to the study of neurotransmitter regulation of LHRH secretion and the complexities inherent in the interpretation of such data. Rather, we focused our attention on a classical neurotransmitter system which, for the past 36 years, has been implicated as a regulator of LHRH secretion. Whether NE secretion is the ultimate regulator of LHRH release through which many of the other neural peptides and transmitters indirectly act to affect LHRH release is not known. Nevertheless, we believe that by measuring turnover rates (an index of secretion) of NE and DA in discretely microdissected nuclei in the hypothalami of a variety of animal models and correlating such changes in CA T/R with the presence or absence of gonadotropin surges we can provide reasonably convincing evidence that NE indeed may be the neural trigger for preovulatory-like surges of LHRH. In our first series of studies in proestrous rats we described an important sequence of events which precedes and accompanies the preovulatory secretion of LH, FSH, and PRL (Fig. 14). These consist of the following: (1) 0900–1200 hours: an increased accumulation of LHRH in the PSTS including ME (Wise *et al.*, 1981c; Rance *et al.*, 1981b); during this interval, NE and DA T/R are low and LH, FSH, and PRL serum levels are basal (Rance *et al.*, 1981b); (2) 1200–1400 hours: increased ME, NE, and DA T/R; (3) 1500–1700 hours: increased NE T/R not only are maintained in ME but are now also evident in the MPN, SCN, and AN. A decline in ME DA T/R also occurs at this time. In these same animals, ME–LHRH declines between 1200 and 1500 hours and LH, FSH, and PRL serum concentrations increase (Rance *et al.*, 1981b). We interpret the increase in hypothalamic NE secretion coupled with the decreases in ME–LHRH and the increase in serum gonadotropins to mean that NE initiates the preovulatory surge of gonadotropins by evoking the release of newly accumulated LHRH from ME axon terminals. If increased NE T/R are blocked by phenobarbital (Rance and Barraclough, 1981) or extinguished 24 hours after P_4 treatment, or after neonatal treatment with androgen (Lookingland *et al.*, 1982; Lookingland and Barraclough, 1982), LH, FSH, and PRL surges do not occur and in ASR the anovulatory persistent estrous syndrome develops (Fig. 14).

Seemingly, the entire sequence of neuroendocrine events which ultimately leads to ovulation depends on the maturation of ovarian follicles which, under the influence of basal concentrations of LH and FSH, increase their secretion of estrogen into blood during diestrous day 2 and proestrous morning. We suggest that estrogen not only may increase the releasable pool size of ME–LHRH (presumably via increased synthesis) but it also is essential for the increased release of NE during the early afternoon of proestrus. These conclusions are based in part on the observations that estrogen treatment of OVX rats results in increased afternoon T/R of hypothalamic NE and gonadotropin surges (Wise *et al.*, 1981b) and that P_4 treatment of E_2-treated OVX rats temporally advances and amplifies the LH surge. Concomitant with these P_4 effects is an increase in ME–LHRH concentrations. Additionally, estrogen-positive feedback effects on gonadotropin secretion are absent in ASR and the hypothalamic noradrenergic system is nonfunctional in these animals. These sequential CNS processes may be genomically programmed events whose expression depends upon adequate concentrations and duration of exposure to endogenous estrogen.

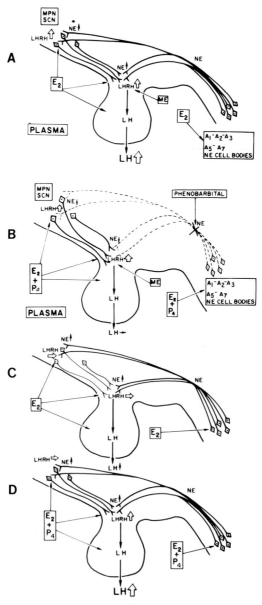

FIG. 14. Diagrammatic representation of the sequence of events which may occur within the hypothalamus to evoke the surge release of LHRH and LH. (A) In proestrous rats, in response to rising serum levels of E_2, an increase in the concentration of LHRH occurs in LHRH neurons between 0900 and 1200 hours. Presumably, LHRH synthesis occurs within the perikarya of the LHRH neuron within the MPN and it is transported and

ACKNOWLEDGMENTS

These studies were supported by Grant HD-02138 to C. A. Barraclough from the National Institutes of Health. Drs. P. M. Wise and M. Selmanoff are recipients of RCDAs AG-0018 and NS-00731, respectively.

REFERENCES

Ahren, K., Fuxe, K., Hamberger, L., and Hökfelt, T. (1971). *Endrocrinology* **88,** 1415–1424.
Aiyer, M. S., and Fink, G. (1974). *J. Endocrinol.* **62,** 553–572.
Banks, J. A., and Freeman, M. E. (1978). *Endocrinology* **102,** 426–432.
Barley, J., Ginsberg, M., MacLusky, N. J., Morris, I. D., and Thomas, P. J. (1977). *Brain Res.* **129,** 309–318.
Barraclough, C. A. (1961). *Endocrinology* **68,** 62–67.
Barraclough, C. A., and Gorski, R. A. (1961). *Endocrinology* **68,** 68–79.
Barraclough, C. A., and Sawyer, C. H. (1957). *Endocrinology* **61,** 341–351.
Barraclough, C. A., and Sawyer, C. H. (1959). *Endocrinology* **65,** 563–571.
Barraclough, C. A., and Wise, P. M. (1982). *Endocrine Rev.* **3,** 91–119.
Blake, C. A. (1977). *Endocrinology* **101,** 1130–1134.

---

stored within ME–LHRH axon terminals (Wise *et al.,* 1981c). E_2 also may directly or indirectly increase the frequency of depolarization of the noradrenergic neurons to increase the release of NE into the vicinity of LHRH neurons and we suggest that the increase in NE T/R which occurs between 1200 and 1700 hours in ME and 1500 and 1700 hours in MPN and SCN serves as the neural trigger for the surge release of LHRH and ultimately of LH into serum. (B) When phenobarbital is administered to proestrous rats, the morning accumulation of LHRH in the ME still occurs but increased afternoon NE T/R in the hypothalamus are blocked (Rance and Barraclough, 1981). Further, if progesterone (P_4) is administered to E_2-primed rats, a similar blockade of increased NE T/R occurs (Rance *et al.,* 1981a). Similarly, if neonatal female rats are sterilized with androgen the preoptico–suprachiasmatic–tuberoinfundibular LHRH system remains functional but the hypothalamic noradrenergic system is permanently disrupted and no increase in NE T/R occurs in response to estrogen (Lookingland *et al.,* 1982; Lookingland and Barraclough, 1982). All of these animal preparations fail to have LH surges in response to estrogen. (C) In OVX rats, the replacement of E_2 to produce a variety of serum E_2 concentrations ranging from 9 to 35 pg/ml results in increases in hypothalamic NE T/R although the LH surges which occur during the afternoon have similar peak concentrations regardless of the serum E_2 concentrations produced. Unlike proestrous rats, there is no significant rise in ME–LHRH concentrations between 0900 and 1200 hours which suggests that E_2 replacement alone is insufficient to replicate those hormonal events which precede and accompany the preovulatory gonadotropin surge on proestrus. (D) When progesterone is administered to E_2-primed OVX rats, a significant increase in ME–LHRH occurs between 0900 and 1200 hours and when increased hypothalamic NE T/R occur there is a marked amplification of LH surge concentrations. Further, NE advances the time at which increased hypothalamic NE T/R occur and it also advances (by 1 hour) the time of the LH surge. Since P_4 does not increase the responsiveness of the pituitary gland to LHRH in E_2-primed rats either greater amounts of NE are released for a more prolonged period to amplify the quantity of LHRH released from the ME axon terminal and/or a greater releasable pool of LHRH exists and is secreted in E_2P_4 versus E_2-treated OVX rats (or both) to account for amplification of the LH surge. (Wise *et al.,* 1981b.)

Blank, M. S., Diez, J. A., and Roberts, D. L. (1983). *Endocrine Soc. Abstr.* No. 143.
Blaustein, J. D., and Feder, H. H. (1979a). *Brain Res.* **169**, 481–497.
Blaustein, J. D., and Feder, H. H. (1979b). *Brain Res.* **177**, 489–498.
Blaustein, J. D., and Feder, H. H. (1980). *Endocrinology* **106**, 1061–1069.
Boverdig, J., Hermann, H. J., and Bajusz, S. (1972). *J. Endocrinol.* **55**, 207–208.
Brittain, R. T., Jack, D., and Ritchie, A. C. (1970). *Adv. Drug Res.* **5**, 197–253.
Brodie, B. B., Costa, E., Dlabac, A., Neff, H., and Smookler, H. H. (1966). *J. Pharmacol. Exp. Ther.* **154**, 493–498.
Caligaris, L., Astrada, J. J., and Taleisnik, S. (1971a). *Endocrinology* **88**, 810–815.
Caligaris, L., Astrada, J. J., and Taleisnik, S. (1971b). *Brain Res.* **192**, 421–432.
Carlsson, A. (1964). *Prog. Brain Res.* **8**, 9–27.
Chappel, S. C., and Barraclough, C. A. (1976). *Biol. Reprod.* **15**, 661–669.
Costa, E., and Neff, N. H. (1970). *Handb. Neurochem.* **4**, 45–90.
Cramer, O. M., Parker, C. R., and Porter, J. C. (1979). *Endocrinology* **105**, 929–933.
DePaolo, L. V., and Barraclough, C. A. (1979a). *Biol. Reprod.* **20**, 1173–1185.
DePaolo, L. V., and Barraclough, C. A. (1979b). *Biol. Reprod.* **21**, 1015–1023.
Etgen, A. M. (1981). *Biol. Reprod.* **25**, 307–313.
Everett, J. W., and Sawyer, C. H. (1950). *Endocrinology* **47**, 198–218.
Everett, J. W., Sawyer, C. H., and Markee, J. E. (1949). *Endocrinology* **44**, 234–250.
Freeman, M. C., Dupke, K. C., and Croteau, C. M. (1976). *Endocrinology* **99**, 223–229.
Fuxe, K., Hokfelt, T., and Nelsson, O. (1972). *Acta Endocrinol. (Copenhagen)* **69**, 625–639.
Fuxe, K., Lofstrom, A., Eneroth, P., Gustafsson, J. A., Skett, P., and Hokfelt, T. (1977). *Psychoneuroendocrinology* **2**, 203–225.
Gorski, R. A. (1971). *In* "Frontiers of Neuroendocrinology" (L. Martini and W. F. Ganong, eds.), pp. 237–290. Oxford Univ. Press, London and New York.
Harlan, R. E., and Gorski, R. A. (1977). *Endocrinology* **101**, 741–749.
Heritage, A. S., Stumpf, W. E., Sar, M., and Grant, L. D. (1980). *Science* **207**, 1377–1380.
Honma, K., and Wuttke, K. (1980). *Endocrinology* **106**, 1848–1853.
Kalra, S. P., and Simpkins, J. W. (1981). *Endocrinology* **109**, 776–782.
Kalra, S. P., Simpkins, J. W., and Kalra, P. S. (1981). *Endocrinology* **108**, 1299–1304.
Killam, K. K. (1962). *Pharmacol. Rev.* **14**, 175–223.
King, J. C., Tobet, S. A., Snavely, F. L., and Arimura, A. A. (1980). *Peptides* **1**, 85–100.
Korf, J., Bunney, B. S., and Aghajanian, G. F. (1974). *Eur. J. Pharmacol.* **25**, 165–169.
Kubo, K., Mennin, S. P., and Gorski, R. A. (1975). *Endocrinology* **96**, 492–500.
Legan, S. J., and Karsch, F. J. (1975). *Endocrinology* **96**, 57–62.
Legan, S. J., Coon, G. A., and Karsch, F. J. (1975). *Endocrinology* **96**, 50–56.
Lindvall, O. and Björklund, A. (1978). *Handb. Psychopharmacol.* **9**, 139–231.
Löfström, A. (1977). *Brain Res.* **120**, 113–131.
Lookingland, K. J., and Barraclough, C. A. (1982). *Biol. Reprod.* **27**, 282–299.
Lookingland, K. J., Wise, P. M., and Barraclough, C. A. (1982). *Biol. Reprod.* **27**, 268–281.
MacLusky, N. J., and McEwen, B. S. (1980). *Endocrinology* **106**, 192–202.
McCann, S. M. (1982). *In* "Neuroendocrine Perspectives" (E. E. Müller and R. M. MacLeod, eds.), pp. 1–22. Elsevier, Amsterdam.
Meites, J., Bruni, J. F., Van Vugt, D. A., and Smith, A. F. (1979). *Life Sci.* **24**, 1325–1336.
Mennin, S. P., and Gorski, R. A. (1975). *Endocrinology* **96**, 486–491.
Mennin, S. P., Kubo, K., and Gorski, R. A. (1974). *Endocrinology* **95**, 412–416.
Meyerson, B. J., and Sawyer, C. H. (1968). *Endocrinology* **83**, 170–176.
Ojeda, S. R., and McCann, S. M. (1978). *Clin. Obstet. Gynecol.* **5**, 283–303.
Palkovits, M. (1982). *Peptides* **3**, 299–303.
Rance, N., and Barraclough, C. A. (1981). *Proc. Soc. Exp. Biol. Med.* **166**, 425–431.

Rance, N., Wise, P. M., and Barraclough, C. A. (1981a). *Endocrinology* **108**, 2194–2199.

Rance, N., Wise, P. M., Selmanoff, M. K., and Barraclough, C. A. (1981b). *Endocrinology* **108**, 1795–1802.

Sawyer, C. H., Markee, J. E., and Hollingshead, W. H. (1947). *Endocrinology* **41**, 395–402.

Sawyer, C. H., Everett, J. W., and Markee, J. W. (1949). *Endocrinology* **44**, 218–233.

Sawyer, C. H., Markee, J. E., and Everett, J. W. (1950). *J. Exp. Zool.* **113**, 659–682.

Sawyer, C. H., Critchlow, B. V., and Barraclough, C. A. (1955). *Endocrinology* **57**, 345–354.

Sawyer, C. H., Radford, H. M., Krieg, R. J., and Carrer, H. F. (1978). *In* "Brain-Endocrine Interaction III. Neural Hormones and Reproduction" (D. E. Scott, G. P. Kozlowski, and A. Weindl, eds.), pp. 263–273. Karger, Basel.

Swanson, H. E., and van der Werff ten Bosch, J. J. (1964). *Acta Endocrinol.* **45**, 1–12.

Van Vugt, D. A., Aylesworth, C. F., Sylvester, P. W., Leung, F. C., and Meites, J. (1981). *Neuroendocrinology* **33**, 261–264.

Weiland, N. G., and Barraclough, C. A. (1983). *Endocrine Soc. Meet.* Abstr. No. 129.

Weiner, N. (1974). *In* "Neuropsychopharmacology of Monoamines" (E. Usdin, ed.)., pp. 143–159. Raven, New York.

Wise, P. M., Camp-Grossman, P., and Barraclough, C. A. (1981a). *Biol. Reprod.* **24**, 820–830.

Wise, P. M., Rance, N., and Barraclough, C. A. (1981b). *Endocrinology* **108**, 2186–2193.

Wise, P. M., Rance, N., Selmanoff, M., and Barraclough, C. A. (1981c). *Endocrinology* **108**, 2179–2185.

DISCUSSION

F. W. Turek: Could you speculate on where you think the trigger is coming from for triggering norepinephrine release or wherever that trigger is originating. Where would it be acting? Would it be acting back in the hind brain on the cell bodies or would it be acting at the axonal terminals in the hypothalamus?

C. A. Barraclough: This is a very obvious question without an obvious answer. First, I do not know what factors are responsible for the increased frequency of depolarization of the catecholaminergic system during the afternoon versus the morning hours in the animal models I discussed. Apparently, this is a biorhythm which is expressed in the presence of estrogen and its timing of onset can be modified by the rat colony lighting schedule. If I might be permitted to speculate, perhaps estrogen on entering the nucleus of the noradrenergic cell body affects membrane ionic transport properties such that threshold potentials change at the level of the cell body. Also, there probably are many higher level influences which are superimposed upon these norepinephrine cells which influence their frequencies of depolarization and these secondary controls also may be modulated by changes in serum estrogen concentrations. An alternative but very real possibility, which you suggest, is that there are factors (hormones, putative transmitters, etc.) which affect the function of hypothalamic noradrenergic terminals. In this scheme, perhaps the firing rates of noradrenergic cells are relatively constant but the amount of NE released is dictated by such modulatory influences within the hypothalamic noradrenergic terminal field.

F. W. Turek: This is an entirely different question. How do you explain Sawyer's recent data which indicate that cutting of the adrenergic fibers from the hindbrain to the hypothalamus does not permanently abolish estrous cyclicity?

C. A. Barraclough: For those of you who may be unfamiliar with these studies, Clifton and Sawyer (*Neuroendocrinology* **28**, 442, 1979; *Endocrinology* **106**, 2889, 1980) bilaterally transected the ascending noradrenergic pathway, allowed the animals to recover, and examined the effects of such transections on the positive feedback effects of estrogen and progesterone on LH release in ovariectomized rats.

Such transections resulted in an 83% depletion of hypothalamic NE. LH surges occurred in such rats in response to steroids and phenoxybenzamine was incapable of blocking LH surges in such animals. Sawyer and Clifton (*Fed. Proc.* **39,** 2889, 1980) conclude that the aminergic innervation of the hypothalamus may influence pituitary secretion in a modulatory manner without being mandatory in the process, and that this is an example of the remarkable plasticity of hypothalamic neuroendocrine mechanisms.

Frankly, the observations of Sawyer and colleagues raise more questions than they answer. For example, what is the origin of the residual 20% NE in the median eminence? Apparently it is not derived from the sympathetic nerves which accompany the blood supply to the ME; also, in destroying the ascending noradrenergic pathway, the major hypothalamic serotoninergic and acetylcholine pathways and perhaps even other afferent systems from midbrain to hypothalamus also are destroyed. What effect does this have on gonadotropin release? Perhaps the normal physiological processes involved in the release of LHRH involve both inhibitory and stimulatory systems which could be modulated during the cycle by estrogen. The destruction of several of these systems may permit an otherwise neutral system to become stimulatory to LH release. Finally, do postsynaptic receptors for NE and DA undergo denervation hypersensitivity after such experimental surgery such that the remaining 20% of the NE is adequate to stimulate LHRH release? The observation that phenoxybenzamine does not block LH release in such animals would argue against this possibility. Obviously, much more information is required before we understand the complex central nervous events which occur to activate the surge release of LHRH.

F. W. Turek: Do you see any increase in neural activity at the time of the LH surge in the cell bodies of the nerves containing norepinephrine?

C. A. Barraclough: We have not measured changes in neural activity in the cell body region of noradrenergic neurons. However, others have reported increased multiunit activity within the arcuate-median eminence region at the time of the LH surge which might represent an increase in frequency of depolarization of the noradrenergic system.

R. Goodman: I have a couple of questions. First, you proposed that estrogen acts in the midbrain to increase norepinephrine turnover and thus induced an LH surge. How do you reconcile this postulate with the data that implants if estradiol into the preoptic area will induce an LH surge in castrate rats?

C. A. Barraclough: We attempted to repeat these types of studies without success for we observed only inhibitory effects of estrogen on LH release. With the advent of highly sensitive RIA procedures, more recent studies from several laboratories have shown that if you implant crystalline estradiol into the hypothalamus, peripheral plasma estradiol increases. Of course once this occurs, estradiol then can affect many other neuroendocrine systems besides the site at which it was originally transplanted. However, your data indicate that estradiol, when implanted into MPN, elicits LH surges, whereas MBH implants are relatively ineffective. I wonder if these extremely high estrogen concentrations, when presented to LHRH perikarya, directly activate LHRH neurons or indirectly affect the noradrenergic system to stimulate LHRH release? Further, since the LHRH perikarya in MPN are being subjected to estrogen concentrations several orders of magnitude greater than would occur via vascular delivery of the steroid, can we attribute the release of LHRH in such animals to the specific action of estrogen?

R. Goodman: Second, would you like to speculate, based on the dopamine data, on the role of a decrease in dopamine in the prolactin surge that occurs on proestrous and in estrogen-treated rats?

C. A. Barraclough: I don't know. In the various animal models I described we observed the following changes in DA turnover rates: (1) proestrus: a rise followed by an abrupt decline in DA in the arcuate-median eminence region during the LH surge; (2) in estrogen plus progesterone-treated OVX rats on day 2 there is no change in DA between morning and afternoon in either the tuberoinfundibular region or in pituitary portal vein blood. So in one model DA initially increases and then declines (proestrus) and in the steroid-treated rat no change in DA turnovers occurs in spite of the fact that both animal models have LH surges.

R. Goodman: But you haven't measured prolactin in that situation?

C. A. Barraclough: On the contrary, we have measured changes in serum prolactin concentrations in every one of these animal models but I didn't have time to show these data. In brief, prolactin surges occur on proestrous and in steroid-treated OVX rats and progesterone amplifies the prolactin surge in estrogen-treated rats in a manner similar to that observed with the LH surge. In day 3 estrogen-treated rats which were treated 24 hours earlier with progesterone there also is a prolactin surge albeit reduced in concentration compared to day 2. Consequently, changes in serum prolactin concentrations parallel the LH surge which occurs during proestrus or in steroid-treated rats in spite of differences in DA turnover in these rat models. These observations argue in favor of the existence of a prolactin releasing factor.

D. Van Vugt: In 1955, I believe that you and Dr. Sawyer demonstrated that morphine administration could block ovulation in the rat.

C. A. Barraclough: Yes, this was a pioneering study.

D. Van Vugt: Have you, as you did with pentobarbital, looked at the effects of morphine on catecholamine turnover, specifically norepinephrine turnover in an attempt to explain how morphine blocks the gonadotropin surge and ovulation?

C. A. Barraclough: We presently are examining the effects of morphine on catecholamine turnover rates in my laboratory. However, there is indirect evidence using the pharmacological approach (Kalra and Simpkins, *Endocrinology* **109**, 776, 1981) which shows that opiates inhibit the positive feedback effects of estrogen and progesterone on LH release via their effects on the noradrenergic system.

C. W. Beattie: I was much interested in your turnover data and your explanation of how estradiol might be affecting the turnover of norepinephrine. About 10 years ago Charles Rogers and I reported on some studies in this area using a model similar to the one you described. What we found was that by following some early work of Costa's group showing that ovariectomized rats had a higher level of hypothalamic tyrosine hydroxylase activity, we ovariectomized rats and looked at the activity of tyrosine hydroxylase in the anterior hypothalamus directly. Ovariectomy increased activity in the hypothalamus. We then put back microgram doses of estradiol and expected to see a decrease in the activity of the enzyme. We did not. In fact activity increased. When we followed estradiol with increasing doses of progesterone we found that the activity of the enzyme decreased. I think these data speak directly to your turnover measurements.

C. A. Barraclough: Yes, thank you.

S. Cohen: You may have already answered my question when you said that there was no change in the metabolism of dopamine in the estrogenized animal. Because I was going to ask whether you thought it might be possible that the estrogen is 2-hydroxylated to a catechol estrogen which can then compete with the dopamine for the inactivating enzyme methyltransferase.

C. A. Barraclough: This a very logical question particularly with the present interest in the CNS actions of the catechol estrogens. We have not worked with the catechol estrogens but from reports in the literature I understand that the 4-hydroxy estradiol has a positive feedback effect and will cause an LH surge. It also binds specifically to brain estrogen nuclear receptors and as such seems to behave as an estrogen rather than as a catechol. In contrast, the 2-hydroxy estradiol has little effect on LH secretion and does not bind to brain estrogen receptors. Consequently, even though estradiol is metabolized to various catechol estrogens in brain, their effects on LH release seem to be via their estrogenic rather than the catechol properties. For such reasons I am not convinced that estrogen has to be converted to a catechol estrogen to have biological activity in the brain.

M. Ferin: You showed us convincing evidence that norepinephrine is involved in the LH surge. Do you have any experimental evidence or is there any information in the literature that norepinephrine or another neurotransmitter is involved in LH pulsatile release?

C. A. Barraclough: We only have examined catecholamine turnovers in the rat, an animal in which LH surges occur rather rapidly (about 270 minutes for the total surge). Because of the methodology required to determine turnover rates which involves adminis-tration of α-methyl-p-tyrosine and brain removal 45 and 90 minutes later, we are unable to specifically determine whether NE turnover rates parallel the pulse discharge of LH which cumulatively accounts for the LH surge profile. In the rat, these events occur too quickly to be measured by the methods we have described.

D. R. Keefe: Swanson found that CRF neurons interrelate cell groups in the hypothala-mus, including the PVN, with the cell groups in the medulla and midbrain which you indicate may mediate LHRH release through norepinephrine. In addition CRF can increase sponta-neous firing of neurons in the locus coeruleus and hippocampus. We know CRF has a diurnal variation, and it may be found in the SCN. Do you think that CRF may be involved in a diurnal rhythm of norepinephrine and thus have a role in mediating the rhythm of the LH surge?

C. A. Barraclough: Thank you for this information. As you know, the locus coeruleus (LC) and its projections have been studied extensively as it is a well-defined noradrenergic system which lends itself to electrophysiological studies. Chu and Bloom (*Brain Res.* **66,** 1, 1974; *J. Neurobiol.* **5,** 527, 1974) recorded LC neuronal activity during sleep and waking behavior in cats. They observed slow tonic discharges during quiet waking stages, somewhat slower activity during slow wave sleep, and more rapid phasic discharges during REM sleep bursts (50–70 Hz). Other LC neurons showed activity during REM sleep which was slower than in waking or slow wave sleep. These cells may tonically inhibit neurons of the pontine reticular fields. These types of studies demonstrate that activity of midbrain noradrenergic neurons can be affected by imput from other brain regions and in turn affect secondary systems via their axonal projections to a variety of terminal fields. Unfortunately, the LC does not send noradrenergic axons to those hypothalamic regions concerned with LHRH release. Whether recordings of changes in spontaneous neuronal activity in the A_1, A_2, A_5, A_7 cell groups can be made remains to be resolved.

R. E. Peter: With John Chang and others in my laboratory, we have been studying the actions of catecholamines on gonadotropin release in the goldfish, using both *in vivo* and *in vitro* approaches. What our results indicate is that dopamine has a direct gonadotropin release inhibitory action in the goldfish. First, it can modulate or block the spontaneous release of gonadotropin. For example, *in vitro* spontaneous release of gonadotropin from dispersed pituitary cells can be reduced or modulated by dopamine, and, *in vivo*, dopamine can modulate the release of gonadotropin from transplanted pituitaries. Results from other experiments support this as well.

Second, dopamine can also modulate the action of the releasing hormone, for example, it will reduce or turn off the secretion that is on-going as a result of injection of releasing hormone, and if you give the fish apomorphine or dopamine before the releasing hormone you can reduce or even block the action of the releasing hormone. *In vivo* if the fish are given pimozide to block the dopamine receptors followed by releasing hormone, the action of the releasing hormone is potentiated as much as 10-fold. From this we think that the gonadotropin cells in goldfish are under the dual regulation of a dopamine release inhibitory action and stimulation by the releasing hormone. For the ovulatory surge of gonadotropin in goldfish, our data suggest that it involves a decrease of the dopamine action, to back off the inhibition, plus a stimulation by the releasing hormone. As a challenge to your statement that dopamine isn't doing anything, perhaps the situation is that you are looking at dopamine in the wrong way, that in fact it may be serving as a release inhibitor factor in the system you have described.

C. A. Barraclough: I think your observations on the effects of dopamine on LHRH release in goldfish are very interesting. In the rat, certain neuroendocrinologists originally advocated a stimulatory role for dopamine on LHRH release. More recent studies from a variety of laboratories conclude that dopamine inhibits or suppresses LHRH release in the rat. Whether it is necessary to reduce such inhibitory dopaminergic influences for norepinephrine to exert a stimulatory action on LHRH secretion is not known. In our steroid-treated rats, DA turnover rates and portal blood DA do not change from morning to afternoon. Rather, only when NE turnover rates increase does an LH surge occur. In the proestrous rat there is a decline in DA turnover rates as LH plasma rises to reach peak plasma concentrations. This could be interpreted as removal of a tonic inhibitory influence on LHRH secretion. Because of these discrepancies in dopamine turnover rates in the two rat models, I am reluctant to assign an inhibitory role of dopamine to the release of LHRH until I have more conclusive evidence.

R. E. Peter: In your turnover studies of dopamine you found an increase in turnover, did you not, toward the end of the proestrous surge?

C. A. Barraclough: The increase in DA turnover in proestrous rats occurred at the beginning of the LH surge. However, as plasma LH continues to rise there seems to be an abrupt shutdown of tuberoinfundibular dopaminergic activity. At this time we observed increases in NE turnovers not only in the preoptic area and suprachiasmatic nuclei but also within the arcuate nucleus. We do not know if the increase in NE turnover in the arcuate nuclei is responsible for the decline in dopamine turnover in the median eminence. Perhaps the reason why median eminence dopamine turnovers decline during proestrous but not in steroid-treated rats is due to the differences in the patterns and concentrations of plasma estradiol and progesterone observed in the two models. In proestrous rats, as plasma LH begins to rise there is a progressive decline in plasma estradiol and a rise in progesterone. In estrogen or estrogen plus progesterone-treated rats, these plasma steroids are maintained as constant stable concentrations due to use of Silastic capsules. We have not examined the possibility that changing the serum steroid profile might also change DA turnover rates in the tuberoinfundibular region.

R. E. Peter: There is literature suggesting that dopamine has a release inhibitory action in rabbits and humans.

C. A. Barraclough: That is correct and similar observations have been reported in rats. However, some investigators still propose that dopamine stimulates LH release in certain rat models.

A. L. Barofsky: I wonder if you have had the opportunity to look at norepinephrine turnover in androgen-sterilized rats that have been induced to ovulate by a mating stimulus?

C. A. Barraclough: No, we have not, so I do not know what would happen.

A. L. Barofsky: It would be interesting to see whether the mating stimulus overrides the block in norepinephrine turnover to induce ovulation.

C. A. Barraclough: Perhaps, and there is some evidence in the literature that rats made persistently estrous by constant light can be induced to ovulate by vaginal cervix stimulation. However, some years ago Gorski and I examined mating behavior in adult sterile rats neonatally treated with low doses of androgen and observed that these animals would accept the male. However, none of these rats ovulated the next day (*J. Endocrinol.* **25**, 175, 1962). What concerns me is the 25–65% reduction in norepinephrine concentrations which we observed in the various components of the preoptico–suprachiasmatic–tuberoinfundibular system in these animals. Since you have so little norepinephrine available for release from the axon terminals I wonder if, on vaginal cervix stimulation, the remaining catechol pool would be adequate to activate LHRH release. Alternatively, such reflex-induced LH surges in androgen-sterilized rats may be due to activation of other neural systems as, for example, the acetylcholine network which also is an essential link in reflexly induced ovulation in the rabbit.

D. Pomerantz: There seems to be a bit of a paradox, perhaps you can help me. You stated that the androgen-sterilized animal is unable to produce an LH surge because it was actually locally produced estradiol that caused the hypothalamic lesion. So the paradox that I see is that in one case, estradiol is preventing LH surges in sterilized females and preventing increases in catecholamine turnover. Yet, in the situation in which you are simply trying to induce an LH surge with estradiol, the estradiol capsule experiment is an example, you have a situation where estradiol certainly does cause an LH surge. It certainly does cause increased catecholamine turnover. Can you sort these two out for me?

C. A. Barraclough: Are you referring to the negative versus positive feedback effects of estradiol on LH release?

D. Pomerantz: They are both positive feedback effects that I am referring to.

C. A. Barraclough: Naftolin and his colleagues as well as others, have provided rather conclusive evidence that the neonatal androgen when presented to the hypothalamus is aromatized to estrogen and it is estrogen rather than androgen which "masculinizes" or "defeminizes" the brain. Normally, during this critical period in brain maturation, estrogen-concentrating neurons are protected from the rather high circulating levels of estrogen observed in neonates by the presence of a serum estrogen binding protein (α-fetal protein). However, if testosterone is presented to the brain via either the normal testicular secretion of androgen in the male or after exogenous administration of this steroid to the female, it can be aromatized to an estrogen. Thereafter, this estrogen binds to specific neuronal nuclear receptors at a time during brain maturation when estrogen seemingly has ultimate disastrous effects. We propose that it is the noradrenergic system which is particularly vulnerable to such neonatal estrogen exposure. Thereafter, this NE system passes through a transition phase of positive responsiveness to estrogen feedback (50–60 days of life) to a permanent state of unresponsiveness to estrogen. The changes which occur in biochemical processes within the neurons which occur with age are unknown. In contrast, in cyclic rats which have developed normally, this loss of responsiveness to the positive feedback effect of estrogen does not occur in young adult rats but it is observed as the animal passes through middle to old age.

N. B. Schwartz: Dr. Rosemary Grady studied negative feedback in the androgen-sterilized rat. She showed that LH and FSH responses to ovariectomy are very much blunted in the androgen-sterilized rat, but the response to the exogenous GnRH stimulus is perfectly normal for both of these hormones. Have you ever measured norepinephrine turnover in an ovariectomized animal before you give estrogen? That is, have you followed the time course of turnover following release from negative feedback? Is it different in the androgen-sterilized rat as well as the normal rat?

C. A. Barraclough: We have examined both NE and DA turnover rates in the morning versus afternoon 9 days after ovariectomy (Wise *et al., Endocrinology* **108**, 2186, 1981). NE turnover rates, average rate constants, and initial concentrations in OVX rats remained constant between morning and afternoon in ME, SCN, and MPN. However, AN NE average rate constants and turnover rates decreased during the afternoon compared to morning values. DA turnover rates were increased in the afternoon compared to morning in the median eminence but were decreased in the AN and MPN in the afternoon in OVX rats. Since such rats are exhibiting pulsatile LH release throughout the day, it is difficult for me to interpret the significance of such catecholamine turnover rates particularly in terms of the pulsatile release of LH. Because of this problem in interpretation, we did not examine catecholamine dynamics in OVX androgen-sterilized rats.

N. B. Schwartz: Do you find that the turnover changes as a function of time after gonadectomy? Since norepinephrine turnover is involved as a causative agent in increasing LH, do you also find changes in turnover when LH increases because of removal of negative feedback?

C. A. Barraclough: How do you remove the negative feedback of estrogen?

N. B. Schwartz: Just removing the ovaries.

C. A. Barraclough: We have not examined changes in catecholamine turnover rates as a function of time after ovariectomy and with the methodology required to measure such turnover rates it is doubtful if we could detect the rapid changes in either NE or DA which precede or accompany each pulse release of LH.

N. B. Schwartz: Is the increased LH secretion associated with removal of negative feedback accompanied by, or preceded by an increase in norepinephrine turnover?

C. A. Barraclough: I do not know.

R. Goodman: Just a comment and one question that is not really related to the comment. We have data in sheep suggesting that dopamine may be involved in suppressing tonic LH secretion in anestrus. A couple of days ago, I presented data that pentobarbital anesthesia increases LH in anestrus ewes. If we inject such animals with pimozide, a dopamine receptor blocker, a similar increase in LH occurs, suggesting that, at least in intact anestrous ewes, dopamine actively inhibits LH. My question relates to your androgen-sterilized model. You suggested that the primary effects of androgen are in the mid brain. Would you then postulate that cutting the neural track from this area to the hypothalamus in androgen-treated females would reinitiate estrous cycles?

C. A. Barraclough: I do not know what would occur if the ascending noradrenergic bundle was transected in androgen-sterilized rats. As I showed in the first slide (Fig. 1), many putative neurotransmitters have been reported to affect LHRH secretion including not only NE and DA but also acetylcholine, serotonin etc. In androgen-sterilized rats, perhaps not only NE but also any or all of these other systems also are affected by neonatal androgen exposure. The same comments apply to the studies of Krieg and Sawyer. Since many of the cell bodies of origin for acetylcholine and serotonin reside in the midbrain, by transecting the central tegmental tract they also are eliminating most of the hypothalamic imput of acetylcholine, serotonin, and perhaps other important modulating influences as well. Since we know little about how these various putative neurotransmitter systems themselves are regulated it would be premature to postulate how their interactions are controlled. Perhaps the noradrenergic system is affected directly or indirectly by these other hypothalamic imputs and it is via the norepinephrine system that LHRH release is affected.

R. B. Billiar: I would like to push you a little more on where the cell bodies of the noradrenergic neurons are derived from that are innervating the SCN, either from your knowledge of the literature or from some studies you have done. It seems to me this is a very crucial point and how this relates to the estradiol-concentrating neurons of the CNS.

C. A. Barraclough: I really don't know which noradrenergic cell bodies project to which regions of the preoptico–hypothalamic system or even if such point-to-point axonal projections exist. My comments related to the turnover rate data we obtained suggest that various components of the noradrenergic system are differentially affected by the various treatment regimes we used in these studies. However, I get the feeling that some neuroanatomical distinction exists between cells projecting to the preoptic area versus those projecting to other hypothalamic regions although I do not know of any experimental evidence that suggests such an arrangement. I wonder if Dr. Martin has any ideas about these possibilities.

J. Martin: I am not aware that those facts are known in detail. However, I did want to interject a point that relates to that. If one generalizes the α-adenergic system in terms of its neuroendocrine control in the rat it is evident that it influences a variety of hormones, as you have already commented. For example, in addition to its known effects on LH secretion and on prolactin, it is the single most important transmitter accounting for the growth hormones surges that we have demonstrated. In addition, there is an α-adenergic control of TSH in the rat and there is probably also an effect on CRF or ACTH control. One has the problem, both anatomically and functionally, of putting together a very small group of neurons (if you actually count the cells in A_1, A_2, A_5, A_7, or even the locus coeruleus, the number of nerve cells present is very small). The projections from them have multiple collaterals to various parts of the brain. The problem is how to put together that rather parsimonious system with a multiple of functions as it must occur at the terminals of those nerve cells. How, in fact, does the system work to regulate independently of each hormone system? I wonder if you have any thoughts about that particular point? It is possible that noradrenergic effects may, in fact, be neuromodulatory, i.e., a permissive system in some way rather than a point-to-point stimulatory system.

C. A. Barraclough: Thank you, I agree with everything you have said and these comments really point out how little we really know about the organization of afferent input to the hypothalamus. For example, we have only superficial knowledge about how the classical central noradrenergic system functions, what turns it on, and what regulates it. Further, not only is somatostatin and perhaps GRH, TRH, and CRF affected by the noradrenergic system but also, 14 neurohormones have been identified by immunocytochemical methods as residing within the median eminence and perhaps superimposed on top of these controls could be the modulatory noradrenergic system.

R. B. Billiar: In your animal model, where you ovariectomized the animal and then you introduced the estrogen capsule and you get these daily LH surges, I assume if you added more estrogen you would get a larger surge. What I am trying to get clear is whether or not you think the control or the site of control of these daily LH surges is the same as the ovulatory surge of LH?

C. A. Barraclough: It is interesting that as we increased plasma estradiol from OVX levels (5 pg/ml) through various concentrations ranging from 7 to 36 pg/ml the peak LH surge concentrations never exceeded 1000 ng/ml (LH-RP-1 standard). In these various groups, median eminence LHRH progressively increased as the high OVX plasma LH concentrations declined which suggests that LHRH release but not synthesis is inhibited by estrogen.

R. B. Billiar: So you believe that the control of these daily LH surges is analogous to or the same as the proestrous LH surge?

C. A. Barraclough: I believe that the estrogen-induced LH release is analogous to the proestrous LH surge. One explanation I can offer to explain the discrepancies between the peak concentrations observed in estrogen-treated OVX and proestrous rats involves changes which occur in the responsiveness of the pituitary gland to LHRH. In proestrous rats, as the LH surge begins it affects the ovarian secretion of estradiol, estrogen declines in serum, and progesterone serum concentrations rise. Some years ago, Turgeon and I (*Endocrinology* **101**, 548, 1977) demonstrated that the decline in serum estrogen which accompanies the LH surge on proestrous dictates the magnitude of the peak in LH achieved during the afternoon and subsequently Turgeon and Waring (*Endocrinology* **108**, 413, 1981) reported that progesterone amplifies pituitary responsiveness to LHRH but only if a decline in estrogen first occurs. In more recent studies with Patricia Camp we observed that as serum estradiol concentrations are increased, pituitary gland responsiveness to LHRH also increases in a dose-responsive manner. These observations suggest that a reciprocal relationship develops between the amount of LHRH released and the responsiveness of the pituitary gonadotrophs to LHRH. As a consequence of these two events, LH surge concentrations do not change when serum E_2 levels are elevated. Also, since serum estrogen concentrations remain constant (due to the Silastic capsule implant) and no progesterone is provided (as occurs in proestrous rats) the amount of LHRH released in response to increased norepinephrine turnovers during the afternoon seems restricted to only that amount which can be discharged in the presence of estrogen.

G. Callard: I have two questions. Did the punched areas in your preoptic samples include the sex dimorphic nuclei of the medial preoptic area?

C. A. Barraclough: Yes, these sexually dimorphic nuclei were removed with our preoptic punches.

G. Callard: Did those fragments also include other, adjacent tissues?

C. A. Barraclough: When we make our medial preoptic punches, we take two 500-μm punches from either side of midline from two 300-μm sections. Consequently, we remove not only the sexually dimorphic nuclei, but most of the MPN tissue.

G. Callard: So the sex dimorphic nucleus is represented in all of your preoptic area punches?

C. A. Barraclough: Yes, absolutely.

G. Callard: Now I have a general question. Viewed in the background of your own research, what do you think is the functional significance of these particular cell clusters?

C. A. Barraclough: I have no idea about the physiological significance of these morphologically identified structures. What I do know is that in androgen-sterilized rats in which these nuclei resemble those observed in males, the preoptico–hypothalamic LHRH system seems to be capable of normal function. These conclusions are based on the observations that (1) LHRH synthesis, transport, and storage can occur normally in steroid-treated OVX androgen-sterilized rats; (2) when depolarizing stimuli are presented to the preoptic area, the serum concentrations of LH released are the same in normal and in androgen-sterilized rats. Also, Everett and Tyrey (*Endocrinology* **111**, 1979, 1982) recently have shown that similar LH surges occur after MPN stimulation in rats treated with pentobarbital, morphine, chlorpromazine, or atropine. All of these observations suggest that the preoptico–hypothalamic LHRH system is not particularly affected by various drugs or neonatal androgen treatment. However, this does not preclude the possibility that the morphological differences in the sexually dimorphic nuclei in MPN are not due to changes in structure and/or function of one or more of the many modulatory influences which affect this final common path (the LHRH neuron).

R. O. Greep: I thought it would be interesting if you would comment just briefly on the extension of this triggering mechanism to an induced ovulator like the rabbit, and to the primate menstrual cycle.

C. A. Barraclough: Over 36 years ago Sawyer and his colleagues implicated the noradrenergic system in copulation-induced ovulation in the rabbit. They observed that dibenamine or SKF-501 (adrenergic receptor blockers) would effectively block ovulation if administered before copulation. Subsequently, Sawyer and his colleagues demonstrated that epinephrine or norepinephrine, when injected into the third ventricle of the rabbit, induced the release of ovulating hormone.

Unfortunately, we have so little information on the role of the catecholamine system in the release of LHRH in the monkey that I cannot make any knowledgeable comments on whether or not this system is important in the surge release of LH in primates.

RECENT PROGRESS IN HORMONE RESEARCH, VOL. 40

Cell Proliferation in the Mammalian Testis: Biology of the Seminiferous Growth Factor (SGF)

ANTHONY R. BELLVÉ AND LARRY A. FEIG*

*Department of Physiology and Biophysics, and the Laboratory of Human Reproduction and Reproductive Biology, and the *Laboratory of Molecular Carcinogenesis, Dana Farber Cancer Institute. Harvard Medical School, Boston, Massachusetts*

I. Introduction

Regulating cell proliferation is primal to the generation of spermatozoa. The complexity of producing vast numbers of germ cells in a precise and coordinative pattern within the seminiferous epithelium requires intricate regulatory mechanisms. The proliferative and differentiative processes of spermatogenesis are dependent, in part, on the two glycoprotein hormones, LH and FSH (Clermont and Morgentaler, 1955; Lostroh, 1969). In the absence of these hormones spermatogenesis does not proceed beyond meiotic prophase, and the divisions of the spermatogonial stem cells may be quantitatively if not qualitatively impaired. However, there is no definitive evidence showing FSH, LH, and/or testosterone act directly to induce germ cell proliferation, rather than having some indirect effect on somatic cell growth and differentiation. It seems reasonable, therefore, to suspect that local mitogenic factors could exist to stimulate germ cell proliferation in the mammalian testis (Bellvé, 1979). Precedence for this concept is provided by contemporary studies regarding the role of erythropoetin in promoting the proliferation of erythroid progenitor cells (Till and McCulloch, 1980), and the action of interleukins 1 and 2 in stimulating the division of resting and differentiating T lymphocytes, respectively (Gillis *et al.*, 1982; Mizel, 1982). The following review discusses the evidence for the existence, biological properties, and potential functions of the seminiferous growth factor, SGF.

II. Proliferation of Somatic Cells during Testicular Development

Formation of the mammalian testis from the initial appearance of the primordial gonads involves the precise temporal proliferation and differentiation of both germinal and somatic cells. Thus, after migrating from

531

the yolk sac endoderm, the primordial germ cells arrive to populate the two gonadal anlagen as the latter start forming at the dorso-medial angle of the celom, immediately adjacent to the mesonephri (for reviews, see Bellvé, 1979; Eddy et al., 1981). At this time, days 11 to 12 of fetal life in the mouse and rat, the somatic elements of the primordial gonads appear to assemble primarily by the rapid proliferation of epithelial cells that migrate from the involuting mesonephric tubules (Jost, 1972; Upadhyay et al., 1979). Additional recruitment of mesonephric cells, and the continued proliferation of the migrating cell population, lead to a substantial enlargement of the sexually indifferent gonad. This massive mobilization of mesonephric cells to provide the initial phase of gonad formation and growth is clearly evident in the developing ram testis (Zamboni and Upadhyay, 1982). Also during this growth phase, a few mesenchyme cells appear dispersed among the epithelial and germinal elements. These cells proliferate rapidly to yield connective tissue, a discrete stromal layer as the progenitor of the tunica albuginea, and a subsurface layer of neoformed capillaries that progressively penetrate the compact gonadal mass. This early organizational phase is heralded by the formation of the seminiferous cords.

Assembly of rat seminiferous cords occurs when the mesonephric cells populating the indifferent gonad differentiate to yield the primordial Sertoli cells on day 13 of fetal life. These proliferating cells envelop the neighboring germ cells and align with interdigitating cytoplasmic processes to form the seminiferous cords, the first obvious indication of sex determination (Magre and Jost, 1980). Cord formation gradually extends into the posterior regions of the primordial gonad. Meanwhile, additional mesonephric cells accumulate at the termini of the cords, in the anteriodorsal region of the gonad, to form the rete testis and efferent ductules (Zamboni and Upadhyay, 1982). During the remainder of fetal development and early postnatal life the Sertoli cells continue to proliferate rapidly (Orth, 1982), thereby enabling the seminiferous cords to expand radially and to lengthen considerably (Huckins and Clermont, 1968). However, following birth the proliferative activity of these epithelial cells diminishes quickly, until by day 16 neither mitotic divisions nor DNA synthesis are detectable (Clermont and Perey, 1957; Hilscher and Makoski, 1968; Steinberger and Steinberger, 1971; Nagy, 1972; Orth, 1982). Thus, the total number of Sertoli cells populating the adult testis is established early in prepuberal development. The cells simply grow in size to accommodate and to sustain the increasing cohorts of differentiating spermatogenic cells (Sapsford, 1963; Flickinger, 1967).

Other cell populations comprising the mammalian testis also exhibit discrete phases of proliferation during their ontogeny. Leydig cells appear in the interstitium simultaneously or secondarily to cord formation in most mammalian species (Gillman, 1948). In the rat at day 14 of gestation, the stellate mesenchyme cells differentiate to form fibroblasts and Leydig cells, the latter having some elementary characteristics of steroid-secreting cells (Black and Christensen, 1969; Merchant, 1975). Within another 24 to 96 hours the Leydig cells increase substantially in number, and soon acquire more extensive arrays of smooth endoplasmic reticulum to facilitate steroidogenesis (Russo and de Rosas, 1971). In man, horse (Gillman, 1948), macaca fascicularis (Fouquet and Dang, 1980), and guinea pig (Black and Christensen, 1969) the Leydig cells attain maximal numbers near mid-term and then decline, while in the mouse, rat (Roosen-Runge and Anderson, 1959), and rabbit (Bjerrgaard et al., 1974) maximal numbers are maintained until birth. Regardless, prior to or just after birth, the Leydig cells undergo a marked regression, leaving only a few survivors that persist throughout the early postnatal period (Roosen-Runge and Anderson, 1959; Gondos et al., 1976). Then later, coincident with the inception of spermatogenesis, the remnant population of Leydig cells enters another proliferative phase, which continues for a prolonged period during puberal development to provide the full, adult complement of these steroidogenic cells.

Finally, during late fetal stages, the fibroblasts in the interstitium actively divide to yield one or more layers of peritubular fibrocytes. Within the first 1 to 3 weeks after birth, depending upon the species, the inner layer of fibrocytes differentiates to form peritubular myocytes and then the myoid cells that eventually endow the seminiferous tubules with contractile properties (Leeson and Leeson, 1963; Ross, 1967; Bustos-Obregon and Courot, 1974; Leeson, 1975; Leeson and Forman, 1981). These particular cells continue to proliferate until late puberty, as the seminiferous tubules increase in length and number.

III. The Inception, Renewal, and Proliferation of Germ Cells

After colonizing the indifferent gonads, the primordial germ cells continue to proliferate, even while being enveloped within the growing seminiferous cords. This proliferative phase is reflected by a high mitotic index and a marked increase in germ cell number (Beaumont and Mandl, 1962, 1963; Chrétien, 1966). In the rat, the original $\sim 5 \times 10^3$ germ cells populating each primordial gonad increase to over 140×10^3 by day 17.5, when the mitotic index declines to minimal levels (Beaumont and Mandl, 1963). Thereafter, the germ cells remain in a quiescent G_1 phase (G_0) of the cell cycle for ~ 8 to 10 days, while growing 4-fold in size (Beaumont and Mandl, 1963; Hilscher and Hilscher, 1976, 1978). Then, between days 3 and 5 after birth, in both the rat and the mouse, the germ cells resume active proliferation and quickly differentiate into transitional primitive type A spermatogonia and then type A spermatogonia (Novi and Saba, 1968; Huckins and Clermont, 1968). Although having some characteristics typical of adult type A spermatogonia, these transitional cells are larger (Bellvé et al., 1977a) and undergo the first sequence of spermatogonial divisions, through to the primary spermatocyte stage, at an accelerated rate (Kluin et al., 1982). Also, many spermatogonia die during this period, perhaps only passing through one or two cell divisions before undergoing cytolysis (Franchi and Mandl, 1964; Huckins and Clermont, 1968).

The surviving type A spermatogonia proceed through a series of mitotic divisions to yield the sequence of differentiating spermatogonia that are responsible for initiating adult spermatogenesis (Clermont and Perey, 1957; Nebel et al., 1961; Bellvé et al., 1977b; Kluin et al., 1982). In the mouse, this proliferative process first yields preleptotene spermatocytes on days 9 to 10, pachytene spermatocytes on days 13 to 14, spermatids (steps 1–2) on day 18, and condensing spermatids (steps 15–16) on days 30 to 32 (Bellvé et al., 1977a,b). During these early stages of mouse development, even until day 30 postnatal, the cycle of the seminiferous epithelium proceeds more rapidly (7.5 days) than in the adult animal (8.6 days) (Kluin et al., 1982). This observation is compatible with an earlier report of shorter cell cycle times occurring in spermatogonia at the onset of rat spermatogenesis (Huckin, 1973). Both observations suggest that the proliferation of the undifferentiated spermatogonia may be modulated by some intragonadal factor(s).

Spermatogenesis in the adult testis involves a continual process of stem cell renewal, a precisely regulated sequence of spermatogonial divisions, and the two meiotic reduction divisions of the primary and secondary spermatocytes (Fig. 1). There is general agreement concerning the sequence of spermatogonial divisions, which in mice, rats, and hamsters involves serial mitoses of type A_{1-4}, intermediate, and type B spermatogonia (for review see Clermont, 1972). However, some contention remains concerning the renewal mechanism of the spermatogonial stem cells (A_s or A_0) (cf. Monesi, 1962; Clermont and Bustos-Obregon, 1968; Clermont and Antar, 1973; Huckins, 1971a–c; Oakberg, 1971a; Huckins and Oakberg, 1978a,b; Bartmanska and Clermont, 1983; Lok and de Rooij, 1983). The experimental evidence now favors a model in which the long cycling stem cells (A_s) undergo a sequence of mitoses to yield a *pair* of spermatogonia (A_{pr}) which remain interconnected by a cytoplasmic bridge, then an *aligned* chain of four spermatogonia (A_{al-4}), and finally a syncytial clone of A_{al-8} and perhaps even A_{al-16} (Huckins and Oakberg,

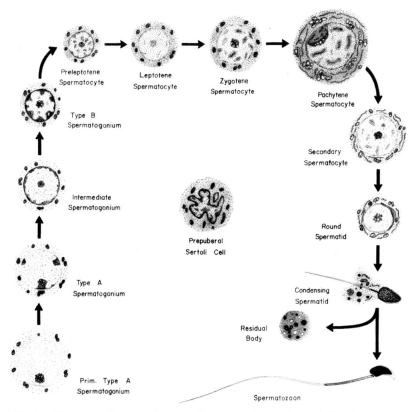

FIG. 1. Schematic diagram of mammalian spermatogenesis, depicting the sequence, relative sizes, and distinctive structural features of the differentiating germ cells. The ascending axis shows the series of types A_{1-4}, intermediate and type B spermatogonia, which expand geometrically in number with successive cell divisions. The primitive type A spermatogonia exist only transiently in neonatal mice and rats, yielding soon after birth the renewing spermatogonial stem cells (A_s/A_0), and the undifferentiated (A_{pr}, A_{al}) (not shown) and the differentiating spermatogonia that initiate prepuberal spermatogenesis. The horizontal axis depicts primary spermatocytes at successive stages of meiotic prophase, while the descending axis shows the two meiotic reduction divisions yielding the secondary spermatocyte and spermatid, respectively. The latter undergoes complicated differentiative processes to form spermatozoa. [Reproduced from Bellvé *et al.* (1977a), with permission of the Editor, *J. Cell Biol.*]

1978a). Either of the latter clones can transform to provide syncytia of type A_1 spermatogonia for entering the differentiating pathway leading to preleptotene spermatocytes (Fig. 1).

The renewal and the differentiative sequence of spermatogonial proliferation must be stringently regulated to ensure constancy between the successive stages of cycle of the seminiferous epithelium (Clermont and Leblond, 1955). Thus, in the Chinese hamster, the undifferentiated spermatogonia (A_s, A_{pr}, and A_{al}), all of which have long cell cycle times of ~87 hours or more, exhibit a peak of mitotic activity during Stages XII to VI (Lok et al., 1983). Many of these cells then become arrested in G_1 (or G_0), until differentiating into A_1 spermatogonia at Stage IX. Once embarking on the differentiative pathway the spermatogonia experience a progressive lengthening in the period of DNA synthesis (S phase) and a commensurate decrease in the G_2 interval (Monesi, 1962; Huckins, 1971a; Lok and de Rooij, 1983). Therefore, within a given species the total cell cycle time (T_c) remains relatively constant, with all cells of a particular clone, and all adjacent, like clones, dividing in synchrony. Thus, even after the initial induction of DNA synthesis in the G_1-arrested, A_1 spermatogonia the subsequent divisions appear to be coordinately controlled, a process that would ensure the recurring regularity in the known cell associations of the seminiferous epithelium.

IV. Factors Regulating Cell Proliferation

The developing and adult testes are derived principally from three progenitor cell types: mesenchymal, epithelial, and germinal cells. Being of such different origins, these respective cell populations are likely to proliferate and to differentiate in response to distinct inductive signals. These most likely involve endocrine, paracrine, and autocrine regulators emanating from both intra- and extragonadal sources. At this time only limited information is available concerning the nature of such "mitogenic factors" that, in some cases, still remain purely hypothetical. Regardless, further consideration of the pertinent evidence can provide valuable leads for identifying a potentially important class of regulatory polypeptides and for defining their respective physiological roles in testicular function.

The rapid and precocious development of the mammalian testis, compared to the ovary, suggests the former may be responsive to specific growth promotors. The enhanced growth rate, detectable early in the ontogeny of the testis (Mittwoch, 1969, 1970), is reflected in part by a rapid onset of cord formation, greater numbers of gonocytes, an early proliferation and differentiation of Leydig cells, and the precocious vascularization of the gonad. While these effects could be ascribed to the intragonadal expression of some undefined product encoded by a gene(s) on the Y chromosome (Mittwoch and Buehr, 1973), there is no direct evidence to support this contention. A "growth factor" having all of the prerequisite properties for enhancing testicular development has not been identified at this time. Nevertheless, a number of possible candidates and sources need to be considered.

Least is known concerning the regulation of cell proliferation in the fetal testis. Only a few conclusions can be drawn. First, since the onset of gonadal growth coincides with the arrival of the primordial germ cells, it has been suggested that they may have an inductive influence. However, the germ cells are not a likely source of a growth factor, as the somatic elements express "normal" growth and differentiation in their near or complete absence (Everett, 1943; Mintz and Russell, 1957; Merchant, 1975). Second, the early differentiation of Leydig cells ensures a source of testosterone, a known promotor of cell proliferation in the efferent ductules, Wolffian ducts, and seminal vesicles after day 16 of development in the rat (Price and Pannabecker, 1959; Price, 1970). Thus, androgens acting in concert, or synergistically with a peptide growth factor could promote gonadal growth. Third, the gonadotropic hormones, FSH and LH, first produced by the fetal pituitary between days 18 and 20 (Tougard et al., 1977; Begeot et al., 1981), may stimulate cell proliferation in the neonatal testis. At this time, however, there is no direct experimental evidence to suggest any of the classical hormones are involved in enhancing the early phase of gonadal growth.

Growth of the puberal and adult testes could be modulated, directly or indirectly, by the pituitary gonadotropins. In the ram, a seasonal breeding species, a positive correlation exists between testicular size and the plasma levels of FSH, LH, and testosterone (Courot and Ortavant, 1981). The highest serum levels of the gonadotropins occur during the fall months when maximal sperm production is required for the breeding period. While much of the associated increase in testis size can be accounted for by somatic cell hypertrophy, some proportion can be ascribed to the greater number of germ cells. Apparently, the efficiency of spermatogonial divisions is enhanced, thereby generating a greater yield of leptotene spermatocytes and a consequential increment in sperm production (Hochereau-de Reviers et al., 1976). Hypophysectomy, while causing a drastic depletion of the advanced germ cells, also reduces the yield of the differentiating type A and type B spermatogonia, many of which cease to divide and soon degenerate (Courot and Ortavant, 1981). Replacement therapy with PMSG, but not hCG or testosterone, is partially effective in maintaining the replicating spermatogonia in hypophysectomized animals. This inferred role for FSH is compatible with the apparent loss of spermatogonia in prepuberal rats following treatment with an anti-FSH antibody (Chemes et al., 1979). Also, in combination with transferrin and insulin, FSH appears to have some beneficial effect in promoting further divisions of the differentiating spermatogonia in the cryptorchid testis cultured *in vitro* (Haneji and Nishimune, 1982). Aside from an indication that FSH may bind directly to these germ cells (Orth and Christensen, 1978), definitive evidence on the hormonal control of spermatogonial proliferation is not available.

Other studies imply the existence of local factors regulating the proliferation of spermatogonia. The depletion of differentiating germ cells from the testis following X-irradiation (Dym and Clermont, 1970; Huckins, 1978a,b) and pituitary ablation (Huckins and Cunningham, 1975) leads to an apparent compensatory increase in the proliferation of the spermatogonial stem cells. This response is probably not mediated by hormones *in vivo,* since the levels of circulating gonadotropins and intratesticular testosterone are not altered following X-irradiation (Huckins and Cunningham, 1978). One alternate explanation invokes the action of a testicular chalone, an inhibitor of cell proliferation (Clermont and Mauger, 1974, 1976; Irons and Clermont, 1979). In this case, "neutralization" of the chalone presumably would release the spermatogonial stem cells from their prolonged G_0 arrest and thereby allow rapid repopulation of the seminiferous epithelium following X-irradiation. Some investigators question the existence of a chalone (Cunningham and Huckins, 1979) and so, while the concept remains interesting, further validation is required.

The inherent maximal limit to sperm production, given an optimal hormonal environment, appears to be primarily a function of the number of Sertoli cells populating the testis (Hochereau-de Reviers and Courot, 1978; de Reviers *et al.,* 1980). The size of the Sertoli cell population is determined during the prepuberal period by the proliferative capacity of these cells, a trait that may be subject to genetic control (de Reviers *et al.,* 1980). Significantly, hemicastration of prepuberal rats (Cunningham *et al.,* 1978), cockerels, lambs, and calves (de Reviers *et al.,* 1980), when undertaken during the period of Sertoli cell proliferation, leads to a compensatory hypertrophy of the remaining testis. This effect is due primarily to an enhanced hyperplasia of the Sertoli cells, and a subsequent commensurate increase in the number of germ cells. This effect has been attributed to the higher circulating levels of FSH that occur in response to hemicastration (Cunningham *et al.,* 1978), a conclusion reinforced by the observation that FSH increases the mitotic index of prepuberal rat Sertoli cells *in vitro* (Griswold *et al.,* 1976, 1977).

V. Identification of a Growth Factor in the Mammalian Testis

The traditional approach toward elucidating the control of mammalian spermatogenesis has been to study the effects of FSH, LH, and testosterone. Such experiments, as discussed above, indicate a possible role for FSH in regulating the proliferation of Sertoli cells and spermatogonia, although the molecular mechanisms remain unknown. Also, an increasing amount of evidence suggests a major part of this control process is mediated locally within the testis, implying the existence of paracrine and/or autocrine regulatory molecules. Based on these concepts, the initial goals of this study have been to determine directly whether the mammalian testis contains putative growth-regulating macromolecules. Initially hindered by the difficulties encountered in culturing testicular cells, the study circumvented such problems by selecting BALB/c 3T3 cells as model target cells. This line of mouse fibroblastic cells has been utilized because (1) they are known to respond to a variety of polypeptide growth factors, (2) they display *in vitro* growth properties comparable to normal cells, such as contact inhibition, and (3) many somatic cell types comprising the testis are of mesenchymal lineage. The standard assay involves quantitating the capacity of testis samples to induce DNA synthesis in confluent, quiescent BALB/c 3T3 cells in the presence of [*methyl*-^{3}H]thymidine (Klagsbrun *et al.*, 1977). Following 48 hours of culture, the 3T3 cells are processed to quantitate the amount of isotopic precursor incorporated into DNA.

The first study undertaken clearly demonstrates the existence of a potent mitogen in the mammalian testis (Feig *et al.*, 1980). Homogenates of testes from adult, CD-1 mice induce a dramatic increase in DNA synthesis among quiescent 3T3 cells, with the half-maximal activity occurring on addition of 400 μg of testis protein per ml. The maximal response is equal to that observed when 3T3 cells are exposed to fresh 20% calf serum, and represents a 90- to 100-fold stimulation in comparison to untreated cells. Similar preparations of isolated seminiferous tubules also stimulate DNA synthesis in confluent 3T3 cells, generating a dose–response curve commensurate and parallel to that observed for testis homogenates (Fig. 2). The proportion of cells responding to the growth factor, as assessed by autoradiography, exceeds 98% at maximal stimulation, with both testis and seminiferous tubule preparations again exhibiting comparable specific activites (Fig. 3). Significantly, seminiferous tubules constitute >90% of the total mass of the adult testis (Roosen-Runge and Anderson, 1959; Reddy and Svoboda, 1967), and so these observations also demonstrate that the bulk of the growth-promoting activity resides within the seminiferous epithelium. Furthermore, seminiferous tubules isolated from rat, guinea pig, and calf testes contain comparable levels of mitogenic activity suggesting the activity may be ubiquitous to mammals (Table I).

Confluent BALB/c 3T3 cells (24 × 10^3 cells/cm^2) undergo multiple divisions, increasing 5-fold in number within 7 days of being maximally

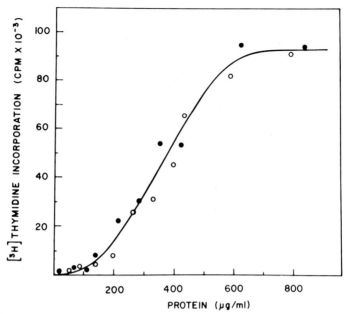

FIG. 2. Dose–response curve for DNA synthesis in confluent, quiescent BALB/c 3T3 cells after being stimulated by the mitogenic activity from mouse testes. Aliquots of either perfused, homogenized testes or seminiferous tubules were added, together with [methyl-³H]thymidine (4 μCi/ml), to the 3T3 cells. Following a further 48-hour culture period, the induction of DNA synthesis was assayed by quantifying the amount of [methyl-³H]thymidine incorporated into TCA-precipitable material. Data points represent the average of duplicate determinations. Testes (○), seminiferous tubules (●). [Reproduced from Feig *et al.* (1980), with permission from the Editor, *Proc. Natl. Acad. Sci. U.S.A.*]

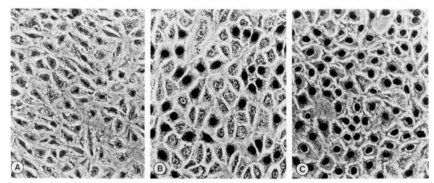

FIG. 3. Autoradiographic analysis of confluent BALB/c 3T3 cells following the induction of DNA synthesis by varying levels of mitogenic activity. The cells were exposed for 48 hours to aliquots of mouse seminiferous tubule cytosol (100,000 *g*) in the presence of [³H]thymidine (4 μCi/ml). The cultures were then fixed and autoradiographed to assess the proportion of cells with labeled nuclei. Similar results were obtained with cytosolic preparations of mouse testes. (A) Untreated control (1% nuclei labeled); (B) 160 μg of protein per ml (40% nuclei labeled); (C) 360 μg of protein per ml (>95% nuclei labeled). [Reproduced from Feig *et al.* (1980), with permission from the Editor, *Proc. Natl. Acad. Sci. U.S.A.*]

TABLE I
Mitogenic Activity in the Seminiferous
Epithelium of Different
Mammalian Species[a]

Species	Mitogenic activity (units/mg protein)
Prepuberal	
Mouse	44.1 ± 5.2
Calf	54.0 ± 6.5
Adult	
Mouse	11.7 ± 0.6
Rat	9.7 ± 0.9
Guinea pig	20.0[b]

[a] Seminiferous tubule homogenates from testes of mouse, rat, guinea pig, and calf were assayed for their ability to stimulate DNA synthesis in confluent cultures of BALB/c 3T3 cells. One unit of mitogenic activity equals the amount of activity required to stimulate half-maximal DNA synthesis among 8×10^3 BALB/c 3T3 cells cultured in a 0.3-cm^2 microtiter well. Data points represent the mean ±SE of repeat determinations on at least four samples, unless indicated otherwise.

[b] Guinea pig data were derived from repeat estimates on a single sample.

stimulated by a single addition of mitogenic activity (Fig. 4). Similarly, cells *sparsely* seeded (5×10^3 cells/cm^2) in limiting concentrations of serum (1.5%, v/v) also respond to the mitogen by increasing 5-fold in number within 6 days (Fig. 5). Thus, by inducing multiple rounds of cell division in both sparse and confluent cell cultures, the mitogenic activity in the mammalian seminiferous epithelium satisfies certain criteria necessary for its classification as a growth factor (Gospodarowicz and Moran, 1976).

VI. Biochemical Characterization of the Seminiferous Growth Factor

The biochemical and biological properties of the mitogenic activity, denoted as the seminiferous growth factor (SGF), have been characterized primarily by using seminiferous tubules from adult mice and seminiferous cords of 2- to 4-week-old calves. Growth factor activities prepared

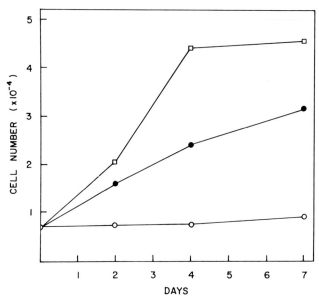

FIG. 4.   Stimulation of cell division in *confluent, quiescent* BALB/c 3T3 cells by mitogenic activity from mouse seminiferous tubules. The 3T3 cells were stimulated at both 0 and 48 hours by adding varying aliquots of homogenates prepared from isolated seminiferous tubules. Following an additional culture period of 0, 2, 4, and 7 days, the 3T3 cells were detached from the substrate with trypsin and then quantified. Treatments included control, 0 μg protein/ml (○), 320 μg/ml (●), and 800 μg/ml (□). [Reproduced from Feig *et al.* (1980), with permission from the Editor, *Proc. Natl. Acad. Sci. U.S.A.*]

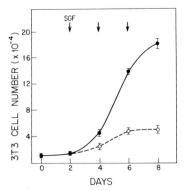

FIG. 5.   Stimulation of cell proliferation in *sparse* cultures of BALB/c 3T3 cells by mitogenic activity partially purified from the adult mouse seminiferous epithelium. The 3T3 cells were plated sparsely on day 0 (5×10^3 cells/cm^2) in DMEM containing 10% calf serum (CS). On day 2, the culture media was replaced with DMEM supplemented with 1.5% CS. At this time and at 48-hour intervals thereafter (arrows), until the cells were harvested, the cultures received either PBS (○) or SGF at 100 μg protein/ml (●). Data points represent the mean $\pm$SE of triplicate determinations.

from these two sources are essentially indistinguishable by biochemical criteria. As a source for characterizing and purifying the factor, calf testes have the advantages of being relatively abundant in supply and of expressing a high specific activity for SGF.

A. STABILITY PROPERTIES

SGF activity is sensitive to protease as determined by the >80% loss of activity occurring on digestion of a tubule extract with a mixture of trypsin and chymotrypsin (each at 200 μg/ml) (Table II). Also, cytosolic preparations (100,000 g) incubated at 100°C for 2 minutes lose all activity.

TABLE II
Stability Properties of SGF

Treatment	Incorporation of [^{3}H]thymidine (cpm)
A.[a]	
Phosphate-buffered saline (PBS)	1,600
Tubule cytosol (TC) + PBS	55,500
TC + trypsin + α-chymotrypsin	5,400
TC + heat inactivated trypsin + α-chymotrypsin	51,100
TC + 5 mM dithiothreitol	65,100
TC + 100°C	2,500
B.[b]	
PBS	2,100
TC, pH 2.4	1,000
TC, pH 3.0	4,100
TC, pH 5.0	53,300
TC, pH 7.0	56,800
TC, pH 9.0	29,100
TC, pH 11.0	11,700

[a] Cytosol was prepared from the seminiferous tubules of adult mice and aliquots were incubated at 37°C for 4 hours with a mixture of trypsin (500 μg/ml) and α-chymotrypsin (500 μg/ml), an equivalent mixture of heat-inactivated trypsin and α-chymotrypsin, or PBS alone. The incubation was terminated by adding soybean trypsin inhibitor (2 mg/ml). Other samples were exposed at 25°C for 2 hours to PBS, to dithiothreitol, or to 100°C for 2 minutes. All samples were tested for their ability to stimulate DNA synthesis in BALB/c 3T3 cells. Data points are the mean of duplicate determinations.

[b] Aliquots of seminiferous tubule cytosol were dissolved in 1.0 M acetic acid that was previously buffered with NH$_4$OH to the pH values indicated. After a 2-hour incubation at 20°C the samples were lyophilized and tested for mitogenic activity.

SGF exhibits maximal activity between pH 5 and 7, but is inactivated by more extreme acidic and basic conditions, and reduction of disulfide bonds during a 2-hour exposure to 5 mM dithiothreitol has no adverse effect (Table II). Collectively, these observations suggest SGF is a polypeptide, whose tertiary structure is not functionally altered in an irreversible manner by disulfide bond reduction.

B. ESTIMATION OF SGF'S MOLECULAR WEIGHT

Mitogenic activity in the cytosol of calf and mouse seminiferous epithelia elutes in the void volume (M_rs > 100,000) when chromatographed by gel filtration in nondissociating conditions (Fig. 6). By contrast, a single, symmetrical peak of mitogenic activity is recovered when extracts are chromatographed on a BioGel P150 column in the presence of high salt (1 M ammonium acetate, pH 7.2). The elution volume corresponds to an

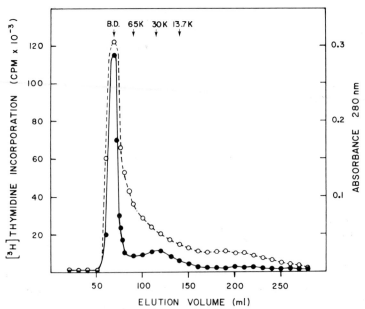

FIG. 6. Exclusion chromatography of mitogenic activity in nondissociating conditions. Seminiferous tubules of adult mice were homogenized in PBS and subjected to centrifugation (100,000 g; 60 minutes) to prepare a cytosolic fraction. An aliquot of cytosol was applied to a BioGel P150 column (5 × 60 cm) and the eluant fractions were lyophilized directly. The samples were solubilized in PBS for testing in the BALB/c 3T3 cell bioassay. In these dissociating conditions, essentially all of the activity elutes in the void volume as high-M_r complexes. Standards include Blue dextran (B.D., $M_r = 2 \times 10^6$), bovine serum albumin (65,000), carbonic anhydrase (30,000), and ribonuclease (13,700). Absorbance 260 nm (○), mitogenic activity (●).

M_r of 14,000–17,000 (Feig *et al.*, 1983). Likewise, a comparable peak of activity having an identical M_r is observed also when cytosol from either species is subjected to gel filtration in completely dissociating conditions, consisting of 6 M guanidine hydrochloride (G·HCl) and 5 mM DTT (Fig. 7). Repeated analyses in these denaturing conditions defines the M_r of SGF to be 15,700 (Feig *et al.*, 1983), as calculated by the procedure of Porath (1963).

C. ISOELECTRIC POINT OF SGF

Calf and mouse growth factor activities, when subjected to preparative isoelectric focusing, are recovered in those fractions having a pH of 3.8 to 4.2 (Fig. 8). Besides this acidic growth factor, the calf sample contains another mitogen that is isoelectric at pH 7.8 to 8.2 and represents ~15%

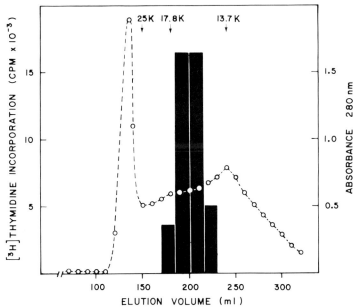

FIG. 7.   Gel filtration chromatography of calf seminiferous tubule cytosol in denaturing conditions. The sample, 1 mg protein in 100 μl of 6 M G · HCl, 5 mM DTT, pH 7.0, was applied to a Spherogel-TSK G3000SW high-performance gel filtration column (0.75 × 60 cm) equilibrated in the same buffer. The eluant fractions (1 ml) were dialyzed extensively against 20 mM ammonium bicarbonate, lyophilized, and assayed for their ability to stimulate DNA synthesis in confluent BALB/c 3T3 cells. The mitogenic activity was eluted as a monomeric polypeptide of 15,700 daltons. Similar results were obtained for the cytosol of adult mouse seminiferous tubules. Standards include Blue dextran (M_r = 2 × 106), ovalbumin (43,000), chymotrypsinogen (25,000), myoglobin (17,800), ribonuclease (13,700), and [³H]leucine (131). Absorbance 260 nm (○). Mitogenic activity (solid bars). [Reproduced from Feig *et al.* (1980), with permission of the Editor, *Proc. Natl. Acad. Sci. U.S.A.*]

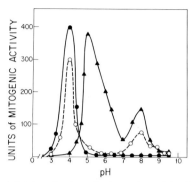

FIG. 8.   Isoelectric point determination of mitogenic activity from mouse and calf semi-niferous tubules under native and denaturing conditions. Both activities were purified by gel filtration chromatography from the cytosol of adult mouse (10 mg protein) and prepuberal calf (4.2 mg protein) seminiferous tubules. The mitogenic activity was applied, either in the presence or absence of 6 M urea, 5 mM DTT, to an isoelectric focusing column that was formed with carrier ampholytes, pH range 3.5 to 10. Eluant fractions were measured for pH, dialyzed, and then assayed for their ability to stimulate DNA synthesis in BALB/c 3T3 cells. Samples include native mouse SGF (●), native calf SGF (○), denatured calf SGF (▲). [Reproduced from Feig *et al.* (1983), with permission of the Editor, *J. Cell Biol.*]

of the total mitogenic activity. Since this cationic growth factor is not detectable in the adult mouse testis, it could be characteristic of prepu-beral animals or it may be unique to the calf seminiferous epithelium. This point has yet to be resolved.

The pH which SGF focuses may not represent the true isoelectric point of SGF for the following reasons. First, in conditions of low ionic strength, the growth factor aggregates and so the observed pI of the mitogenic activity may reflect some multimer or aggregate of the polypep-tide. Second, many proteins in their native conformation contain ioniz-able groups displaying abnormal dissociation constants. Such groups could be buried within the interior of the molecule or participating in strong intramolecular bonds (Tanford, 1962). These two possibilities have been examined by undertaking preparative isoelectric focusing in the presence of 6 M urea, an agent capable of dissociating oligimers and exposing buried ionizable groups (Ui, 1971). In these conditions, the calf preparation still yields two peaks of mitogenic activity, but the major peak is now isoelectric at pH 4.5 to 5.5, representing a basic shift of 1.0 pH unit (Fig. 8). By contrast, the minor peak is still isoelectric at pH 7.8 to 8.2. This difference in the apparent pIs in nondenaturing and denaturing con-ditions suggests the anionic growth factor associates with an acidic mole-cule or that ionizable groups are buried within the polypeptide's tertiary structure. These two possibilities can be distinguished by undertaking

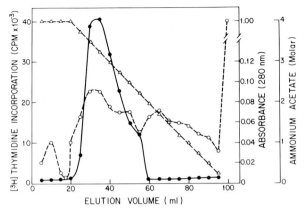

FIG. 9. Fractionation of the calf SGF by hydrophobic chromatography on dodecyl-agarose. Mitogenic activity, recovered following gel filtration in dissociating conditions (Feig *et al.*, 1983), was concentrated and then increased in ionic strength by adding solid ammonium acetate to a final concentration of 4.0 M. This sample, 5 mg protein in 10 ml, was applied to a dodecyl-agarose (1.5 × 1.7 cm) column that was previously equilibrated in the same buffer. SGF activity was eluted by applying a decreasing, linear gradient (75 ml) of 4.0 to 0 M ammonium acetate, pH 7.2. Eluted fractions were lyophilized and assayed for their ability to stimulate DNA synthesis in confluent cultures of BALB/c 3T3 cells. Mitogenic activity (●); absorbance, 280 nm (○); ammonium acetate concentration (△). [Reproduced from Feig *et al.* (1983), with permission of the Editor, *J. Cell Biol.*]

similar experiments once purified SGF is available. A comparable difference in p*I* is observed when pure thyroglobulin is exposed to similar conditions (Ui, 1971).

D. HYDROPHOBIC CHROMATOGRAPHY

SGF can be separated from many other proteins in the seminiferous epithelium on the basis of its hydrophilic properties. Thus, mouse and calf activities both elute from dodecyl-agarose at 3.0 to 1.5 M ammonium acetate after applying a decreasing, linear, salt gradient (Fig. 9). By contrast, >90% of testicular proteins are strongly hydrophobic in these conditions and therefore remain bound to the dodecyl-agarose.

E. SUMMATION OF THE BIOCHEMICAL PROPERTIES OF SGF

Calf and mouse SGF are heat sensitive proteins, having an M_r of 15,700 and a p*I* of 4.5 to 5.5 in dissociating conditions. Both polypeptides appear to have few exposed hydrophobic domains, yet they display strong tendencies to aggregate. Thus, SGF activities from these two sources are similar in their biochemical and biological properties. Comparable mitogenic activity has been observed in the seminiferous epithelium of all mammalian species tested. These common biochemical properties also demonstrate that SGF is distinct from other well-characterized growth factors such as EGF (Carpenter and Cohen, 1979), PDGF (Ross and Vogel, 1978), and the somatomedins (Van Wyk and Underwood, 1978). Another growth factor capable of stimulating BALB/c 3T3 cell proliferation has been discovered in rete testis fluid of rams (Brown et al., 1982), but based on current evidence it, too, appears to be biochemically distinct. However, an endothelial cell growth factor derived from bovine brain may be related to SGF since it has a similar M_r and pI (Maciag et al., 1982).

VII. Scheme for the Partial Purification of SGF

Seminiferous tubules of prepuberal calves have been used as a source for purifying SGF because of their availability, high specific activity,

TABLE III
Partial Purification of SGF from Calf Seminiferous Epithelium

Procedure	Protein recovered (mg)	Activity recovered (units × 10^{-3})[a]	Activity recovered (%)[b]	Purification factor[c]	Half maximal activity (μg/ml)[d]
Crude homogenate	12,000	300	100	—	160
Cytosol	6,000	270	90	1.8	89
Ammonium sulfate	2,225	200	66.7	3.6	44.0
DEAE ion exchange	400	95	31.7	9.5	16.8
P150 gel filtration	38.0	71	23.7	76.2	2.1
Dodecyl-agarose	4.30	35.5	11.8	333.3	0.48
HPLC gel filtration	0.45	4.0	1.3	355.6	0.45

[a] One unit of mitogenic activity is defined as the amount of activity necessary to induce half-maximal DNA synthesis in one microtiter well (250 μl) of confluent 3T3 cells (8 × 10^3 cells/0.33 cm^2).
[b] Activity recovered is expressed as the percentage of the activity in the original crude homogenate.
[c] The purification factor is the ratio of the specific mitogenic activity (units/mg protein) measured after each purification step to the specific mitogenic activity measured in the crude homogenate.
[d] Half-maximal activity is the protein concentration at which the pooled, active fractions stimulate half-maximal DNA synthesis in confluent cultures of BALB/c 3T3 cells.

and the similar biochemical properties of the calf and mouse polypeptides. Routinely, seminiferous cords are first recovered (Price, 1978) from 400 to 1000 calf testes to remove growth factors present in the interstitium and blood tissue. SGF then is partially purified by using the scheme outlined in Table III, and as detailed previously (Feig et al., 1983).

Briefly, most nonmitogenic proteins are precipitated from the seminiferous tubule cytosol with 40% saturated ammonium sulfate. Soluble constituents are recovered and fractionated by DEAE ion-exchange chromatography. Consistent with its pI, the anionic SGF elutes from DEAE cellulose at 75 to 125 mM NaCl in the presence of 10 mM sodium phosphate (pH 6.1). The eluted activity peak is equilibrated in 1 M ammonium acetate and subjected to gel filtration chromatography followed by hydrophobic chromatography on dodecyl-agarose. Finally, the activity is resolved by high-performance liquid chromatography (HPLC) in 6 M G·HCl. While a considerable proportion of the activity is lost in this latter separation, primarily due to an irreversible denaturation of SGF, several major contaminating proteins are removed successfully. The progressive purification of SGF is revealed by SDS–PAGE analysis of the successive preparations. These demonstrate a marked reduction in protein complexity through to the final preparation of seven polypeptide bands (Fig. 10). Unfortunately, attempts to recover SGF following SDS–PAGE have not been successful, and so the identity of the polypeptide band having activity remains to be determined.

The final preparation of SGF stimulates half-maximal DNA synthesis in BALB/c 3T3 cells at 450 ng/ml. The purity of this preparation can be estimated by comparing the specific mitogenic activity with that expected for a pure growth factor. After allowing for the known extent ($\sim$80%) of irreversible denaturation during the last purification step, the specific activity of SGF may approximate 90 ng protein/ml. However, pure SGF, if comparable to other growth factors, should stimulate 3T3 cell proliferation at protein concentrations of 1 to 10 ng/ml (Gospodarowicz and Moran, 1976). On this basis, the present preparation of SGF has a purity of 1–10%.

Further purification of SGF will require additional high resolution fractionation techniques. For this reason the purified preparation is being used as an immunogen to generate a series of hybridoma lines for selecting monoclonal antibodies directed against the polypeptide. Optimistically, by selecting specifically for switch antibodies, these monospecific reagents may be useful as immunoaffinity ligands for purifying SGF to homogeneity.

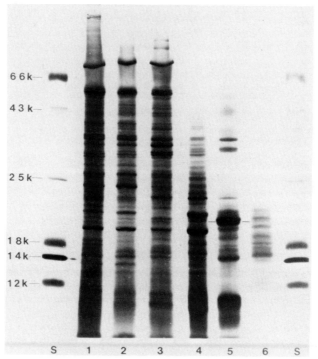

FIG. 10. SDS–PAGE analysis of proteins recovered at successive steps of purifying calf SGF. Aliquots of activity pooled at each purification step were analyzed by SDS–PAGE (Laemmli, 1970) and silver staining (Oakley *et al.,* 1980). The sample lanes include protein from crude cytosol (1); ammonium sulfate precipitate (2); and the pooled activity following chromatography on DEAE (3); gel filtration in 1.0 *M* ammonium acetate (4); dodecyl-agarose (5); and HPLC under dissociating conditions (6). Standards (S) include bovine serum albumin (66,300), ovalbumin (43,000), chymotrypsinogen (25,000), myoglobin (17,800), lysozyme (14,300), and cytochrome *c* (12,400). [Reproduced from Feig *et al.* (1983), with permission of the Editor, *J. Cell Biol.*]

VIII. Biological Properties of SGF

A. LOCALIZATION OF SGF WITHIN THE MAMMALIAN SEMINIFEROUS EPITHELIUM

The seminiferous epithelium consists of two classes of cells, the sustentacular Sertoli cells and both the renewing and differentiating spermatogenic cells. In the mouse, at 6 days after birth, the epithelium is comprised solely of the mitotically proliferating spermatogonia (~16%) and Sertoli cells (~84%) (Bellvé *et al.,* 1977a,b). However, during the

TABLE IV

Temporal Appearance of Spermatogenic Cells during Development of the Mouse Testis[a]

Cell type	Days after birth								
	6	8	10	12	14	16	18	20	84
Primitive type A spermatogonia	16								
Type A spermatogonia		17	7	7	6	9	3	4	1
Type B spermatogonia		10	11	8	6	8	7	6	3
Preleptotene spermatocytes			15	11	9	5	10	7	2
Leptotene spermatocytes			15	12	13	5	5	9	2
Zygotene spermatocytes				23	14	7	8	8	2
Pachytene spermatocytes					15	27	36	33	15
Secondary spermatocytes							1	1	1
Round spermatids							1	4	31
Condensing spermatids									40
Sertoli cells	84	73	52	39	37	39	29	28	3

[a] Data are expressed as a percentage of total cells in the seminiferous epithelium of prepuberal and adult mice. The cell counts were determined by classifying nuclei present in 50 cross-sections chosen at random after sectioning the testes of three mice killed at each designated age. Degenerating and unidentified cells (2–4%) are not included in these data. For simplicity the data have been corrected to the nearest integer. Round spermatids include steps 1–8, condensing spermatids steps 9–16. (After Bellvé et al., 1977a, reproduced by permission of the Editor, J. Cell Biol.)

second and third week of development the meiotic spermatocytes and haploid spermatids appear in increasing numbers, until they become the dominant cell types (93%) in the adult seminiferous epithelium (Table IV) (Bellvé et al., 1977b). Consequently, a study of growth factor activity in the developing seminiferous epithelium can indicate the most likely source(s) of SGF.

Quantifying the growth factor in the seminiferous tubules of mice at successive stages of postnatal development shows the highest specific activity to occur 6 days after birth (Fig. 11). Thereafter, the specific mitogenic activity declines substantially; compared to the levels observed at day 6, the specific activity reduces to one-third at day 20, and to one-fifth in the adult testis. This apparent dilution of activity correlates with the temporal appearance and the gradual but substantial accumulation of meiotic and postmeiotic germ cells (cf. Table IV; Bellvé et al., 1977a,b). These data, therefore, strongly suggest the growth factor resides in Sertoli cells and/or spermatogonia, rather than in the more differentiated germ cells.

Localization of SGF within the seminiferous epithelium can be resolved more directly by isolating discrete populations of specific cell types. This

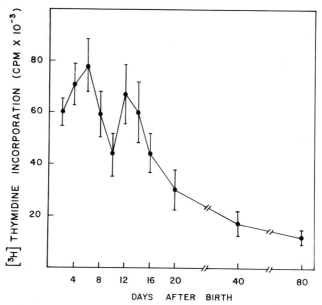

FIG. 11.   Mitogenic activity in the seminiferous epithelium during postnatal development of the mouse. Seminiferous tubules were isolated from testes of individual mice at various ages after birth. Multiple aliquots of cytosolic protein (25 μg) were tested for mitogenic activity on confluent BALB/c 3T3 cells. [Reproduced from Feig *et al.* (1980), by permission of the Editor, *Proc. Natl. Acad. Sci. U.S.A.*]

is accomplished by using differential sedimentation velocity at unit gravity (Romrell *et al.,* 1976; Bellvé *et al.,* 1977a,b). When cytosolic preparations of the isolated cells, including Sertoli cells (>99% pure) and the respective spermatogenic cells, are tested for mitogenic activity on confluent BALB/c 3T3 cells substantial differences are observed. Prepuberal Sertoli cells contain by far the greatest concentration of activity, with lesser but still significant amounts occurring in both primitive type A spermatogonia and preleptotene spermatocytes (Fig. 12). By contrast, no activity is detected in type A or type B spermatogonia, leptotene, zygotene, or pachytene spermatocytes, spermatids, or residual bodies.

These results show Sertoli cells to be the major source of mitogenic activity in the seminiferous epithelium of the prepuberal mouse testis. An important question still remaining is whether the nondividing, Sertoli cells of the adult testis also contain the growth factor. This possibility could be resolved by directly assaying Sertoli cells isolated from adult mice. Unfortunately, monodisperse suspensions of adult Sertoli cells are difficult to generate because the extensive array of intercellular, tight junctions resist dissociation by enzymes. Thus, sedimentation velocity at unit gravity is not applicable for purifying these cells.

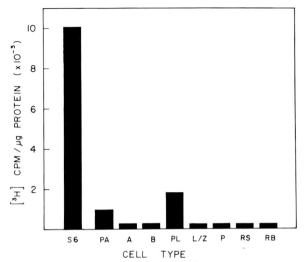

FIG. 12.   Growth factor activity in cells isolated from the mouse seminiferous epithelium. The respective cell types were purified from the seminiferous epithelia of prepuberal
and adult mice by using sedimentation velocity at unit gravity (Bellvé *et al.*, 1977a,b). The
cells were homogenized and aliquots tested for activity on confluent BALB/c 3T3 cells. The
cell types tested include Sertoli cells from 6-day-old mice (S6); primitive type A (PA), type A
spermatogonia (A), type B spermatogonia (B); preleptotene spermatocytes (PL), leptotene/
zygotene spermatocytes (L/Z), pachytene spermatocytes (P), round spermatids (RS), and
residual bodies (RB). [Reproduced from Feig *et al.* (1980), with permission of the Editor,
Proc. Natl. Acad. Sci. U.S.A.]

These problems can be circumvented, in part, by utilizing testes of
germ cell-depleted mice. Homozygous mice of the genotype W/W^v are
characterized by severe anemia, coat color spotting, and infertility due to
the absence of germ cells (Mintz and Russell, 1955, 1957). In this case, it
is feasible to prepare purified (>90%) populations of Sertoli cells from the
seminiferous tubules of W/W^v adult testes by a brief collagenase dissociation. Notably, homogenates of these cells stimulate DNA synthesis in 3T3
cells to half-maximal levels at a protein concentration of 92 ± 10 μg/ml.
Similarly, homogenates prepared from the germ cell-depleted seminiferous tubules of hypophysectomized, adult mice stimulate half-maximal
DNA synthesis in confluent 3T3 cells at a similar protein concentration of
80 ± 15 μg/ml. By contrast, comparable preparations of heterozygous
(W^v/+) and wild type (+/+) seminiferous tubules, both containing
normal complements of germ cells, stimulate half-maximal DNA synthesis at 400 ± 9.0 μg protein/ml. Thus, the specific mitogenic activity of the
"Sertoli cell only" tubules is 4-fold greater than seminiferous tubules of
normal adult mice. Since these epithelial cells represent some ~25% of
the total cell volume of the normal, adult seminiferous epithelium (Cavic-

chia and Dym, 1977), these results are consistent with Sertoli cells being the major source of mitogenic activity throughout postnatal development.

The existence of a mitogenic factor in Sertoli cells suggests the polypeptide may have a role in regulating spermatogenesis. Sertoli cells, in forming the seminiferous epithelium, may serve many functions in spermatogenesis, including (1) acting as target cells through which FSH and testosterone influence spermatogenesis (review; Fawcett, 1977), (2) providing pyruvate and lactate as an energy source for germ cell metabolism, and (3) possibly creating a unique microenvironment for germ cell differentiation. Also, Sertoli cells cease to proliferate during prepuberal development implying that the mitogen may be targeted for neighboring cells in the testis. A paracrine role for SGF is consistent with earlier evidence indicating locally produced "factors" may promote the proliferation of spermatogonia. Moreover, Sertoli cells are known to synthesize transferrin (Skinner and Griswold, 1980), an iron-transporting protein that enables cells to traverse the G_2 phase of the cell cycle (Rudland *et al.*, 1977). Therefore, it is plausible that SGF, by inducing cells to proceed through the G_1 phase of the cell cycle, acts coordinately with transferrin to promote spermatogonial proliferation. The partial restoration of spermatogonial divisions by the synergistic effects of transferrin, insulin, and FSH (Haneji and Nishimune, 1982) is consistent with this idea. Finally, SGF may act external to the seminiferous epithelium. Some evidence already exists to suggest "factors" from the epithelial compartment may influence cells locally in the interstitium of the testis (Aoki and Fawcett, 1978) and perhaps in the caput epididymis (Fawcett and Hoffer, 1979). The factor(s) and the mechanisms involved in these various physiological responses are still being elucidated by contemporary studies.

B. DEPENDENCE OF SGF ACTIVITY ON THE PITUITARY AND GONADOTROPIN HORMONES

Synthesis of SGF, even in Sertoli cell cultures, cannot be demonstrated definitively in the absence of highly specific and sensitive probes. It is plausible, however, that the levels of activity in Sertoli cells may be dependent on the presence of a functional pituitary, either as a source of the polypeptide or by being regulated by the gonadotrophic hormones, FSH and/or LH. These two possibilities have been examined by assaying for SGF activity in the seminiferous tubules of mice 30 days posthypophysectomy.

Removal of the pituitary causes a 4-fold increase in the specific mitogenic activity (units/mg protein) of testis homogenates. This apparent increase, in part, is due to the selective depletion of spermatocytes and spermatids from the seminiferous epithelium (Clermont and Morgentaler,

TABLE V
Growth Factor Activity in the Adult Mouse Testis following Hypophysectomy[a]

Sample	Specific activity (units/mg protein)	Total protein (mg/testis)	Total activity (units/testis)
Control	11.8 ± 0.6	11.5 ± 0.9	137 ± 11.3
Hypox[b]	47.7 ± 6.1	2.1 ± 0.3	90 ± 4.9

[a]Testes were recovered separately from five normal adult mice and seven adult mice 30 days posthypophysectomy. The protein content, specific mitogenic activity (units/mg protein), and the total activity/testis were determined for the two groups of experimental animals. Data represent mean ± SE.

[b]All values are significantly different ($p < 0.002$) from the corresponding control values, as determined by two-sample t tests.

1955; Russell and Clermont, 1976), which causes a 6-fold decrease in total testicular protein (Table V). After accounting for these changes, the total mitogenic activity per testis actually decreases 35% ($p < 0.002$) in response to hypophysectomy. This decrement is modest compared to the 1000-fold decrease in ABP levels (Sanborn et al., 1977) and the 10-fold reduction in FSH binding sites (Thanki and Steinberger, 1978) in Sertoli cells. Similarly, two other growth factors, EGF in the salivary gland (Byyny et al., 1972) and somatomedins in blood (Stiles et al., 1979) decline 14-fold and 20-fold, respectively, following hypophysectomy. Moreover, the levels of mitogenic activity of Sertoli cells of hypophysectomized, adult mice are comparable to those of mice with normal pituitary function. Based on this evidence, the pituitary does not seem to be a major regulator of SGF levels in the seminiferous epithelium. This conclusion does not negate the possibility of changes in SGF activity occurring at earlier times after hypophysectomy. More detailed experiments are required to resolve this issue.

C. STIMULATION OF SERTOLI CELL PROLIFERATION *IN VITRO* BY SGF

The ability of SGF to induce proliferation of confluent BALB/c 3T3 cells has enabled the discovery, characterization, and partial purification of the polypeptide. However, this assay does not provide direct information concerning the mitogen's physiological function in the mammalian testis. Therefore, a search for testicular cells capable of responding to SGF has been initiated. Sertoli cells can be maintained in primary culture for moderate periods of time, and therefore can be tested directly (Steinberger *et al.,* 1975; Dorrington *et al.,* 1975). These cells are isolated routinely from 6-day-old mice by sedimentation velocity and then seeded in minimal Eagle's medium (MEM), supplemented with 10% calf serum (CS). After the cells firmly adhere to the culture dish (~12 hours), the MEM-CS is replaced by a chemically defined medium consisting of Hams F12 and Dulbecco's modified Eagle's medium (DMEM) (1:1 v/v), supplemented with $NaHCO_3$ (1.2 ng/liter), HEPES (15 mM), glutamine (2 mM), insulin (10 μg/ml), transferrin (5 ng/ml), retinoic acid (50 ng/ml), gentimycin sulfate (50 μg/ml), and fungizone (2.5 μg/ml) (Bottenstein *et al.,* 1979). Compared to control cells in these conditions, partially purified SGF at 30 μg protein/ml promotes an additional 2.5-fold increase in cell number within 6 days (Fig. 13).

The ability of SGF to induce Sertoli cell proliferation is mimicked by partially purified cartilage derived-growth factor (CDGF, 100 μg/ml) (Klagsbrun and Smith, 1980). By contrast, pure epidermal growth factor (EGF, 50 ng/ml) and partially purified platelet-derived growth factor (PDGF, 1 μg/ml) do not have a mitogenic effect (Fig. 13), even though at these same concentrations all growth factor preparations maximally stimulate DNA synthesis in confluent BALB/c 3T3 cells. Likewise, FSH (10

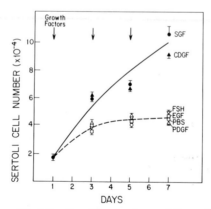

FIG. 13. Stimulation of Sertoli cell proliferation by partially purified mouse SGF. Prepuberal Sertoli cells were purified by velocity sedimentation at unit gravity from testes of 6-day-old mice and seeded at moderately sparse densities (9×10^3 cells/cm^2) in MEM containing 10% calf serum. The cells were cultured for 14 hours to allow attachment to the substratum, at which time the serum-containing medium was removed by washing. At 14 hours and at every subsequent 48 hours, until the cells were harvested for counting, fresh medium and growth factors (arrows) were added. Data represent the mean ± SE of triplicate determinations. Potential mitogens tested include SGF, partially purified from adult mouse seminiferous tubules, 30 μg protein/ml (●); CDGF, cartilage extract, 100 μg/ml (▲); PDGF, purified by ion-exchange chromatography and gel filtrations, 1 μg/ml (△); pure EGF, 50 ng/ml (□); rat FSH, 10 μg/ml (▽); and PBS, control (○).

μg/ml) did not have a significant effect on Sertoli cell proliferation. This latter result contrasts with the reports of Griswold *et al.* (1976, 1977), who claim FSH stimulates both [^{3}H]thymidine incorporation into DNA and cell division, as determined by an increased mitotic index in primary cultures of rat Sertoli cells. This apparent discrepancy may be due to a species difference or to the dissimilar experimental procedures.

Regardless, SGF is considerably more effective than FSH in promoting the *in vitro* proliferation of prepuberal mouse Sertoli cells. Moreover, the growth factor activity is greatest in the seminiferous epithelium of postnatal mice (Fig. 11), during a period when the Sertoli cells are proliferating maximally (Nagy, 1972; Steinberger and Steinberger, 1971; Orth, 1982). An analogous autocrine stimulation also appears to occur *in vitro* for CDGF (Klagsbrun *et al.*, 1977) and nerve growth factor (Sherwin *et al.*, 1979). In this regard it is interesting that Sertoli cells cease dividing during prepuberal development (Steinberger and Steinberger, 1971; Nagy, 1972), and yet the differentiated cells still contain considerable amounts of mitogenic activity. One possibility presently under investigation is whether Sertoli cells lose the ability to respond to SGF after acquiring their differentiated functions, or whether the mitogenic response is simply "uncoupled" from the pathways involved in expressing the cells' other physiological functions.

IX. Discussion

The seminiferous growth factor, SGF, is an anionic, hydrophilic polypeptide having a monomeric M_r of 15,700. This mitogenic protein, being distinct from other well-characterized growth factors, is presumed to play fundamental roles in testicular physiology. First, SGF appears to be ubiquitous to mammalian species, implying that it is phylogenetically conserved and therefore must serve an essential function, at least in regulating cell proliferation, if not in modulating the expression of some differentiative process. Second, the polypeptide is localized primarily to Sertoli cells, the "sustentacular" cells of the seminiferous epithelium. These epithelial cells are responsive to FSH and testosterone (Means *et al.*, 1976) and, therefore, are considered to have a central role in regulating spermatogenesis. Their ability to synthesize and secrete transferrin (Skinner and Griswold, 1980) and lactate, a preferred metabolic substrate of germ cells (Robinson and Fritz, 1981; Nakamura *et al.*, 1981), supports this idea. Thus, Sertoli cells may direct SGF, as required, to promote spermatogonial proliferation in the basal compartment or to induce the two meiotic reduction divisions that occur in the avascular, central compartment of the seminiferous epithelium. Third, SGF's property of inducing DNA synthesis and cell proliferation among prepuberal Sertoli cells and the fibroblastic BALB/c 3T3 cells suggests a major role for the polypeptide in promoting testicular development. Simply by enhancing the proliferation of cells of epithelial and mesenchymal origin, SGF could act as a major determinant of gonadal growth and differentiation. The potential implications of SGF foster continuing current efforts to purify the polypeptide to homogeneity. This approach will facilitate future studies designed to resolve the physiological functions of the seminiferous growth factor in promoting mammalian spermatogenesis.

ACKNOWLEDGMENTS

The preparation of this review article was funded, in part, by a research grant from Emtek Corp. The authors extend their appreciation to Mrs. Barbara Lewis for help in preparing the manuscript and to Steven Borack for photographic services rendered.

REFERENCES

Aoki, A., and Fawcett, D. W. (1978). *Biol. Reprod.* **19**, 144.

Bartmanska, J., and Clermont, Y. (1983). *Cell Tissue Kinet.* **16**, 135.

Beaumont, H. M., and Mandl, A. M. (1962). *Proc. R. Soc. Ser. B* **155**, 557.

Beaumont, H. M., and Mandl, A. M. (1963). *J. Embryol. Exp. Morphol.* **11**, 715.

Begeot, M., Dupouy, J. P., Dubois, M. P., and Dubois, P. M. (1981). *Neuroendocrinology* **32**, 285.

Bellvé, A. R. (1979). *In* "Oxford Reviews of Reproductive Biology" (C. A. Finn, ed.), pp. 159–261. Oxford Univ. Press, London and New York.

Bellvé, A. R., Cavicchia, J. C., Millette, C. F., O'Brien, D. A., Bhatnagar, Y. M., and Dym, M. (1977a). *J. Cell Biol.* **74**, 68.

Bellvé, A. R., Millette, C. F., Bhatnagar, Y. M., and O'Brien, D. A. (1977b). *J. Histochem. Cytochem.* **25**, 480.

Bennet, D. (1956). *J. Morphol.* **98**, 199.

Bjerregaard, P., Bro-Rasmussen, F., and Reumert, T. (1974). *Z. Zellforsch.* **147**, 401.

Black, V. H., and Christensen, A. K. (1969). *Am. J. Anat.* **124**, 211.

Bottenstein, I., Hayashi, I., Hutchings, S., Masui, H., Mather, J., McClure, D. B., O'Hara, S., Rozzino, A., Sato, G., Serrero, G., Wolf, R., and Wu, R. (1979). *In* "Methods in Enzymology" (W. B. Jakoby and I. N. Pastan, eds.), pp. 94–109. Academic Press, New York.

Brown, K. D., Blakeley, D. M., Henville, A., and Setchell, B. P. (1982). *Biochem. Biophys. Res. Commun.* **105**, 391.

Bustos-Obregon, E., and Courot, M. (1974). *Cell Tissue Res.* **150**, 481.

Bynny, R. C., Orth, D. N., and Cohen, S. (1972). *Endocrinology* **90**, 1251.

Carpenter, G., and Cohen, S. (1979). *Annu. Rev. Biochem.* **48**, 193.

Cavicchia, J. C., and Dym, M. (1977). *Am. J. Anat.* **150**, 501.

Chemes, H. D., Dym, M., and Raj, H. G. M. (1979). *Biol. Reprod.* **21**, 241.

Chrétien, F. C. (1966). *J. Embryol. Exp. Morphol.* **16**, 591.

Clermont, Y. (1972). *Physiol. Rev.* **52**, 198.

Clermont, Y., and Antar, M. (1973). *Am. J. Anat.* **136**, 153.

Clermont, Y., and Bustos-Obregon, E. (1968). *Am. J. Anat.* **122,** 237.

Clermont, Y., and Leblond, C. P. (1955). *Am. J. Anat.* **96,** 229.

Clermont, Y., and Mauger, A. (1974). *Cell. Tissue Kinet.* **7,** 165.

Clermont, Y., and Mauger, A. (1976). *Cell. Tissue Kinet.* **9,** 99.

Clermont, Y., and Morgentaler, H. (1955). *Endocrinology* **57,** 369.

Clermont, Y., and Perey, B. (1957). *Am. J. Anat.* **100,** 241.

Courot, M., and Ortavant, R. (1981). *J. Reprod. Fertil. Suppl.* **30,** 47.

Cunningham, G. R., and Huckins, C. (1979). *Cell. Tissue Kinet.* **12,** 81.

Cunningham, G. R., Tindall, D. J., Huckins, C.,and Means, A. R. (1978). *Endocrinology* **102,** 16.

de Reviers, M., Hochereau-de Reviers, M.-T., Blanc, M. R., Brillard, P., Courot, M., and Pelletier, J. (1980). *Reprod. Nutr. Dev.* **20,** 241.

Dorrington, J. H., Roller, N. F., and Fritz, I. B. (1975). *Mol. Cell. Endocrinol.* **3,** 57.

Dym, M., and Clermont, Y. (1970). *Am. J. Anat.* **128,** 265.

Eddy, E. M., Clark, J. M., Gong, D., and Fenderson, B. A. (1981). *Gamete Res.* **4,** 333.

Everett, N. B. (1943). *J. Exp. Zool.* **92,** 49.

Fawcett, D. W. (1977). *In* "Frontiers in Reproduction and Fertility Control" (R. O. Greep and M. A. Koblinsky, eds.), pp. 302–320. MIT Press, Cambridge, Massachusetts.

Fawcett, D. W., and Hoffer, A. P. (1979). *Biol. Reprod.* **20,** 167.

Feig, L. A. (1982). Ph.D. thesis, Harvard University, pp. 1–157.

Feig, L. A., Bellvé, A. R., Horbach-Erickson, N., and Klagsbrun, M. (1980). *Proc. Natl. Acad. Sci. U.S.A.* **77,** 4774.

Feig, L. A., Klagsbrun, M., and Bellvé, A. R. (1983). *J. Cell Biol.* **97,** 1435.

Flickinger, C. J. (1967). *Z. Zellforsch.* **78,** 92.

Fouquet, J. P., and Dang, D. C. (1980). *Reprod. Nutr. Dev.* **20,** 1439.

Franchi, L. L., and Mandl, A. M. (1964). *J. Embryol. Exp. Morphol.* **12,** 289.

Gillis, S., Mochizvki, D. Y., Conlon, P. J., Hefeneider, S. H., Ramthun, C. A., Gillis, A. E., Frank, M. A., Henney, C. S., and Watson, J. D. (1982). *Immunol. Rev.* **63,** 167.

Gillman, J. (1948). *Contrib. Embryol. Carnegie Inst.* **32,** 82.

Gondos, B., Renston, R. H., and Goldstein, D. A. (1976). *Am. J. Anat.* **145,** 167.

Gospodarowicz, D., and Moran, J. S. (1976). *Annu. Rev. Biochem.* **45,** 531.

Griswold, M. D., Mably, E. R., and Fritz, I. B. (1976). *Mol. Cell. Endocrinol.* **4,** 139.

Griswold, M. D., Solari, A., Tung, P. S., and Fritz, I. B. (1977). *Mol. Cell. Endocrinol.* **7,** 151.

Handel, M. A., and Eppig, J. (1979). *Biol. Reprod.* **20,** 1031.

Haneji, T., and Nishimune, Y. (1982). *J. Endocrinol.* **94,** 43.

Hilscher, B., and Hilscher, W. (1978). *Cell Tissue Res.* **190,** 61.

Hilscher, W., and Hilscher, B. (1976). *Andrologia* **8,** 105.

Hilscher, W., and Makoski, H. B. (1968). *Z. Zellforsch.* **86,** 327.

Hochereau-de Reviers, M.-T., and Courot, M. (1978). *Ann. Biol. Anim. Biochem. Biophys.* **18,** 573.

Hochereau-de Reviers, M.-T., Loir, M., and Pelletier, J. (1976). *J. Reprod. Fertil.* **46,** 203.

Huckins, C. (1971a). *Cell Tissue Kinet.* **4,** 139.

Huckins, C. (1971b). *Anat. Rec.* **169,** 533.

Huckins, C. (1971c). *Cell Tissue Kinet.* **4,** 313.

Huckins, C. (1973). *Anat. Rec.* **175,** 347 (Abstr.).

Huckins, C. (1978a). *Biol. Reprod.* **19,** 313.

Huckins, C. (1978b). *Biol. Reprod.* **19,** 747.

Huckins, C., and Clermont, Y. (1968). *Arch. Anat. Morphol. Exp.* **69,** 297.

Huckins, C., and Cunningham, G. R. (1975). *Anat. Rec.* **181,** 380a.

Huckins, C., and Cunningham, G. R. (1978). *Radiat. Res.* **76,** 331.

Huckins, C., and Oakberg, E. F. (1978a). *Anat. Rec.* **192,** 519.
Huckins, C., and Oakberg, E. F. (1978b). *Anat. Rec.* **192,** 529.
Irons, M. J., and Clermont, Y. (1979). *Cell Tissue Kinet.* **12,** 425.
Jost, A. (1972). *Arch. Anat. Microsc. Morphol. Exp.* **61,** 415.
Klagsbrun, M., and Smith, S. (1980). *J. Biol. Chem.* **255,** 10859–10866.
Klagsbrun, M., Langer, R., Levenson, R., Smith, S., and Lillehei, C. (1977). *Exp. Cell Res.* **105,** 99.
Kluin, Ph. M., Kramer, M. F., and de Rooij, D. G. (1982). *Int. J. Androl.* **5,** 282.
Laemmli, U. K. (1970). *Nature (London)* **227,** 680.
Leeson, C. R., and Forman, D. E. (1981). *J. Anat.* **132,** 491.
Leeson, C. R., and Leeson, T. S. (1963). *Anat. Rec.* **147,** 243.
Leeson, T. S. (1975). *J. Morphol.* **147,** 171.
Lok, D., and de Rooij, D. G. (1983). *Cell Tissue Kinet.* **16,** 7.
Lok, D., Jansen, M. T., and de Rooij, D. G. (1983). *Cell Tissue Kinet.* **16,** 19.
Lostroh, A. J. (1969). *Endocrinology* **85,** 438.
Maciag, T., Hoover, G. A., and Weinstein, R. (1982). *J. Biol. Chem.* **257,** 5333.
Magre, S., and Jost, A. (1980). *Arch. Anat. Microsc. Morphol. Exp.* **69,** 297.
Means, A. R., Fakunding, J. L., Huckins, C., Tindall, D. J., and Vitale, R. (1976). *Recent Prog. Horm. Res.* **32,** 477.
Merchant, H. (1975). *Dev. Biol.* **44,** 1.
Mintz, B., and Russell, E. S. (1955). *Anat. Rec.* **122,** 443.
Mintz, B., and Russell, E. S. (1957). *J. Exp. Zool.* **134,** 207.
Mittwoch, U. (1969). *Nature (London)* **221,** 446.
Mittwoch, U. (1970). *Philos. Trans. R. Soc. London Ser. B* **259,** 113.
Mittwoch, U., and Buehr, M. L. (1973). *Differentiation* **1,** 219.
Mizel, S. B. (1982). *Immunol. Rev.* **63,** 51.
Monesi, V. (1962). *J. Cell Biol.* **14,** 1.
Nagy, F. (1972). *J. Reprod. Fertil.* **28,** 389.
Nakamura, M., Hino, A., Yasumasu, I., and Kato, J. (1981). *J. Biochem.* **89,** 1309.
Nebel, B. R., Amarose, A. P., and Hackett, E. M. (1961). *Science* **134,** 832.
Novi, A. M., and Saba, P. (1968). *Z. Zellforsch.* **86,** 313.
Oakberg, E. F. (1971a). *Anat. Rec.* **169,** 515.
Oakberg, E. F. (1971b). *Mutat. Res.* **11,** 1.
Oakley, B. R., Kirsch, D. R., and Morris, N. R. (1980). *Anal. Biochem.* **105,** 361.
Orth, J. (1982). *Anat. Rec.* **203,** 485.
Orth, J., and Christensen, A. K. (1978). *Endocrinology* **103,** 1944.
Porath, J. (1963). *Pure Appl. Chem.* **6,** 233.
Price, D. (1970). *Philos. Trans. R. Soc. London Ser. B* **259,** 133.
Price, J. M. (1978). *Am. J. Anat.* **156,** 147.
Price, D., and Pannabercer, R. (1959). *Arch. Anat. Microsc. Morphol. Exp.* **48,** 223.
Reddy, K. J., and Svoboda, D. T. (1967). *Arch. Pathol.* **84,** 376.
Robinson, R., and Fritz, I. (1981). *Biol. Reprod.* **24,** 1032.
Romrell, L. J., Bellvé, A. R., and Fawcett, D. W. (1976). *Dev. Biol.* **49,** 119.
Rooij, D. G., de (1973). *Cell Tissue Kinet.* **6,** 287.
Roosen-Runge, E. C., and Anderson, D. (1959). *Acta Anat.* **37,** 125.
Ross, M. H. (1967). *Am. J. Anat.* **121,** 523.
Ross, R., and Vogel, A. (1978). *Cell* **14,** 203.
Rudland, P. S., Durbin, H., Clingan, D., and De Asua, L. J. (1977). *Biochem. Biophys. Res. Commun.* **75,** 556.
Russell, L. D., and Clermont, Y. (1976). *Anat. Rec.* **187,** 347.

Russo, J., and de Rosas, J. C. (1971). *Am. J. Anat.* **130**, 461.

Sanborn, B. M., Steinberger, A., Tcholakian, R. K., and Steinberger, E. (1977). *Steroids* **29**, 493.

Sapsford, C. S. (1963). *J. Anat. (London)* **97**, 225.

Skinner, M. K., and Griswold, M. D. (1980). *J. Biol. Chem.* **255**, 9523.

Steinberger, A., and Steinberger, E. (1971). *Biol. Reprod.* **4**, 84.

Steinberger, A., Heindel, J. J., Lindsey, J. N., Elkington, J. S. H., Sanborn, B. M., and Steinberger, E. (1975). *Endocrine Res. Commun.* **2**, 261.

Stiles, C. D., Capone, G. T., Scher, C. D., Antionades, H. N., Van Wyk, J. J., and Pledger, W. J. (1979). *Proc. Natl. Acad. Sci. U.S.A.* **76**, 1279.

Tanford, C. (1962). *Adv. Protein Chem.* **17**, 69.

Thanki, K. H., and Steinberger, A. (1978). *Andrologia* **20**, 195.

Thumann, A., and Bustos-Obregon, E. (1978). *Andrologia* **14**, 35.

Till, J. E., and McCulloch, E. A. (1980). *Biochim. Biophys. Acta* **605**, 431.

Tougard, C., Picart, R., and Tixier-Vidal, A. (1977). *Dev. Biol.* **58**, 148.

Ui, N. (1971). *Biochim. Biophys. Acta* **229**, 567.

Upadhyay, S., Luciani, J. M., and Zamboni, L. (1979). *Ann. Biol. Anim. Biochem. Biophys.* **19**, 1179.

Upadhyay, S., Luciani, J. M., and Zamboni, L. (1981). *In* "Development and Function of Reproductive Organs" (A. G. Byskov and H. Peters, eds.), pp. 18–27. Excerpta Medica, Intern. Congr. Ser., Amsterdam.

Van Wyk, J. J., and Underwood, L. E. (1978). *In* "Biochemical Actions of Hormones" (G. Litwaek, ed.), pp. 101–114. Academic Press, New York.

Zamboni, L., and Upadhyay, S. (1982). *Am. J. Anat.* **165**, 339.

DISCUSSION

B. Posner: In your purification scheme it seemed that the last step, the HPLC step, did not add anything to the extent of purification although it did result in a very substantial loss of protein. I think you ended up with one-tenth the amount of protein and the specific activity did not change. So, I imagine you will not continue with that last step.

A. R. Bellvé: Correct. While the isocratic HPLC step was important for resolving the mitogenic activity from among the other polypeptides, pooling the active peak gave only a marginal improvement in the specific activity of SGF. This procedure did facilitate the removal of a major contaminating protein ($M_r \sim 22,500$), but the increased purity was offset by an apparent denaturation of SGF in the presence of 6 M G · HCl, the column eluant. Recent efforts have been directed toward applying alternate procedures for purifying SGF by HPLC, including isocratic, ion-exchange, and reverse-phase methods.

B. Posner: The second question is that your assay looks at mitogenic activity in cultured cells. Have you tried injecting this material into the testis to see whether it stimulates tritiated thymidine incorporation into cells in the testis? You could use one testis as a control for the other, perhaps.

A. R. Bellvé: No, that particular experiment has not been attempted. We have considered undertaking comparable experiments using partially purified preparations of the mitogen. But, until pure SGF is available the ensuing data would be equivocal. The results could be confounded by the presence of other mitogens or by the "chalone," an inhibitor of spermatogonial DNA synthesis purportedly present in testicular extracts [see Irons, M. J., and Clermont, Y. (1979). *Cell Tissue Kinet.* **12**, 425–433]. Interestingly, Hochereau-de-Reviers and colleagues have observed a marginal increase in the number of type A spermatogonia (Stages 3, A_0–A_3) in adult rat testes after administering an extract of prepuberal testis [Hochereau-de Reviers *et al.* (1982). *Andrologia* **14**, 297–305]. This effect may not be due to SGF, however, since the authors used an acidified acetone extract of crude testicular cytosol, a procedure that would be expected to irreversibly denature most of the SGF activity.

J. F. Roser: Can you expand on the idea of FSH being an activator for SGF?

A. R. Bellvé: Not really, as we do not have any direct evidence to support this notion. The testicular levels of SGF activity decline to ~65% of control values by 30 days following hypophysectomy, but these limited data should not be interpreted as evidence for a role of FSH in promoting SGF synthesis, secretion, or effects on target cells. Definitive experiments on the possible gonadotropin regulation of SGF levels in the testis will be feasible when a specific and sensitive immunoassay is developed for the polypeptide.

S-Y. Ying: In the study on hypophysectomized mice would you conclude that the pituitary is involved in regulating the expression of SGF? Have you attempted to restore testicular SGF activity in hypophysectomized animals by administering LH or FSH?

A. R. Bellvé: The hypophysectomy experiment was performed primarily to determine whether testicular SGF originates from the pituitary, perhaps as a mitogenic component of prolactin, FSH, LH, or GH. Since the testis still contains ~65% of the original levels of activity at 30 days posthypophysectomy, this possibility now seems most unlikely. In reference to the original question, the hypophysectomy data should not be misconstrued as evidence for SGF levels being regulated by the pituitary. In fact, none of the pituitary polypeptide hormones have yet been directly implicated in controlling either the synthesis or the expression of SGF. Since pituitary extracts are usually contaminated with growth factors, experiments involving hormone replacement therapy will need to utilize pure preparations of the gonadotropins and other polypeptide hormones. Such experiments also should be undertaken using an assay specific for SGF. Two reasonable approaches would be to use a "Sertoli cell" bioassay, which is responsive to perhaps only one other growth factor, and/ or a highly sensitive and monospecific immunoassay.

S-Y. Ying: The second question is whether similar activity exists in the ovary?

A. R. Bellvé: Preliminary experiments suggest comparable activity is not detectable in isolated rat granulosa cells. Instead, the ovary appears to contain a basic growth factor having properties quite different from those defined for SGF [see Makris *et al.* (1984). *Biol. Reprod.* **29**, 1135–1141].

D. L. Foster: You indicated that Sertoli cells cease division in the adult and that Sertoli cell derived growth factor (SGF) is low compared to the levels found in prepuberal males. However, in adults of seasonally breeding species, regression and regrowth of the testes occur annually. Have you examined SDGF during the phase of testicular regrowth in adult seasonal breeders? I wonder if increased production of SGF during testicular maturation occurs only during initial testicular maturation.

A. R. Bellvé: Expression of SGF is not restricted solely to the developing testis. The specific mitogenic activity is highest in the early postnatal testis, but considerable amounts of activity also exist in Sertoli cells of the adult animal. Yes; SGF levels may vary with the reproductive status of seasonal breeders, but the appropriate experiments to prove this point have yet to be undertaken. It is an intriguing possibility.

J. A. Dias: You mentioned that the specific activity of your preparations was highest in the immature animal and interestingly enough, of course, the receptor concentration or the specificity activity of FSH receptor is highest in the immature animal compared to the mature animal. However, if the calculations are based on the total testicular weight it turns out that the picture is somewhat different. Thus, FSH receptor number appears to rise with age. Have you performed your calculations of the total yield or theoretical yield of activity in the different ages of animals in terms of the mitogenic factor and what can you tell us about that. Is the total testes activity actually less or higher in the immature animal compared to the mature?

A. R. Bellvé: Yes; the *total* amount of SGF activity in each Sertoli cell, and hence in the whole testis, increases as development proceeds. Presumably, SGF also has important functions in regulating spermatogenesis in the adult animal.

A. H. Payne: What ages were your hypophysectomized animals and how long after hypophysectomy did you measure the amount of Sertoli cell growth factor per testis?

A. R. Bellvé: The animals used in those particular experiments were adult mice, 84- to 110-days old, at 30 days posthypophysectomy.

A. H. Payne: Do the numbers of Sertoli cells decrease following hypophysectomy? Could the decrease in total activity that you observed, which is not a very marked decrease, actually be due to a decrease in the number of Sertoli cells?

A. R. Bellvé: This would be true for adult animals. However, hypophysectomy in prepuberal rats and lambs apparently does cause a reduction in the total number of Sertoli cells that eventually populate the adult testes [see de Reviers *et al.* (1980). *Reprod. Nutr. Develop.* **20**, 241–249]. Also, compensatory testicular hypertrophy, which occurs after unilateral orchidectomy, occurs only in prepuberal animals [Cunningham *et al.* (1978). *Endocrinology* **102**, 16–23]. It seems reasonable to speculate that SGF may be involved in both processes.

H. G. Raj: Sertoli cells are exposed to high concentrations of testosterone and to the many autoantigens present in the luminal fluids. Are adult Sertoli cells responsive to high concentrations of the growth factor? Does SGF show cellular specificity?

A. R. Bellvé: The possible responses of adult Sertoli cells to SGF have not been examined thoroughly. Since these cells usually do not proliferate, their responses could include synthesis of specific proteins or glycoproteins. Other testicular targets may include spermatogonia, Leydig, and peritubular cells. Epithelial cells in the caput region of the epididymis also may respond.

D. Pomerantz: Can you speculate further about the possibility of SGF having access to cells in the interstitial compartment?

A. R. Bellvé: SGF may be secreted from the basal surface of the Sertoli cell, thereby bypassing the extensive intercellular Sertoli junctions that form during prepuberal development. FSH is internalized via its receptors across this basal plasma membrane, but whether polypeptides, such as SGF and ABP, are ''secreted'' in the opposite direction has not been demonstrated. Regardless, Leydig cells are one of the more likely targets for SGF action.

G. P. Budzik: Can you detect SGF either in medium from cultures of Sertoli cells or in medium from incubation of whole tissue? If you can, why did you not use that as a starting material for your purification instead of homogenates?

A. R. Bellvé: SGF is detectable at high specific activities in spent medium that is collected from Sertoli cell cultures every 48 hours during the first 10-day period after the initial seeding. However, since these are primary cultures, it would be prohibitively expensive to collect sufficient spent medium for the preparative purification of SGF.

G. P. Budzik: Is SGF a glycoprotein?

A. R. Bellvé: This is not known; there may be a low proportion of carbohydrate. SGF does not bind to concanavalin A, but other lectins still need to be tested.

G. P. Budzik: Is there any precedent of any other growth factors, for example, EGF or platelet derived growth factor for stimulating the cell from which they are synthesized as SGF appears to potentiate growth in Sertoli cells?

A. R. Bellvé: This is an important question. Most of the well-characterized growth factors do not have a known autocrine function. The two exceptions are SGF and the cartilage-derived growth factor (CDGF). The latter originates from chondrocytes and stimulates chondrocyte proliferation, in addition to promoting the division of fibroblasts and endothelial cells populating cartilaginous tissue. The respective origins and target cells of many other growth factors have not been completely defined. In this regard, spermatogenesis provides an excellent model system, since it involves an active and continuous proliferation of stem cells, the process is subject to endocrine control, and the differentiating germ cells can be isolated and identified. Moreover, the endocrine contributions of the supporting somatic elements, principally the Leydig and Sertoli cells, have been adequately defined. This comprehensive knowledge undoubtedly will facilitate future studies on the role of endogenous growth factors in promoting testicular development and in regulating spermatogenesis.

R. A. Huseby: Some years ago we described the rapid (~24 hours) induction of localized angiogenesis by a mouse testis that had been transplanted to a subcutaneous site in the rabbit. This observation suggested that the testis contains an "angiogenesis factor." Have you by chance had an opportunity to test a preparation of SGF against normal endothelial cells?

A. R. Bellvé: Yes; partially purified preparations of SGF are very effective in stimulating the proliferation of human umbilical vein endothelial cells in primary culture. Whether the induction of angiogenesis is another property of SGF, or due to some other macromolecule in the testis, can be ascertained only when the former polypeptide is purified. Meanwhile, it is intriguing to consider the possibility that SGF may be responsible for the precocious capillarization of the developing gonad in the male rodent fetus.

B. A. Littlefield: There is probably a good reason why others have not asked this particular question. Is there any evidence for the existence of a growth factor in the ejaculate?

A. R. Bellvé: Yes; abundant quantities of nerve growth factor (NGF) exist in the seminal secretions of several mammalian species. In the bovine, 100 ml of semen contains ~10 mg of NGF, making seminal plasma one of the richest known sources for this polypeptide [Harper et al. (1982). J. Biol. Chem. **257**, 8541–8548]. While a mitogenic protein has been reported to exist in rete testis fluid [Brown et al. (1982). Biochem. Biophys. Res. Commun. **105**, 391–397], there is no evidence to suggest that either this polypeptide or SGF exist in seminal plasma.

S. L. Cohen: Practically any tissue, except nervous tissue, will regrow following injury. Now, many growth factors have been identified, but does this mean that there is one specific for every tissue in the body?

A. R. Bellvé: At this time it is possible to respond with only a speculative answer to your question. A few years ago a limited number of growth factors had been identified, notably NGF, EGF, FGF, and PDGF. This number has since expanded considerably as new growth factors have been identified. Whether each tissue contains a specific growth factor(s) that influences single or multiple cell types, or even multiple tissues, can be resolved only with further research. It also seems reasonable to expect that each cell type in a particular tissue could be responsive to multiple growth factors, perhaps acting sequentially, in concert, and/or synergistically. In turn, the various cell populations comprising a tissue may modulate their responses by varying receptor numbers to the respective growth factors. The Sertoli cell could control cell proliferation in its immediate environment by regulating SGF synthesis and secretion into adjacent compartments of the testis.

P. K. Donahoe: Can you characterize and describe the source of the TR-ST tumor line?

A. R. Bellvé: Dr. J. P. Mather and colleagues (Population Council, New York) isolated the TR-ST cell line from a rat having a spontaneous testicular tumor. These transformed cells, while exhibiting some morphological characteristics typical of Sertoli cells, also proliferate rapidly with a cell cycle time of ~9 hours in the presence of serum and ~24 hours in defined medium. The important question for our purposes is whether TR-ST cells become contact inhibited at confluency, in the absence of serum, and then show renewed proliferation in response to SGF.

P. W. Concannon: The implications of SGF existing in Sertoli cell tumors seem obvious. Have you had an opportunity to determine whether such tumors contain or are responsive to SGF?

A. R. Bellvé: Not at this time, although we would be willing to assay any available samples. Spontaneous Sertoli cell tumors primarily occur in the canine and equine species.

P. W. Concannon: I think the incidence of Sertoli cell tumors is higher in both dogs and horses than in other species. Another question, Dr. Bellvé, you indicated a single application of SDGF would cause mitogenic activity in the 3T3 cells within 2 to 4 days. In a subsequent experiment you were repeatedly adding the factor. Do you have information on how brief a period of exposure will subsequently give you mitogenic activity?

A. R. Bellvé: This is another important question which needs to be resolved as soon as pure SGF is available.

C. S. Nicoll: Do you believe there is any relationship between SGF and the Müllerian duct inhibiting substance (MIS)?

A. R. Bellvé: The biochemical characteristics of these two polypeptides are quite different. Monomeric MIS appears to be a glycoprotein of M_r 35,000–40,000. Possibly, Drs. Donahoe or Budzik may wish to respond directly to your question.

C. S. Nicoll: Perhaps you should consider the possibility of SGF being a peptide fragment of MIS?

G. R. Budzik: Comparing your data on SGF and our data on Müllerian inhibiting substance (MIS), at least at this point, the two factors look quite different. MIS is a high-molecular-weight, glycoprotein dimer of 74,000 molecular weight subunits, linked by a disulfide(s). I think the idea that SDGF may be related somehow to MIS, as a processing product perhaps is intriguing and may bear some further work.

A. R. Bellvé: Several recent reports suggest that either a proteolytic product or the intact molecule of certain polypeptide hormones can have mitogenic properties. A proteolytic fragment of prolactin may be mitogenic for mammary epithelial cells, and growth hormone appears to stimulate the proliferation of preadipocyte fibroblasts. There is limited evidence to suggest FSH is able to promote the *in vitro* proliferation of prepuberal rat Sertoli cells [Griswold *et al.* (1977). *Mol. Cell. Endocrinol.* **7**, 151–165]. However, we were unable to confirm this earlier observation. To resolve whether a proteolytic fragment of MIS, LH, GH, or prolactin is capable of stimulating Sertoli cell proliferation will require a careful, in-depth study.

A. L. Barofsky: The *in vitro* proliferation of Sertoli cells in response to the cartilage-derived growth factor (CDGF) suggests the two polypeptides may share biochemical properties. Do you have evidence for or against this possibility?

A. R. Bellvé: CDGF purified by Dr. M. Klagsbrun of Childrens Hospital Medical Center, Boston, appears to be a unique polypeptide having an M_r of 18,000 and a $pI = 9.8$. The physiological significance of Sertoli cells proliferating in response to CDGF, and whether the two polypeptides recognize the same cell surface receptor, is unknown.

H. G. Raj: Can you elaborate on the possible synergism of SGF with insulin or the insulin-like growth factors, IGF_1 and IGF_2?

A. R. Bellvé: Insulin is not mitogenic for BALB/c 3T3 cells, except at high concentrations when it may cross-react with somatomedin receptors. However, in the presence of insulin, the mitogenic effect of SGF on the confluent, quiescent 3T3 cells is potentiated ~5-fold. A similar response has been observed previously for certain other growth factors.

P. K. Donahoe: I was intrigued with Dr. Cohen's question as I often am, about the general phenomenon of a cell, and in this particular case the Sertoli cell producing its own stimulator. Probably every cell type has both its own stimulator and inhibitor. Autocrine control, if we can predict, will become increasingly important as we delve further into the study of factors such as these.

A. R. Bellvé: The probable existence of a "chalone" in the mammalian testis is compatible with a notion of a negative control for germ cell proliferation.

G. Callard: As you know, in the mammalian ovary, proliferation of oogonia occurs at a much earlier point in development than in the testis, and I wonder when you looked at ovaries for this mitogenic factor, did you look during that time, that is, in the fetal ovary?

A. R. Bellvé: A comparison of SGF expression in developing ovaries and testes undoubtedly will be the first and perhaps the most important experiment we shall undertake once a sensitive and specific biological and/or immunoassay is available. Incidentally, I believe it is the testis, not the ovary, that undergoes precocious growth early in fetal development.

G. Callard: I am not clear whether you are leaning toward the idea that this factor causes proliferation of Sertoli cells or of the somatic cells in the testis?

A. R. Bellvé: Existing evidence suggests that SGF causes Sertoli cells, the somatic epithelial cells, to proliferate. This does not preclude a role for the polypeptide in stimulating the division of certain spermatogonial stem cells. Both possibilities need to be examined experimentally.

R. E. Peter: Comparative endocrinologists are aware of the limitations and potential problems of using heterologous bioassays and radioimmunoassays. As a philosophical question, how do you justify using BALB/c 3T3 cells, a fibroblastic cell line to detect a testicular growth factor?

A. R. Bellvé: The difficulties encountered in isolating and culturing testicular cells of both somatic and germ cell origin have severely hindered research efforts to define the mechanisms regulating cell proliferation. A few somatic cell lines have been established recently, but attempts to culture the germ cells are still foundering. In an effort to circumvent these limitations, we utilized the simpler BALB/c 3T3 cell bioassay for the initial search. This seemed a reasonable first approach, particularly since confluent, quiescent 3T3 cells are known to respond to several different growth factors. Perhaps other model systems may reveal additional testicular growth factors.

R. E. Peter: But, after identifying a particular growth factor and its testicular target cell, you must still have the continual problem of retesting against this cell type to ensure the correct identity of the purified product.

A. R. Bellvé: This is a good point. In the case of SGF, the characterization and purification of the polypeptide are accomplished primarily by using the BALB/c 3T3 cell assay. Therefore, by testing only periodically against Sertoli cells in primary culture, a considerable amount of time and unnecessary expenditure are saved. The retesting process is essential, however.

F. S. French: As you probably know, Drs. E. Martin Ritzen and colleagues, Karolinska Institute, Stockholm, have detected somatomedin A in the spent medium of Sertoli cell cultures [E. M. Ritzen et al. (1982). *Program, Inter. Diabetes Fed., 11th Congress, Nairobi, Kenya*, p. 58]. Somatomedin A is similar to and may be identical to somatomedin C (IGF$_1$). This observation has been confirmed recently by Drs. L. Tres et al. [*J. Cell. Biol.* (1983). **97**, 18a], University of North Carolina, Chapel Hill, who used a monoclonal antibody against somatomedin C to localize minor amounts of immunoreactive material in Sertoli cells. It seems that this "somatomedin C-like" material is stimulated by GH rather than by FSH. Of course, GH is known to stimulate somatomedin C production in chondrocytes and thereby promotes bone growth. In the presence of a progression factor, somatomedin C also stimulates BALB/c 3T3 proliferation. SGF and somatomedin C have distinct biochemical and biological properties and therefore must be different entities. Still, it would be interesting to know whether SGF is distributed in other tissues. Have you assayed any other tissues for the presence of SGF?

A. R. Bellvé: The biochemical evidence demonstrating that SGF is a distinct polypeptide is compelling. However, SGF's apparent synergistic action with insulin is a property also characteristic of IGF_1. Clearly, it is essential to determine unambiguously whether the IGF_1 monoclonal antibody has any cross-reactivity with SGF. Since IGF_1 may occur in the ovary for promoting meiotic maturation, comparable activity (or SGF) could serve a comparable function in the mammalian testis.

A model biological assay, using Sertoli cells rather than the BALB/c 3T3, could provide the specificity needed to screen for SGF activity in other tissues. Thus, Sertoli cells in primary culture do not proliferate in response to PDGF, EGF, FGF, or FSH. A search is being made now to identify a transformed cell line of testicular origin that exhibits comparable specificity.

A. R. Means: We probably need to exert some caution about what we call growth factors, and mitogens, because when you really think about it, we do not know very much about what controls cell proliferation. When someone considers a substance to be a mitogen or a growth factor, it is not because you can take a cell population and a balanced salt solution, add this one substance and get those cells to proliferate. Rather it is because there are sufficient other permissive substances present, that when one additional compound is added cell growth occurs. If one looks hard enough one could probably find that a great number of proteins that you can buy from Sigma would in fact be "growth factors" if you have the proper other substances already in the solution. As Tony begged earlier in this discussion, until an antibody to this testis substance can be made it is not possible to accurately determine where it is produced, where it appears following secretion, and whether it is species specific. Only after extensive studies of this nature can we determine whether, in fact, this truly is a growth factor or a mitogen in the classic sense of the word.

A. R. Bellvé: This cautionary note is well taken. Complete characterization of SGF and its functions within the testis will require judicious use of the purified polypeptide and specific monoclonal antibodies. When available, these reagents must be applied to prove that SGF, acting at concentrations of approximately 10^{-10} M, can (1) induce confluent, quiescent cells to undergo DNA synthesis and cell proliferation; (2) promote clonal growth of sparsely seeded cells; and (3) interact with specific surface receptors to cause a characteristic physiological response. Finally, it will be necessary through peptide mapping and gene sequencing to identify SGF as a unique entity with a characteristic set of biological functions for promoting testicular development and/or spermatogenesis.

Endocytosis and Membrane Traffic in Cultured Cells

MARK C. WILLINGHAM AND IRA PASTAN

*Laboratory of Molecular Biology, National Cancer Institute,
National Institutes of Health, Bethesda, Maryland*

I. Summary

Animal cells internalize many different macromolecules from their environment. A large percentage of these materials, including many polypeptide hormones, are selected from the surrounding medium by binding to specific receptors on the cell surface. The internalization of these receptor-bound molecules is rapid and highly specific. The general pathway of entry involves assembly of clusters of ligand–receptor complexes in clathrin-coated pits of the plasma membrane, formation of intracellular endocytic vesicles called receptosomes (or endosomes) from these coated pits, saltatory movement of these vesicles to the Golgi system, selective fusion of these receptosomes with the trans-reticular elements of the Golgi, and routing by as yet unknown mechanisms either to lysosomes, or back out of the cell by constitutive exocytosis. Some receptors accompany the ligand into lysosomes where they are degraded, whereas others appear to separate from the ligand and are recycled back to the cell surface; ligands such as transferrin are not delivered to lysosomes, but appear to accompany the receptor back to the cell exterior. Similar processes may be involved in the intracellular routing of materials synthesized in the endoplasmic reticulum. Intracellular traffic control may be in some ways analogous to traffic control at the cell surface in the requirement for specific receptors, and the use of clathrin-coated regions of membrane. Certain disease-causing substances, such as bacterial toxins and viruses, have taken advantage of this pathway to gain entrance to the cell. The endocytic pathway probably has a significant role in hormone action either directly or indirectly by the regulation of surface receptor numbers, or the transport of carrier molecules or other molecules involved in the mechanisms of action of hormones.

II. Introduction

In recent years, studies on the entry of macromolecules from the external environment of animal cells have enjoyed considerable interest. The use of new techniques of cytochemistry and biochemistry has allowed careful examination of these events. One recent realization has been that the processes of endocytosis via coated pits and intracellular molecular movements can be very rapid, in many cases occurring in a few seconds. A number of recent articles have comprehensively reviewed this area (Anderson *et al.*, 1982; Pastan and Willingham, 1981, 1983; Steinman *et al.*, 1983; Helenius *et al.*, 1983); this article will attempt to highlight certain parts of this process, concentrating mainly on investigations in our own laboratory that utilize cultured cells. The subjects covered will be subdivided into (1) the events at the plasma membrane including specific receptor binding and clustering in clathrin-coated pits; (2) the formation of receptosomes (endosomes) from coated pits and their characteristics; (3) the role of the Golgi system in the control of macromolecular traffic; and (4) the use of parts of these systems by pathologic agents such as viruses and toxins. A diagrammatic summary of the organelles involved in this morphologic pathway is shown in Fig. 1.

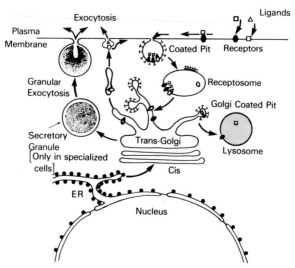

FIG. 1.   Diagrammatic summary of the pathways of endocytosis and exocytosis in animal cells. The (open square) ligand corresponds to epidermal growth factor which binds to a specific receptor (closed) that is delivered into lysosomes along with the ligand. The (triangular) ligand binds to the (open) receptor and corresponds to transferrin, in which the receptor and ligand both recycle to the cell surface. ER, Endoplasmic reticulum.

III. The Role of the Plasma Membrane and Clathrin-Coated Pits

The plasma membrane of most animal cells contains a variety of specific receptors for external macromolecules (Kahn, 1976). Some of these ligands function in a hormonal role, such as insulin or triiodothyronine (Carpentier *et al.*, 1979; Cheng, 1983); others serve an apparent metabolic function, such as LDL or lysosomal enzymes (Goldstein *et al.*, 1979; Neufeld and Ashwell, 1979); others are involved in removal of altered proteins from the blood (α_2-macroglobulin or asialoglycoproteins) (Willingham *et al.*, 1979; Wall *et al.*, 1980); still others are pathologic agents, such as bacterial toxins and viruses (Pappenheimer, 1977; Simons *et al.*, 1982). Other ligands, such as plant lectins or cationized ferritin, also enter the cell through coated pits and are useful to study the general mechanisms involved, without a specific physiological consequence (Gonatas *et al.*, 1980; Ottosen *et al.*, 1980).

Many, but not all, surface receptors are glycoproteins. The receptor for cholera toxin is a glycolipid and that for vesicular stomatitis virus may be a phospholipid (Schlegel *et al.*, 1983). Other materials which do not have receptors of high specificity can enter cells by the same pathway; however, materials, such as horseradish peroxidase, are not selectively concentrated from the environment as those that bind to specific receptors (Ryser *et al.*, 1982).

The surfaces of almost all animal cells have specialized regions which are demarcated by a fuzzy, cytoplasmic coat made predominantly of a protein called clathrin (Pearse, 1976). These coated regions, or "coated pits," serve as foci at which specific surface receptors cluster prior to endocytosis (Anderson *et al.*, 1976). Each cell may have from 500 to 1500 of these structures on its surface. A second population of smaller coated pits occurs inside the cell in the Golgi system (Friend and Farquhar, 1967). Studies on cell surface receptors indicate that the clustering of receptors into these pit regions appears to be a passive process, in the sense that lateral thermal diffusion of these receptors in the plane of the membrane accounts for their mobility through these coated regions. The coated pits act as traps to immobilize the receptor. The mechanism of this immobilization is not clear. Some drugs are able to prevent much of this clustering process (Davies *et al.*, 1980); the most potent of these is dansylcadaverine.

The immobilization of receptors in coated pits seems to be dependent on occupancy of the receptor with ligand in some cases (such as the receptor for epidermal growth factor) (Willingham and Pastan, 1982), but not in others (such as for LDL) (McGookey *et al.*, 1983). Receptors for lysosomal enzymes (phosphomannosyl receptor) and for transferrin are found clustered in coated pits without added exogenous ligand, but the true state of occupancy of these receptors is not easily determined because the cells themselves often contain either previously internalized transferrin or many different lysosomal enzymes that could result in receptor occupancy (Willingham *et al.,* 1983b, 1984). Receptors for viruses such as Semliki Forest virus or Vesicular Stomatitis virus are probably normally unoccupied, and these receptors are diffusely distributed over the entire plasma membrane (Helenius *et al.,* 1980; Schlegel *et al.,* 1983). Thus, it is possible that receptor clustering in coated regions may be either ligand dependent or independent. Once immobilized in coated pits, however, the internalization process that follows is the same for all of these materials.

Coated pits do not appear to discriminate between different ligand–receptor complexes. In many double-label experiments, two receptor–ligand systems share the same coated pits (Pastan and Willingham, 1981). By both fluorescence light microscopy and electron microscopy, two different ligands (e.g., α_2-macroglobulin and EGF) can be followed from the same coated pits into the same endocytic vesicles together (Willingham *et al.,* 1983a).

The process of transfer from coated pits into endocytic vesicles is very rapid. Quantitative estimates of the internalization of α_2-macroglobulin in cultured fibroblasts suggest that each coated pit can transfer its content into an endocytic vesicle (receptosome) once every 20 seconds at 37°C (Pastan and Willingham, 1981). Considering that there are perhaps 1000 coated pits/cell and the entry of a ligand such as α_2-macroglobulin is a continuous process, the amount of cell surface internalized via coated pits corresponds to roughly the total amount of plasma membrane that is constantly turned over. Thus, the coated pit system is probably responsible for the turnover of the entire membrane (with a $t_{\frac{1}{2}}$) of 30–60 minutes. Therefore, not only receptor-bound clustered materials are internalized through coated pits, but also other components of the membrane are brought in by this process, such as plasma membrane lipids.

The understanding of the character of coated pits has to a great extent been derived from the interpretation of morphologic images. These structures were originally seen in the process of mediating the uptake of ferritin in erythroblastic cells by Bessis and co-workers (Bessis, 1963), although they did not recognize the characteristics of the coat itself. Gray described the coat structure in neuronal cells (Gray, 1961), and a number of other studies described them in insect cells, liver cells, kidney, and other tissues (reviewed in Bowers, 1964). Roth and Porter (1964) described these structures in liver and insect oocytes, and coined the term "bristle-coated pits." They and others suggested their involvement in endocytosis. Part of the original description included the observation that these structures frequently appeared as isolated vesicles in thin sections, and the hypothesis that these pits pinched off to form isolated coated vesicles inside cells has been accepted as fact for the ensuing 20 years. However, there is morphologic evidence now that this conclusion may not be correct (Willingham *et al.*, 1981a,b; Wehland *et al.*, 1981; Willingham and Pastan, 1983). Virtually all of the coated vesicular profiles seen near the plasma membrane in cultured cells are almost certainly coated pits connected to the cell surface. These structures can undergo elaborate infoldings and changes in shape that make their surface connections very difficult to resolve. Serial section analysis, impermeant marker labeling, and microinjection experiments have suggested strongly that the evidence previously cited for the character of isolated coated vesicles is not sufficient to establish their existence (Willingham and Pastan, 1983). While it is possible such vesicles form for very brief periods of time during the endocytosis process, there is no compelling evidence that this occurs. The bulk of the recent morphologic evidence does not support such a process.

The coat protein was isolated from purified coated membrane preparations by Pearse and named "clathrin," from the Latin "clathra-" meaning "lattice" (Pearse, 1976). The structure of the clathrin coat is that of a basketwork or lattice that is most clearly shown using surface replica techniques in intact cells (Heuser and Evans, 1980), or by negative staining in isolated vesicle preparations (Keen *et al.*, 1979). The predominant protein in the lattice is a 185,000 M_r clathrin "heavy chain," along with smaller amounts of "light chains" around 35,000 in M_r (Kirchhausen and Harrison, 1981). These proteins will self-assemble in the test tube to form the characteristic pentagon–hexagon clathrin lattice (a pattern similar to the surface of a soccer ball) (Keen *et al.*, 1979). It is not likely that such an assembly process actually occurs on the rapid time scale of the endocytic event, but this may reflect how newly synthesized clathrin becomes associated with coated pits.

Helenius *et al.* (1983) have recently reviewed the evidence that coated pits pinch off to form isolated coated vesicles. In this formulation coated vesicles exist only for very short times (less than a few seconds), and the clathrin latticework disassembles and reassociates with the plasma membrane, producing an isolated uncoated vesicle. Since electron microscopic immunocytochemistry has suggested that there is very little, if any, soluble clathrin in the cytosol of living cells (Willingham *et al.*, 1981a), the assembly process would require a selective compartmentalization of clathrin in these regions of the membrane to allow assembly to take place. This has not been demonstrated.

Transitional images at plasma membrane regions adjacent to the coated pits have suggested that the endocytic vesicles derived from coated pits (receptosomes) may form by a ballooning-out of membranes, rather than requiring the pinching-off of intact clathrin-coated vesicles (Willingham and Pastan, 1980). The size and composition of these vesicles also suggest that they could not form only as an uncoating of pinched-off isolated coated vesicles. The ballooning process may be dependent on an ion pump in the membrane of the coated pit which produces a hydrostatic pressure to drive the increase in vesicle size prior to pinching-off of an "uncoated" vesicle (receptosome) (Dickson *et al.*, 1982). There is no evidence to suggest that receptosomes form selectively from regions other than those associated with coated pits; they do not represent random endocytic vesicle formation at other areas of the plasma membrane. There is also no evidence that the endocytosis through coated pits is necessarily driven by the presence of ligand–receptor complexes in them. It is likely that this process is constitutive and will occur no matter whether the pits are full or empty.

IV. Receptosomes

It has been a general observation that the rapid endocytosis of materials from the cell surface, no matter what ligand or what cell type has been studied, involves the formation of an intermediate endocytic vesicle which we termed a "receptosome" (Willingham and Pastan, 1980), and others have termed an "endosome," "endocytic vacuole," or other terms (Helenius *et al.*, 1983). All of these vesicles have essentially the same appearance. The formation of these structures is very rapid at 37°C, usually less than 20 seconds in continuous incubations, or less than 2 minutes when cells are warmed to 37°C from a prior incubation at 4°C (Pastan and Willingham, 1981). These vesicles are initially 200–300 nm in diameter, have a clear almost empty appearance by electron microscopy, often contain a single small intralumenal vesicular structure, and have a fuzzy cytoplasmic border along a straightened edge of the membrane (Willingham and Pastan, 1980). Their initial identification as a special organelle was based on their content of clustered receptor-bound ligand that had just previously been located in coated pits of the plasma membrane. They have recently been isolated in a highly purified form and analyzed biochemically. They have been shown to have a considerable amount of cholesterol and not to have significant amounts of clathrin or lysosomal enzyme activities (Dickson *et al.*, 1983). The pH of these vesicles has been measured directly in living cells, and within a few minutes of their formation, their internal pH approaches that of lysosomes (near pH

5.0) (Tycko and Maxfield, 1982). Receptosomes are known to be isolated vesicles in living cells because, when labeled with internalized fluorescent ligand, they can be seen to move by saltatory motion on intracellular microtubule tracks in the cytoplasm (Pastan and Willingham, 1981). Receptosomes have been directly observed in living cells to fuse with each other (Willingham and Pastan, 1984). One of their hallmark features is that they do not fuse directly with mature lysosomes in the cytoplasm, but only fuse with each other or the trans-reticular elements of the Golgi system. Some of the ligands which are internalized in receptosomes go on to be degraded in lysosomes; some others, such as transferrin, do not. Thus, these organelles are not prelysosomes. Receptors for some ligands have been localized to receptosomes by biochemical and immunocytochemical techniques; these include the epidermal growth factor receptor, the transferrin receptor, and the phosphomannosyl receptor (Beguinot *et al.*, 1984; Willingham *et al.*, 1983b, 1984). Thus, these organelles represent distinct specialized isolated vesicles which form exclusively from clathrin-coated regions at the plasma membrane and deliver their contents to trans-Golgi elements. During this transit they acquire an acidic pH and do not fuse with lysosomes.

The time of transit of receptosomes from the cell surface to the Golgi elements is variable depending in part on cell shape. In very flattened cells there are relatively long distances between a peripheral portion of the plasma membrane and the Golgi system. In rounded cells the distance is much shorter between these elements, often less than 1 or 2 μm. Thus, the life time of a receptosome, from its formation at a coated pit to its eventual fusion with the Golgi, can be from 5 minutes or less to 1–2 hours, depending on the cell type. Because receptosomes fuse with each other, the number containing a newly ingested ligand decreases as fusions progress. In many cell types, the static number visible may be only a few hundred/cell. The membranes of the receptosomes are presumably donated to the overall Golgi system, which in turn is constantly delivering membrane to the plasma membrane and lysosomes.

V. The Role of the Golgi in Macromolecular Traffic

It is not entirely clear today which organelles Camillo Golgi may have described in 1898 (Golgi, 1898). Studies subsequent to his work demonstrated a network of vesicular, tubular, and stack-like structures in almost all cells (reviewed in Goldfischer, 1982). The stack structures are, of course, involved in the transport and processing of proteins synthesized in the endoplasmic reticulum destined for either exocytosis or lysosomal delivery (Farquhar and Palade, 1981). A major portion of the "Golgi," however, is composed of a less well defined network of tubules referred to as the trans-reticular (TR) Golgi system. These structures can be closely associated with the trans stack structures, or can be extensively distributed throughout the cytoplasm originating at the trans stacks. It is these tubular structures that contain the clathrin-coated pits of the Golgi system. These pits are smaller in size than the ones at the plasma membrane (60–70 nm). This area of the Golgi has also been called the GERL, in reference to its role in delivery of lysosomal enzymes to lysosomes (Novikoff *et al.*, 1980), or CURL, in reference to its role in receipt of incoming endocytic ligands and receptors (Geuze *et al.*, 1983).

Ligands, receptors, and other materials internalized into receptosomes are selectively delivered to the trans-reticular Golgi. In the case of asialoglycoproteins, α_2-macroglobulin, LDL, EGF, lysosomal enzymes, and many other ligands, this delivery results in their eventual transfer into lysosomes. Transferrin, IgA in hepatocytes, or maternal IgG in neonatal gut enter cells in the same receptosomes as ligands destined for lysosomes, but are returned back to the cell surface (Willingham *et al.*, 1984; Courtoy *et al.*, 1982; Abrahamson and Rodewald, 1981). The last place at which all these ligands are found in common prior to their separation and delivery to different destinations is the trans-reticular Golgi, and it is here that one would look for mechanisms of sorting and traffic control. There is preliminary evidence to suggest that materials destined for exocytosis that have been synthesized in endoplasmic reticulum and processed through the Golgi stacks may also be found in these trans-reticular elements (Wehland *et al.*, 1982). Also, lysosomal enzymes after proceeding through the Golgi stacks also are present in these structures (Novikoff *et al.*, 1980). Thus, the Golgi system receives materials from the endocytosis pathway or the endoplasmic reticulum, and efficiently transfers them to either exocytosis or lysosomes. The site at which this control of traffic occurs may well be the trans-reticular elements. The exact mechanism that mediates these events is not yet understood. However, there is some evidence to suggest that the coated pits of the Golgi may in some ways mimic the plasma membrane's ability to select materials from the external environment and deliver them into the interior of the cell.

For example, the delivery of lysosomal enzymes from Golgi to lysosomes seems to require the presence of the phosphomannosyl recognition marker on all lysosomal enzymes which interacts with a specific receptor in the trans-reticular Golgi (Willingham *et al.*, 1983b; Sly and Stahl, 1978). I-cell disease is a human genetic disorder in which the recognition marker is not properly synthesized and a majority of the synthesized lysosomal enzymes are secreted out of the cell, rather than being delivered to lysosomes (Sly *et al.*, 1981). This suggests that receptor-dependent processes, something like those on the cell surface, could be involved in traffic control in the Golgi.

When the uptake of EGF coupled to horseradish peroxidase was examined, the transfer of EGF to lysosomes from the trans-reticular Golgi was preceded by clustering of EGF in the coated pits of the Golgi, analogous to the clustering in the coated pits on the cell surface (Willingham and Pastan, 1982). When the uptake of transferrin-peroxidase was studied, which is delivered to the cell surface rather than to lysosomes, it did not efficiently cluster in these same pits (Willingham *et al.*, 1984).

These studies cause one to speculate that the Golgi uses its coated pits in a manner analogous to the sorting of ligand–receptor complexes that occurs at the cell surface, and that similar biochemical mechanisms may be involved.

VI. Toxins, Viruses, and Other Effects

Using electron microscopy, Dales and co-workers studied the internalization of different viruses by animal cells during the infection process (reviewed in Dales, 1973). Usually, virus particles are found bound to receptors on the cell surface, and can also be found in coated pits on the plasma membrane and in receptosomes in the cytoplasm. For non-membrane-limited viruses, such as adenovirus, intact viral particles subsequently can be found in the cytosol, outside of membrane-limited vesicles (Chardonnet and Dales, 1970). This release of viruses into the cytosol probably occurs due to lysis of receptosomes containing virus particles (FitzGerald *et al.*, 1983). The virus induces this lysis.

Membrane-limited viruses also have been found to enter by coated pits and receptosomes (Helenius *et al.*, 1980; Dickson *et al.*, 1981). The escape of the viral nucleoid into the cytoplasm occurs through a membrane fusion event that is stimulated greatly by the acidic environment present in receptosomes (Helenius and Marsh, 1982). Inhibition of the endocytosis or the acidification of these intracellular compartments blocks the infectivity of these membrane-limited viruses (Schlegel *et al.*, 1982; Helenius *et al.*, 1980). Thus, the infectivity of many different viruses may require the endocytosis process and the unique environment in the receptosome.

Bacterial toxins such as *Diphtheria* or *Pseudomonas* toxin exert their effects in the cytosol through inhibition of protein synthesis (Sandvig and Olsnes, 1980; Pappenheimer, 1977). To gain access to the cytosol, *Pseudomonas* toxin binds to a specific receptor on the plasma membrane, can be found in coated pits, and is internalized into receptosomes (FitzGerald *et al.*, 1980). From this site, *Pseudomonas* toxin somehow escapes into the cytosol. Such a membrane transport event has been described for *Diphtheria* toxin and appears to be enhanced by an acidic environment, such as that present in receptosomes (Sandvig and Olsnes, 1980). By combining the receptosome lysis ability of adenovirus and the toxin effects of *Pseudomonas* toxin coupled to EGF, FitzGerald *et al.* (1983) showed that the presence of adenovirus dramatically enhanced the toxicity of this growth factor–toxin conjugate. The mechanism of enhancement seemed to be the lysis of receptosomes by adenovirus, coupled with the presence of viral particles and the EGF–PE conjugate in the same receptosomes.

Since the endocytosis process is ubiquitous among virtually all functioning cells, other processes have been examined for their requirement for this pathway to achieve their effect. There is good evidence to suggest that the action of some hormones may be influenced by the endocytosis process by regulation of receptor numbers on the cell surface. As yet, there are no clear examples in which it has been conclusively shown that the endocytosis process directly mediates the primary action of hormones. However, dansylcadaverine treatment of GH₃ cells has been shown to inhibit triiodothyronine accumulation in the nucleus. Interferon is internalized into cells through the coated pit pathway, but it is not clear that its action depends on this process (Zoon *et al.*, 1983). Hormones such as hCG, which stay on the cell surface for many hours without internalization (Ahmed *et al.*, 1981), probably do not require endocytosis for their tropic effects. Interestingly, one early effect of insulin, the stimulation of glucose transport, may involve membrane compartment transport processes in the placement of glucose carriers on the cell surface, and their subsequent removal from the surface after the removal of insulin from the medium (Cushman and Wardzala, 1980). These types of protein movement from one compartment to another may not be uncommon in hormone action.

VII. Conclusions

The morphologic structures involved in endocytosis and exocytosis have recently been investigated in great detail. It has become clear that the clathrin-coated pits of the cell surface, receptosomes, and the trans-reticular Golgi and its coated pits play very precise roles in the selective delivery of materials from the cell surface to the interior of the cell. In the TR Golgi the cell can direct the traffic of some materials to lysosomes and others back to the cell surface. This occurs in a very precise manner. The same portion of the Golgi system seems to be involved in the routing of materials synthesized within the cell and transported to the TR Golgi via the Golgi stacks. A few of the biochemical elements of these events are known; most are still under investigation. Some pathologic substances such as viruses and bacterial toxins utilize some of the elements of this system. These traffic control events appear to be highly conserved through evolution and are of central importance in cell function. An understanding of the mechanism involved will certainly have far-reaching implications for the clear understanding of animal cell functions and their alterations in disease.

ACKNOWLEDGMENTS

The authors wish to thank A. V. Rutherford, M. G. Gallo, and E. T. Lovelace for expert technical assistance. Also, we thank Drs. D. J. P. FitzGerald, J. H. Hanover, R. B. Dickson, and S.-y. Cheng for helpful discussion, R. L. Steinberg for photographic help, and R. M. Coggin for typing and editing the manuscript.

REFERENCES

Abrahamson, D. R., and Rodewald, R. (1981). *J. Cell Biol.* **91,** 270.

Ahmed, C. E., Sawyer, H. R., and Niswender, G. D. (1981). *Endocrinology* **109,** 1380.

Anderson, R. G. W., Brown, M. S., and Goldstein, J. L. (1976). *Proc. Natl. Acad. Sci. U.S.A.* **73,** 2434.

Anderson, R. G. W., Brown, M. S., Beisiegel, U., and Goldstein, J. L. (1982). *J. Cell Biol.* **93,** 523.

Beguinot, L., Lyall, R., Waterfield, M. D., Willingham, M. C., and Pastan, I. (1984). *Proc. Natl. Acad. Sci. U.S.A.* (in press).

Bessis, M. (1963). *Harvey Lect. Ser.* **58,** 125.

Bowers, B. (1964). *Protoplasma* **59,** 351.

Carpentier, J.-L., Gorden, P., Barazzone, P., Freychet, P., LeCam, A., and Orci, L. (1979). *Proc. Natl. Acad. Sci. U.S.A.* **76,** 2803.

Chardonnet, Y., and Dales, S. (1970). *Virology* **40,** 462.

Cheng, S.-Y. (1983). *Endocrinology* **112,** 1754.

Courtoy, P. J., Quintart, J., and Baudhuin, P. (1982). *J. Cell Biol.* **95,** 424a.

Cushman, S. W., and Wardzala, L. J. (1980). *J. Biol. Chem.* **255,** 4758.

Dales, S. (1973). *Bacteriol. Rev.* **37,** 103.

Davies, P. J. A., Davies, D. R., Levitzki, A., Maxfield, F. R., Milhaud, P., Willingham, M. C., and Pastan, I. H. (1980). *Nature (London)* **283,** 162.

Dickson, R. B., Willingham, M. C., and Pastan, I. (1981). *J. Cell Biol.* **89,** 29.

Dickson, R. B., Schlegel, R., Willingham, M. C., and Pastan, I. (1982). *Exp. Cell Res.* **142,** 127.

Dickson, R. B., Beguinot, L., Hanover, J. H., Richert, N. D., Willingham, M. C., and Pastan, I. (1983). *Proc. Natl. Acad. Sci. U.S.A.* **80,** 5335.

Farquhar, M. G., and Palade, G. E. (1981). *J. Cell Biol.* **91,** 77s.

FitzGerald, D. J. P., Morris, R. E., and Saelinger, C. B. (1980). *Cell* **21,** 867.

FitzGerald, D. J. P., Padmanabhan, R., Pastan, I., and Willingham, M. C. (1983). *Cell* **32,** 607.

Friend, D. S., and Farquhar, M. G. (1967). *J. Cell Biol.* **35,** 357.

Geuze, H. J., Slot, J. W., Strous, G. J. A. M., Lodish, H. F., and Schwartz, A. L. (1983). *Cell* **32,** 277.

Goldfischer, S. (1982). *J. Histochem. Cytochem.* **30,** 717.

Goldstein, J. L., Anderson, R. G. W., and Brown, M. S. (1979). *Nature (London)* **279,** 679.

Golgi, C. (1898). *Arch. Ital. Biol.* **30,** 60.
Gonatas, J., Steiber, S., Olsnes, S., and Gonatas, N. K. (1980). *J. Cell Biol.* **87,** 579.
Gray, E. G. (1961). *J. Anat.* **95,** 345.
Helenius, A., and Marsh, M. (1982). *Ciba Symp.* **92,** 59.
Helenius, A., Kartenbeck, J., Simons, K., and Fries, E. (1980). *J. Cell Biol.* **84,** 404.
Helenius, A., Mellman, I., Wall, D., and Hubbard, A. (1983). *Trends Biochem. Sci.* **8,** 245.
Heuser, J., and Evans, L. (1980). *J. Cell Biol.* **84,** 560.
Kahn, C. R. (1976). *J. Cell Biol.* **70,** 261.
Keen, J. H., Willingham, M. C., and Pastan, I. H. (1979). *Cell* **16,** 303.
Kirchhausen, T., and Harrison, S. C. (1981). *Cell* **23,** 755.
McGookey, D. J., Fagerberg, K., and Anderson, R. G. W. (1983). *J. Cell Biol.* **96,** 1273.
Neufeld, E., and Ashwell, G. (1979). *In* "Biochemistry of Glycoproteins and Proteogly-cans" (W. Lennarz, ed.), pp. 241–266. Plenum, New York.
Novikoff, A. B., Novikoff, P. M., Rosen, O. M., and Rubin, C. S. (1980). *J. Cell Biol.* **87,** 180.
Ottosen, P. D., Courtoy, P. J., and Farquhar, M. G. (1980). *J. Exp. Med.* **152,** 1.
Pappenheimer, A. M. (1977). *Annu. Rev. Biochem.* **46,** 60.
Pastan, I. H., and Willingham, M. C. (1981). *Science* **214,** 504.
Pastan, I. H., and Willingman, M. C. (1983). *Trends Biochem. Sci.* **8,** 250.
Pearse, B. M. F. (1976). *Proc. Natl. Acad. Sci. U.S.A.* **73,** 1255.
Ryser, H. J.-P., Drummond, I., and Shen, W.-C. (1982). *J. Cell. Physiol.* **113,** 167.
Roth, T. F., and Porter, K. R. (1964). *J. Cell Biol.* **20,** 313.
Sandvig, K., and Olsnes, S. (1980). *J. Cell Biol.* **87,** 828.
Schlegel, C. R., Dickson, R. B., Willingham, M. C., and Pastan, I. (1982). *Proc. Natl. Acad. Sci. U.S.A.* **79,** 2291.
Schlegel, R., Tralka, T. S., Willingham, M. C., and Pastan, I. (1983). *Cell* **32,** 639.
Simons, K., Garoff, H., and Helenius, A. (1982). *Sci. Am.* **246,** 58.
Sly, W. S., and Stahl, P. (1978). *In* "Transport of Molecules in Cellular Systems" (S. C. Silverstein, ed.), pp. 229–244. Dahlem Konferenzen, Berlin.
Sly, W. S., Natowisz, M., Gonzalez-Noriega, A., Grubb, J. H., and Fischer, H. D. (1981). *In* "Lysosomes and Lysosomal Storage Diseases" (J. W. Callahan and J. A. Low-den, eds.), pp. 131–146. Raven, New York.
Steinman, R. M., Mellman, I. S., Muller, W. A., and Cohn, Z. A. (1983). *J. Cell Biol.* **96,** 1.
Tycko, B., and Maxfield, F. R. (1982). *Cell* **28,** 643.
Wall, D. A., Wilson, G., and Hubbard, A. L. (1980). *Cell* **21,** 79.
Wehland, J., Willingham, M. C., Dickson, R. B., and Pastan, I. (1981). *Cell* **25,** 105.
Wehland, J., Willingham, M. C., Gallo, M. G., and Pastan, I. (1982). *Cell* **28,** 831.
Willingham, M. C., and Pastan, I. (1980). *Cell* **21,** 67.
Willingham, M. C., and Pastan, I. H. (1982). *J. Cell Biol.* **94,** 207.
Willingham, M. C., and Pastan, I. H. (1983). *Proc. Natl. Acad. Sci. U.S.A.* **80,** 5617.
Willingham, M. C., and Pastan, I. H. (1984). In preparation.
Willingham, M. C., Maxfield, F. R., and Pastan, I. (1979). *J. Cell Biol.* **82,** 614.
Willingham, M. C., Keen, J. H., and Pastan, I. (1981a). *Exp. Cell Res.* **132,** 329.
Willingham, M. C., Rutherford, A. V., Gallo, M. G., Wehland, J., Dickson, R. B., Schlegel, R., and Pastan, I. (1981b). *J. Histochem. Cytochem.* **29,** 1003.
Willingham, M. C., Haigler, H. T., FitzGerald, D. J. P., Gallo, M. G., Rutherford, A. V., and Pastan, I. H. (1983a). *Exp. Cell Res.* **146,** 163.
Willingham, M. C., Pastan, I. H., and Sahagian, G. G. (1983b). *J. Histochem. Cytochem.* **31,** 1.
Willingham, M. C., Hanover, J. H., Dickson, R. B., and Pastan, I. (1984). *Proc. Natl. Acad. Sci. U.S.A.* **81,** 175.

Zoon, K. C., Arnheiter, H., Zur Nedden, D., FitzGerald, D. J. P., and Willingham, M. C. (1983). *Virology* **130**, 195.

DISCUSSION

J. H. Oppenheimer: You and your colleague, especially Dr. Cheng, have published rather extensively about the possibility that T3 enters the cell by receptor-mediated endocytosis. Although you did not discuss T3 in your presentation I assume that your position remains the same. If T3 enters by this pathway, how does it leave the cell? In the case of liver, the exchange process is extremely fast and in intact animal, the equilibrium between plasma and hepatic T3 is established within 1 minute. Also, do you have any data regarding the mean to transit time in the various systems which you have used? Lastly, I wonder how sensitive your system is to general metabolic poisons such as cyanide and oligomycin? Could you give us some indication about the energy requirements for the transfer?

M. C. Willingham: Needless to say, the lack of data on T3 is not for want of trying; T3 is a very difficult system. Jane Cheng (Sheue-yann Cheng) has made some monumental efforts in trying to study the process. As yet, we don't have a good marker for T3 for electron microscopy. Cheng and co-workers have now followed the entry of T3 by affinity-labeling and have identified a plasma membrane receptor using bromacetyl-T3. In the cultured cells that she has been working with, there is a major 55K plasma membrane receptor. The appearance of T3 in the nuclear fraction, which takes some time in these cultured cell systems, is dependent on this endocytosis process, in the sense that if one inhibits it with some of the inhibitors of endocytosis (such as dansylcadaverine) one does not find T3 in the nuclear fraction.

J. H. Oppenheimer: Have you or your associate had the opportunity to study T3 binding by isolated receptosomes?

M. C. Willingham: You mean after they are isolated as a fraction?

J. H. Oppenheimer: Yes.

M. C. Willingham: I don't know whether Jane has done that kind of incubation experiment. Measuring receptor inside cells is really not a trivial matter.

J. H. Oppenheimer: What about the energy requirement of the endocytic process?

M. C. Willingham: The endocytosis appears to be energy-dependent.

J. H. Oppenheimer: How quickly is endocytosis shut off after treatment with oligomycin?

M. C. Willingham: Jane has done experiments using rotenone, for example, and other inhibitors that shut off ATP synthesis, and that has a dramatic effect on the total entry of T3 measured in cell homogenates. At least the preliminary data make it look like it is an energy-dependent process.

J. A. Dias: The rate of entry and exit of proteins into "coated pits" is fairly rapid (a matter of seconds). You mentioned that some sort of a conformational change in the ligand may occur prior to localization in the coated pit, but following binding to receptor. It wasn't clear to me if you were suggesting that it was necessary for the ligand to have this conformational change prior to stabilization in the coated pit? If that is correct, then I was wondering what your current thinking is in terms of the driving forces that may induce the conformational change or stabilize it and whether you think these driving forces are covalent or noncovalent interactions. Finally, in terms of a charge effect, do you think that there may be a role for endogenously present charged substances such as polyamines which may modulate the effects that you are postulating?

M. C. Willingham: You mean in terms of the proton gradients? I haven't the faintest idea what the effect of polyamines would be on this system. All of the acidified compartments in the cell apparently respond in the same way to these monovalent ionophores, at least those that have proton specificity such as nigericin and monensin. They do many strange things themselves, such as swelling of the Golgi and changing the processing of proteins. They also interfere with the initial internalization event. Whether that is anything to get excited about or not is not clear. As for as the conformational changes, what I was thinking of is the conformation of the receptors in response to ligands. There is really no hard evidence at all that such a thing takes place. One would expect that many of these receptors which cluster together in very small coated pits presumably would use a single mechanism for this process, and therefore should have some commonality in their structure on their cytosol membrane surface, but there really is no direct evidence that such a commonality exists. It is certainly possible that one can imagine receptors which already have clicked into the right conformation independent of whether the ligand is present or not, whereas there might be others that will never click into the right conformation because they don't have the proper structure. Then there are others that are completely ligand-dependent. All possibilities in between probably exist, so it is simply a hypothesis, noting the commonality of the clustering mechanism in terms of morphologic position. We would like to think that there is a common biochemical mechanism, but we have no direct evidence for it.

J. A. Dias: Have you determined if the size of the receptor in the isolated receptosome is different from the size of the receptor in the plasma membrane?

M. C. Willingham: Yes, and there are not gross molecular weight differences.

J. E. Rall: Thank you for a map of a very complicated traffic pattern which I always have difficulty understanding and which does, I must say, seem to change from year to year. May I offer a succinct comment and a rather vague question. The comment is that transferin is actually an ambivalent molecule because it is a ligand when it binds iron and the other type of ligand when it is bound by a receptor. My question concerns clathrin which you showed us hooked on to some of the Golgi-type vesicle and also attached to the coated pits. Do you suppose the clathrin exchanges between these locations, but there should be free clathrin in the cytosol.

M. C. Willingham: First about transferrin: I probably did not mention it, but obviously the major reason cells bother to have transferrin receptors and take it up is that they need iron to grow. The transferrin system actually is a very interesting one from this standpoint, because the cell has taken advantage of the acidified nature of the receptor in some compartment to do two very specific things: (1) it does not want to degrade the transferrin, and so it recycles it out to the surface intact, and (2) it also wants to be able to get the iron off before it gets out. It so happens that transferrin binding of iron is quite pH-dependent, and it dissociates at pH 5, whereas transferrin's interaction with its receptor is the reverse, it gets even tighter at low pH. This is a very unusual ligand. As you know, most ligand–receptor binding is quite acid-sensitive. The transferrin is a receptor for iron and the cell has a receptor for transferrin. It is a very clever mechanism, but an analogous situation is, in a way, α_2-macroglobulin (α_2-M). α_2-M has a specific receptor on the cell, but α_2-M itself is a "receptor" for a wide variety of proteases. You could think of α_2-M as a protease receptor, and then the cell has a receptor for α_2-M. Presumably, there may be other systems that have evolved which use this piggyback-receptor approach. These really are quite clever.

The reason that we are so impressed that there was so little detectable clathrin in the cytosol in cells is because when one talks about the endocytic event, and realizes the speed with which it operates, in order to have these rapid events in a few seconds with disassembly and reassembly over the entire cell (1000 coated pits per cell), significant concentrations of the precursor (free clathrin) would have to be present. On the other hand, if you think of the synthesis of a protein and its assembly as a cytoskeletal element, then one does not require a high concentration in the cytosol. If you look for free concentrations of some of the other cytoskeletal proteins such as intermediate filaments, they are very low in the cytosol, yet there are many intermediate filaments in the cell, presumably because the reaction favors the formation of the structure. Tubulin, on the other hand, which can assemble and disassemble readily has a major pool of free tubulin in the cytosol. That is the reason we think of clathrin as being a stable cytoskeletal element; it is stable in terms of seconds, but this doesn't mitigate its turnover with the usual characteristics of other stable cytoplasmic proteins of many hours. We would like to think that the assembly–disassembly process that is seen *in vitro* is important for the formation of these structures, both in the Golgi and the plasma membrane. Some of these workers suggest that there are specific binding sites which recognize parts of the clathrin complex that make it assemble there and not somewhere else. I am not particularly concerned about the lack of a high concentration in the cytosol (high enough that we could detect it by immunocytochemistry). This low concentration would be that expected for a relatively stable cytoskeletal element that did not undergo very rapid and reversible assembly events, which is the model of clathrin-mediated endocytosis we favor. There is no evidence that I know of that there is a major interplay between the Golgi-coated structures and those at the plasma membrane. I think of these as two independent stable structures, which happen to share a common cytosol precursor from the synthetic standpoint, but not from the standpoint of rapid turnover.

K. Yoshinaga: Dr. Michael Conn of Duke University has been working on the mechanism of action of GnRH. He reports that the initial microaggregation of receptor is probably important for the GnRH action, but later capping and internalization are not essential for the action of GnRH. Does this apply to the other peptidal hormones? Can we hear your concept on the relationship between the mechanism of hormone action and those steps you have described here?

M. C. Willingham: Many of the ligands that we've worked with are not really hormones, in the sense that they are macromolecular things that bind for other reasons. I would think as a general rule that present evidence (forgetting T3 for the moment) that internalization is involved in tropic action of a hormone is much weaker than for the role of internalization in receptor regulation. Many of the actions of these hormones occur when they are on the cell surface. For example, EGF produces dramatic morphologic structural changes in the cell type A-431 independent of mitogenic effects. Clearly, it probably does not require internalization for that event to occur. Our general thinking is that internalization is important for regulation of receptor numbers on the cell surface (which population of receptors might be there) but it doesn't necessarily imply that the internalization event itself is a positive required step in the action of hormones; in fact, it's more often probably a negative step when it removes hormones from the cell surface. That's our general thinking. In the microaggregation events, it's really not clear that the coated pit is the mediator of the aggregation, because they are two entirely different types of events. Microaggregation of receptors can occur anywhere on the membrane and not have anything to do with coated pits. In coated pits, we are dealing with many molecules (10, 20, 30) being together in one tiny spot, and then very rapidly disappearing from the cell surface, whereas things such as capping and patching are relatively longer term events requiring many minutes.

P. Wynn: I was interested in your comments earlier that you have studied the frog erythrocyte provided by Lefkowitz's group. They reported that down-regulation was accompanied by a quantitative recovery of receptors in a light vesicle fraction of cell cytosol which is not associated with the cell surface. Are these vesicles associated with membrane receptor internalization or are they part of a separate system in this particular cell? If they are, would you comment on the functional significance of having two different classes of vesicles?

M. C. Willingham: The results that I was referring to is a very preliminary one. We were particularly interested in whether those cells had a coated pit system in them or not, or whether endocytosis in those cells would involve a different system. Those cells are extremely difficult to deal with on a morphologic basis by electron microscopy, because they are filled with hemoglobin, but it turns out that they do have coated pits and they do have structures that resemble receptosomes. Whether that has anything to do with the regulation of receptors on the cell surface is not clear. Certainly, the time course of regulation in that system is very long compared to that in epithelial and fibroblastic mammalian cells in culture. It is not at all clear what the significance of these coated pits is; I just mentioned it to show the rather ubiquitous distribution of these structures in all kinds of cells.

P. Wynn: So you do not know how important these vesicles are in contributing to the down-regulatory process?

M. C. Willingham: That is correct, we do not know.

B. I. Posner: How did you determine the extent of purification of your receptosome preparation? What was the marker that you used and how did you express it?

M. C. Willingham: We've had a little difficulty in knowing how to express those data. The basis for the isolation was the purification of internalized EGF, i.e., the number of counts of ^{125}I-labeled EGF in these cell fractions per milligram of protein. It's clear that that must be somewhat of an underestimate because of the amount of protein that's there that relates to total cell rather than specific membrane protein. That was the way it was expressed, and I really don't know any better way to express that purification.

B. I. Posner: So your marker was ^{125}I-labeled EGF and you expressed extent of purification as specific activity of the homogenate?

M. C. Willingham: Right, it was ^{125}I-labeled EGF that had been internalized by a warm-up protocol 8 minutes before, and at very precise times it was put back in the cold and was homogenized at that point.

B. I. Posner: And you are getting 30- to 40-fold augmentation of ^{125}I-labeled EGF concentration over that in homogenate?

M. C. Willingham: Yes.

B. I. Posner: Second, you seem to point out that there is a pathway for exocytosis of endocytosed material which bypasses the secretory pathway. A number of investigators, including our own group, have shown that endocytosed material enters the secretory pathway. For examples, GnPH has been shown to enter secretory granules of the pituitary (G. Pelletier *et al., Endocrinology* **111**, 1068, 1982) and insulin enters secretory granules of the acinar pancreas (J. Cruz *et al.,* submitted for publication). It is therefore possible that the two exocytotic pathways to which you refer may represent branch points from a common pathway.

M. C. Willingham: Most of those studies refer to ligands being found in secretory granules. Of course, in the cells that we work with we don't have a secretory granule population. The way I would like to think about that is that there is a common Golgi-mediated step which is responsible for the formation of secretory granules as well as any other constitutive pathway. If something is internalized into that common area, then it is very easy for them to appear in both pathways. Marilyn Farquhar did one of these experiments years ago with cationized ferritin, showing entry into Golgi stacks and also appearing in secretory granules. I would like to think that there is a common element in the trans part of the Golgi where all these things mix together, and then the Golgi somehow determines where they are going to go. I would not be surprised if a secretory granule concentrated some component and also contained another one that might not necessarily be concentrated efficiently. The two might mix together in the same spot, a little of one and alot of another, and it wouldn't have to be a perfectly efficient system of separation.

B. I. Posner: Finally, I would like to comment that of the many groups studying internalization your group and our group agree most closely on the pathways involved.

K. Sterling: I wanted to draw your attention again to the T3 receptors of the plasma membrane. I have followed the work of S.-Y. Cheng, especially the rhodamine-labeled T3, which is clearly seen in these coated pits; the entry of the hormone into the cell seems to be an energy-dependent process minimal at 4°C; warming either to 37°C or even room temperature activates the process and Dr. Cheng has told me that it can be poisoned by cyanide. Now the question is the relation to some of the other work on plasma membrane receptors. I am think of Ora Goldfine's studies and those of Segal and Ingbar which have demonstrated by extracts the existence of in plasma membrane of a rather convincing T3 binder with a reasonably strong association constant and displacement from the binding sites by nonradioactive T3. The physiologic effect of T3 binding is to increase the inward movement of hexose and other substrates probably. I am just wondering whether this is not a separate and distinct receptor from the coated pit binder that presumably functions to get T3 into the cell where it can interact with nuclei, mitochondria, and so on, and whether the direct effects throughout the plasma membrane may not be required to allow accelerated transport processes. I wonder if you have any thoughts about this?

M. C. Willingham: Jane Cheng should be the one to answer that question, but unfortunately she is not here. The kinetics and binding characteristics of this plasma membrane receptor correspond fairly closely to what has been described for the other T3 receptors in other sites, so that from those criteria it does not seem to be abnormal. The molecular weight of this plasma membrane receptor by affinity labeling is about the same as has been described for other T3 receptors. Actually, the number of receptors in the cell surface for T3 is rather high, perhaps hundreds of thousands per cell. This makes it a fairly significant uptake and binding process. Of course, as you know, the association–dissociation aspects of this receptor are such that it is very difficult to do those experiments. It does not associate well in the cold, for example, where one would like to do most of these experiments. The nonspecific component is higher than for many other ligands. I am just not sure what the real answer to your question is. When we're looking at the uptake of rhodamine-labeled T3 where one can show specificity of binding by competition experiments, we can be fairly sure that the labeled vesicles are receptosomes, which we know by analogy only arise from coated pits; but we don't have good markers yet for T3 at the electron microscopic level, where we could really say something definitive about what compartment the label was in. I really don't know the answer.

J. Djiane: You reported several years ago that amines like methylamine or bacitracin and inhibitors of phospholipase A2 are able to inhibit the internalization of hormone receptor complexes. We have tested all these compounds for prolactin receptors in the mammary cell model without success. What are your thoughts today about inhibitors of internalization? And second, are you able to modify the internalization process with antibody against clathrin?

M. C. Willingham: The second part of that question first: the antibodies to clathrin that have been microinjected had no effect on the internalization process. Of course, one has to microinject these antibodies because clathrin is not exposed on the cell surface. In spite of the fact that the antibodies go into the cytoplasm, bind to the clathrin that's on coated pits, and there is excess antibody available in the cytosol, there is no effect on endocytosis, there is no effect on the rate of formation of endocytic vesicles, or anything else, as far as we can tell. The inhibitor studies are just that—they are pharmacologic inhibitor studies, the specificity of which is not always terribly clear. There are, as you point out, different classes of these kinds of inhibitors of the transglutaminase system, and others which have nothing to do with transglutaminases which affect other enzyme systems. It is really not clear what the biochemical mechanisms are that mediate these events at the plasma membrane. There are, in fact, multiple classes of drugs which inhibit the clustering process, and then there are other classes which inhibit things beyond the clustering process (such as monovalent ionophores which have no effect on clustering). For what it's worth, the most potent of those inhibitors of the transglutaminase type is dansylcadaverine, which is effective at 10 μM in some cells. It, of course, does other things to cells. It interferes with phospholipid metabolism, among other things. So it is very hard to know what those pharmacologic studies tell us. There has not been further biochemical purification of the enzyme(s) that might be involved.

C. Sonnenschein: From the answer you gave to a previous question, are you implying that the most important function of transferrin is that of serving as an iron pump? According to data you presented, transferrin is not metabolized at all.

M. C. Willingham: Right, but when transferrin gets into the low pH environment of the receptosome, it loses its iron and the iron presumably then is made available by this mechanism to get into the cytosol. Then, the transferrin is recycled intact, without iron on it.

C. Sonnenschein: Therefore, transferring functions like an iron pump?

M. C. Willingham: That is right, it is an iron pump.

C. Sonnenschein: I recognize that your slides are schematic, but could you provide us with any clues regarding how EGF effects cell multiplication?

M. C. Willingham: These are very hard experiments to figure out. The cell multiplication effects, the growth factor effects of things like EGF (which by the way is a fairly poor mitogen), is a very long-term effect. In order to get initiation of DNA synthesis from a G_1-arrested cell population, you have to expose it to EGF for many hours, during which time there is a dramatic down-regulation of receptor numbers on the cell surface. That implies that the initial internalization that one sees for EGF and its receptor may have nothing to do with the mitogenic response. There is one early rapid effect of EGF that is seen in A-431 cells where there is a stimulation of surface ruffling activity, a rather aberrant form of ruffle which is a very slow wave of ruffling. That is an unusual cell type because it has about 3 million receptors per cell and the ruffling response is clearly not related to overall internalization. So I would think that it is not at all clear that internalization of EGF, for example, is involved in the mitogenic signal. The experiments to show that are very difficult to do. If you try to inhibit internalization, the cells get sick after awhile, and you can't keep inhibitors present for a day in order to find out whether mitogenesis has occurred, because the cells will die from the drugs. In another context, the internalization pathway is probably responsible for the turnover of the entire cell surface membrane and probably has a very major physiological function. The cell needs to replace its surface membrane components frequently, and that may be the reason that it has been so difficult to isolate mutations in this general pathway.

G. D. Aurbach: Mark, could you fill us in on what is known about the mechanism of adenovirus potentiation in the internalization of receptor complexes. Is there any knowledge about the chemistry of the virus and its interaction with the cell membrane?

M. C. Willingham: We have been very interested to know what the biochemical mechanisms are that account for the adenovirus effects. It is not just specific for one type of adenovirus. Whether this function is present on other non-membrane-limited viruses we don't know yet. Prem Seth and David FitzGerald in our laboratory have been trying to identify the components of the virus responsible for this lytic activity. At the moment, all we know is that is appears to be partially pH dependent. That is, when cells are treated with drugs that dissipate the acidic gradients in receptosomes, the potentiation effect is markedly inhibited. It shares that in common with the fusion events seen with membrane-limited viruses. We are trying to isolate the proteins of the virus, make antibodies to them, and look for enzymatic activity that might explain this lytic property. It appears to be independent of viral replication, since UV-inactivated virus shows the same property.

P. Wynn: How much credence do you put on the use of dansylcadaverine as an inhibitor of internalization. Our studies with the GnRH receptor have shown no dose-dependent inhibition of internalization but that once a threshold concentration is reached, internalization is completely inhibited; does this mean that the cells are just dying from the toxic effects of this inhibitor?

M. C. Willingham: The internalization is inhibited?

P. Wynn: Yes, internalization is inhibited by 90% using micromolar concentrations whereas lower concentrations show no inhibitory effects at all.

M. C. Willingham: One of the problems is the kind of experiments one can do with such an inhibitor. One can do very short-term experiments where toxicity is not a severe problem, where one is dealing with 15-minute incubations. There you can show direct effects on one event, e.g., internalization, but when one tries to put this inhibitor in for a longer period of time, other forms of toxicity become manifest. It becomes very hard to interpret a result that might require many hours to be measured. Dansylcadaverine is a very toxic drug; there is no question that we can use it in short-term experiments on internalization, and its effects are reversible and the cells survive. However, as you say, if you leave it in long enough, the cells will start dying because it affects many other systems. If the effect you are trying to measure takes a long time, then such an experiment is not easily interpreted.

Hereditary Resistance to 1,25-Dihydroxyvitamin D

STEPHEN J. MARX,* URI A. LIBERMAN,*,† CHAS EIL,‡
GEORGE T. GAMBLIN,‡ DONALD A. DEGRANGE,* AND SONIA BALSAN§

*Metabolic Diseases Branch, NIADDK, Bethesda, Maryland, †Beilinson Medical Center
and Tel Aviv University Medical School, Tel Aviv, Israel, ‡Endocrinology Branch, Naval
Hospital Bethesda, USUHS, Bethesda, Maryland,[1] and §Calcified Tissue Laboratory,
Hopital des Enfants Malades, Paris, France

I. Introduction

Prior to 1920, rickets and osteomalacia were widespread problems in temperate zones. The discovery of and subsequent prophylactic use of vitamin D (D refers to D_2 and/or D_3) have remained among the most dramatic accomplishments in the fields of medical research and public health. By 1930 rickets and osteomalacia had become rare problems in the United States; however, occasional cases resistant to commonly used doses of vitamin D began to come to attention at that time. In 1937 Fuller Albright and co-workers published the first detailed analysis of one such patient with typical radiographic features of rickets resistant to the usual doses of vitamin D (Albright *et al.*, 1937). This patient exhibited hypophosphatemia but not the hypocalcemia typical of nutritional deficiency of vitamin D; these features are typical of the commonest variant of hereditary rickets, X-linked hypophosphatemia (Scriver *et al.*, 1982). With our present understanding of the hormonal nature of the calciferol system, Albright's discription can be considered the first detailed report of pathological resistance to a hormone or vitamin in man. In 1961 Prader and co-workers described cases with hypocalcemia and rickets resistant to vitamin D (van Creveld and Arons, 1949, 1954; Prader *et al.*, 1961). Because of the greater resemblance of the cases with hypocalcemia to nutritional rickets, the terms pseudo-vitamin D deficiency or vitamin D dependency have been used. Insight into the mechanisms of these disorders was not possible until the steps leading to bone mineralization, including the pathways of calciferol action, were clarified.

---

[1] The opinions expressed herein are those of the authors and are not to be construed as reflecting the views of the Navy Department, of the Naval Service at large, or of the Department of Defense.

589

II. Normal Vitamin D Action

Vitamin D is produced from cholesterol-like precursors by radiation-induced opening of the B-ring. The open ring classifies the calciferols as seco-steroids. Vitamin D_3 (cholecalciferol) is produced from 7-dehydro-cholesterol in epidermis, and vitamin D_2 (ergocalciferol) is a synthetic product derived from ergosterol, a plant sterol. Vitamin D_2 enters the body as a food supplement; vitamin D_3 enters the body either as a food component, a food supplement, or as an endogenous metabolite in skin. Vitamin D is inactive in calciferol target tissues *in vitro;* its activation usually requires two hydroxylation reactions (Marx *et al.,* 1983). Vitamin D is taken up by hepatocytes and hydroxylated at carbon-25. 25(OH)D can then be converted to $1,25(OH)_2D$ or to other metabolites of uncertain importance. $1,25(OH)_2D$ is the most potent natural calciferol metabolite. Its principal site of production is the renal proximal convoluted tubule. The activity of the 25(OH)D 1-α-hydroxylase (1-hydroxylase) is stimulated by parathyroid hormone and inhibited by $1,25(OH)_2D$, phosphorus, and (perhaps) calcium in serum (Trechsel *et al.,* 1979, 1980; Omdahl *et al.,* 1980).

$1,25(OH)_2D$ acts by a mechanism analogous to that of the steroid hormones. It is transported in blood by an α-globulin with preferential affinity for 25(OH)D (transcalciferin), and it binds in target cells to receptors with preferential affinity for $1,25(OH)_2D$. The hormone–receptor complex in the nucleus of target cells initiates changes in cellular levels of selected mRNAs. mRNA for a calcium-binding protein, structurally related to calmodulin and troponin-C, has been studied in greatest detail (Norman *et al.,* 1982; Hunziker *et al.,* 1983), but the translated protein has unknown function (Feher, 1983) and is unlikely to account for all the actions of $1,25(OH)_2D$. Like true steroids, $1,25(OH)_2D$ may also have effects through genome-independent pathways.

By its nuclear interaction, $1,25(OH)_2D$ initiates at least four different types of process (Table I). First, $1,25(OH)_2D$, by acting upon intestinal mucosa, bone resorbing surfaces, or renal tubules, stimulates translocation of calcium and other minerals (magnesium and phosphorus) into the blood (Marx *et al.,* 1983). Second, $1,25(OH)_2D$, acting through its receptors, affects the calciferol metabolic pathways; it increases accumulation of 7-dehydrocholesterol in skin (Esvelt *et al.,* 1980), it inhibits 1-hydroxylase, and it stimulates 25(OH)D 24-hydroxylase (24-hydroxylase) (Trechsel *et al.,* 1979; Omdahl *et al.,* 1980; Colston and Feldman, 1982). Third, it modulates secretion of several proteins; in osteoblasts (as assessed in whole calvaria or in cultured osteoblast-like osteosarcoma cells) collagen secretion is decreased (Rowe and Kream, 1982) and osteocalcin secretion is increased (Price and Baukol, 1980), and in cultured pituitary cells pro-

TABLE I

Actions of 1,25(OH)$_2$D^a

Type of action	Comment
Increase calcium flux to plasma	Intestinal mucosa
	Bone resorbing surface
	Renal distal tubule
Modulate calciferol metabolism	Increase 7-dehydrocholesterol in skin
	Decrease 1-hydroxylase in kidney^b
	Increase 24-hydroxylase in kidney^b
Modulate protein secretion	Decrease collagen from osteoblast
	Increase osteocalcin from osteoblast
	Increase prolactin from pituitary
Regulate cell differentiation	Monocyte toward macrophage

^{a} References are cited in Section II.

^{b} 1-Hydroxylase and 24-hydroxylase have been identified in extrarenal sites. In some cases, the extrarenal calciferol hydroxylases have been shown to have regulation similar to the renal hydroxylases.

lactin secretion is increased (Wark and Tashjian, 1982). Fourth, it can modulate differentiation of certain cells; for example, it causes malignant (Abe *et al.*, 1981) or normal (Provvedini *et al.*, 1983) monocytes to express features of differentiated macrophages.

Some tissues, not known to respond in any of the above four ways, possess components of the effector system for 1,25(OH)$_2$D. Both receptors for 1,25(OH)$_2$D (Pike *et al.*, 1980; Colston *et al.*, 1980; Stumpf *et al.*, 1981) and immunoreactive vitamin D-dependent calcium-binding protein (Christakos *et al.*, 1979; Norman *et al.*, 1982; Thomasset *et al.*, 1982) are present, for example, in the brain, the pancreatic β cell, and the parathyroid gland of some species.

III. Resistance to Calciferols: Definitions

We define resistance to a factor as the combination of a subnormal biologic effect with normal levels of the factor at relevant sites (Kahn, 1978; Marx, 1984). This definition has three important components that require identification: the factor, the location of the factor, and the biologic effect. Among the calciferols, the principal factors to consider are vitamin D, 25(OH)D, and 1,25(OH)$_2$D. Marked resistance to a distal metabolite [1,25(OH)$_2$D] usually implies resistance to the proximal metabolites, but the reverse need not be true. For example, a selective deficiency of 1-hydroxylase (vitamin D dependency type 1) causes resistance to D and 25(OH)D but not to 1,25(OH)$_2$D (Fraser *et al.*, 1973). This discussion will focus upon resistance to 1,25(OH)$_2$D.

The most relevant site to assess 1,25(OH)$_2$D level is a distal point in its path of action, i.e., in the nucleus of target tissues, but this is not possible in humans. The level of 1,25(OH)$_2$D in target tissue nuclei correlates with the 1,25(OH)$_2$D level in other locations including nuclei or cytoplasm of tissues that are not known targets, plasma, and the level in diet [the latter being an index of 1,25(OH)$_2$D turnover in patients receiving high dose therapy with oral 1,25(OH)$_2$D$_3$]. The level of 1,25(OH)$_2$D in target tissue nuclei *in vivo* may also correlate with the intrinsic properties of the genes controlling the receptors themselves.

Since 1,25(OH)$_2$D has a broad spectrum of biologic effects, any one could be used in assessing hormone resistance. The different actions are not equivalent. The mineral transport effects particularly at the level of the intestine give to 1,25(OH)$_2$D all or most of its antirachitic effect. Defects in calcium-transport response to 1,25(OH)$_2$D are associated with serum levels that are low for calcium and high for PTH (Arnaud *et al.*, 1970). However, there are variants of rickets resistant to 1,25(OH)$_2$D in which the serum (and presumably target tissue) levels of calcium, phosphorus, PTH, and 1,25(OH)$_2$D are normal (e.g., hereditary hypophosphatasia, a defect in cellular mediation of bone mineralization). The remainder of this discussion will deal with defects in the calcium transport response to 1,25(OH)$_2$D *in vivo* as assessed by tests of intestinal absorption of calcium, calcium in serum, or PTH in serum (as an index of ionized calcium). For studies *in vitro,* we shall discuss the response of 25(OH)D-24-hydroxylase (24-hydroxylase) to 1,25(OH)$_2$D.

The above definition of resistance to 1,25(OH)$_2$D can be refined further by considering the relation between a range of 1,25(OH)$_2$D levels and their biologic effects. Resistance can be subdivided into defects in sensitivity, defects in responsiveness, and defects that are mixed or indeterminate (Fig. 1) (Kahn, 1978; Marx, 1984). Deficient sensitivity is defined as an increase in the level of 1,25(OH)$_2$D required to produce a half-maximal bioeffect. Deficient responsiveness is defined as inability to attain the normal maximal bioeffect even at extremely high levels of 1,25(OH)$_2$D. A series of theoretical calciferol dose–response curves can be constructed to illustrate application of the above terms to the calcemic bioeffect of the factors D and 1,25(OH)$_2$D (Fig. 2).

IV. Calcium Deficiency Resistant to 1,25(OH)$_2$D: Acquired

Several variants of calcium deficiency resistant to 1,25(OH)$_2$D that are not hereditary have been recognized in man and in other species.

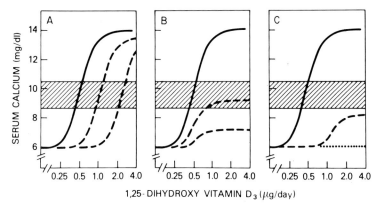

FIG. 1. Variants in resistance of serum calcium to 1,25(OH)₂D₃. Stippled zone indicates
normal level of calcium. Solid line, normal response (assuming constant calcium intake and
a baseline of vitamin D deficiency). (A) Dashed lines, two grades of decrease in sensitivity to
1,25(OH)₂D₃. (B) Dashed lines, two grades of decrease in responsiveness to 1,25(OH)₂D₃.
(C) Dashed line, combination of decrease in sensitivity and decrease in responsiveness to
1,25(OH)₂D₃. Dotted line, unmeasurable response; this can reflect unmeasurable sensitivity,
unmeasurable response, or combinations of the two. The extension of the response curves
to high serum calcium concentrations is theoretical; testing *in vivo* at this range of serum
calcium is not possible, and responses would be unstable because of calcium toxicity. (From
Marx, 1984).

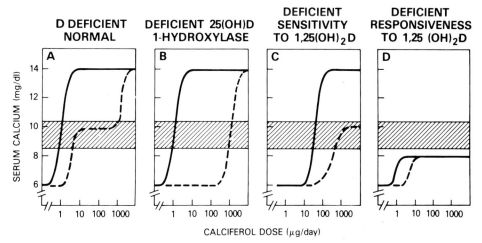

FIG. 2. Theoretical effects of a range of maintenance doses of calciferols [1,25(OH)₂D₃,
solid lines; vitamin D₂, dashed lines] in four (A–D) conditions. All curves assume constant
calcium intake and a baseline of vitamin D deficiency. Stippled zone indicates normal level
of calcium. Note in particular, the special consequences of regulated conversion of D₂ to
1,25(OH)₂D₂ in A. (From Marx, 1984.)

The intestine of the fetal rat does not show induction of a calcium transport response to 1,25(OH)$_2$D *in vitro* (Halloran and DeLuca, 1980). This is directly attributable to an absence of receptors for 1,25(OH)$_2$D in this tissue, and both receptors for 1,25(OH)$_2$D and inducibility of the calcium-transport response to 1,25(OH)$_2$D appear together at 2 weeks postpartum (Halloran and DeLuca, 1981). This example indicates that the tissue content of receptors for 1,25(OH)$_2$D can be regulated in significant fashion.

During adolescent growth in humans, ingestion of a diet severely deficient in calcium can result in skeletal deficiency of calcium (osteomalacia), mild hypocalcemia, secondary hyperparathyroidism, and high serum levels of 1,25(OH)$_2$D (Pettifor *et al.*, 1981).

During the treatment phase of nutritional deficiency of vitamin D, serum levels of 25(OH)D begin to rise at a time when skeletal remineralization results in a continued hypocalcemic stimulus to the parathyroids; serum levels of 1,25(OH)$_2$D may rise to several hundred pg/ml (nl 20–60) at this time (Papapoulos *et al.*, 1980; Stanbury *et al.*, 1981; Garabedian *et al.*, 1983). In the latter two examples the target cells for 1,25(OH)$_2$D are presumed to respond normally but calcium pools and fluxes outside 1,25(OH)$_2$D target cells of intestinal epithelium maintain the state of calcium deficiency in plasma.

A fourth example may combine features of cellular and extracellular deficiencies in calcemic response to 1,25(OH)$_2$D. Survivors of extremely premature birth exhibit hypocalcemia, rickets, and elevated plasma levels of 1,25(OH)$_2$D (Steichen *et al.*, 1981; Chesney *et al.*, 1981). This might reflect a combination of transiently deficient target cell response (as in the intestine of neonatal rat) plus high skeletal demands for mineral; the high skeletal demands are related to the fact that the human fetal skeleton normally would accumulate 300 mg of calcium per day via placental transfer during the third trimester.

V. Calcium Deficiency Resistant to 1,25(OH)$_2$D: Hereditary

Fourteen reported kindreds show clinical features suggestive of hereditary calcium deficiency resistant to 1,25(OH)$_2$D (vitamin D dependency type 2 or pseudo-vitamin D deficiency type 2).[2] Because of the variable expression between kindreds and because of the spectrum of techniques used to study these kindreds, there are few features common to all. The only common features, when these have been assessed, are secondary hyperparathyroidism and high levels of 1,25(OH)$_2$D during therapy.

---

[2] An additional kindred was described in a preliminary report (Yoshikawa *et al.*, 1982), but the diagnosis was revised subsequently to deficiency of 25(OH)D 1-hydroxylase (S. Yoshikawa, personal communication).

TABLE II

Clinical Data from Cases of Hereditary Calcium Deficiency Resistant to 1,25(OH)$_2$D

Case[a]	Total affected siblings (n)	Consan- guinity	Age at onset[b] (years)	Alo- pecia	Serum level of 1,25(OH)$_2$D		References
					Before therapy (pg/ml)	During therapy[c] (pg/ml)	
—	1	?	15	0	137	297	Brooks et al. (1978)
1A	2	0	2	0	213	270	Marx et al. (1978)
1B	2	0	0.5	0	280	640	Marx et al. (1978)
—	?	?	2	0	212	189	Zerwekh et al. (1979)
A	2	0	9	0	93	?	Adams et al. (1979)
B	2	0	2	0	54	?	Adams et al. (1979)
—	1	?	45	0	?	?	Fujita et al. (1980)
—	1	0	12	0	143	?	Kudoh et al. (1981)
2A	2	+	2	+	169	?	Rosen et al. (1979)
2B	2	+	1	+	142	800	Rosen et al. (1979)
3	2	+	1	+	710	?	Liberman et al. (1980)
—	1	?	1.5	+	>200	?	Sockalosky et al. (1980)
KN	?	+	1.5	+	?	4800	Tsuchiya et al. (1980)
IH	2	+	1	+	108	?	Feldman et al. (1982)
4	2	+	0.8	+	66	?	Balsan et al. (1983)
5	4	+	0.6	+	?	1400	Balsan et al. (1983)
6	1	—	3	+	916	?	Beer et al. (1981)

[a] For kindreds 1 through 6 members of whose cells we evaluated (Liberman et al., 1983a), identification symbol is derived from that study. Several cases are described in more than one report; the most recent or most comprehensive is cited.

[b] Age at onset is considered to be age at first recognition of metabolic bone disease (rickets, osteomalacia, or fracture diathesis).

[c] Serum levels of 1,25(OH)$_2$D during therapy are tabulated only during normocalcemia induced by D$_2$, 25(OH)$_2$D$_3$, or 1α(OH)D$_3$. Levels fluctuate rapidly during therapy with 1,25(OH)$_2$D$_3$ so data during this therapy are excluded. Thus the tabulated data are indices of steady-state hormone levels to give comparable calcemic responses.

Among the 14 kindreds, the family pattern was consistent with autosomal recessive transmission in each; there were affected siblings in 6 kindreds and parental consanguinity in 6 (Table II). We have evaluated cells from members of six of these kindreds and will describe the relation between data from these patients *in vivo* and from their cells *in vitro*. The heterogeneity in major clinical features has been striking and will be illustrated by several examples. A similar resistance to 1,25(OH)$_2$D has been suggested to characterize the marmoset, a New World monkey (Shinki et al., 1983).

VI. Interactions with Calciferols *in Vivo*: Alopecia

Half of reported kindreds with hereditary calcium deficiency resistant to $1,25(OH)_2D$ have shown total alopecia in affected members (Table II). Among seven kindreds with multiple affected siblings per kindred, each kindred has been consistent with regard to alopecia (five kindreds) (Fig. 3) (Rosen *et al.*, 1979; Liberman *et al.*, 1980; Feldman *et al.*, 1982; Balsan *et al.*, 1983) or normal hair growth (two kindreds) (Marx *et al.*, 1978; Adams *et al.*, 1979).

In patients with alopecia, there are features suggesting that the underlying disorder is more severe than in those with normal hair. Thus, the alopecic cases show earlier age of onset of metabolic bone disease (1.5 versus 11 years) and higher serum level of $1,25(OH)_2D$ associated with attainment of normocalcemia (2330 versus 349 pg/ml) (Table II).

Alopecia is probably a direct consequence of resistance to $1,25(OH)_2D$.

1. High affinity uptake of $[^3H]1,25(OH)_2D_3$ occurs in the nucleus of the outer root sheath cells of the hair follicle in the rat (Stumpf *et al.*, 1981).

2. The epidermis and hair follicles contain a calcium-binding protein with some similarities to the intestinal vitamin D-dependent calcium-binding protein (Saurat *et al.*, 1981; Rinaldi *et al.*, 1982).

3. $1,25(OH)_2D_3$ administered to vitamin D-deficient rats results in selective accumulation of 7-dehydrocholesterol in skin (Esvelt *et al.*, 1980).

4. The consistency of the association of alopecia with severe resistance to $1,25(OH)_2D$ is the strongest argument that the association is not fortuitous.

What remains puzzling is that abnormalities of the epidermal appendages have not been noted with deficiency of $1,25(OH)_2D$ secondary to deficiency of D, of $25(OH)D$, or of 1-hydroxylase. The alopecia associated with hypoparathyroidism in the polyglandular autoimmune deficiency syndrome is a unique exception (Neufeld *et al.*, 1981); alopecia is not seen in other variants of hypoparathyroidism (such as resistance to parathyroid hormone or postparathyroidectomy). Several explanations for the association of alopecia and hereditary calcium deficiency resistant to $1,25(OH)_2D$ can be considered. First the deficiency in calciferol action may be more severe in cases with clinically manifested hereditary resistance to $1,25(OH)_2D$. Second the deficiency in calciferol action may be expressed very early in cases with resistance to $1,25(OH)_2D$. Hereditary resistance to $1,25(OH)_2D$ in a fetus is associated with an outwardly completely normal gestation. White hypocalcemia and rickets do not develop *in utero* because of normal placental function, actions of $1,25(OH)_2D$ in

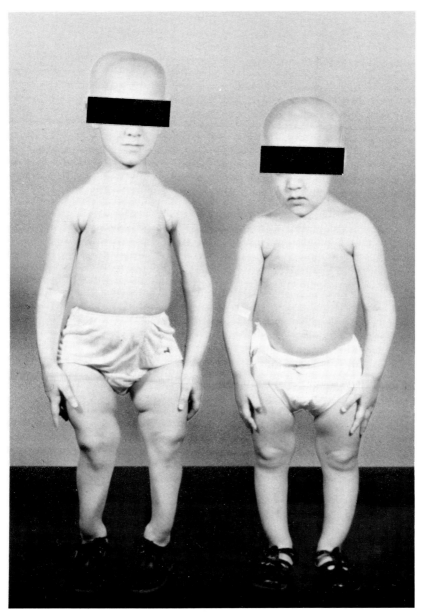

FIG. 3.   Patients 2A (right side, age 3 years) and 2B (left side, age 7 years). (Courtesy of Dr. J. F. Rosen.)

the fetus unrelated to mineral transport may be defective at this stage. It seems possible that 1,25(OH)$_2$D stimulates differentiation of the hair follicle. Third, the alopecia might be a direct consequence of high serum levels of 1,25(OH)$_2$D; this would imply some bioeffect of 1,25(OH)$_2$D not mediated by the classical receptor for 1,25(OH)$_2$D.

VII. Interactions with Calciferols *in Vivo*: Variability between Kindreds

Patient 1B presented with rickets at age 5 months in 1952 (Marx *et al.*, 1978). She was the third of four siblings from nonconsanguineous parents. Two siblings are normal but an older brother also had shown rickets resistant to D$_2$. She and her affected brother had normal hair growth. During childhood she had responded to high doses of D$_2$. When evaluated without therapy at age 18, she exhibited hypocalcemia and secondary hyperparathyroidism. For the next 6 years she was normocalcemic receiving a maintenance dose of D$_2$ of 0.5 mg/day. At age 24 therapy was changed to 1,25(OH)$_2$D$_3$ orally. She required a maintenance dose of 17–18 μg/day (with supplemental calcium 800 mg/day orally) to maintain serum calcium in the normal range (Fig. 4). During the second and third trimesters of pregnancy still higher dosages of 1,25(OH)$_2$D$_3$ were required to normalize her serum calcium (corrected for albumin concentration in serum) (Marx *et al.*, 1980). Of particular note, following delivery of a normal child, she became mildly hypercalcemic on the same dose of 1,25(OH)$_2$D$_3$ that she had required prior to delivery. Analysis of the relation of serum calcium response to oral 1,25(OH)$_2$D5 is consistent with decreased sensi-

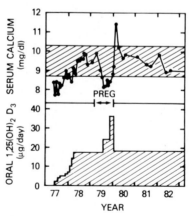

FIG. 4. Calcemic effect of 1,25(OH)$_2$D$_3$ orally in patient 1B. Stippled zone indicates normal level of calcium in upper panel. PREG, Pregnancy.

tivity to the hormone (Fig. 5). The dose of $1,25(OH)_2D_3$ for half-maximal calcemic response is shifted upward. Though the curve extends to the hypercalcemic range, it is not possible to determine *in vivo* if the maximal calcemic response to $1,25(OH)_2D$ is normal. Thus, her calcemic resistance could be a defect in sensitivity to $1,25(OH)_2D$ or a combination of defects in sensitivity and responsiveness to $1,25(OH)_2D$. Analysis of stored serum showed that, at age 18, when she had not received any calciferols for approximately 7 years, her serum level of $1,25(OH)_2D$ had been 280 pg/ml (nl 23–62) (Table II).

Patient 4 showed almost total alopecia at age 40 days in 1977 and signs of rickets at age 8 months (Balsan *et al.*, 1983). She was the offspring of consanguineous parents, the fifth child in a sibship of five; three sibs were apparently normal but an older brother had died at age of 3 years with alopecia and rickets resistant to high doses of D_2. On detailed evaluation at age of 2 years and 7 months she showed hypocalcemia and secondary hyperparathyroidism. Various calciferol analogs at high dosage (with supplemental calcium 1000 mg/day orally) were administered over the ensuing 2 years without any consistent change in the hypocalcemia or the secondary hyperparathyroidism (Fig. 6). During this time elevated levels

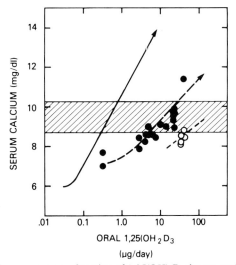

FIG. 5.   Calcemic response as a function of $1,25(OH)_2D_3$ dosage orally in patient 1B (see Fig. 4). Stippled zone indicates normal level of calcium. Solid line, normal curve (theoretical) assuming zero calciferol intake at baseline and not specifying an upper limit to the calcemic response (see also legend of Fig. 1). Dashed lines, patient 1B when not pregnant (●, large dashes) and during second half of pregnancy (○, small dashes).

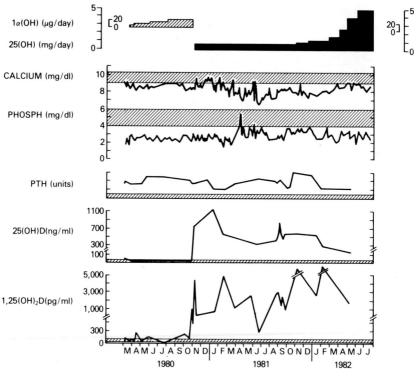

FIG. 6.   Absent calcemic response to calciferols. Treatment regimens and serum levels of electrolytes and calciferols in patient 4 (Balsan *et al.*, 1983). 1α(OH) refers to 1α(OH)D₃ or 1α,25(OH)₂D₃ given orally. 25(OH) refers to 25(OH)D₃ given orally. Stippled zones indicate normal ranges.

of 1,25(OH)₂D₃ in serum were documented on multiple occasions (in the fasting state prior to receipt of medication) with values as high as 10,500 pg/ml (nl 20–110).

In this patient there was no clear change in serum calcium in response to striking elevation of the serum level of 1,25(OH)₂D₃. We shall return later to a discussion of why serum calcium in this patient was generally not depressed below 8 mg/dl.

While striking differences in calcemic response to calciferols are evident between kindreds, within kindreds the differences have been very mild. In fact, multiple affected members have been evaluated in detail in only two kindreds (Marx *et al.*, 1978; Rosen *et al.*, 1979; Eil *et al.*, 1981). Within each kindred calcemic responses were present, and similar doses of calciferols were effective in siblings.

VIII. Interactions with Calciferols *in Vivo*: Temporal Variation within a Patient

The degree of resistance of serum calcium to 1,25(OH)$_2$D can vary over time within a subject. This was clearly shown in patient 1B, when pregnancy increased her resistance (Figs. 4 and 5). During that time, the extra calcium requirements of gestation probably accounted for a shift in the relation between 1,25(OH)$_2$D$_3$ dose and the calcemic response.

Patient 3 presented at age 10 months in 1963 with alopecia, rickets, and hypocalcemia (Liberman *et al.*, 1980). Her parents were consanguineous; a younger sister born in 1964 died at age 10 months with alopecia and rickets. She exhibited no response to D$_2$ at 20 mg/day over 4 months. When evaluated at age 13 for hypocalcemic convulsions, her only treatment was calcium supplementation. She exhibited normal levels of 25(OH)D, very high levels of 1,25(OH)$_2$D, and undetectable levels of 24,25(OH)$_2$D (below detection limit of 0.39 ng/ml on four occasions) (Fig. 7). When she failed to respond to 1α(OH)D$_3$ orally up to 8 μg/day for 2 months or 1,25(OH)$_2$D$_3$ 5 μg/day for 3 months, a brief trial of oral treatment with 24,24(OH)$_2$D$_3$ 2 μg/day was given. Immediately after her serum level of 24,25(OH)$_2$D reached the normal range, serum calcium normalized and serum levels of 1,25(OH)$_2$D decreased though not to the normal range (Fig. 7). Nine months after stopping 24,25(OH)$_2$D$_3$ therapy, the biochemical improvement persisted.

In this patient with undetectable serum levels of 24,25(OH)$_2$D prior to therapy, a profound change in the relation of serum calcium and serum 1,25(OH)$_2$D occurred at the time of iatrogenic elevation of serum level of 24,25(OH)$_2$D. It is not certain that 24,25(OH)$_2$D$_3$ caused this change as further therapeutic trials have not yet been described in this patient or in other similar patients.

In another example, the cause for temporal variation in resistance to 1,25(OH)$_2$D is not known. Patient 5 was born to consanguineous parents in 1974 (Balsan *et al.*, 1983). Three of seven siblings had died previously between ages 2 and 3 with alopecia and severe rickets. Alopecia was documented at age 11 days, and radiographs first showed rickets at age of 7 months. Evaluation at age 22 months showed hypocalcemia and secondary hyperparathyroidism. Over a period of 6 years the child received high dosages of calciferol analogs. Her course could be categorized into three phases (Fig. 8). During the initial 9 months rickets was active (first phase). However, during therapy with high dosage 25(OH)D$_3$ there was symptomatic improvement followed by healing of rickets and resolution of hypocalcemia and secondary hyperparathyroidism. Over the next 2 years, calcium deficiency was in recovery (second phase) with therapy of 4–8

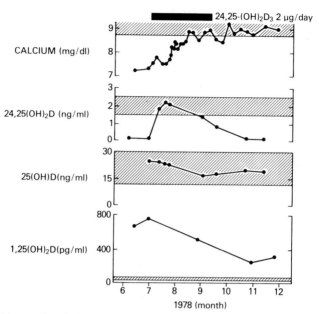

FIG. 7. Temporal variation in calcemic response to calciferols. Serum levels of electrolytes and calciferol metabolites around time of therapy with 24,25(OH)₂D₃ in patient 3 (Liberman *et al.*, 1980). Stippled zones indicate normal ranges.

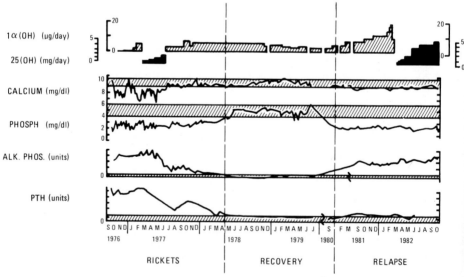

FIG. 8. Temporal variation in calcemic response to calciferols. Treatment regimens and serum components in patient 5 (Balsan *et al.*, 1983). 1α(OH) refers to 1α(OH)D₃ or 1α,25(OH)₂D₃ given orally. 25(OH) refers to 25(OH)D₃ given orally. Stippled zones indicate normal ranges.

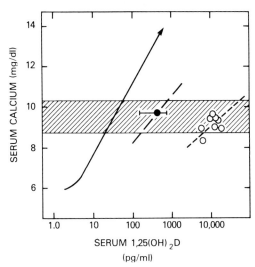

FIG. 9.   Calcemic response as a function of 1,25(OH)₂D level in plasma during recovery and relapse phases (see Fig. 8) in patient 5. Stippled zone indicates normal level of calcium. Solid line, normal curve (theoretical) assuming zero calciferol intake at baseline and not specifying an upper limit to the calcemic response (see also legend of Fig. 1). (●), Long dashes, recovery phase. (○), Short dashes, relapse phase.

μg/day of 1α(OH)D$_3$. By August 1981 she again showed hypophosphatemia and radiographic rickets. This relapse (third phase) continued over the ensuing two years despite administration of high doses of various calciferols. Hypocalcemia persisted during therapy with 25(OH)D$_3$ at 4–5 mg/day and associated with serum 1,25(OH)$_2$D$_3$ levels of 13,000 pg/ml (mean of seven).

Evaluation of the relation of serum calcium and serum 1,25(OH)$_2$D indicates a striking change between the periods of recovery and relapse (Fig. 9). The explanation for this change is not known. There was no associated major change in external calcium flux, and linear (and skeletal) growth was proceeding parallel to the normal curve.

IX. Calciferol Metabolism *in Vivo:* 25(OH)D 1-Hydroxylase

Patients with hereditary calcium deficiency resistant to 1,25(OH)$_2$D show the highest peripheral serum levels of 1,25(OH)$_2$D found in any living systems. These patients can sustain the combination of hypocalcemia, secondary hyperparathyroidism, hypophosphatemia, and high serum levels of 25(OH)D. Thus three potential stimulators of 1-hydroxylase can synergize in the presence of high levels of 25(OH)D substrate for the enzyme.

Patient 5 was studied in detail at the Hôpital des Enfants Malades at a time when her disease was in recovery phase (Fig. 8) (Balsan *et al.*, 1983). At this time the serum concentrations of calcium, PTH, and phosphorus were all normal. A brief change of therapy from $1\alpha(OH)D_3$ to $25(OH)D_3$ resulted in extremely high levels of $1,25(OH)_2D_3$ in serum, necessarily derived from endogenous production (Fig. 10). While the levels of $25(OH)D_3$ substrate for the 1-hydroxylase were higher than normal, this alone could not account for the high levels of $1,25(OH)_2D_3$ in serum. It seems likely that, under the test conditions, the patient exhibited the consequence of defective feedback inhibition of 1-hydroxylase by $1,25(OH)_2D$ action on its receptor in the proximal tubule of the kidney. Such "aberrant" regulation of 1-hydroxylase might in fact be beneficial to patients with hereditary calcium deficiency resistant to $1,25(OH)_2D$. Several others, such as patient 1B (described above), have sustained prolonged remissions of hypocalcemia based upon endogenous production of $1,25(OH)_2D$ (Marx *et al.*, 1978; Brooks *et al.*, 1978, 1980; Zerwekh *et al.*, 1979; Tsuchiya *et al.*, 1980).

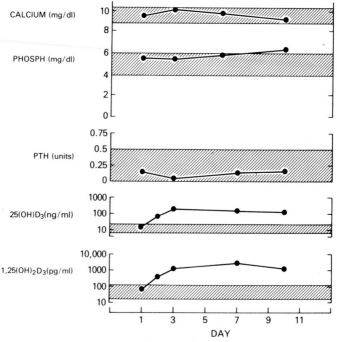

FIG. 10.   Abnormal regulation of $1,25(OH)_2D$ level in serum. Effects of $25(OH)D_3$ orally during recovery phase in patient 5 (Balsan *et al.*, 1983). Therapy with $1\alpha(OH)D_3$ 5 μg/day was stopped 2 days before day zero (June 30, 1979, see Fig. 8). Stippled zones indicate normal ranges. Note logarithmic scales for calciferol metabolites.

X. Calciferol Metabolism *in Vivo*: 25(OH)D-24-Hydroxylase

Serum levels of 24,25(OH)$_2$D are thought to be regulated less tightly than those of 1,25(OH)$_2$D, and there has been no clear relation between the serum level of 24,25(OH)$_2$D and PTH (reflected by status of serum calcium), 25(OH)D, or 1,25(OH)$_2$D in patients with hereditary calcium deficiency resistant to 1,25(OH)$_2$D (Table III). Most of these patients have had serum levels of 24,25(OH)$_2$D at the lower range of normal, including during periods with high levels of 25(OH)D due to therapy with D$_2$ or 25(OH)D$_3$. Though 1,25(OH)$_2$D is a potent inducer of 24-hydroxylase *in vitro*, even extremely high serum levels of 1,25(OH)$_2$D in these patients do not cause high levels of 24,25(OH)$_2$D.

There are several possible explanations for the paucity of high serum levels of 24,25(OH)$_2$D among these patients. Accelerated clearance of 24,25(OH)$_2$D seems unlikely: the principal excretory route is the biliary tree (Kumar *et al.*, 1982) and there is no evidence of hepatobiliary dysfunction in this group. Decreased synthesis seems more likely. Decreased synthesis could reflect deficiency of the enzyme or abnormal regulation of the enzyme. In patient 3, described above, a primary deficiency of 24-

TABLE III

Serum Levels of 24,25(OH)$_2$D and Several Determinants of Those Levels[a]

Case	Therapy	Calcium	25(OH)D (ng/ml)	24,25(OH)$_2$D (ng/ml)	1,25(OH)$_2$D (pg/ml)	References
				Concentration in serum		
1A	0	Low	21	1	213	Marx *et al.* (1978)
1B	0	Low	26	2.5	280	Marx *et al.* (1978)
3	0	Low	21	<0.4	710	Liberman *et al.* (1980)
4	1α(OH)D$_3$	Low	19	1	100	Balsan *et al.* (1983)
4	25(OH)D$_3$	Low	550	4.0	2730	Balsan *et al.* (1983)
5	1α(OH)D$_3$	Low	12	1.7	330	Balsan *et al.* (1983)
5	25(OH)D$_3$	Low	790	1.8	13000	Balsan *et al.* (1983)
6	D$_2$	Low	130	1.0	916	Beer *et al.* (1981)
1B	1,25(OH)$_2$D$_3$	NL	26	0.8	220	Marx *et al.* (1978)
1B	D$_2$	NL	130	3.6	640	Marx *et al.* (1978)
5	1α(OH)D$_3$	NL	7	5.0	430	Marx *et al.* (1978)
5	25(OH)D$_3$	NL	175	4.0	1400	Balsan *et al.* (1983)

[a] Normal ranges: 25(OH)D (10–50 ng/ml), 24,25(OH)$_2$D (0.8–3 ng/ml), and 1,25(OH)$_2$D (20–110 pg/ml age 0–15, 23–62 pg/ml age 15+). Only patients 1A and 1B were older than 15 years at times of these analyses. These data are derived from several laboratories, and normal ranges vary slightly from the above in some cases.

hydroxylase seems possible as administration of 24,25(OH)$_2$D seemed to ameliorate some of the other clinical features. For most other cases, defective induction of 24-hydroxylase by 1,25(OH)$_2$D seems more likely (see Section XIV).

XI. Interactions with Calciferols *in Vitro:* Cell Culture and Analysis of 1,25(OH)$_2$D Binding with Soluble Extract of Skin Fibroblasts

While features of these patients *in vivo* point strongly to deficiencies in target actions of 1,25(OH)$_2$D, the classical target tissues are not readily accessible for analysis. Three laboratories, working independently, first reported the presence of components of the 1,25(OH)$_2$D effector system in skin (Simpson and DeLuca, 1980; Colston *et al.*, 1980; Eil and Marx, 1981). Our approach is outlined briefly below (Eil *et al.*, 1980; Eil and Marx, 1981; Liberman *et al.*, 1983a). We obtain a 4-mm punch biopsy of the skin (from the forearm, thigh, or mons pubis). The biopsy specimen is finely minced and then incubated in a medium containing collagenase. After 24 hours the collagenase is removed, and cells are grown as monolayers. Confluent cells are harvested with 0.05% trypsin–0.02% EDTA and transferred to progressively larger flasks. Sufficient cells for analyses are generally obtained after 6–8 weeks, and analyses are done during passages 4–20. For 48 hours prior to any analyses, cells are incubated in serum-free medium to elimate calciferol metabolites and calciferol binders derived from serum-containing culture media.

For analysis of [^{3}H]1,25(OH)$_2$D$_3$ binding with soluble extracts all subsequent procedures are performed at 0–4°C. Dispersed cells are sonicated in a buffer containing 300 mM KCl, 10 mM sodium molybdate, and 1 mM dithiothreitol. The supernate after centrifugation at 100,000 g for 60 minutes is termed soluble extract (the conventional term is cytosol but the high ionic strength buffer used in this procedure probably solubilizes components from all cell compartments). The soluble extract is then incubated for 15 hours with varying concentrations of [^{3}H]1,25(OH)$_2$D$_3$ with or without excess 1,25(OH)$_2$D$_3$; bound and unbound radioligand are separated with hydroxylapatite. Data are analyzed by the method of Scatchard (Scatchard 1949).

Analysis of [^{3}H]1,25(OH)$_2$D$_3$ binding with soluble extracts from skin fibroblasts cultured from members of six kindreds with hereditary calcium deficiency resistant to 1,25(OH)$_2$D showed normal binding in three and abnormal binding in three (Table IV) (Liberman *et al.*, 1983a). For two kindreds, no hormone binding was measurable while one showed binding that was normal in affinity but 90 percent deficient in capacity (Fig. 11). For the four kindreds, whose cultured cells showed measurable hormone

TABLE IV

Interactions with 1,25(OH)$_2$D in Vitro and in Vivo for Six Kindreds with Calcium Deficiency Resistant to 1,25(OH)$_2$D[a]

	1,25(OH)$_2$D interaction[b] in cultured skin fibroblasts		Remission of hypocalcemia with high doses of calciferol analogs
Case(s)	Soluble extract binding	Nuclear uptake	
3	Normal	Normal	No[c]
1A, 1B	Normal	UM[d]	Yes
2A, 2B	Normal	UM	Yes
4	10% capacity	10% capacity	No
5	UM	UM	Yes, transient
6	UM	UM	No

[a] Marx *et al.* (1978), Rosen *et al.* (1979), Liberman *et al.* (1980, 1983a), Eil *et al.* (1981), Beer *et al.* (1981), Balsan *et al.* (1983).

[b] Values with fibroblasts cultured from normal skin are as follows: capacity of binding in soluble extract, 8900 sites per cell; affinity of binding in soluble extract, 0.13 nM; capacity of nuclear uptake, 10,300 sites per cell; affinity of nuclear uptake, 0.5 nM.

[c] This patient showed no response to high doses of D$_2$, 1a(OH)D$_3$, or 1,25(OH)$_2$D, but showed amelioration of resistance to 1,25(OH)$_2$D during and following a trial with "physiologic" doses of 24,25(OH)$_2$D (see Section VIII and Fig. 7).

[d] UM, Unmeasurable.

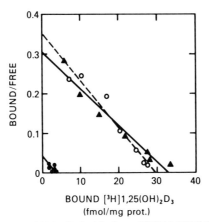

FIG. 11.   Scatchard plot of high affinity binding of [^{3}H]1,25(OH)$_2$D$_3$ with soluble extracts of cultured skin fibroblasts. (○), Dashed line, normal. (▲), Solid line, patient 3. (●), Solid line, patient 4. (From Liberman *et al.*, 1983a.)

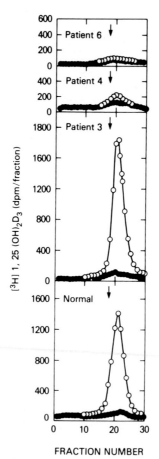

FIG. 12. Sedimentation of radioligand in sucrose density gradients after incubation with soluble extract from cultured skin fibroblasts. Arrow marks position of [^{14}C]ovalbumin (3.7 S). Solid symbols represent binding obtained during coincubation with excess 1,25(OH)$_2$D$_3$. (From Liberman *et al.*, 1983a.)

binding with soluble extract, analysis of the bound radioligand by sedimentation in sucrose density gradients containing 300 mM KCl, showed a sedimentation velocity of approximately 3.7 S identical to that for the "receptor" from normal fibroblasts (Fig. 12).

XII. Interactions with Calciferols *in Vitro:* Nuclear Uptake of 1,25(OH)$_2$D

To study receptor-mediated nuclear uptake of hormone, cells are cultured and dispersed as above, and then incubated intact with varying

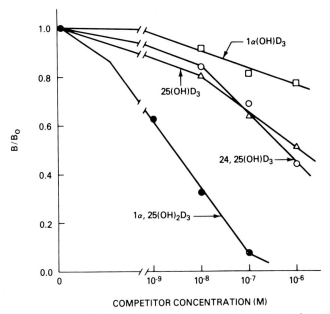

COMPETITOR CONCENTRATION (M)

FIG. 13. Hormonal specificity of competition for nuclear uptake of [³H]1,25(OH)₂D₃. The competitors are (●) 1,25(OH)₂D₃, (△) 25(OH)₂D₃, (○) 24,25(OH)₂D₃, and (□) 1α(OH)D₃. (From Eil and Marx, 1981.)

concentrations of [³H]1,25(OH)₂D₃ with or without excess 1,25(OH)₂D₃ for 45 minutes at 37°C. They are then centrifuged, lysed with an isotonic buffer containing Triton X-100, and nuclei and collected by centrifugation.

Nuclear uptake of hormone showed features of receptor mediation; it showed high affinity, low capacity, and hormonal specificity (Fig. 13) (Eil and Marx, 1981). Cells from the three kindreds with deficient binding of hormone in soluble extract exhibited parallel deficiencies in nuclear uptake (Liberman *et al.*, 1983a; Balsan *et al.*, 1983). However, among the three kindreds with apparently normal binding in soluble extract, two showed no measurable nuclear uptake (Table IV). Sucrose density gradient analysis was also performed with bound radioligand from nuclei of cells with detectable nuclear uptake, and the sedimentation position of ³H on the gradient was normal in both cases. The evaluations of cultured skin fibroblasts with radioligand have shown four patterns: (1) normal binding with soluble extracts and normal nuclear uptake in dispersed cells ("receptor normal" defect), (2) hormone binding with soluble extract that is normal in capacity, affinity, and sedimentation velocity but that is undetectable in nuclei from intact cells ("cytosol-to-nucleus translocation" defect), (3) normal affinity and sedimentation velocity of hormone with soluble extract and nuclei but only 10% of normal maximal capacity with both ("receptor capacity" defect), and (4) unmeasurable binding of hormone to soluble extract or to nuclei of intact cells ("receptor negative" defect).

XIII. Interactions with Calciferols *in Vitro:* Cells from Bone

The demonstration of striking abnormalities in cultured fibroblasts from members of five of the six kindreds suggests that the fibroblasts are a valid index of the genes controlling the actions of $1,25(OH)_2D$ in target tissues. An independent assessment was made by culturing cells from bone of patient 2B at the time of elective tibial osteotomy for rachitic deformity (Liberman *et al.*, 1983b). Cells were derived from cleaned bone explants. They grew with a fibroblastic morphology but showed greater levels of alkaline phosphatase than shown by fibroblasts from skin; this suggested that the cultures were derived, at least in part, from osteoblasts. As with the cells cultured from her skin, the cells cultured from bone of patient 2B showed normal binding in soluble extract but no measurable nuclear uptake of hormone in intact cells.

XIV. Interactions with Calciferols *in Vitro:* Bioeffects on Cultured Skin Fibroblasts

$1,25(OH)_2D$ may not have important actions in skin fibroblasts *in vivo*. However, bioeffects of $1,25(OH)_2D$ *in vitro* may prove to be useful correlates with bioeffects of $1,25(OH)_2D$ *in vivo*. Two bioeffects of $1,25(OH)_2D_3$ have been reported with cultured skin fibroblasts, stimulation of 24-hydroxylase (Chandler, 1984; Griffin *et al.*, 1983; Feldman *et al.*, 1982; Gamblin *et al.*, 1983), and inhibition of proliferation (Clemens *et al.*, 1983). For both bioeffects, the apparent affinity (measured by concentration for half maximal response) and the specificity have been suggestive of mediation by the receptor for $1,25(OH)_2D$. Furthermore, fibroblasts from affected members of seven kindreds with hereditary resistance to $1,25(OH)_2D$ all showed defective or absent bioeffect of $1,25(OH)_2D_3$ *in vitro*. Preliminary analyses (Gamblin *et al.*, 1983) suggest that, in patients with calcemic response to calciferols in *in vivo*, $1,25(OH)_2D$ can induce 24-hydroxylase *in vitro* [though the 24-hydroxylase response shows resistance to $1,25(OH)_2D$], and $1,25(OH)_2D$ shows no induction of 24-hydroxylase in cells of patients lacking calcemic response to calciferols *in vivo*. Furthermore, among patients with detectible induction of 24-hydroxylase, the $1,25(OH)_2D$ dose for half maximal induction may be a valid index of sensitivity to $1,25(OH)_2D$ *in vivo*.

XV. Comparisons of 1,25(OH)$_2$D Interactions *in Vivo* and *in Vitro*

The principal data obtained *in vivo* and *in vitro* show marked heterogeneity of the disorder in six kindreds we have studied (Table IV). Since each kindred appears unique, we shall consider each briefly.

In kindred 3, 1,25(OH)$_2$D interactions with soluble extract of cells and nucleus of intact cells appeared normal yet there was no calcemic response to high doses of D$_2$ or 1-hydroxy analogs of calciferol *in vivo*. There are several possible explanations. First there may be a defect in 1,25(OH)$_2$D interaction distal to nuclear uptake. In one other case with much milder resistance to 1,25(OH)$_2$D (bone disease was mild, normocalcemia occurred without calciferol therapy, and there was no alopecia) a "postreceptor" defect was suggested by the combination of normal nuclear uptake but defective induction of 24-hydroxylase *in vitro* (Griffin *et al.*, 1983). Alternatively, the cultured fibroblasts from patient 3 may not express the defect present *in vivo* in target tissues.

In kindred 1, receptor binding was normal with soluble extract from cultured skin fibroblasts, but nuclear translocation of hormone was not measurable *in vitro*. However, an adequate calcemic response occurred with high doses of 1,25(OH)$_2$D$_3$. It seems unlikely that a calcemic response to 1,25(OH)$_2$D$_3$ would occur without nuclear translocation of hormone in target cells *in vivo*.

In kindred 2, principal biochemical features were similar to those in kindred 1: however, both affected members of kindred 1 show normal hair while both affected members of kindred 2 have total alopecia (Fig. 3). We have recently observed *in vitro* that 1,25(OH)$_2$D$_3$ can induce 24-hydroxylase in cells from patients 1A and 2B, but the apparent affinity of the 24-hydroxylase system for 1,25(OH)$_2$D is decreased (Gamblin *et al.*, 1983). It is not technically feasible to analyze nuclear uptake of [^{3}H]1,25(OH)$_2$D$_3$ with medium concentrations of hormone increased above the usual method. We believe that the cellular defects in these two kindreds are similar in location but different in severity.

In cells from kindred 4, affinity of binding to soluble extract and nuclear uptake are normal, but the capacity of both processes was only 10% of normal. Of particular note, the tested patient showed no calcemic response to prolonged therapy with high doses of calciferols (Fig. 6). It is also noteworthy that this patient never exhibited severe hypocalcemia. We suggest that her calcemic response to 1,25(OH)$_2$D$_3$ follows a relation similar to that for 1,25(OH)$_2$D interaction with soluble extract or nucleus *in vitro* and as illustrated in Fig. 2D. Prior to therapy, high endogenous levels of 1,25(OH)$_2$D would result in expression of a maximal level of 1,25(OH)$_2$D-related calcium transport by intestinal cells. This explanation is consistent with studies *in vitro* showing a linear relation between occupancy of the receptor for 1,25(OH)$_2$D and bioresponse as measured by levels of vitamin D-dependent calcium binding protein in intestine or levels of collagen in osteosarcoma cells.

In cells from kindred 5 no saturable interaction with 1,25(OH)$_2$D was measurable. However, a transient calcemic response during administration of calciferol analogs was documented. Explanations analogous to those suggested for bioresponse in kindreds 1 and 2 seem plausible. Preliminary studies with cells from three kindreds without measurable 1,25(OH)$_2$D$_3$ interactions *in vitro* have shown normal or near-normal concentrations of receptor for 1,25(OH)$_2$D (cross-reacting material), when assessed with a monoclonal antibody to the receptor (Pike *et al.*, 1984). Thus absence of measurable receptors with a hormone-binding technique need not imply total absence of receptor protein in vitro or of capacity to show a bioresponse *in vivo*. The transient nature of the calcemic response in patient 5 remains unexplained. Perhaps, like in the intestine of the neonatal rat (Halloran and DeLuca, 1981), receptor levels in the target tissues undergo temporal variation that has exaggerated consequences in a defective effector system.

In cells from kindred 6 no interaction with 1,25(OH)$_2$D has been measurable *in vitro* or *in vivo*. For affected patients from kindreds such as this one, the only effective therapy may be oral calcium at high dosages. While high doses of calcium orally are inconvenient, they offer the potential to move calcium into plasma by passive absorption in sufficient amounts to ameliorate secondary hyperparathyroidism and PTH-induced renal wasting of phosphorus (Marx, 1983).

XVI. Synthesis

Evaluations of patients with hereditary calcium deficiency resistant to 1,25(OH)$_2$D have revealed an unanticipated degree of heterogeneity. Many features can be explained from our current understanding of the 1,25(OH)$_2$D effector system. In some kindreds with hereditary resistance to 1,25(OH)$_2$D the receptor abnormality allows a calcemic response to certain calciferol analogs, while in others such responses have not been possible (when patients receive supplementation with modest doses of calcium orally). The relations between serum calcium and levels of 1,25(OH)$_2$D (as oral dosage level or as serum level) can shift either because of primary changes in calcium fluxes or because of other changes that may involve directly the target cells for 1,25(OH)$_2$D. In patients with hereditary calcium deficiency resistant to 1,25(OH)$_2$D serum levels of 1,25(OH)$_2$D are often extraordinarily high while levels of 24,25(OH)$_2$D are often low; the abnormal levels of both metabolites usually reflect defective function of the receptor for 1,25(OH)$_2$D (in tissues where it is coupled to the calciferol hydroxylase systems). In some cases high activity of 1-hydroxylase can support remission of hypocalcemia during therapy with 25(OH)D or its precursors. Alopecia is frequently associated with hereditary calcium deficiency resistant to 1,25(OH)$_2$D; this association is strong evidence that 1,25(OH)$_2$D has important actions in man beyond its traditionally recognized target tissues.

The studies of interactions with 1,25(OH)$_2$D *in vitro* have provided explanations for much of the heterogeneity *in vivo*. In the near future, it may be possible to use assays *in vitro* to plan clinical therapy for these patients. In particular, it may be possible to predict which patients would show limited or absent capacity to respond to 1,25(OH)$_2$D *in vivo*. Such patients could be spared the physical discomfort and expense of long therapeutic trials. Further studies of cells expressing mutations in the effector system for 1,25(OH)$_2$D should clarify important steps in the mechanism of action of secosteroid and steroid hormones.

REFERENCES

Abe, E., Miyaura, C., Sakagami, H., Takeda, M., Konno, K., Yamazaki, T., Yoshikawa, S., and Suda, T. (1981). *Proc. Natl. Acad. Sci. U.S.A.* **78,** 4990–4994.

Adams, J. S., Wahl, T. O., Moore, W. V., Horton, W. A., and Lukert, B. P. (1979). *Annu. Meet. Endocrine Soc., 61st,* 767 (Abstr.).

Albright, F., Butler, A. M., Bloomberg, E. (1937). *Am. J. Dis. Child.* **54,** 531–547.

Arnaud, C., Maijer, R., Reade, T., Scriver, C. R., and Whelan, D. T. (1970). *Pediatrics* **46,** 871–879.

Balsan, S., Garabedian, M., Liberman, U. A., Eil, C., Bourdeau, A., Guillozo, H., Grimberg, R., Le Deunff, M. J., Lieberherr, M., Guimbaud, P., Broyer, M., and Marx, S. J. (1983). *J. Clin. Endocrinol. Metab.* **57,** 803–811.

Beer, S., Tieder, M., Kohelet, D., Liberman, U. A., Vure, E., Bar-Joseph, G., Gabizon, D., Borochowitz, V., Varon, M., and Modai, D. (1981). *Clin. Endocrinol.* **14,** 395–402.

Brooks, M. H., Bell, N. H., Love, L., Stern, P. H., Orfei, E., Queener, S. F., Hamstra, A. J., and DeLuca, H. F. (1978). *N. Engl. J. Med.* **298,** 996–999.

Brooks, M. H., Stern, P. H., and Bell, N. H. (1980). *N. Engl. J. Med.* **302,** 810.

Chandler, J. S., Chandler, S. K., Pike, J. W., and Haussler, M. R. (1984). *J. Biol. Chem.* **259,** 2214–2222.

Chesney, R. W., Hamstra, A. J., and DeLuca, H. F. (1981). *Am. J. Dis. Child.* **135,** 34–37.

Christakos, S., Friedlander, E. J., Frandsen, B. R., and Norman, A. W. (1979). *Endocrinology* **104,** 1495–1503.

Clemens, T. L., Adams, J. S., Horiuchi, N., Gilchrest, B. A., Cho, H., Tsuchiya, Y., Matsuo, N., Suda, T., and Holick, M. F. (1983). *J. Clin. Endocrinol. Metab.* **56,** 824–830.

Colston, K., and Feldman, D. (1982). *J. Biol. Chem.* **257,** 2504–2508.

Colston, K., Hirst, M., and Feldman, D. (1980). *Endocrinology* **107,** 1916–1922.

Eil, C., and Marx, S. J. (1981). *Proc. Natl. Acad. Sci. U.S.A.* **78,** 2562–2566.

Eil, C., Lippman, M. E., and Loriaux, D. L. (1980). *Steroids* **34**, 389–404.

Eil, C., Liberman, U. A., Rosen, J. F., and Marx, S. J. (1981). *N. Engl. J. Med.* **304**, 1588–1591.

Esvelt, R. P., DeLuca, H. F., Wichman, J. K., Yoshizawa, S., Zurcher, J., Sar, M., and Stumpf, W. E. (1980). *Biochemistry* **19**, 6158–6161.

Feher, J. J. (1983). *Am. J. Physiol.* **244** C303.

Feldman, D., Chen, T., Hirst, M., Colston, K., Karasek, K., and Cone, C. (1980). *J. Clin. Endocrinol. Metab.* **51**, 1463–1465.

Feldman, D., Chen, T., Cone, C., Hirst, M., Shani, S., Benderli, A., and Hochberg, Z. (1982). *J. Clin. Endocrinol.* **55**, 1020–1022.

Fraser, D., Kooh, S. W., Kind, H. P., Holick, M. F., Tanaka, Y., and DeLuca, H. F. (1973). *N. Engl. J. Med.* **289**, 817–822.

Fujita, T., Nomura, M., Okajima, S., and Furuya, H. (1980). *J. Clin. Endocrinol. Metab.* **50**, 927–931.

Gamblin, G. T., Liberman, U. A., DeGrange, D. A., Downs, R. W., Jr., Eil, C., and Marx, S. J. (1983). *Clin. Res.* **31**, 693A.

Garabedian, M., Vainsel, M., Mallet, E., Guillozo, H., Toppet, M., Grimberg, R., NGuyen, T. M., and Balsam, S. (1983). *J. Pediatr.* **103**, 381–386.

Griffin, J. E., and Zerwekh, J. E. (1983). *J. Clin. Invest.* **72**, 1190–1199.

Halloran, B. P., and DeLuca, H. F. (1980). *Am. J. Physiol.* **239**, G473.

Halloran, B. P., and DeLuca, H. F. (1981). *J. Biol. Chem.* **256**, 7338–7342.

Hunziker, W., Siebert, P. D., King, M. W., Stucki, P., Dugaiczyk, A., and Norman, A. W. (1983). *Proc. Natl. Acad. Sci. U.S.A.* **80**, 4228–4232.

Kahn, C. R. (1978). *Metabolism* **27** (Suppl. 2), 1893–1902.

Kudoh, T., Kumagai, T., Uetsuji, N., Tsugawa, S., Oyanagi, K., Chiba, Y., Minami, R., and Nakao, T. (1981). *Eur. J. Pediatr.* **137**, 307–311.

Kumar, R., Wiesner, R., Scott, M., and Go, V. L. W. (1982). *Am. J. Physiol.* **243**, E370–E374.

Liberman, U. A., Samuel, R., Halabe, A., Kauli, R., Edelstein, S., Weisman, Y., Papapoulos, S. E., Clemens, T. L., Fraher, L. J., and O'Riordan, J. L. H. (1980). *Lancet* **1**, 504–507.

Liberman, U. A., Eil, C., and Marx, S. J. (1983a). *J. Clin. Invest.* **71**, 192–200.

Liberman, U. A., Eil, C., Holst, P., Rosen, J. F., and Marx, S. J. (1983b). *J. Clin. Endocrinol. Metab.* **57**, 958–961.

Marx, S. J. (1983a). *In* "Current Therapy" (H. F. Conn, ed.), pp. 451–456. Saunders, Philadelphia, Pennsylvania.

Marx, S. J. (1984). *In* "Vitamin D Metabolism: Basic and Clinical Aspects" (R. Kumar, ed.), pp. 721–746. Nijhof, The Hague.

Marx, S. J., Spiegel, A. M., Brown, E. M., Gardner, D. G., Downs, R. W., Jr., Attie, M., Hamstra, A. J., and DeLuca, H. F. (1978). *J. Clin. Endocrinol. Metab.* **47**, 1303–1310.

Marx, S. J., Swart, E. G., Jr., Hamstra, A. J., and DeLuca, H. F. (1980). *J. Clin. Endocrinol. Metab.* **51**, 1138–1142.

Marx, S. J., Liberman, U. A., and Eil, C. (1983). *Vitam. Horm.* **40**, 235–238.

Neufeld, M., Maclaren, N. K., and Blizzard, R. M. (1981). *Medicine* **60**, 335–362.

Norman, A. W., Roth, J., and Orci, L. (1982). *Endocrine Rev.* **3**, 331.

Omdahl, J. L., Hunsaker, L. A., Evan, A. P., and Torrez, P. (1980). *J. Biol. Chem.* **255**, 7460–7466.

Papapoulos, S. E., Clemens, T. J., Fraher, L. J., Gleed, J., and O'Riorday, J. L. H. (1980). *Lancet* **3**, 612–615.

Pettifor, J. M., Ross, F. P., Travers, R., Glorieux, F. H., and DeLuca, H. F. (1981). *Metab. Bone Dis. Relat. Res.* **2**, 301–305.

Pike, J. W., Gooze, L. L., and Haussler, M. R. (1980). *Life Sci.* **26**, 407–414.

Pike, J. W., Dokoh, S., Haussler, M. R., Liberman, U. A., Marx, S. J., and Eil, C. (1984). *Science,* in press.

Prader, V. A., Illig, R., Heidi, E. (1961). *Helv. Paed. Acta* **5/6**, 452–468.

Price, P. A., and Baukol, S. A. (1980). *J. Biol. Chem.* **255**, 11660–11663.

Provvedini, D. M., Tsoukas, C. D., Deftos, L. J., and Manolagas, S. C. (1983). *Science* **221**, 1181–1183.

Rinaldi, M. L., Haiech, J., Pavlovich, J., Rizk, M., Ferraz, C., Derancourt, J., and Demaille, J. G. (1982). *Biochemistry* **21**, 4805–4810.

Rosen, J. F., Fleischman, A. R., Finberg, L., Hamstra, A., and DeLuca, H. F. (1979). *J. Pediatr.* **94**, 729–735.

Rowe, D. W., and Kream, B. E. (1982). *J. Biol. Chem.* **257**, 8009–8015.

Saurat, J. H., Didierjean, L., Pavlovitch, J. H., Laouri, D., and Balsan, S. (1981). *J. Invest. Dermatol,* **76**, 221–230.

Scatchard, G. (1949). *Ann. N.Y. Acad. Sci.* **51**, 660–672.

Scriver, C. R., Reade, T. M., DeLuca, H. F., and Hamstra, A. J. (1978). *N. Engl. J. Med.* **299**, 976–979.

Scriver, C. R., Fraser, D., and Kooh, S. W. (1942). *In* "Calcium Disorders" (D. A. Heath and S. J. Marx, eds.); pp. 1–46. Butterworths, London.

Shinki, T., Shiina, Y., Takahashi, N., Tanioka, Y., Koizumi, H., and Suda, T. (1983). *Biochem. Biophys. Res. Commun.* **114**, 452–457.

Simpson, R. U., and DeLuca, H. F. (1980). *Proc. Natl. Acad. Sci. U.S.A.* **77**, 5822–5826.

Sockalosky, J. J., Ulstrom, R. A., DeLuca, H. F., and Brown, D. M. (1980). *J. Pediatr.* **96**, 701–703.

Stanbury, S. W., Taylor, C. M., Lumb, G. A., Mawer, E. B., Berry, J., Hann, J., and Wallace, J. (1981). *Min. Electrolyte Metab.* **5**, 212–227.

Steichen, J. J., Tsang, R. C., Greer, F. R., Ho, M., and Hug, G. (1981). *J. Pediatr.* **99**, 293–297.

Stumpf, W. E., Sar, M., and DeLuca, H. F. (1981). *In* "Hormonal Control of Calcium Metabolism" (D. V. Cohn, R. V. Talmage, and J. L. Matthews, eds.), pp. 222–229. Excerpta Medica, Amsterdam.

Thomasset, M., Desplan, C., and Parkes, O. (1982). *In* "Vitamin D: Chemical, Biochemical and Clinical Endocrinology of Calcium Metabolism" (A. W. Norman, K. Schaefer, D. v. Herrath, and H. G. Grigoleit, eds.), pp. 197–202. de Gruyter, New York.

Trechsel, U., Bonjour, J. P., and Fleisch, H. (1979). *J. Clin. Invest.* **64**, 206–217.

Trechsel, U., Eisman, J. A., Fischer, J. A., Bonjour, J. P., and Fleisch, H. (1980). *Am. J. Physiol.* **239**, E119–E124.

Tsuchiya, Y., Matsuo, N., Cho, H., Kumagai, M., Yasaka, T., Suda, T., Orimo, H., and Shimaki, M. (1980). *J. Clin. Endocrinol. Metab.* **51**, 685–690.

van Creveld, S., and Arons, P. (1949). *Ann. Paediatr.* **173**, 299–313.

van Creveld, S., and Arons, P. (1954). *Ann. Paeditr.* **182**, 191–202.

Wark, J. D., and Tashjian, A. H. (1977). *Endocrinology* **111**, 1755–1757.

Yoshikawa, S., Nakamura, T., and Nishii, Y. (1982). *In* "Vitamin D, Biochemical and Clinical Endocrinology of Calcium Metabolism" (A. W. Norman, K. Schaefer, D. v. Herrath, and H. G. Grigoleit, eds.), pp. 1001–1003. de Gruyter, New York.

Zerwekh, J. E., Glass, K., Jowsey, J., and Pak, C. Y. C. (1979). *J. Clin. Endocrinol. Metab.* **49**, 171–175.

DISCUSSION

G. Slaughter: Do you think that these patients have genes that have hot spots in them, that is, areas where you get a very high rate of independent mutation. Therefore, they tend to mutate differently so that within even one family the disease is expressed by different characteristics?

U. A. Liberman: I don't know, it might be. I may add two features: (1) almost all of these patients originate from one geographical region, and (2) there is a high frequency of parental consanguinity.

J. H. Oppenheimer: There appears to be a very interesting analogy between the problem of vitamin D resistance and the problem T3 resistance inasmuch as some patients in both categories have an absence of nuclear sites whereas others do not. Have you considered the possibility of determining whether or not the fibroblasts can respond to vitamin D by looking at the mRNA activity profiles? Dr. Tophss in our laboratory has successfully demonstrated that the responsiveness of hepatocyte mDNA preparations to T3 can be demonstrated in such a fashion. If any one of 200–300 mRNAs would respond you could infer vitamin D responsivity.

U. A. Liberman: It is obvious that this is one of the techniques to be used in the near future. The problem that we face is the limited number of fibroblasts and the limited life span of these cells. Therefore, one must choose what experiments to perform in order of preference.

J. H. Oppenheimer: With the use of total RNA to program the reticulocyte lysate translational system, we were able to use exceedingly small quantities of RNA. Have you excluded an extra nuclear pathway?

C. Eil: I would like to make a comment in that regard that might help clarify the situation. The time course of induction is consistent with mRNA synthesis, namely about 15 hours, and, second, the process is inhibitable by cyclohexamide.

U. A. Liberman: Dr. John Chandler showed in other cell systems that the induction of the enzyme 25-hydroxyvitamin D 24-hydroxylase by $1,25\text{-}(OH)_2D_3$ is mediated through its specific receptor and that transcriptional and translational processes are involved. The earliest time that we could detect induction of the enzyme in our system was 4 hours.

P. Wynn: With reference to the alopecia patients, have you studied the morphology of hair follicles in skin biopsies derived from these patients? Is the number of follicles reduced, do they resemble primordial follicles morphologically, or do they have an intent inner and outer root sheath and dermal papilla?

U. A. Liberman: Very few skin biopsies, about three or four, have been evaluated from these patients. As I recall, the histology showed marked reduction in the number of follicles and atrophic changes.

P. Wynn: I did notice that there were some hairs on one of the patients that you showed.

U. A. Liberman: This is a typical feature. These patients have some hair when born and lose most of it usually during the first year of life.

P. Wynn: One further question. Have you been able to detect the presence of vitamin D receptors on cells from these hair follicles?

U. A. Liberman: Dr. Marx mentioned the work of Stumpf et al. that demonstrated by autoradiographic techniques specific upttake of 1,25-dihydroxyvitamin D around the hair follicles. The group of Dr. Feldman demonstrated the existence of receptors in cultured keratinocytes, and Laouari et al. found a calcium-binding protein that is possibly vitamin D-dependent in rat skin.

J. Geller: There seem to be three patients who all had absent nuclear receptor who became normocalcemic on calciferol therapy. I think you mentioned that all three of these patients showed 24-hydroxylase responses to high doses of calciferol. I was wondering therefore if you would draw a general conclusion from this experimental data that judging sensitivity of target organs to hormone is probably better done by measurement of either the messenger RNA or translational products rather than receptor which seems sometimes to give wrong information.

U. A. Liberman: The three patients with a calcemic response to 1,25-dihydroxyvitamin D *in vivo* and no nuclear uptake of the hormone into their cultured fibroblasts *in vitro* can be divided into two groups. In one patient, we could not demonstrate a specific receptor in soluble extract. One can speculate that we are dealing with a decrease in affinity that could not be demonstrated in the *in vitro* system due to technical limitations in achieving high enough concentrations of 1,25-dihydroxyvitamin D. In the two other patients, absent nuclear uptake of the hormone was associated with a normal receptor in the soluble extract fraction prepared from the same cultured fibroblasts. However, one has to remember that the whole cell nuclear uptake of 1,25-dihydroxyvitamin D is carried at 37°C for 45 minutes, while equilibrium binding of the hormone with the cytosol is performed at 0–7°C for 15 hours. Thus, we have a combination of a normal extracted receptor for 1,25(OH)₂D with an absent nuclear uptake, an induction of the 25-hydroxyvitamin D 25-hydroxylase enzyme *in vitro*, and a calcemic response *in vivo*. We believe that the hormone gets into the nuclei of these cells and our inability to demonstrate nuclear uptake *in vitro* may point toward the possible molecular defect in the target cells of these patients with end organ resistance to 1,25(OH)₂D. I fully agree that the sensitivity of target organs to a hormone is best measured by the physiological effects on a translational product that will mark the distal effect of the hormone; however, as I tried to point out, the receptor studies give us additional and different information on more proximal events and may help in elucidating the possible pathogenic mechanism.

G. W. Moll, Jr.: In trying to recall rare forms of dwarfism, I am struck by some similarities in the pictures of your patients and those of chondroectodermal dysplasia patients which appear in a few texts. Is it possible that some chondroectodermal dysplasias form part of the spectrum of your variable vitamin D resistance disorder?

U. A. Liberman: It is difficult to answer, but I would assume that if vitamin D resistance occurs in epidermal dysplasia, you would expect these patients to show clinical features of rickets or osteomalacia and I am not aware that this is the case. We measured receptors for 1,25-(OH)₂D in cultured skin fibroblasts from a child with total alopacia and primary hypoparathyroidism and they are normal. It seems to be, therefore, that not all alopecias are connected with abnormalities in intracellular receptors for 1,25-(OH)₂D.

S. Marx: We have not yet evaluated the possibility for localized deficiency of receptors for 1,25(OH)₂D in either the ectodermal dysplasias or in the bone and cartilage dysplasias, some of which look superficially like rickets. The evidence to date suggests that all hereditary defects in the effector system for 1,25(OH)₂D are generalized, and in fact the ability to model an intestinal defect by using skin cells is certainly one logical extension of that. However, there is a precedent for tissue-specific regulation of receptors for 1,25(OH)₂D in that the intestine of the fetal rat does not show receptors for 1,25(OH)₂D, and the receptors and vitamin D-dependent calcium transport appear only post-natally in the intestine (Halloran and DeLuca, 1981).

G. W. Moll, Jr.: With regard to your described vitamin D-dependent calcium-binding protein, could its distribution in brain and other areas of the body explain the peculiar distribution of ectopic calcifications noted in psuedohypoparathyroidism and idiopathic hypoparathyroidism?

S. J. Marx: The calcificaion in question is principally in the basal ganglia. The vitamin D-dependent calcium-binding protein has a different distribution.

M. R. Walters: As you know, we are among those who think that the widespread tissue distribution of the $1,25(OH)_2D_3$ receptor indicates that there might be a very fundamental role for $1,25(OH)_2D_3$ and its receptor in cell function, cell differentiation, cell development, etc. One of the major criticisms of that concept has been the question of whether these are clinical aberrations in other physiological systems in your patients or patients who have nutritional vitamin D deficiency. I wonder if you have looked at these patients to see whether other systems are normal. And in conjunction with that, whether you have any information on whether there is an abnormal rate of spontaneous abortion in patients who do try to carry pregnancies.

U. A. Liberman: We would like to believe that $1,25(OH)_2D$ may have some fundamental function in every cell and that the effect of the hormone on net transcellular transport is just an extension of what happens in every cell regardless of its function. In the patients we do not have, however, any evidence for additional abnormalities other than transepithelial calcium transport. In some patients every endocrine axis was measured and was normal; there is no evidence for cardiovascular defects. Two female patients are menstruating normally and two gave birth to a normal child. One adult male has a normal child, so except from the skeletal deformities and alopecia. I cannot recall any other abnormalities.

S. J. Marx: The association of alopecia with the syndrome is, in fact, the first demonstration that vitamin D does have some important physiologic role outside of its classical target tissue. These patients do offer a very interesting model to test the kinds of questions that you are asking. In vitamin D deficiency the pathologic state takes a long, long time to evolve; patients show hypocalcemia and many secondary changes. In patients with hereditary resistance to $1,25(OH)_2D_3$, there is the opportunity for chronic therapy with high doses of $1,25(OH)_2D_3$, completely normal calcium homeostasis, and then abrupt withdrawal of $1,25(OH)_2D_3$. Since this hormone has a very short half time on its receptor, it then becomes possible to analyze the consequences of the specific deficiency in the absence of secondary changes. This kind of testing has not been done yet.

M. R. Walters: I really want to try to understand this because it has been causing some problems for us—is it that you think that the absence perhaps of clinical aberrations in other systems in your patients is because in a large number of them you are giving them effective replacement therapy? That is, that in order to establish whether there are other problems you would then have to withdraw them?

S. J. Marx: Yes, I would agree with that. Most of these patients are very well maintained on vitamin D analogs. Some may be treated with vitamin D or 25-hydroxy vitamin D which allows regulation of endogenous production of $1,25(OH)_2D$. Others may require constant high doses of $1,25(OH)_2D_3$ or $1\alpha(OH)D_3$; with this therapy they cannot regulate their endogenous levels of $1,25(OH)_2D$ but they seem to have adequate mineral homeostasis because they have parathyroid hormone at least as the back-up system for regulation.

M. R. Walters: What about the question of the general fertility of the families of these patients?

U. A. Liberman: I may add that a few of our patients were tested before therapy began and at least in one of them insulin secretion was normal. You may argue, of course, that because the patients maintain such a high level of $1,25(OH)_2D$, it may be enough to keep all other $1,25(OH)_2D$-dependent systems normal while it is not enough for the systems in which net calcium transport occurs.

M. R. Walters: Okay. And the fertility question?

U. A. Liberman: Do you ask about the fertility in the family or of the patients?

M. R. Walters: Both.

U. A. Liberman: In the parents there is no fertility problem. In some of these families there are up to eight children. As far as the patients are concerned, very few already achieved maturity, but, as mentioned before, three have normal children; in one woman there was a need to increase the dose of vitamin D during pregnancy.

B. Little: What do they die of?

U. A. Liberman: They die during infancy mainly because of pulmonary complications from bony deformity of the chest and perhaps from some other effects.

R. Chatterton: I was curious about why you chose to use the T47D mammary tumor cell line to look for vitamin D receptors. Of course calcium is transported across the mammary epithelium and this is an important component of lactation, but do you have evidence that vitamin D is necessary for this process?

U. A. Liberman: We used the T47D cell line as well as the MCF-7. Because of its convenience those cells are proliferating at a very high rate and one can get a lot of cells in a short time. If I recall correctly, there is some recent work showing that $1,25(OH)_2D_3$ affects calcium transport across mamillary ducts. I assume that Dr. Walters will know more about it.

M. R. Walters: As I recall the work started out with the observation of receptors for $1,25(OH)_2D_3$ in a variety of species in normal mammary glands as well as in mammary tumors and the MCF-7 cell line. I believe that there is some evidence now for one or more of the calcium-binding proteins. The problem with calcium-binding protein, of course, is that now there is a family of these proteins and we do not yet know which one to look for in what tissue.

C. Eil: I would like to make an extension of that. The MCF-7 cell line has been shown to have a 24-hydroxylase enzyme which is also inducible by $1,25(OH)_2D_3$.

D. Schulster: I wonder if you can tell me about the relationship between the tissue distribution of vitamin D receptors and PTH receptors? As we have recently shown PTH responsiveness in adrenocortical cells [Refferty *et al.* (1983). *Endocrinology* **113,** in press), might it be worthwhile evaluating vitamin D responsiveness?

S. J. Marx: Basically I think there is very little relation. PTH receptors have been identified in the kidney, in bone, on hepatocytes, and in certain cultured cells such as lymphocytes. $1,25(OH)_2D$ receptors and $1,25(OH)_2D$ effector protein have been found in many, many sites. Basically the receptors are distributed very differently. There is some evidence for reciprocal regulation of responsiveness between these two hormones.

M. R. Walters: I would like to make a comment about that. I think in all fairness to the PTH field that we have been looking very hard among a number of tissues using very sensitive assays for the steroid receptors for $1,25(OH)_2D_3$; and perhaps the PTH receptor has not been looked at in as many tissues quite as extensively.

K. von Werder: What is the placental transfer of the 1,25-dihydroxy-cholecalciferol? If this vitamin D_3 metabolite passes the placenta, would you expect abnormalities in the children who have normal receptor sites when they receive large amounts of $1,25(OH)_2D_3$ from their mothers who are treated with very high dosages?

U. A. Liberman: The placenta itself is a source of $1,25-(OH)_2D$ and $24,25-(OH)_2D$. As Dr. Marx mentioned two women with the disease had a child with no abnormalities in mineral metabolism.

S. J. Marx: We followed one of these patients very carefully because we were terribly worried about this when the woman first became pregnant. We shared Dr. Werder's concern because independent of treatment, she was certain to have very high serum levels of $1,25(OH)_2D$ throughout pregnancy. Basically what happened was she had a normal child

(Marx *et al.*, 1980). We measured 1,25(OH)$_2$D concentration in cord blood; it was very high. Serum calcium levels were normal in mother and umbilical cord. The baby showed mild hypercalcemia for 2 days. Our interpretation was that *in utero* serum calcium, phosphorous, and 1,25(OH)$_2$D were driven by the maternal levels of each, and abnormal 1,25(OH)$_2$D levels *in utero* did not have major consequences. We do not know what the fetal serum levels of 1,25(OH)$_2$D were prior to parturition.

INDEX

A

A23187, Ca mobilization in platelets, 315–320

Adenovirus, 586

Adenylate cyclase, role in action of GRF, 257–261

Adrenocorticotropin, 233

Alopecia, 596

Amino acid analysis, of GRF, 242

Arachidonic acid, 301, 302
  release, 323–329
  role in signal transduction, 328

Arcuate nucleus, CA turnover rates, 492–494, 504–506

B

Blindness, effects on reproductive cycle, 205–207, 226–227

Bovine papilloma virus, 132–133

BPV, see Bovine papilloma virus

Breast cancer cell, human, estrogen-inducible gene in, 28–35

Bromocriptine treatment, 108–110, 117

C

Calciferols, see also 1,25-Dihydroxyvitamin D
  binding to fibroblast extract, 606–607
  in vitro interactions, 606–610
  in vivo interactions, 596–606
    alopecia, 596–598
    temporal variation in individual, 601–603
    variability between kindreds, 598–600
  in vivo metabolism, 603–606
  resistance to, 591–592

Calcium deficiency resistance to 1,25(OH)₂D
  acquired, 592–594
  hereditary, 594–605

Calcium ion, role in action of GRF, 257, 258

Calcium-mediated response system, 302

Calcium mobilization, 311
  protein kinase C activation and, 315–320

Capsite, 7

Cartilage-derived growth factor, 564, 565

β-Casein gene, transcription of, 417–427

CAT activity assay, see Chloramphenicol acetyltransferase activity assay

Catecholamine
  determination of activity in brain, 489–490
  turnover rates, effect of estradiol on, 500–502
    effect of phenobarbital on, 495–497
    effect of progesterone on, 500–502
    gonadotropin and, 490–502
    progesterone negative feedback on, 503–507

Catecholaminergic system, hypothalamic, function of, 507–516

5'-CCPuCCC-3' consensus sequence, 7

CDGF, see Cartilage-derived growth factor

Cerebrospinal fluid, collection from third ventricle, 452

CG, see Chorionic gonadotropin

Chimeric recombinants, 22–23

Chloramphenicol acetyltransferase activity assay, 125
  applications, 125–127

Chlorpromazine, 321, 322, 323, 487

Cholera toxin, 253, 257–258, 260

Chorionic gonadotropin
  mechanism of action, 76–78
  structure, 43–44
  α subunit gene, 45–51
  β subunit gene, 51–55
    evolution of, 66–71, 75–76
    expression of, 64–66
    isolation, 51–55
    multiple copies of, 55–60, 76–77
    nucleotide sequences, 60–64

Chromatin, modification in response to hormone action, 136–138

Circadian rhythmicity, 144
  physiological significance of, 147–149

Circadian system, role in reproductive phenomena, 143–183

Clathrin, 573, 582–583
Clathrin-coated pit, 571–572, 576
Coated pit, *see* Clathrin-coated pit
Coated vesicle, 573–574
Collagen, 302, 309–311, 317
Complementary deoxyribonucleic acid, for TSH subunits, cloning of, 88–91
Conalbumin gene promoter region, 21–28
Corticotropin-releasing factor, 233, 475
CRF, *see* Corticotropin-releasing factor
Cyanogen bromide digestion, of GRF, 242–243, 245
Cyclic adenosine monophosphate, role in action of GRF, 257–261
Cyclic adenosine monophosphate system, 302
Cyclic guanosine monophosphate
  as negative intracellular messenger, 325
  receptor response system and, 323–329, 336–337
Cyclic nucleotide, receptor stimulation and, 323–329, 336–337

D

Dansylcadaverine, 586–587
Delayed anovulatory syndrome, 510–512
Dexamethasone, 125
Diacylglycerol, 303, 305
  calcium mobilization and, 315–320
  protein kinase C activation and, 311–315, 317
  role in signal transduction, 328
Diarachidonin, 306
Dibenamine, 487
Dibucaine, 321, 322, 323
1,25-Dihydroxyvitamin D
  binding to fibroblast extract, 606–608
  biological activities, 590–591
  calcium deficiency resistance to, 592–595
  nuclear uptake, 608–610
  site of action, 590
Dilinolein, 306
Diolein, 305, 306
Dipalmitin, 306
Diphtheria toxin, 578
Distearin, 306
Dopamine
  determination of activity in brain, 489–490

turnover rate, hormonal surges and, 490–502

E

Edman degradation, of GRF, 242
Endocytosis, 569–587
  pathways in, 570
β-Endorphin, 233, *see also* Opioid peptides
  modulation by ovarian steroids, 461–463
  origin and localization, 455–458
  role in menstrual cycle, 463–467, 471–475
  site of action, 467–471
Enhancer elements, 8–21
  entry-site model, 9–10
  open window function, 10–16
  regulation of transcription by, 19–21
Entry-site hypothesis, 9–10
Estradiol
  diurnal patterns in levels of, 144–149
  effect on catecholamine turnover rates, 500–502
  on LH secretion, 190–195, 197–199, 204–206, 210, 211, 447–449, 497–499
  inhibitory feedback control, 447–449
  level of, during proestrus, 491
  modulation of β-endorphin by, 461–463
  pS2 RNA production and, 29–35
Estrogen
  induction of gene in human breast cancer cell, 28–35
  regulation of gene expression, 21–28
Estrogen-sensitive protein, 28–35, 41–42
Estrous cycle, *see also* Menstrual cycle; Ovarian cycle
  circadian timed events of, 149–158
  LH pulse generator and, 190–195
  photoperiodic regulation, 189–201
Exocytosis, pathways in, 570, 584
External coincidence model, 162

F

Fibroblast, cultured, effects of calciferols on, 610
Follicle stimulating hormone
  diurnal patterns in levels of, 144–149
  function, 43
  level of, during proestrus, 491

secretion, effect of opiates on, 458–459
structure, 43–44
α subunit gene, 45–51
Forskolin, 253, 257–258, 261
FSH, *see* Follicle stimulating hormone

G

Gene transfer, for localization of glucocorticoid regulatory element, 125–127, 140
Germ cell, inception, renewal, and proliferation of, 533–536
5'-GGGCGG-3' consensus sequence, 7
5'-GGPyCAA$_A^T$CT-3' consensus sequence, 7
Glucocorticoids, action on mammary gland, 380, 381
Glucocorticoid regulation
    identification of regulatory sequences, 124
    localization of regulatory sequences, 125–127
    mouse mammary tumor virus model of, 121–124
    response assays, 124–125
Glycoprotein hormone, 43, 79–80, *see also* specific hormone
    biosynthetic mechanisms, evolution of, 74–76
    structure, 43–44, 79
    α subunit gene, 45–51
    subunit synthesis, 82–88
Glycosylation, 78
Golgi complex
    role in macromolecular traffic, 575–577
    trans-reticular system, 576
Gonadal steroid, diurnal variations in levels of, 144–149
Gonadotropin, 43, *see also* Luteinizing hormone pulse
    diurnal variations in levels of, 144–149
    pulsatile release, 442–447
    secretion, effects of opiates on, 458–461, 482–483
        effect of phenobarbital on, 495–497
        model for control of, 514–518
        progesterone negative feedback on, 503–507
    SGF activity and, 554–555

Gonadotropin-releasing hormone, *see also* Luteinizing hormone-releasing hormone
    estrous cycle and, 189–195
    modulation of secretion, 451–454, 467–471
    pulsatile release, 441–443
    role in menstrual cycle, 471–475, 480–481
Gonadotropin-releasing hormone neuron, distribution in hypothalamus, 449–451, 482
GRF, *see* Somatocrinin
Growth hormone, 77, 233
Growth hormone releasing factor, *see* Somatocrinin

H

hCG, *see* Chorionic gonadotropin
Hexose transport, insulin and, 362–366
High-pressure liquid chromatography, for analysis of GRFs, 243–245
Hogness–Goldberg box, 6–7
Hormone, polypeptide, mechanism of biosynthesis, evolution of, 74–75
Hormone action
    analysis on minichromosomes, 130–138
    internalization and, 583, 585
Hormone responsive sequence, mapping techniques, 124–125
HSAB, *see* N-Hydroxysuccinimidyl-4-azidobenzoate
Hydrophobic chromatography, 547
N-Hydroxysuccinimidyl-4-azidobenzoate, 400–402
25-Hydroxyvitamin D 1-hydroxylase, 590, 603–604
25-Hydroxyvitamin D 24-hydroxylase, 590, 605–606, 610
Hypothalamus
    catecholamine turnover rates in, 487–529
    GRF-containing cells in, 278–281
    ovarian steroid effects on, 447–449

I

IBMX, *see* 3-Isobutyl-1-methylxanthine
IGF, *see* Insulin-like growth factor
Imipramine, 321

Inositol phospholipid, *see also* Phospholipid
structure, 302
turnover, 301–337
Insulin
effect on insulin-like growth factor receptors, 366–368
hexose transport and, 362–366
mechanism of action, 347–377
regulation of membrane components by, 362–368
Insulin intracellular mediator, similarity to prolactin mediator, 430, 437
Insulin-like growth factor, 354–358, 373–374, 376–377
Insulin-like growth factor receptor, insulin modulation of, 366–368
Insulin receptor complex
biosynthesis, 351
intersubunit disulfides, 349–350
mediating actions of, 368–370
oligosaccharide units, 351
proteolytic nicking of, 349–351
regulation of function of, 358–362
similar receptor structures, 354–358
subunits, 348–349
tyrosine kinase activity of, 351–354
Internal coincidence model, 162
3-Isobutyl-1-methylxanthine, 253, 257, 260
Isoproterenol, 359, 360

L

LH, *see* Luteinizing hormone
LHRH, *see* Luteinizing hormone-releasing hormone
Lipid, neutral, activation of protein kinase C by, 305, 306
Locomotor activity, ovarian cycle and, 151–158
Long terminal repeat
deletion experiments, 125–127
naturally occurring mutations in, 127–130
nucleosomes and, 140
promotor region, regulation of, 133–136
replication of minichromosome carrying, 132–133
LRF, 233, 280, 287
LTR, *see* Long terminal repeat

L-T$_3$ treatment, 104–108, 118–119
Lunar cycle, influence on reproductive cycle, 227–228
Luteinizing hormone
diurnal patterns in levels of, 144–149
function, 43
level of, during proestrus, 491
mechanism of action, 76–78
ovulation and, 149–151, 180–181
structure, 43–44
α subunit gene, 45–51
β subunit gene, 54
comparative restrictive enzyme analysis, 56–60
nucleotide sequence, 60–64
Luteinizing hormone pulse, *see also* Gonadotropin, secretion
characteristics of, 442–447
effect of estradiol and progesterone on, 497–499
of opiates on, 458–461
β-endorphin and, 463–467
model for control of, 514–518
progesterone negative feedback and, 503–507
Luteinizing hormone pulse generator
estrous cycle and, 190–195
melatonin and, 220–221, 225
photoperiodic pathway to, 202–220
photoperiodic regulation of, 196–199
Luteinizing hormone-releasing hormone
level of, during proestrus, 491
secretion, catecholamines and, 489–518
historical overview, 487–489
inhibitors of, 488
stimulators of, 488
Luteinizing hormone-releasing hormone neuron, 488
Lysosomes, 576–577

M

Macromolecular traffic, 569–587
role of Golgi in, 575
Mammary gland, hormones acting on, 380
MCF-7 cells, 29–35
Medial basal hypothalamus, 441, 447–448, 450, 456
Medial preoptic nucleus, 157
CA turnover rates in, 492–494, 504–506

Median eminence, CA turnover rates in, 492–494, 504–506

Melatonin
daylength coding by, 217–220, 227, 228
effect on response to GnRH, 229–230
LH pulse generator, 220–221, 225, 230–231
reproductive arrest and, 216–217
reproductive induction and, 214–216
timekeeping function, 210–214

Membrane
regulation of components of, by insulin, 362–368
role in endocytosis, 571

Menstrual cycle, *see also* Estrous cycle; Ovarian cycle
β-endorphin and, 463–467, 471–475
hypothalamic control of, 441–485

Messenger ribonucleic acid, for TSH subunits, 87–88, 97–98, 110–113, 117

Minichromosome
hormone action on, 130–138
nuclear proteins on, 141

MIS, *see* Müllerian inhibiting substance

Monoolein, 306

Monopalmitin, 306

Morphine, effect on gonadotropin secretion, 458–459, 468

Mouse mammary tumor virus model, 121–124

Müllerian inhibiting substance, 565

Myosin light chain kinase, 311

N

Naloxone, 455, 459–461, 465–467, 481–482

Night-interruption experiment, 165–169

Norepinephrine
determination of activity in brain, 489–490
turnover rate, hormonal surges and, 490–502

Nucleosome gap, 14–16

Nucleosome phasing, 140

O

1-Oleoyl-2-acetyl-glycerol, 312, 314, 316–319

1-Oleoyl-2-stearoyl-glycerol, 306

Open window generation, 10–16

Opioid peptide, *see also* β-Endorphin
physiological role, 454–475

Organum vasculosum lamina terminalis, 157, 449, 450

ORI region, cuts in, 10–16

Ovalbumin gene promoter region, 21–28

Ovarian cycle, *see also* Estrous cycle; Menstrual cycle
circadian rhythm of locomotor activity and, 151–158
neural events and, 156–158
photoperiodic control of, model for, 199–201
role of pineal gland, 208–210

Ovarian steroid
modulation of β-endorphin, 461–463
site of feedback action, 447–449

Ovulation, circadian nature of timing of, 149

P

Paraventricular nucleus, 202

Phenobarbital, 495–497

Phorbol-12,13-dibutyrate, 329
protein kinase C activation by, 329–335

Phorbol ester, protein kinase C activation by, 329–335

Phosphatidic acid, 303

Phosphatidylcholine, 306, 307

Phosphatidylethanolamine, 305, 306, 307

Phosphatidylinositol, 306, 307

Phosphatidylinositol biphosphate, 301, 302

Phosphatidylserine, 305, 306, 307

Phospholipid, activation of protein kinase C by, 305–307

Phospholipid turnover, 301–345

Photoperiod
model for regulation of ovarian cycle by, 199–201
role in reproductive cycles, 160–172, 187–189

Photoperiodic time measurement, 161–169

Photoreceptor, location, 202–207

Pineal gland, 170–172, 208–210, 221, 232

Pituitary
glycoprotein hormones in, 81–82
hypothyroid, TSH secretion, regulation of, 108–110

TSH mRNA ratios in, 110–113
Pituitary hormones, SGF activity and,
    554–555
Placental lactogen, 77
Platelet, activation studies, 309
Pregnancy, circadian system and, 159–160
Premenstrual syndrome, 483
Preoptico-suprachiasmatic area, role in
    gonadotropin secretion, 514–515
prepro-GRF, structure, 241–242
Pribnow box, 6
Progesterone
    action on mammary gland, 380, 381
    effect on LH surge, 497–499
    level of, during proestrus, 491
    LH pulse and, 190–195
    modulation of β-endorphin by, 461–463
    negative feedback, 503–507
    regulation of gene expression, 21–28
Prolactin, 233, see also Prolactin receptor
    binding inhibition by antireceptor serum,
        405–406
    dissociation from receptor, 382–384
    fast and slow components of, 382–384
    intracellular mediator for, 416–430
    level of, during proestrus, 491
    mechanism of action, 431–432, 437
Prolactin mediator
    assay, 419–424
    identification, 417–419
    mechanism of action on nucleus, 427–
        430
    physiochemical characteristics, 427
    release from membrane, 424–427
    similarity to insulin mediator, 430
Prolactin receptor
    affinity labeling, 400–402
    antibody preparation, 405
    dissociation of prolactin from, 382–384
    down-regulation, 385–389, 439
    electrophoretic analysis, 397–399
    hormonal responses after occupancy of,
        393–394
    intracellular, 389–393
    photoaffinity labeling, 402–405
    purification, 394–397
    up-regulation, 384–385
Prolactin receptor antiserum
    inhibitory and stimulatory actions, 405–
        411

monovalent and bivalent fragments, 411–
    416
    preparation, 405
Promoter elements
    distal upstream, 7–8
    eukaryotic, 3–21
Promoter region, 4
Proopiomelanocortin, 455–457
Prostaglandin E_2, mechanism of action,
    261–262
Prostaglandins, 328
Protein kinase A, activity in platelets, 312–
    313
Protein kinase C, 303
    activation, 304–307
        calcium mobilization and, 315–320
        by phorbol esters, 329–335
        protein phosphorylation and, 309–315
        by TPA, 329
    activity in platelets, 312–313
    inhibitors of, 321
    properties, 307–309
    substrate specificity, 321–323
Protein phosphorylation
    inhibitors of, 321–323
    by insulin receptor complex, 351–354
    protein kinase C activation and, 309–315
Pseudomonas toxin, 577–578
pS2 RNA, 29–35

R

Ram effect, 205, 226–227, 229
Rat
    androgen-sterilized, 507–513
    ovariectomized model, 497–499
Receptor, 571
    classes of, 326–327
    model of stimulation of, 336–337
    phosphorylation of, 351–354
Receptosome, 574–575
Reproduction, role of circadian systems in,
    143–183
Reproduction, seasonal
    model for neuroendocrine basis of, 221
    strategy of, 185–186
Reproductive arrest, role of melatonin in,
    216–217
Reproductive cycle, role of photoperiod in,
    160–172, 187–189

Reproductive induction, role of melatonin in, 214–216
Reserpine, 487
Resistance, definition, 591–592, 593
Resonance experiments, 162–164
Retinohypothalamic tract, 202, 207–208
Retrovirus, life cycle, 122–124
RNA tumor virus, life cycle, 122–124
RNA polymerase, classes of, 4–5
RNA polymerase B(II), 2

S

SDGF, *see* Sertoli cell-derived growth factor
Seminiferous epithelium, SGF in, 550–554
Seminiferous growth factor
  biochemical properties, 547–548
  biological properties, 550–557
  gonadotropins and, 554–555
  identification of, 538–541
  isoelectric point, 545–547
  localization within seminiferous epithelium, 550–554
  molecular weight estimation, 544–545
  partial purification, 548–550
  pituitary hormones and, 554–555
  separation by hydrophobic chromatography, 547
  stability properties, 543–544
Sertoli cell, stimulation of proliferation, 555–557
Sertoli cell-derived growth factor, 562–563
72 bp repeat region, 10–19, 40–41
SGF, *see* Seminiferous growth factor
Signal translation, model, 304, 328, 329
SKF-501, 487
Somatic cell, proliferation during testicular development, 531–533
Somatocrinin, 233–299
  antagonism of somatostatin by, 263–271
  clinical studies with, 281–282
  CNBr fragment, carboxyl terminus of, 247–248
  discovery and isolation, 233–237
  dose-response relationships, 253, 256–257
  effect on pituitary secretions, 288–290
  hypothalamic, isolation of, 240–241
    primary structure, 242–248

localization in neural tissues, 278–281
mechanism of action, 251–252
pancreatic, structure of precursor, 241–242
prostaglandin E_2 and, 261–262
radioimmunoassays, 252
rapidity of action, 262–263
role of adenylate cyclase-cAMP system in action of, 257–261
  of extracellular Ca^{2+} on action of, 257, 258
sex differences in response to, 291
species specificity, 292
specificity of action, 253–255
synthetic replicates, biological activity, 292–295
in vivo studies with, 271–277
structure-activity relationships, 248–251
tumor-derived, isolation of, 237–239
  primary structure, 242–248
Somatostatin, 233
  antagonism of GRF by, 263–271
Somatostatin A, 566
Somatostatin C, 566–567
Sperm, *see* Germ cell
Spermatogenesis, 534–535
Sphingomyelin, 306, 307
Stable transformation assay, 125
  applications, 125–127
1-Stearoyl-2-oleoyl-glycerol, 306
Suprachiasmatic nucleus, 157–158, 169–170, 178–179, 182, 202, 221, 231–232
  CA turnover rates in, 492–494, 504
  role in gonadotropin secretion, 514–515
SV40 early promoter element, 8
SV40 enhancer, 10–19

T

T_3
  endocytosis of, 581, 584–585
  treatment with, 104–108, 118–119
TATA box, 6–7
Testis, mammalian
  formation, 531–533
  regulation of cellular proliferation in, 536–538
  somatic cell proliferation and, 531–533

Testosterone, diurnal patterns in levels of, 144–149
12-O-Tetradecanoylphorbol-13-acetate, 304, 329–335
T experiments, 164–165
−35 region, 7
Thrombin, 302, 309–314, 316
Thyroid stimulating hormone
  biosynthesis, 82–88
  cDNA for subunit genes, 88–91
  clinical studies of subunits of, 80–82
  extrapituitary, 102–103
  function, 43
  glycosylation of subunits, 85–87
  mRNAs for, 87–88
  secretion of, regulation by thyroid hormones, 103–110
  structure, 43–44, 79
  α subunit, leader sequences, 94–95
  α subunit gene, 45–51
    chromosomal location, 98–99
    map of, 100–102
  α subunit mRNA, 97–98
  β subunit, amino acid sequence, 93
  β subunit gene, chromosomal location, 98–99
    map of, 100–102
    nucleotide sequence, 92, 96
  β subunit mRNA, 97–98
Thyroid stimulating hormone-secreting tumor
  hormone secretion, regulation of, 103–108

TSH mRNA ratios in, 110–113
Thyrotropin, 233
Thyrotropin releasing factor, 233
Toxin, endocytosis of, 577–578
TPA, see 12-O-Tetradecanoylphorbol-13-acetate
Transcriptional activity, assays for, 124–125
Transcriptional control, 2
Transferrin, 582, 586
Transient expression assay, 125
Transport, traffic control in, 569–587
TRF, see Thyrotropin releasing factor
Trifluoperazine, 321
Triolein, 306
Tripalmitin, 306
TSH, see Thyroid stimulating hormone
Tumor promotion, 329–336
21 bp repeat region, 11, 13
Tyrosine kinase activity, of insulin receptor complex, 351–354, 361, 375

U

U3 sequence, 122
U5 sequence, 122

V

Virus particle, endocytosis of, 577